My Life as a COMMERCIAL DIVER

PETER ATKEY

Published by AquaPress Ltd, 25 Farriers Way, Temple Farm Industrial Estate, Southend-on-Sea, Essex, SS2 5RY, United Kingdom.

First Published 2024

AquaPress and the AquaPress Logo are Trademarks of AquaPress Ltd.

A CIP catalogue record for this book is available from the British Library.

For information on all other AquaPress titles visit www.aquapress.co.uk

ISBN: 978-1-905492-50-3

Contents

Part Six **401**

Part One

CHAPTER ONE

Getting Started

Looking back over the past sixty-five years it is clear that I have been a very lucky chap! Of course, I often didn't realise this but with the benefit of hindsight it's true. It has become clear that I seem to have had a bit of a talent for being in the right place at the right time.

I was born into a lovely family who while not rich were comfortable, I came into this world at six o'clock in the evening of the 28th April 1956, I was born at home in a small semi-detached house in Morden, Surrey. I had a sister who was two and a half years my senior, my early years were spent in this wonderful suburban environment, my parents were able to take us on holidays most years and I remember, or have been told that we went to France when I was three, Switzerland and France again when I was six and Italy when I was nine.

One of these trips we actually went by air in a propellor driven aircraft and believe it or not we even took our car on the flight with us! I can't really remember much of this but do have a vague memory of being in the plane, and I have some photographs of our car being loaded onto the plane at an airport in England.

My earliest recollection is of a field in France where we were meeting my uncle and Grandmother who were lending us their caravan for our holiday, I was three. Another memory of our holidays is somewhat more traumatic and this took place when I was six in France on a beach in Nice, as was normal when we were on a beach my dad used to like to go off and take a long swim. It seems that I was not happy being left on the beach and so decided to go with him, I mean, how hard can it be? I followed but was too far behind dad for him to know I was coming along.

Of course, at the age of six I was yet to master the skills required to swim and so before I had gone any distance I was in trouble and, it seems was on the verge of drowning! I am told that I had to be rescued by a very kind French man who although I may well owe my life to him, I have no real memory of and certainly didn't know his name. Still this event put me off the water for quite a considerable time and indeed dad was not able to tempt me back into the water until I was ten when he finally managed to teach me to swim! If he hadn't managed to convince me that I was missing out on a lot of fun and get me into the water then my diving career would not have taken off at all, so there you go, I was lucky to have a great dad and indeed to have survived unscathed from the incident on that French beach.

Schooling was not something that I ever really wanted to be involved with, I remember at the age of five being dragged kicking and screaming to the primary school just around the corner from my home by my mum. I had worked myself up to such an extent that I puked in the playground, not a particularly good start. I was given no quarter and had to go to school anyway and of course that was a good thing, I just didn't see it that way at the time.

My family decided to move to Devon when I was still quite young and so I found myself growing up in Torquay housed in a lovely Victoria Villa which my mum ran as a holiday letting business while dad got a job with a local garage handling their accounts. Having now learned to swim and to an extent as was normal in those days being left to my own devices during school holidays, I spent most of my days on beaches with friends having a wonderful time. This is how things went for my first thirteen years, but then it all started to get serious.

Fourteen years of age I was impressed by the likes of Black Sabbath and Deep Purple, I felt their music was great and this has continued to be my genre of choice. Fourteen is a very impressionable age, as a teenager I would always watch the Frenchman Jacques Cousteau and his undersea world on the television every week, this for me was absolutely magical, I could not really see me in an office doing a paperwork job all day and neither, it has to be said could any of my school masters, I'm sure.

However, when careers information lectures started at school such as they were in those days, I was asked, "What do you want to do with your life boy?" I answered with, "I'm going to be a diver!" Well, this was greeted with derision and I was told "Don't be so ridiculous, grow up and look to applying yourself to getting a proper job", (This was a sentiment with which my wife would be in complete in agreement). "But sir, I replied, all I ever wanted to do was to go diving!" It was clear that my career at school was anything but outstanding and indeed when I was in my fifth year, I was put into a class with the other boys who I think they had really given up on. The normal numbering system for the classes was 5a, 5b, 5c… however our class was given the number 5Z2! My English teacher even went to the extent of telling me I would never make anything of myself as I was as thick as twelve lavatory seats, his assessment of my capabilities was that I would be lucky to be sweeping streets!

Well, being stubborn and not at all sure that I could apply myself in the way I was evidently meant to, I decided the only path left open to me would be rebellion. I duly left school as one of Torquay Boys Grammar schools less remarkable pupils and indeed if truth be told I think they were probably as glad to see the back of me as I was to be leaving.

This was in 1971 and I was fifteen years old. Having failed most of my GCE O'Levels, in fact I had just one O'Level in Geography and one grade one CSE in Woodwork. My parents decided to send me to a different school for re-tests. My opinion was not sought in the discussions on this point as nobody seemed to be in the least bit interested in my point of view, had my parents asked I would probably not have opted for more schooling, as all I really wanted to do was go diving.

Anyway, in the September of that year I was enrolled at Kingsbridge comprehensive sixth form college as my parents had taken on the running of a pub in Modbury near Plymouth, by this time I was not in the least interested in school or the things that could be learned from it. The school however had different ideas, and again if we are being truthful here, they were proven to be right to persevere as I did finally achieve some qualifications in Maths and Physics, this I think surprised everybody almost as much as it did me, so it was that armed with my immensely improved future prospects I left school midway through 1972. During my time at Kingsbridge, I found a new circle of friends who introduced me to music such as Pink Floyd with Meddle (especially the track on side two 'Echoes'), I loved it and again continue to follow their music still enjoying their albums today; I also found Led Zeppelin as well, what a great era for music.

In April of 1973 I was finally seventeen this meant I could get my driving licence my parents were still running the Red Devon pub in Modbury so my life was good. I was a young guy living in a pub with a great circle of friends and now I was going to be able to drive, what could be better? Anyway, on the afternoon of the twenty-eighth of April I had my provisional licence and my mum decided I should be given my first driving lesson, she would sit next to me while I drove from Modbury to Bigbury-on-Sea; I was so excited, I mean how hard could it be? I had already been taken to car parks where I had in my mind mastered clutch control etc., so I was definitely ready!

I was taken to mums Hillman Hunter estate car where I was installed in the driver's seat; I knew how to adjust the driving position and being as mum was likely to be critical I really took my time. Eventually, I was settled and ready, I looked across to mum, she looked somewhat apprehensive but told me to drive off. Everything started OK, as I drove out of Modbury on a two-lane road which was clearly wide enough, I was a little apprehensive when other vehicles approached going in the opposite direction but, I didn't hit anything. Then, we turned right onto the B3392 towards Bigbury, well this was a completely different kettle of fish! Now there were sections where there were no lines at all in the middle of the road, how wide was the road? Was there enough room for two cars? In a particularly narrow section, there were hedges on either side of me and I was faced with a car coming straight towards me; I wasn't sure whether there was room to get through! Mum just said, "Go on there's plenty of room?" Well, it didn't look that way to me so I stopped; the chap following was not amused at all and stood on his horn, gesticulating at me through his windscreen.

My confidence was shaken but I carried on as soon as the path was again clear; eventually, we arrived in Bigbury-on-Sea, I was not exactly shaking but I was worn out and I had only driven a few miles! Over the coming months things improved with me learning how wide the car was and where I could fit it, I didn't hit anything so my confidence grew, it was great.

Anyway, in early summer having left school I was freed up to do what I really wanted .... Go to the beach, and become gainfully employed Surfing, Swimming and generally doing all the things that a young lad wants to do. It was a great summer, I spent the majority of it during the days as part of the surf life-saving club at Bigbury beach talking to girls and in the evenings going to disco's where great music from Deep Purple, Black Sabbath, Led Zeppelin and other heavy metal bands would feature; and of course, there were more girls, it was brilliant. Problem was it soon became evident that I was expected to either go on to further education or to somehow earn some money; this quite quickly started to get in the way of things, impeding my leisure activities in particular.

After looking around and with some guidance from my dad, I decided to follow his lead (he had been a radio operator on convoys during the war. Very brave and to my chagrin I never told him how brave I felt he had been during this time!). I was therefore enrolled at a college in Plymouth to become a marine radio and radar operator/technician; this took the pressure off for the summer so that I could carry on with all the things I had been enjoying for the last couple of months.

In September I duly arrived in Plymouth to commence three years of training. As my parents had now moved back to Torbay by this time I had to go into 'digs' in Plymouth during the week and to travel home at weekends; I had a Yamaha 125 cc (YAS1) motorcycle which allowed me to have a little independence but I didn't have much money so couldn't afford to buy much fuel or anything else really. I had wanted a motorcycle principally as most of the friends from school had already bought bikes but, it did make perfect sense as they were cheap to run. My parents were not really keen on my having a bike but as dad used to ride them, he really couldn't object too strenuously; anyway, I was going to have one as far as I was concerned.

The local motorcycle sales shop was Torre Motorcycles, as the name suggested this was in a Torre; on Union Street, on the day I was due to pick up the bike I arrived at the shop with dad; as we walked into the showroom, I was blown away by all these beautiful high-powered bikes; there must have been thirty or more in this tiny showroom. Anyway, we made our way past rows of bikes on show to the counter where dad completed the paperwork and of course paid the money over.

Dad then had to go on to work and so I was left on my own to pick up the bike; in 1973 there was no requirement for any formal training before being allowed out on the road on a motorcycle so long as it was no larger than 250cc. I had ridden bicycles and a few very small mopeds of 50cc before but they were automatic and didn't require any gear changing at all, so although I understood balance and the front brake, I just had absolutely no idea about gears or how to apply the rear brake etc. The only stipulation mum had put on the purchase was that I had to agree to always wear a crash helmet although in those days even this was not a legal requirement!

Mark, the chap behind the counter told me to go upstairs to the workshop and ask for Steve who would show me the ropes. The staircase up to the workshop was off to the left of the shop counter, it was very narrow with greasy hand prints on the wall, the stair treads were not covered in anything other than ground in oil and grease. Gripping my brand-new full-face helmet (another requirement of mum's) I started to climb the stairs only to meet someone coming down at high speed, there was not room to pass so I backtracked to let him past. He was wearing dark blue overalls which again were covered in grease and oil, I took it that he was one of the mechanics who was probably coming down to pick up a spare part or something and I certainly didn't want to get in the way of his work.

As I reached the top of the stairs, I found myself in the workshop, there were bikes in various stages of repair all over the place. I don't know how many mechanics were there but I could see at least three plus the one who I had seen coming down the stairs. The workshop was well lit by sun coming through skylights in the ceiling, it was a hive of activity, I asked the first chap I saw where I could find Steve. He pointed to another blue overalled individual who was working on a bike over to the left near the rear door; I thanked the mechanic who didn't really acknowledge me at all and made my way over to Steve.

I started off by trying to introduce myself but just as I started one of the mechanics behind me started a very noisy bike up and commenced revving it up, maybe he was testing something but it was just as likely he wanted to make me look stupid. I really didn't need much help in that department though, I was completely out of my depth; eventually Steve glared at the mechanic and beckoned for me to follow him outside.

As we emerged from the workshop, I found myself on a small back street behind the row of shops of which Torre Motorcycles was just one, the back lane was grandly named Southlands Road but it was really just a lane behind the shops and actually led nowhere. There standing by the side of the road was my new bike, well, it wasn't new but it was new to me. The bike had been customised by the previous owner and sported a racing style petrol tank and seat both made of fibre glass painted brilliant white, it looked great. The

YAS1 had a twin cylinder 125cc engine that was started using a kick start, there was no such thing as electric start in those days either.

Steve was clearly used to giving this training to new and extremely green individuals like me, he was very patient explaining all the controls to me. It went something like this: "this is the front brake, this is the clutch, this is the key, this is the rear brake and this is the gear lever!" Each time he spoke he would point at the relevant lever or point of interest; I was trying to take it all in but no sooner had he finished his first run around the bike than he was on to the next lesson. "The gears are one down and four up with neutral between first and second", he demonstrated this by pushing the gear lever down once and then pulling it up several times before returning the lever to where he told me neutral was! He went on with "you start it like this." He turned the key; a few lights came on in the speedometer, he then sat astride the bike and pulled the kick starter out into its ready position before placing his foot onto it and pushing down; the engine sparked into life and sat there merrily burbling away, he turned off the ignition, climbed off handing me the keys.

While I had understood everything, he had told me I was not absolutely sure I would remember anything. Anyway, he looked at me and said "happy?" I of course didn't want to sound stupid so told him that yes, I was happy, he invited me to sit on and get it started. I climbed on sitting astride the seat, I had by now put my helmet on and was ready for the off; I went through the same sequence he had used by turning the key until I saw the lights in the speedo then I pulled the kick starter out and jumped onto it. I was surprised by how little force was needed to push it down and by the time it had reached the bottom of its travel the motor was running.

Steve then told me to pull in the clutch lever which I did, then he told me to press the gear lever down, the gear lever was on the left of the bike just in front of the foot-rest; I felt a slight jolt which indicated I had selected first gear, then he told me to give a bit of a twist of the throttle with my right hand while feeding the clutch lever out. Of course, the first couple of times I just stalled the engine; on the third time I was off, although a bit unsteady. After about fifteen metres I reached the end of the road where I would need to turn either left or right; I had pulled the clutch lever in so the engine was still running, I went through the process of pulling away again while also turning left to go down the hill. Phew I had managed to get around the corner where I wobbled down the road until I arrived at Union Street where I had to stop again. This must have been painful to watch as I really hadn't mastered anything yet, but I did manage to pull away onto Union Street without hitting anything and then for the first time I had some space to settle down into riding along a flat straight road, that was much better.

I took my time but rode around Torquay for the next couple of hours learning how to control the bike; I had several near misses but didn't hit anything or fall off so this was a result as far as I was concerned. I must confess that many years later I was very relieved that when my son bought his first bike he was required to go through mandatory training before he could take the bike out on the road for the first time.

Anyway, I survived that first day and from then on improved my skills without hurting myself although I did go on to fall off from time to time, I never really hurt myself until some four years later when I broke my leg but even then, I was not driving, I was a pillion passenger when that happened.

In September of 1973 I made my way to Plymouth for my course, I was required to wear the uniform of the merchant navy which meant for the first time since I left the grammar school I was in uniform. Mum told me I looked very good but then she was biased; I had been required to cut my hair so for the first time again since leaving school I had a very short back and sides. Anyway, the first three months of my course went well and I started to enjoy the subjects such as morse code, electronics and the like, indeed the prospect of travelling the world as a radio operator in the merchant navy had begun to look quite tasty to me.

In September I had my car driving test booked, I was again quite nervous as although I had previously had lessons, I had not had one for two months. My test was scheduled for the fourth of September, in Newton Abbot; as I didn't have a current driving instructor, I was to take the test in my mum's Hillman Hunter estate car. This was a big car but was the one I had been practicing with so all should be OK, I arrived at the test centre which at the time was right next to Courtney Park in the centre of Newton Abbot. The examiner spent a few minutes testing my eyesight and ability to recognise road signs before taking me out for the practical part (there was no theory test in those days). We turned right out of the test centre and I was directed to drive here, there and everywhere for a good half hour; in that time, I was instructed to carry out an emergency stop, reverse around a corner, carry out a three-point-turn and other things designed to demonstrate my skills.

When we arrived back at the test centre, I was not at all sure I had done enough, the instructor told me to park up and then proceeded to ask me a few more questions before turning to me and telling me to get out of the car and take the 'L'-plates off before I drove home; yes, I had passed first time! Yippee that was great!

Unfortunately, my euphoria was relatively short lived as has often been the case in my life my plans were about to go a bit awry! My sister had enrolled in the RAF and was engaged in her basic training, this meant that her car was at home and therefore was not getting used at all, this seemed a great shame to me, given my new skill of being a qualified car driver. On this particular weekend as usual I had travelled home from Plymouth on the Friday evening in the pouring rain arriving very wet and cold; the next morning I was going out to see some of my friends and looking at the weather I felt that it would be nice to be able to have the use of a car! Anyway, as I said my sister's little mini was at home and had not been used for the past month or so, well, surely, I would be doing her a favour to give it a run, this would charge up the battery again and of course would make sure that the car was still running nicely for when she came home on leave which was due to be the following weekend.

So, off I went, enjoying this lovely little car, especially as it started to rain again almost as soon as I left home. All went well for the first couple of miles but then as I negotiated a corner that I had driven many times before it all went pear shaped. I was driving well within the speed limit but halfway around the corner the rear of the car started to drift out of line, everything seemed to speed up and before I knew it, I had mounted the pavement and crashed through a stone wall. When the car came to a halt, I found that I was not injured, getting out of the car I went to inspect the damage, my sister's pride and joy was now somewhat modified to the point that it couldn't be driven. This of course was in the days before mobile phones so I decided that the best plan of attack would be for me to lean against the car and consider my options.

I didn't have long to wait before a police car turned up, the officer proceeded to take my details and a statement, while this was going on a specialist team arrived. It seemed that this team would test the road surface to see if there was a reason why I lost control, I thought this was clutching at straws but as they told me that if this could be proven I would not be prosecuted I was completely in favour of them conducting whatever tests they felt could prove me innocent; after a few minutes they had finished their tests and had found diesel fuel had been spilt on the road making it very slippery. The police seemed content that I was a victim of this spillage and so there would be no prosecution, I was of course happy about this but this was of course not the end of my problems.

My sister's car was damaged to the point of being written off! The car was third party insured meaning that she would get no replacement from them; I would need to replace her pride and joy as quickly as possible. I also had to pay for the wall to be repaired, I of course had no income and no way of paying these huge sums; my options were very limited, it was clear that I would need to review my life plan.

After due consideration and in consultation with my parents it was decided I had to leave college and find a job pronto! Luckily, at this time there were no shortage of jobs, therefore sooner than planned I embarked on my first career; I was to become a central heating engineer. Not quite what I had in mind of course, but by now I had discovered motorcycles and yes that most expensive pastime, the opposite sex. The company on which I was to be inflicted was based in Torquay; "Interheat" was a small family run firm who had about four or five fitters working for them.

On my first day I was introduced to Fred with whom I would be working, of course at this time I was completely useless to him, and I think he felt that he must have done something wrong to have this duty thrust upon him. After about three months of this I was just starting to find my feet and Fred had actually let me solder a few of the less important joints together. It was then that I had my first real stroke of luck as far as employment went.

In 1973 my dad worked as an accountant for a firm selling cars, and one day out of the blue in walks a chap who worked for Imperial Chemical Industries (ICI) in Brixham, it turns out they were looking for someone of my age group to train as a laboratory technician, not my first choice but it seemed that part of the job would entail diver training and eventually diving to survey pipelines etc. When dad told me that evening, I was dumbstruck, I just couldn't believe it, I applied for the job immediately. ICI obviously took a good look at my impressive academic achievements but despite this they gave me an interview. This turned out to be an all-day affair at their facility at Brixham.

At this time ICI were using the Brixham site for environmental research into the effects of effluent and chemicals, it looked much more my cup of tea than central heating, they must have thought so too as they offered me a job at the princely sum of twelve pounds per week (2 pounds less than I was currently earning with Interheat), I don't think anyone was more surprised than me I can tell you. I started a week before Christmas 1973, so the first thing that happened was I was given several days off, this was evidently my kind of job.

In February 1974 I was scheduled to take my motorcycle test and as with the car test there was no pre-theory test to take so, on the day all I had to do was turn up on a bike. At this time, I no longer had my Yamaha 125 as it had been returned to the shop after proving extremely unreliable, it kept breaking down culminating in the engine seizing up and throwing me up the road one evening when I was riding home from Bigbury-on-Sea. It seemed that the previous owner had carried out some engine modifications that didn't work very well; the first I knew of this was that the spark plugs would suddenly melt causing the engine to misfire. When this happened, I would need to change the plug before being able to get going again; this happened a lot and my dad and I were constantly back at the shop asking them to put it right. Eventually, they supplied me with some 'racing' plugs with tungsten electrodes, they told me there was absolutely no way that these would melt. As it turned out they were correct, the plug's electrodes didn't melt, the piston did! As I say this caused the engine to seize throwing me down the road; the bike was returned with dad getting a full refund.

But the upshot of this was that I had no bike on which to take my test; luckily, I was able to borrow one from a friend who at the time was running a 200cc Yamaha which he offered to me for the test. So, I turned up at the same test centre in Newton Abbot on a bike that was unfamiliar to me but not so very different to the one I was used to riding. In those days the bike test involved the applicant driving around Courtney Park with the examiner walking through the park and leaping out from time to time to make sure the applicant was following all the rules of the road. This included the emergency stop where the examiner would jump out in front of the applicant holding is hand up, the applicant then had to come to a halt as quickly as possible in a controlled fashion; this must have led to some interesting times for the examiners for sure. But I managed everything OK and was again told to remove the 'L'-plates before I drove home; passed first time again.

I immediately took the bike back to my friend, from there I walked up to another friend's house where I paid him three hundred and fifty pounds for his 350cc Yamaha (YR3), this was another good day.

CHAPTER TWO

First Steps as a Commercial Diver for ICI – 1974 to 1975

Over the next couple of years, I was employed "looking after" a variety of very unfortunate fish which were to be the subjects of the experiments, I say unfortunate fish not especially because of the experiments that they would be subjected to, although obviously being chosen to take part in experiments of this nature is not a plus point in a fish's life. No really, I felt sorry for them because I don't think I was really all that good at fish husbandry and they seemed to take great delight in dying at the most inopportune moments. Consequently, ICI decided that I would be better employed as a maintenance fitter and at long last this would mean that I could be spared for offsite survey work including … Diving.

Before being properly trained, it was decided to see if I actually had the aptitude for the job, so I was entrusted to the lead diver of their unit John Yersin, who was instructed to "Take him in and see if he's got what it takes". I still couldn't believe my luck and so consequently, I was in seventh heaven when on one cold and very windy morning we took all the necessary equipment to a seawater swimming pool on the outskirts of Brixham into which I was to make my very first deep, dark and of course very dangerous dive using breathing apparatus. I was extremely excited but being a teenage boy could not bring myself to show it, I spent the whole time helping (Or should that be hindering) John in the setting up the equipment with what must have seemed a very strange expression on my face.

When John had eventually sorted out all of the myriad of valves, bottles, weights and all of the other associated equipment, I was given an extensive briefing for this complex business, it went something like this. "Don't forget to keep breathing, don't hold your breath at any time, if you do, I'll hit you very hard in the stomach!" It seemed that there were to be several previously un-thought of dangers, anyway we were to go into this pool, sit on the bottom and breathe for a few minutes, this it seemed would tell him whether I was going to make a good diver? We lowered ourselves into the water, which I have to say, was a great relief as I was by this time very hot; due to the levels of clothing and suits which all of the other "helpful" divers had suggested I wear for this extended foray into the deep. Also, the weight of the equipment seemed excessive to me.

When we were standing on the bottom with my head just out of the water, John who was facing me started to tell me about the oncoming adventure, I just wanted to get on with it! Finally, it was time and as instructed I spat into my facemask and wiped it around with my finger before washing the resulting mess out with seawater, why? I didn't really know but John did it so it must be necessary, later I found out that this helps to keep the mask from steaming up. We put our masks on and with a thumbs up knelt down. The first shock I had was that I couldn't see much at all! It was not at all like Cousteau had shown it would be. It turned out that the chosen venue for my initial leap into the diving world, Shoalstone pool was topped up by the sea breaking over the wall, and today the sea was taking this project very seriously bringing a lot of sand and dirt into the pool with the water.

Anyway, after the initial shock I found that I could move around and breathe without difficulty and although I was only in about one and a half metres of water, to me it was pure magic, I was hooked. After forty-five minutes, seemed more like just five minutes to me, I was dragged out and told that this was enough. We stripped down the gear and packed it all back into the van, mostly in near silence, I thought that I must have made mistakes and that John was not impressed, so it was with some degree of gloom that we returned to the lab. Over a cup of coffee, it was decided that in fact, I would do and that I should be sent for formal training. I was completely ecstatic, I was shortly to become a commercial diver, not only that but ICI were even going to pay for it!

So, it was that again with a degree of trepidation I embarked on my extensive training at the beginning of 1975, this was to be carried out at Fort Bovisand Underwater Centre, Bovisand is close to Plymouth and so I did not have very far to travel. The training period was to be a full week, at the end of which I assumed I would be fully qualified! The whole week was spent in a whirl of theory and practical exercises, designed to inform me of all the problems possible together with the necessary solutions, precautions and procedures. In fact, it seemed that the main thing was to avoid being shouted at by the instructors who may have been chosen specifically for their ability to go from being rational and reasonable human beings to fire breathing demons threatening to tear my arms off before beating me with the soggy ends in the twinkle of an eye. After five days of this treatment, the report I received was non-committal, it seemed that I had the right aptitude and would benefit from further training. In the meantime I would be acceptable for use as a working diver ..... Success!

Back at Brixham, diving as it turned out would be a very small part of my job, most of the time I was to be employed fixing pipework and painting things, this was not the plan as far as I was concerned. However, my plan seemed of little interest to the powers that be, we embarked on a refit of the whole area, as I know now, this exercise proved to be a great grounding for my career in the diving industry, it just didn't feel like it at the time.

ICIs laboratory in Brixham was not only employed doing environmental research at the time I was there, they also used to have a paint testing department, ICI were making new compounds of paints all the time, and these needed to be tested for weathering, and sometimes this would involve the placing of painted panels on rafts, these rafts were anchored in Brixham harbour. Some of the panels placed on the rafts would be coated with Anti-fouling paints, for use in the prevention of marine growth accumulation on boats, these panels would be suspended in the water, on a frame under the raft.

This is where I came in. Sometimes in bad weather, the frames holding the submerged sample plates would become dislodged and fall off, the paints department would then contact us "The Divers" to go and find them. The very first time this happened after I was trained, the team decided that I should be the diver to go and locate the lost panel, this I assured them would be no problem as I had been trained to do this very task most effectively during my exhaustive training period at Bovisand. On the day in question the weather was not at all bad, the sun was shining and the wind had dropped away to a gentle breeze, I thought that this would be no problem for a diver of my obvious and proven abilities. There were three of us in the team, Yersin was to be the supervisor, Eric Stathes would be my tender and safety standby diver and of course I would be the search diver.

We all three prepared our equipment for the coming plunge to adventure, my equipment included a "Poseidon Uni-suit", which was a very expensive "Dry suit", specifically designed to keep the water out allowing the diver to wear normal warm clothing underneath, this clothing would then keep him or her warm. At this time, I was under the impression that a dry suit would do just that, however I was soon to discover that some dry suits seem to be "designed" to allow water in and having done this keep that water inside. The only reason I can imagine for these being given the name "dry suit" must be for their ability to keep the deck of your boat slightly drier when you emerge from the sea although this doesn't seem to work either, baffling really.

The dive was to be carried out using Self-Contained Underwater Breathing Apparatus, (SCUBA), subsequently I was supplied with the equipment necessary for this, which was a mask that covers your eyes and nose but not the mouth, this is commonly known as a half-mask, in addition I was given an air cylinder holding compressed air at a pressure of two hundred times the pressure of the atmosphere, this pressurised air is then allowed to come to your mouth only when you require it and is triggered by the action of breathing in, the system of valves which allow this is called a demand valve, an invention credited to one Jacques Cousteau, my particular valve was also made by "Poseidon". In addition, I had various other pieces of equipment, namely a pair of "Fins" (never flippers!) to allow me to speed "effortlessly" through the water, a "quick release" weight belt with weights attached thus ensuring that when I jump in the water I can actually submerge, this is necessary owing to the buoyancy given by the dry suit.

Strapped to my wrists were a compass to allow me to find my way whilst on the bottom, a depth gauge to let me know the depth to which I had descended and a watch so that I could work out my decompression thus allowing safe return to the surface and last but by no means least was the "Divers Dagger!" A huge knife which was to be strapped to the diver's leg in case of sea monster attack or perhaps some more mundane problem such as the diver becoming entangled in rope while underwater. For this dive I would also be taking two ropes, one would be used as a "Distance line" to help with a logical search pattern, and a work line this line would be attached to the offending paint panel when (Not if, but when) I found it, so allowing recovery to the surface.

After dressing in the equipment and carrying out all required safety checks ensuring the equipment was working properly, I was sitting on the side of the boat completely covered in equipment from head to foot. John gave me the thumbs up to enter the water, we had already dropped a "Shot line" from the boat, this is a rope with a large weight tied to it, the weight is lowered to the seabed, the line was then tied off to the boat on the surface, this gives the diver a rope to descend and also it can be used as an aid to the ascent at the end of the dive and gives a fixed reference point (datum point) for the search pattern.

The normal method for entering the water is for the diver to hold their facemask and the demand valve in the mouth with one hand and then to roll backwards into the water. Now as I rolled off the boat the two ropes in my hand were perfectly under control, somehow though when I entered the water upside down these ropes managed to become entangled around me, my fins and my bottle. When I came up, I must have looked like a bowl of spaghetti. With a little help from my tender who was by this time having an almost uncontrollable fit of laughter, I managed to get the ropes back under control and was then ready to leave surface.

When I was positioned on the shot-line I noted the time on my brand-new diver's watch, and with a last look at the perfect blue sky I submerged, this time as I descended the visibility was excellent, at least four metres. Travelling down the line, I could see the bottom coming up to meet me and suddenly I was down there! Horror of horrors I had landed at such a rate that the soft mud around me had been disturbed and was now in a cloud all around me, no more visibility. The depth gauge read twenty-two feet (6.7 metres), and I remember thinking "No decompression problems then", this is because if the dive is less than thirty-three feet (10 metres) the diver can stay there almost indefinitely without having to stop on the way up to allow the extra gasses dissolved in their bloodstream and tissues absorbed during the dive to be breathed out in a safe and controlled fashion. If the diving depth is deeper than ten metres the diver may be required to stop at intervals on the way back to the surface to allow the accumulated gas to come out of the bloodstream safely, these stops are termed "decompression stops".

Anyway, back to my first commercial dive, quite soon it became evident that there was a small current, this soon took the disturbed mud away from me and I was again able to see. The plan had been for me to tie the distance line onto the shot weight, I would then move out along the line to a point at which I could still see the shot weight, then swim in a circle around the shot searching as I went, this is termed a 'circular search' and this is where the compass came in.

When I was in position next to the shot weight, I took a bearing on the compass which happened to show due east, as I swam in a circle around the shot the compass bearing would change, so I would know when I had completed a circle around the shot when the compass showed due east again. I tied the distance line onto the shot weight, moved out to a distance of about two and a half metres, at this distance I could still see the shot weight. The paint panel I was looking for was quite a bit bigger than the shot so I should be easily able to see it if it was between me and the shot weight. Once in position I pulled the distance line taut and set off, trying to keep the distance line taut to the shot looking at the compass and searching while also dragging the work line around with me, I remember thinking that this may not be as easy as I had been led to believe, especially when the seabed consisted of mud, the consistency of which was similar to a substance normally found in a cow shed.

During my first circle the visibility very soon returned to zero, I found that I had to peer through the gloom conducting the search with my hands. Even seeing the compass had become almost impossible. Now when searching underwater in zero visibility your mind and imagination can play tricks on you, so that even though I knew that I was in Brixham harbour and the most dangerous thing in there (apart from me) was probably an inquisitive flatfish, most of which had probably seen all of this before and therefore would be quite bored by the machinations of this bumbling idiot, I found that my heart was going rather quickly, so much so that when my hand touched something hard in the gloom and murk I recoiled from it ......just in case, you understand. As I returned to it in order to explore further, I found that it was in fact not anything sinister, it was in fact the shot weight, I had spiralled in onto it in the murk.

Feeling a bit embarrassed and more than a little bit glad that no one else would ever know of my reactions I moved out away from the shot again until the distance line was properly taut and resolved to ensure I kept the line taut. I again checked the bearing on the compass, and set off again, once I had completed the first circle, I moved out along the distance line another metre, turned around and started back to complete another circle; I carried out this second circle moving in the opposite direction, thus ensuring the work line which was being tended on the surface by my trusty standby diver stayed free and useable, as one circuit would tie it around the shot line, the next circuit going the opposite way would unwind it again. At the end of the second circuit still I had found nothing, this went on for another three circuits by then I was feeling pretty good and indeed was beginning to enjoy myself, so much so that I couldn't believe that someone was paying me to do this.

Anyway, while feeling my way through the gloom, something hit me on the head, I started to feel all around the seabed and oh joy! I had found a tubular steel item, I was sure this had to be the paint panel; actually, I remember being quite chuffed that I had found it. All that remained for me to do was to tie the work line onto it and return triumphantly to the surface. Another dilemma now, which knot was the right one to use? Well! Never mind that, what seemed to be more to the point was which knot could I tie underwater bearing in mind that I was wearing big thick neoprene rubber gloves and could not see anything at all, whichever knot I chose would also need to have a reasonable expectation of still being tied when the rope was pulled up to the surface.

Finally, I settled on a round turn and two half hitches, which I tied with absolute confidence! Once this was done, I signalled four pulls on my safety life line indicating that I was ready to leave bottom and come to surface, on receiving the answering signal I started to ascend being careful not to come up too quickly as this could be dangerous. As I neared the surface the water again became clearer and lighter, then as I broke surface back into the sunlight, I felt great, a job well done, or so I thought.

When we had established that I was still breathing and felt in good spirits, the team in the boat helped to remove most of my equipment to bring me inboard. Eric then started to heave up the paint panel from its resting place, both John and I looked on, soon the panel loomed into view and was pulled onto the boat. I thought that it looked great but not at all what I had been expecting; it was old, rusty and somewhat strangely shaped, however this was vindication that I was indeed going to make the grade as a commercial diver. However, the other faces in the boat did not mirror my obvious delight, it seemed that my "Panel" was in fact part of the frame from an old wheel barrow, oh dear!

Eric was duly dressed into his gear and dropped over the side, I was demoted to his tender and took to this task with a black cloud hanging over my head, after another half-hour I received a signal on the work line, Eric was on his way back up. When he surfaced, we removed his diving gear and pulled him into the boat. I then pulled up the work line, which was indeed tied quite firmly to the offending paint panel, again I felt fairly gloomy during the trip back to base.

CHAPTER THREE

First Trip Away as a Commercial Diver – 1975

After this particularly inauspicious start to my diving career things thankfully improved, soon I was looked upon as a valued member of our small team. Over the next few months, we were called upon to look for several more of the cursed paint panels, and I even managed to find some of them. So it was that during June of that year I was included as part of the team that would be travelling to Whitby in Yorkshire for two weeks diving on some outfalls carrying effluent from a Potash mine at Boulby, this was some way north from Whitby.

On the day of departure, we loaded the company Ford Transit van with all the equipment we would need for this expedition, this included an inflatable boat complete with outboard motor, miles of rope, a myriad of plastic buoys, a heap of boxes and bottles for the samples we were to collect, and of course our diving gear. By the time we had loaded everything the van was absolutely full to the brim.

Leaving Brixham the sun was again shining and all the holiday makers were enjoying a splendid day by the seaside, we however had a job to do at the other end of the country. The journey took most of the day, finally we arrived in Whitby at about seven in the evening.

Whitby was a very picturesque fishing village; nestling in a steep valley at the mouth of the river Esk, the harbour was protected from the worst of the winter's storms by a rather strange looking pier on the Southside of the harbour entrance, perhaps one of Whitby's major claims to fame is that Abraham (Bram) Stoker wrote Dracula while staying there. It was at the time of my visit, home to a busy little fishing fleet, most of which seemed to be in port that evening, this resulted in the harbour looking very congested, this caused some concern, the worry was that we may have to lug our gear across several boats to get to the one we were to use. I thought that this may not be a problem as surely, they would all go to sea, looking for fish in the morning leaving us a clear quayside, and since we had been travelling all day, we would simply find our hotel and unload the van in the morning from a clear and deserted quay. However, John was having none of that; we drove straight down to the dockside to look for our hired vessel.

The boat we were to be using was a fairly small motor fishing vessel (MFV) called the "Achieve", sure enough the crew were waiting for us and luckily the boat was alongside the quay ready for us to load our gear. My task during this operation was to carry the equipment from the van to the loading point; it turned out that the van could not be taken quite far enough onto the quayside as it was too heavy for the quay. This meant that I would have to carry the equipment a distance of about forty or fifty feet (about 12 metres). This doesn't sound very far but with the amount of equipment we had I can assure you it was far enough. Eric was to be stationed in the boats fish room where the equipment would be stored. Having never been in a trawlers fish room at this point I thought Eric had the better end of the deal, I now know differently. John was busy off-loading the van, much faster than I could deal with, so a pile of equipment accumulated behind the van.

It took a couple of hours for all of the equipment to be loaded and stowed properly in the hold, and for the inflatable boat to be pumped up, readied and launched. By this time, I was ready for a bit of rest and relaxation, but this was still not to be, it seemed that we now had to discuss with the skipper what would be required for the next morning. After another hour we were finally ready to leave the boat crew to secure the vessel and we could go to our hotel.

We had been booked into the "Royal hotel" standing at the top of the cliffs with a splendid view of the harbour and the ruined abbey sitting on the headland on the other side of the river, a relic of Henry the eighth no doubt. We climbed the path to the top of the headland where we passed a set of whale's jawbones set as a feature standing in testament to Whitby's whaling past. In the hotel we were given twin rooms which were certainly as good as anything in which I had stayed up to this point, by the time we were installed the time was a little after eleven o'clock and I was ready for my bed, we were to be given a lay in the next day so the wakeup call was to be for a very luxurious five-thirty AM, with a view to leaving the hotel at six.

The alarm seemed to sound slightly before my head touched the pillow, so a very tired and it has to be said, slightly grumpy Peter arrived in the lobby, everyone else seemed in very good spirits, most strange I thought. We had been joined by the fourth member of our troop another John, John Tap. Tap was in fact the boss of the diving unit who had been on holiday in the area, John's main claim to fame seemed to be that he could and frequently would eat an ice cream at every kiosk he passed on the way from the boat to the hotel, and then have more at the subsequent dinner.

We made our way down to the boat; just a short walk down the hill. The weather was absolutely idyllic, this lifted my spirits dramatically, I was really looking forward to doing some real diving. Once on the boat the crew cast off and we headed for the open sea, one of the crew a very large chap I later found to be called "Jimmy" came up from below and started to speak to me, the language he was speaking was totally incomprehensible to me, I thought he was speaking English but I still couldn't understand him. Eric came to my aid and translated for me; it seemed that Jimmy wanted to know if I took sugar in my tea! Obviously, I was going to have a bit of learning to do in order to fit in here.

The position of the outfalls we had come to inspect were, just off the cliffs at Boulby a few miles north of Whitby so, during the steam up there we started to set up our gear, I was sent into the fish room to pass up the equipment, it was now that I realised that Eric had done me a favour last night by being stationed here. The smell was horrendous, it was a heady mix of fish guts, diesel fumes and smoke from the coal fired cooking stove which was positioned just forward of the fish hold, so with our forward movement all the smoke produced seemed to accumulate in the hold. Our gear was shifted out of that hold at an extremely rapid rate I can tell you.

When we arrived on site the first task was to mark the position of the outfalls, this was carried out with the help of a couple of surveyors stationed on top of the cliffs equipped with theodolites and radios. We steamed directly in towards one of the surveyors from a position out at sea and dropped the buoys when given the signal from the other surveyor, onto what we hoped would be the exact location of the outfalls, after this we made ready to dive. The first dive was to be carried out by the John Tap and Eric, with John Yersin and myself as surface support. I had already learnt that a tidy site is a safe site and that seemed to be especially true on a small fishing trawler where deck space was limited; I made it my job to ensure everything was stowed tidily and I resolved to ensure the decks were kept clear and tidy.

I have always made every effort to work with this principle as I have seen people hurt quite badly when there has been poor housekeeping on site. While we were preparing ourselves the crew of the Achieve anchored the vessel in a location close to the inshore buoy, this was apparently in about thirty feet (about 9 metres) of water. Once they had done this their days work seemed to be finished, apart that is from supplying us with copious quantities of food, tea and coffee both of the latter being made with condensed milk, this gives a very distinctive taste and to some extent the taste for this type of beverage must be acquired. At this time, I definitely had not acquired it and found it rather unpleasant to say the least, as I remember though I did not convey my dislike to Jimmy who stood watching me drink my first cup before nodding sagely and then disappearing below.

The first dive went very well, with Tap surfacing after about thirty minutes having moved the buoy line onto the outfall, this it turned out had been easy as the shot had landed only about fifteen feet from it and with visibility of thirty feet or more they could easily complete their task, there was lots of talk about the dive and how the area had changed from last year, as this was an annual event, they were able to describe the seabed with ease and even had names for certain features such as "Lobster rock", a rock which apparently housed a monster Lobster.

Now it was our turn, we were to carry out the same task on the other outfall which was positioned some distance further out from the beach. After returning to the Achieve to exchange air bottles and personal diving gear, before setting off in the inflatable boat, I was quite nervous as this was my first real test and this was after all, the infamous North Sea! Yersin was very patient as we discussed the coming dive and our respective roles; I was to follow him and be prepared to help whenever he needed it. This I thought I could manage; we dressed in our gear and carried out our checks. As the marker buoy was not in fact attached to anything of much substance, just a fifty-six-pound weight, it was decided that the boat would run up to the buoy and rather than tie up to it they would just drop us off, we would then swim to the buoy and go down on the buoy line.

John Tap was coxswain of the boat for this dive, he brought the boat up to within a few metres of the buoy, we were already sitting on the side of the boat ready, as soon as Eric tapped me on the shoulder I rolled backwards over the side, I surfaced and found Yersin in the water next to me, we both signalled to the boat that we were OK and then started to make our way to the buoy. Swimming on the surface with all of this diving gear was not at all easy and really should be avoided at all costs, so even though the distance was not great it was with some relief when we reached the buoy, we did not want to hang onto the buoy in case we were dragged away from the outfall, so as soon as we were both at the buoy, we looked at one another and John signalled to leave surface.

As we descended, I could see that John was having some trouble equalising the pressure in his ears with the rising pressure produced by the increasing water depth, we had to stop a couple of times for him to hold his nose and pump air into his ears, this is rather like the problem any of us may have when travelling up a large hill while we are suffering from a head cold. Eventually we reached the bottom at forty-three feet (just over 13 metres), I looked around and found I could see about ten metres, the seabed here was amazing, it consisted of a large flat plateau stretching as far as I could see. In some areas there were depressions the edges of which consisted of very thin flat planes extending out from the main plateau into the depression, they seemed to be suspended midwater and did not look strong enough to support their own weight, some of these planes extended a metre or more out over the depression, I found that I could swim under them but if I touched them, they would just crumble.

The whole area reminded me of Roger Dean's artwork from the Yessongs record album cover used by a band called "Yes", I followed John who seemed to know exactly where to go, we moved up onto the plateau and within five minutes had located the outfall. I had tied a distance line onto the shot before we moved away from it, John now indicated that he would hold the distance line and I should go back to the shot and move it in onto the outfall. This I did with some puffing and panting as the shot consisted of a block of steel weighing fifty-six pounds (25Kg), and unfortunately in the process some of the dramatic scenery was destroyed. When back at the outfall we secured the buoy line to the outfall and started to have a look around.

The Cleveland Potash outfalls were constructed by tunnelling out from the beach below the seabed, when at the desired distance a vertical shaft had been constructed; this allowed the outfall pipe to be completely protected from the elements which could apparently be fearsome in that part of the world. This meant that the only part of the whole system to be exposed on the seabed were the diffusers. After securing the shot I found myself looking at one of these diffusers, it was a cylindrical object having a diameter of something approaching two metres, it was sticking up out of the seabed by about three metres, the top the cylinder was closed by a dome and in this dome there were two nozzles protruding by about one hundred and fifty millimetres, they had the appearance of two short stubby horns, each nozzle had a hole about two hundred millimetres in diameter, these were pointing upwards at an angle of about forty five degrees, they were arranged so that they were spaced about thirty degrees apart around the dome.

Later I found out that when the diffuser was working the effluent would be forced upwards and outwards from these nozzles at a velocity of about seventy miles per hour, this helped the effluent to be dispersed quickly and efficiently. After a good look around, we returned to the buoy line which was now securely attached to the outfall, with a final look around we exchanged signals and left bottom. When two divers ascend on the same rope, they should ascend facing one another, this allows each diver to see over the top of the others head, that way if there were to be any overhead obstructions above either diver, the ascent could be halted before it became dangerous.

As we came up the air in my dry suit started to expand, I found that after rising a few feet the air in the suit expanded enough so that I was able to stop finning and just rise effortlessly up the line. As we neared the surface, I had to let some of the air out of the suit through my cuff to stop my ascent becoming uncontrolled but this was easy, so when we broke surface, I was in fine spirits, this was definitely the life for me. The boat was just a few metres away from us, the weather was fine and all was well in my world. So, after signalling that we were fit and well with a thumbs up, we swam towards the inflatable boat. Arriving back aboard "Achieve" there was a welcome cup of coffee albeit made with the cursed evaporated milk and some lunch, we then had to relax for a couple of hours, this was necessary in order to allow the extra Nitrogen taken into our bodies during the dive to be breathed out naturally, in order to avoid decompression sickness "The Bends" when we undertake our second dive of the day, to facilitate this we all graduated to different parts of the boat and once there fell over and snoozed for a couple of hours, this seemed to me to be absolutely fitting for a gladiator of the deep.

During the afternoon the first team was to carry out some sampling of the sea bed around the inshore outfall, this involved collecting samples of mud which would be taken back to the lab in Brixham where they would be dried and sieved, the result would then be examined to find out what species of animal or plant life was resident and how many or each were living there.

Our task as team two would be to attack the actual outfall. At this time my hobby was photography, so when the tasks were originally being allocated for the trip while back at the lab in Brixham, I volunteered to be the photographer, at the time I didn't realise that no one else wanted to do it, but this suited me. The camera we would be using was a Nikonos Calypso Mk II, a camera made by Nikon in Japan; lighting was supplied by an electronic 'strobe' flash unit. I had not actually used this type of camera before but this did not seem to matter, all Yersin said was "Just take lots of pictures and something is bound to come out", of course this was well before the advent of digital photography and therefore I was limited to a maximum of thirty-six shots per roll of film, anyway I hoped his optimism would not be misplaced. Initially I had been quite confident, but now as the time approached, I was beginning to have some doubts as to my ability to come up with the goods.

We duly readied ourselves for our dive, the boat crew had now moved the "Achieve" closer to the buoy, this would allow us to dive from the big boat leaving the inflatable for safety cover. By this time I had checked the camera was loaded and that there were batteries in the Strobe for about the fifteenth time, and taken a couple of pictures on the surface of a board indicating the date and the subject of the following pictures on the film together with a colour reference band which would allow us to ensure that when the pictures were developed the colour balance would be correct, soon the first team had completed their dive and it was again our turn.

There would be a requirement for me to record details of each shot taken and this necessitated the use of a very high-tech piece of kit! In those days there was no such thing as voice communications systems for use with SCUBA so, it would be necessary for me to record all details by writing them down; now clearly this couldn't be done using pen and paper so instead we used a 'scratchboard' and pencil. Pencils are great, they write very well underwater and clearly are cheap, the main issue is that the glue used to join the two sides of the pencil encasing the graphite (lead) was not waterproof! We got over this problem by wrapping the pencil in plastic electrical tape this kept the water out keeping the pencil from splitting apart. Next, we needed something to write on, this was solved by using rigid plastic sheeting normally grey or white, we attached the pencil to the plastic sheet using thin twine to stop the pencil floating away; I had also attached another length of twine to a carabiner that I could clip it onto my gear. While this system worked very well, it was not easy to write clearly due to the gloves we had to wear and the physical difficulties with working underwater in the sea having to cope with tide and swells moving us about. Still, it was what we had and it did work so long as I concentrated and took my time.

Arriving on the bottom of the buoy line we spent a couple of minutes sorting ourselves out before getting on with our respective jobs, John was to take some measurements of the build-up of sediment around the outfall while I was to photograph the seabed in the area, as well as the outfall itself. I spent some time arranging the strobe ensuring that all the distances were correct before taking the pictures, as I say the pictures all had to be logged using my scratchboard. Writing everything down was not nearly as simple as you may think it should be, when looking at the board after taking six shots, I was astounded to see that the information I had meticulously noted down seemed to have been rearranged by some mysterious force. Luckily, I could remember what was needed and so I made the notes again, more carefully this time. By the time I had taken thirty odd shots and logged them all, I found that I only had about ten minutes dive time remaining, I went in search of Yersin.

He was around the other side of the outfall, as I swum towards him all I could see were a couple of legs and a backside sticking out of a hole in the seabed, perhaps he had decided that as he was by the seaside, he would dig a hole, just like being at the beach. Eventually he wriggled back out and indicated to me that I should take a photograph of his hole complete with a tape measure in it to show how deep he had managed to dig in such a short time, he was clearly quite proud of it. This seemed a strange request but he was the boss and since I still had a few shots left, I obliged taking shots from slightly different angles, once done I looked at him and he seemed very happy. We then arranged ourselves at the bottom of the buoy line and when ready both left bottom; once on the surface we made our way to the boat and were helped on board by the crew.

As soon as I was dry, I removed the film from the camera and transferred all of the information from the scratchboard into a notebook I had brought along for the purpose. We then started to derig all of the diving gear in readiness for recharging the bottles which had to be done ashore in the evening of the third day. While we were doing this, I found that contrary to what I had been thinking John had in fact been digging down to find the point on the outfall where the original seabed was located, so I had been photographing the hole with a tape measure in it in order to show how much sediment had been deposited around the outfall, just as well I never said anything.

Over the next couple of days, we each dived twice a day, measuring, sampling and photographing the area around the outfalls. During this time, we had established a line running along the seabed called a jackstay, this stretched from one outfall to the other, we could use this line to swim easily between the outfalls. On the third day it was decided that Yersin and I would photograph the outfall while it was working. The plan was for us to go down onto the offshore outfall which would be switched off, we would then swim along the line between the two and when at the inshore one which would be working, I would take photographs of the outfall in action. This seemed to be no problem to me although I felt that it may be a little pointless, as there would probably be a lot of sediment in the water and I wondered if we would be able to see anything, anyway when we were ready it was established that only the inshore outfall was working, we dropped down onto the outer one as planned.

When on the bottom we started out along the jackstay, approaching the inner outfall, I could hear a deep rumbling and roaring sound, it was loud seeming to come from all around me. This unnerved me a little, as we came up to the outfall I looked up and saw the twin horns of the outfall belching out effluent at a tremendous rate, so whereas previously the task had seemed no problem I found that I was beginning to have second thoughts. Looking up I decided to take some shots of the dual plume in silhouette against the light coming from above, this I did twice with the flash and twice without. We then climbed up the outfall towards the horns of the outfall, Yersin had brought a pole fifty centimetres long with ten-centimetre graduations on it, he positioned himself so that he could place the end of the pole into the rush of effluent coming out of one horn, this gave scale in the finished photograph. I then took a succession of photographs changing settings on the camera to ensure that we did actually end up with a photograph that the client would find useful.

Once this was done, I finished the film taking general shots of the outfall in action, before making our way back along the jackstay to the offshore outfall and subsequently back up to the boat. When on board again I was very careful to rewind the film and log the photographs properly as I had been told that we would not be able to repeat this dive owing to the fact that the plant was going to be on shutdown from now on so there would be no effluent available for us to try again.

Having stowed the diving equipment in the hold ready for the trip back to Whitby, we all went our separate ways, (well as much as you can on a small fishing boat bobbing around in the middle of the North Sea) I found myself on the stern of the boat behind the wheelhouse. This was one of my favourite places as it was always out of the wind when the boat was under way, this evening was absolutely splendid, there was almost no wind so the sea was flat calm and the cliffs were bathed in early evening sunlight. I was listening to the radio and a wonderful song was playing that seemed to be just perfect for the day, it was Johnny Nash, I can see clearly now, brilliant. As we approached Whitby, I could see the beach to the North of the harbour was still packed with holiday makers and day trippers all making the most of the sunshine. Rounding the pier head there was a crowd of people waving and eating ice creams, all having fun but I thought they must all be envious of me because I still just couldn't believe that anyone would pay me to enjoy myself this much.

This evening, we had an additional task, once the boat was tied up close to the harbour wall, we unloaded the air bottles; we had brought twenty-five bottles from Brixham and now they were all empty. We did not have a compressor with us so we would have to take them to a dive shop for refill, the chosen shop was in Redcar some twenty miles up the coast. Once we had loaded the bottles into the van, John Yersin was driving and I accompanied him. We drove off along the coast road, this road wound along the coast up over the cliffs past Boulby where the potash mine was positioned, the evening was still very bright and quite warm. After about forty-five minutes we reached the little shop on the sea-front in Redcar.

Redcar is a small Victorian holiday town at the mouth of the river Tees, I had never been there before but it was just as I imagined a Northern seaside town should be, there were lots of people milling about eating the inevitable ice cream or doughnuts, there was a wide expanse of sandy beach. We took the bottles into the shop, there would inevitably be a wait before they would be ready, so we went for a walk along the front having a couple of ice creams, we sauntered around heading back to the shop about an hour later, the bottles were ready for us so we started to carry them all back out to the van. This took a few minutes, it was not until I had finished that I realised Yersin had not been loading them into the van as had been planned, in fact when I tried the back door it was locked, very strange. There were some strange sounds coming from the front passenger side of the van so I went to have a look and found John apparently trying to break into the van, it seemed the keys to the van had become locked inside and could be seen still in the ignition.

Neither of us were particularly well versed in the art of breaking into a Ford Transit van, I have since been told that this can be achieved in just a few seconds with the right equipment which apparently consisted of a piece of flat steel about forty centimetres long. Anyway, we didn't know this at the time, so after about half an hour of deliberating about what to do, it was decided to remove one of the small quarter-light windows from the front passenger door. This seemed the best option and since we had a knife, we thought that this should not take long.... Wrong! It took us about another half-hour and several near misses with the knife before we eventually managed to pry out the glass and reach into the lock thus unlocking the door. During this time and despite our appearance which must have been quite a sight considering we had spent all day on a trawler and were both still in our working gear not a single person paid us any attention, apart that is from one small lad of about seven years old who probably knew exactly how to break in but decided that there was more sport to be had watching a couple of amateurs struggle, I'm surprised he didn't sell tickets.

Once inside the van we quickly retrieved the keys opening the back doors, loading the bottles, making our getaway before the police arrived. I remember spending most of the journey back to Whitby trying to replace the window in the door; not very successfully it must be said.

We spent the rest of the fortnight diving all day, and relaxing during the evenings, it was a thoroughly satisfying way to spend a couple of weeks, and to make it all worthwhile the photographs came out well thus justifying my appointment as photo technician. We returned to Brixham somewhat fitter and more sun-tanned than when we left, and personally I was firmly convinced that my future lay in diving for a living.

CHAPTER FOUR

Continued work with ICI 1976 to 1979

Over the next few years, I was involved in a number of diving projects throughout the UK we were tasked with several surveys of ICI outfalls and others owned by third parties dotted around the coastline of Britain. Sometimes we were employed to survey locations where proposed pipelines were to be placed, these were at locations such as Aberystwyth and Criccieth in Wales.

However, a good deal of our work was in and around Devon such as in early 1977 we were called to inspect a sewer pipe in Dawlish, this pipe had sprung a leak and needed repair. This pipeline attracted lots of very good-sized plaice a tasty flatfish, during one of the dives I managed to bag four of these which we took home for tea that evening. When I got them home, I presented them to my long-suffering mother, mum was very happy until I turned them out onto the draining board and one of them clearly was still alive and started flapping! I was told in no uncertain terms that I was only to bring things home that were actually dead!

Additionally, we were involved in a lot of dives to collect or photograph marine life on or around many of ICI's various outfalls and indeed at some other companies or local authority facilities.

I remember one episode in particular during September 1979, we were tasked with inspecting a twin set of 36-inch outfall pipelines lying in the Firth of the Forth, Scotland; these pipelines had been set on the river bed to carry effluent produced by the ICI Grangemouth dye works. We started by observing waste from the dye process being forced through the pipe's diffusers to see how they were performing, we then had to remove the pipe end plates to take core samples of the sediment inside. During this week we also had to collect crabs for analysis back at our base in Brixham; you've got to have some sympathy for these poor creatures, not only did these poor crabs have to scrape a living while existing alongside this pipe being immersed in whatever floated down the Firth of Forth and probably drink a certain amount of the effluent but some of the ones who managed to do this were then going to be plucked from their home by us so that we could see how much they had been affected, poor things, not much of a life.

Then one day while they were minding their own business all of a sudden, this ogre in a red rubber suit blowing bubbles turns up to spoil it for them. The job was not that taxing as the depth was very shallow but of course being in an estuary diving had to be done at 'slack water'.

When diving in estuaries the plan is always to dive during neap tides so that the effect of water flow is minimised less height variation means less water will be moved in and out; the rate of flow can be worked out fairly well by use of tide tables and an admiralty chart where tidal flows are indicated by 'tidal diamonds' these give a likely flow coupled with the direction of flow at a given time. Also generally tides obey the 'rule of twelfths'; meaning the peak flow will be mid-way between high and low water. Anyway, divers will normally be most productive when diving during the 'slack water' periods around high and low water.

Coupled with this problem of water flow is the amount of silt suspended in the water, in estuaries it is normal for there to be very little visibility or 'viz'; the Firth of Forth is no exception! It was black as your hat (as the saying goes). This of course is not a major problem for a lot of diving tasks as divers quickly learn to build up a mental image of the worksite by touch and feel; this is very effective and once you get used to it you can find your way around very effectively and achieve complex tasks without too much of a problem.

As I say the final task was to remove the end caps from the pipelines so that they could be inspected internally, the pipelines were made of GRP and so were quite susceptible to damage. To reduce and hopefully prevent damage the pipelines had been covered with rock armour during installation, offering protection from impact damage and helping to keep the pipes in place on the seabed. Each of the pipes had diffusers at intervals along their length, each of these poked out of the rock armour to a length of about eighteen inches (450 mm); when the outfalls were in operation the effluent would be emitted from these diffusers to be carried away on the outgoing tide.

When we had all completed our dives for the day, we made our way back to Grangemouth for the night; once back at the hotel we were of course very hungry, we dispersed to our rooms to get cleaned up and then met in the bar to have a swift beverage before dinner; well, one turned into two or three and by the time we made our way into dinner we were all very happy, reliving the day's work with the waiting staff who seemed in awe of our prowess! Of course, very likely they couldn't wait for these boring Englishmen to finish eating and leave them alone but we didn't get that feeling at the time. Having finished our meal, we decamped back to the bar for a nightcap or two which turned into a few more, well a lot more really. There was no thought about the next day when we would of course need to go back to work and even less about the effect of alcohol on diving. It is very bad to drink before diving as this can lead to an increase in the likelihood of decompression illness (DCI).

All divers know of this problem but unfortunately the demon drink got the better of us, especially as I remember it tequila sunrises went down exceptionally well! We finally wandered off to our rooms about three thirty with an alarm call already placed for six thirty to dive a tide when the diving window (slack water) began at eight thirty. When this call came it was quite frankly unwelcome! I dragged myself out of bed feeling a little second-hand, that last drink must have been off! When I made my way downstairs it seemed that the others weren't much better than me, we were all suffering from the beery vino virus! Anyway, off we went to the boat and joy of joys the wind had got up overnight, it was too much for us to be out in the Firth diving today, of course we were gutted not to be going to work! It was decided to go and find some breakfast and to return at ten o'clock to see if things had improved before the diving window for this tide closed. When we returned, we were all feeling a little better after our full English with lots of tea or coffee but I have to say that I was still hoping the day's diving would be scrapped.

Well, the wind had dropped, the tide had turned and the sun had come out so it was decided we should go for it; we made our way out to the buoy tying the boat up, there was still a bit of a breeze and a nasty chop to the water but now that we were there we had to go diving. As I say the dive was very shallow and we all survived without any incidents but I learned a lesson that day and have never again intentionally drunk too much before diving or indeed going out in a little rubber boat either. However, there was one notable exception to this when I was in France which I will get back to later.

ICI Brixham did not always need divers for their survey jobs, from time to time the divers would go on these 'surface' jobs, these normally required taking water samples, measuring tide and current flow using current meters, measuring water temperature at various depths using specialist sampling equipment. We would also sample seabed material using 'grabs'; the grab of choice was the Smith-McIntyre grab; these grabs would be 'primed; while on deck, this was achieved by opening the bucket pushing two loading bars upwards, this action compressed heavy springs. The bucket was then latched in the open position; at the base of the frame there were two trigger plates, once the grab landed on the seabed or anywhere else the trigger plates would be pushed upwards thus releasing the springs forcing the bucket closed scooping a chunk of whatever lay beneath the grab.

In normal use the grab would be suspended by a rope and lowered onto the seabed, sampling material wherever it landed; the action of the trigger plate touching the seabed would release the spring-loaded bucket, the bucket would then close with considerable force scooping up a section of the seabed. The grab would be winched back to the surface being brought back on deck where it would be placed back into its frame allowing access to the sample for us to collect; all very controlled normally but, if there was movement of the boat due to wave action this could become less controlled.

These grabs are fearsome beasts, once primed, if the trigger plates come into contact with anything the grab will operate closing the bucket. I remember one episode where the dangers of operating these grabs were brought home to us; we were sampling in Tees Bay where we nearly destroyed the boat's wheelhouse.

Tees Bay is just North of Whitby we were again using MFV Achieve. On the day in question the weather was poor, with squally rain coming in pulses; for some of the time the rain would stop completely, making it quite pleasant almost immediately we would see another squall marching across the sea towards us. When squalls arrived, they would be accompanied by strong winds and heavy rain! During one of the frequent squalls, the rain started again accompanied by strong gusts of wind, there was already a bit of a swell running and the squalls made it very difficult to launch the grab.

I was working with a friend Dave Smyth priming the grab and manhandling it while it was lifted or lowered; we were to guide the grab over the side as soon as it had been raised enough making sure it cleared the boat's side as it was lowered. When the grab returned to surface, we would do our best to make sure that it again was brought inboard over the rail, where we would settle it into its frame. On this occasion the primed grab had been raised, we swung it out over the rail, just at the wrong time a squall arrived pushing broadside to the swell, she started to roll unexpectedly, the grab swung out a long way from the boat, of course once it reached the zenith of its swing it started to return at speed.

This was not unusual and normally the winch operator would just drop the grab into the sea harmlessly however the rope got hooked up on this occasion and the winch operator couldn't drop the grab. We could see what was going to happen; I looked at Dave and could see that he had the same idea as I did; we both decided the best place for us to be was somewhere else, we both got out of the way as fast as possible, my escape route was to move around the aft deck to the stern and Dave went the opposite way heading toward the bow. This meant that when the grab returned to the boat moving very rapidly and with nobody there to stop its swing it carried on until it connected with the wheelhouse! The grabs trigger plate contacted the wheelhouse firing the grab; there was an almighty crash with wood and glass splintering but this was nothing to the noise the skipper made when he vented his anger at the winch operator! Luckily nobody was hurt and the damage to the wheelhouse was purely superficial so no real harm done.

CHAPTER FIVE

Overseas Work Begins in 1976

It was on one of these trips when I got my first taste of working overseas; in 1976 ICI were contracted to go to Bilbao in Spain to carry out an extensive survey during two sets of tidal periods. This involved the team flying out to Spain where we stayed for two weeks at a time, we then came home returning a month or so later to finish the job. As I said before, I had been on holiday three times with my family when I was quite small and so had been to France, Italy and Switzerland but of course this was a completely different experience, some of it was great but other parts I could definitely have done without!

The Ria Del Nervión O de Bilbao is the main river running through Bilbao and at the time was in a similar state to a lot of our own rivers such as the Tees in the North East of England, there was a lot of heavy engineering alongside the river, we were there to help find out what effect this was having on water quality. Initially we arrived in the early evening going straight to our hotel which was on El Castañal Kalea, it was quite nice but very different from anything I had stayed in before, we were shown to our rooms and then went out to find something to eat. There was a bar just across the street which suited our purposes very well they served a very nice range of tortilla and various omelettes. Of course, they also served lots of drinks, I decided to stick with a rather nice Spanish beer but a few of the others got heavily into Cuba Libra! Bacardi and Coke to you and me, of course the measures were somewhat larger and cheaper than you would find being served up in an English pub but they were going down very well. After a couple of hours, we all found our way back to our hotel and went to bed.

We were awoken at six thirty with breakfast being served at seven; the breakfast was again not what I was used too but it certainly filled a gap, I was very glad that I had just had a few beers the night before as some of the others certainly looked a bit the worse for wear.

During the first morning we all had to go to the local government facility where we would be issued with the necessary work permits; this took most of the morning and was quite an involved procedure. In 1976 Spain was nowhere near as accessible as it is now, there were very tight controls on people coming to work in Spain; it was a different world back then and indeed even though you could find British newspapers some of them had been doctored to make them acceptable to Spanish authorities. An instance of this was page 3 of the Sun newspaper, at the time page 3 in the Sun included a large photograph of a topless lady model, this had been about for a while in the UK but in Spain it was not felt acceptable for women to be seen topless; the model was still there but had a bikini top painted on to the picture in order to hide their attributes; unfortunately, if you held the page up to the light you could see through the bikini anyway so it wasn't very effective.

The afternoon was to be used to check all the equipment that had been shipped out from England but we were told that before then we had a couple of hours to ourselves; so, three of us decided to take a bit of a detour and see a bit of the area. This was fine for a while we were walking along the river and it seemed we strayed into a sensitive area as a police car screeched up alongside us, two officers leaped out with drawn guns and started to quiz us in very rapid and to us incomprehensible Spanish. Luckily, we had our work permits with us and after a lot of gesticulating they eventually pointed us in the right direction which was back the way we had come. Certainly, focuses your attention when people start pointing guns at you! We were a little more careful to stay on the busier thoroughfares after that.

We eventually found our way back down to the river to meet our respective boatmen and their craft; the river was approached by walking down a small access road leading to a harbour clearly used by local fishing boats. I was again in my element, I couldn't get enough of all these new experiences, the sights, sounds and smells were wonderful to me. When we arrived at the quayside I was paired off with Pedro; our leader Rod Hill felt this was very amusing, Pete being paired with Pedro (the 2 Petes Hilarious!).

Pedro had no English and I of course had no Spanish so communication was going to be challenging to say the least; Pedro's boat had probably been blue at some time in the distant past but now it looked more like something that might win the Turner prize, it was a relatively small open fishing boat with a small wheelhouse near the bow, it was about 35 feet long and maybe 8 feet wide, as we were working in a river this was plenty big enough. We loaded all the various equipment onto our respective boats; I had a water sampler, a PH meter used to measure the level of acid or alkalinity in the river water, I also had a meter that measured the dissolved oxygen concentration, a thermometer and a small current meter. Once we were all loaded, we headed off to our sampling locations, my location was mid river about a mile upstream; arriving on location Pedro dropped anchor and raised the appropriate flags to show that we could not move, this would inform all others that they had to avoid us changing course when necessary.

My job was to take a set of readings every thirty minutes throughout a complete tidal cycle; this meant we were going to be at our current location for thirteen hours. During the first and second days all went very well, the weather was extremely hot and sunny which suited me down to the ground. Rod and another of the team were tasked with keeping the fixed location boats supplied with food and water so from time to time we would see them running up and down the river, it all worked very well.

On day five we were at our location happily sampling away when one of the Harbour Master's vessels came alongside and it was clear that they wanted us to move; I didn't really understand the reasons but Pedro managed to get through to me by pointing and using sign language that there was going to be a ship launched and we were in the way. We moved to the far bank and sat to watch the spectacle, and it really was a spectacle, the ship was a bulk carrier that had been built in a yard on the western bank of the river; it was decked out with flags and a brass band was playing. We didn't see the breaking of the champagne bottle if there was one as we were too far away but we did see her slip into the river to cheers from the assembled workers; she was then taken under tow by a number of tugs that shepherded her alongside the shipyard's quayside for the next phase of her construction or fitting out. This was a welcome distraction from the days sampling but after about an hour and a half we were back on location sampling again.

Over the next few days, we settled into a routine with me sampling every half hour, between samples I would lie in the bottom of the boat and read my book, this time it was Peter Benchley's Jaws. Pedro would sit in his wheelhouse and doze for most of the day; as I say things were fine until around quarter to four in the afternoon, I had finished my sampling and was settling down with my book for another session of ten minutes or so. I don't know what made me look up but what I saw galvanised me into action, bearing down on us at a rate of knots was a huge steel ship's bow rising some twenty feet or so above me, when I first saw the ship, it was no more than five feet away from our boat. The ship was travelling at 4 or 5 knots, when it hit us about amidships pushing the gunnel down until water started to come inboard, this was obviously not a good thing and I thought our boat was about to capsize or at least be damaged to the point of sinking.

That is to say if I had had time to think anything that is probably what I would have thought, anyway as soon as I saw the bow and realised it was going to hit us I launched myself towards the far side of our boat with an aim of going overboard, as luck would have it the action of the ship pushing the gunnel down on the port side meant that the starboard rail I had launched myself towards was now raised up considerably and caught me, I hit the rail and clung on, this was actually just as well because as I say I was already half way over the other side trying to abandon ship. If that hadn't happened, I would have been in the water with the ship about to run over me, that would very likely not have ended well for me.

The ship pushed our boat some distance down river, the port side rail being pushed down, dirty brown river water gushing over the gunnel into the boat but, thankfully then our anchor caught and we were pushed aside, I remember sitting in the bottom of the boat in a pool of water watching the ship's side scrape alongside us until we were left in its wake. I was OK, I just had a few bruised ribs and some lost skin on my knuckles; I was not so sure about Pedro, when the ship hit us the gunnel that he was leaning against had been pushed in by a few inches, this had the result of breaking glass in the wheelhouse some of which had drawn blood from Pedro's head and ear. I spent the next few minutes tending to his cuts with the first aid kit we had brought with us, in fact I spent the next few minutes chasing a very irate Pedro around the deck as he was incandescent with rage shouting with raised fists at the receding ship.

I didn't know any Spanish but I can be fairly certain about the sentiments Pedro was expressing; there were a couple of deck hands leaning on the stern rail of the ship, they smiled and waved; this had the predictable effect on Pedro, I thought he was going to have a coronary! For me I was feeling that I had used up one of my proverbial cat's nine lives and I was only twenty years old!

Once Pedro had calmed down a bit, we made our way back to the quayside as I certainly felt there was enough damage to make it sensible for us to have a good look in case there was more damage than we realised. I was transferred to another boat for the next couple of days as Pedro's boat did need a bit of work and I didn't see him again until we returned for our second trip a few weeks later.

When we returned for our second trip I was again billeted on Pedro's boat and we greeted each other like long lost friends even though we still couldn't talk to one another. We spent the next couple of weeks sampling as before but this was punctuated by periods of screaming when Pedro caught sight of the same ship that had rammed us. It was a fairly small coaster, something of maybe 1,000 tonnes plus I would say; it may have been quite a small ship but it hadn't been a fair fight as our boat was nowhere near a match for it.

As far as I know there was no comeback on the ship but it certainly seemed to brighten Pedro's day whenever he saw this particular coaster. I put it down as another of those experiences I wouldn't want to repeat and it shows that even if you fly all the correct signals, you can't be certain that anyone else will see them or if they do then perhaps, they don't know what they mean. From that time on I always made sure to either keep an eye on what was going on around a boat or ship I was on or to be assured that there were sufficient watch keepers to ensure there would be no repeat of that day.

1976 continued to be a great year for me, firstly, I moved out of the family home in Compton, just outside of Torquay as my parents were about to move to Plymouth; I therefore moved into my first flat with a good friend Ash Nichols, the flat was a modest one-bedroom place in Abbey Road, Torquay, it was great to have freedom and to feel I could come and go as I pleased. Not that I had been really restricted at home but of course when you are just twenty years old even knowing your parents are aware of your comings and goings was enough. I had now been qualified as a diver for well over a year and had really got my feet under the table with the dive team which was great; the summer that year was terrific lasting some six months from March until September and it was hot, somewhere in the UK was over twenty-five degrees Celsius from the twenty-second of June through to sixteenth of July.

Generally, it was fine and dry for the whole period; I spent a lot of that summer working in Wales, firstly diving off of Aberystwyth where we were surveying the seabed for a proposed pipeline to replace a sewer pipe that had been found to be leaking and later carrying out tidal survey work in Criccieth, north Wales. We spent a lot of time between dives water-skiing behind the inflatable dive boat, it was pure hell for a twenty-year old lad as I'm sure you can imagine.

CHAPTER SIX

Motorbikes Can be Bad for Your Health – 1977

1977 however was not such a great year for me, in May the front wheel bearing of my motorbike had to be replaced which was taking some time as I had to wait to be able to afford to have it done. During the time my bike was off the road I cadged a lift to and from work with a colleague Peter Nicholson, at the time Pete ran a beautiful five-hundred cc Triumph, Daytona motorbike, he agreed to pick me up in the morning and drop me back in the evenings. Pete used to wear the brightest set of waterproof clothing you could imagine, they were fluorescent orange, you could certainly see him coming or so I thought. One evening on the way home from work, the weather was perfect, it was dry with the sun shining down and being May it was starting to warm up very nicely.

Travelling along the A379 Dartmouth Road, I was daydreaming about what I would do that evening when suddenly as we approached the junction with Goodrington Road Pete slammed on all the brakes. A car that had been travelling in the opposite direction along the Dartmouth Road had decided to turn right into Goodrington Road crossing our path. There was nothing Pete could have done he was well within the speed limit but the driver of the car gave him no warning of their actions. We ran straight into the front of the car, Pete bore the brunt of the impact which almost took his right leg off, it was some six months before he was sure he wouldn't lose it. I also hit the car with my right leg and suffered a nasty broken tibia and fibula, I really don't remember much about it other than being thrown forward into Pete's back by the sudden braking and then being in the middle of the road in pain.

All I could hear was a woman screaming "I didn't see them" over and over again, she must have been blind to miss Pete's Fluorescence! It subsequently turned out she was a learner driver driving without L-pates and was not accompanied by a qualified driver; luckily though she had paid for insurance. We were taken to Torbay hospital where I was X-Rayed and ultimately had my right leg put into a full-length plaster. My boss Brian Maddock turned up in casualty to find out what had happened which was very nice of him, he then telephoned my parents to tell them what had happened and to confirm how I was, after he had done this, he left me and went home. As I was effectively living on my own, I was kept in hospital over-night, so there I was in the hospital bed at about eight o'clock when in walks Ash who tells me he had heard about the crash and thought he would come to see me. That was very nice but he somehow had thought I had been taken to hospital in Plymouth? I imagine that my dad must have given him that impression but it meant he had gone all the way to Plymouth looking for me only to have to come back to Torbay hospital; it was very nice to see him though.

Anyway, I was due to be discharged the next day and mum had told me that she would come to pick me up, I would be taken back to their house in Plymouth for my convalescence! In the morning after I had been seen by the doctor, I was given instructions to visit the outpatient fracture clinic the following Friday and was moved into the day room to await my collection. The nurses did everything they could to move me carefully but the pain in my leg was awful to the point that when they left me in a wheelchair in the day room my vision blacked out completely. After some time, my vision returned but it really does happen that people black out from pain!

The break in my Tibia proved to be worse than I had been led to believe and after a very painful trip down to my parent's house in Elburton, near Plymouth I found that I just couldn't get comfortable and didn't sleep a wink that night or the next; I was very worried. When I attended the fracture clinic, I had another X-Ray; the doctor then informed me that a triangular section of bone had been punched out of the Tibia, this had then managed to turn through ninety degrees and was currently wedged back in an awkward position which explained the pain. He advised me to have an operation to correct this; I really didn't see any other option so agreed to the op. I was taken into Freedom Fields hospital in Plymouth where the operation was completed, it involved my having a metal plate inserted into my leg to help the bone heal properly.

To my immense relief this did fix the problem and after a few days I started to feel better, the pain disappeared and I started to look forward to getting back to full fitness. Unfortunately, due to a number of factors I was in plaster for eight months! This was due in no small part to my being unable to be a good patient, I kept trying to do too much resulting in falls that broke the bone again. It was a dismal summer, my parents were great but, after some six weeks of being at home with them it was clear my mood was not improving. Mum suggested she take me back to the flat in Torquay for the weekends, the flat was on the ground floor so I wouldn't have to deal with stairs, this seemed like a great idea to me and Ash agreed to look after me so all was agreed. On Fridays mum would take me back to the flat and would pick me up again on Monday so that I spent the weekends in Torquay with my friends. This whole time though of course I could not work and clearly even when I did return to work there was some considerable time before I could again take part in diving operations; I was very lucky that ICI were such a good employer and were prepared to wait.

CHAPTER SEVEN

By 1979 I had been diving with ICI for some 4 years, I was beginning to feel that I needed to move on to the next step; at this time the North Sea oil boom was in full swing, there was a need for divers to maintain the structures; I felt that was for me. I was again very lucky with my timing as the Manpower Services Commission (MSC) a Government Department were funding training for areas where shortages existed and yes, you've guessed it commercial diving was one of these areas; I applied to them for funding in mid-1979.

Coincidentally the BBC made a documentary at Fort Bovisand called Inside Story: Diver, focusing on the very course I had applied for; this was screened in the autumn of 1979 and of course I was glued to it. I watched it with a few of my motorcycling friends who all knew what I did for a living but didn't know I had applied for that course; the documentary was a real eye opener, it looked like hell! Sixteen students commenced the course and over the next 12 weeks this was whittled down to just four who passed! What had I let myself in for?

My place on the Basic Air Diving (BAD) course was due to start at Fort Bovisand at the beginning of the following January, this was confirmed by post in early October, that evening I was in a pub called Coombe Cellars with my best friend Phil Pope. I told him about the course and my hopes for the future. I explained that my plan was of course to pass the course and then to work offshore as a diver; I am not sure he could in any way see the attraction but he was I know pleased for me. At this time my plan was to work offshore for between five and ten years; I certainly didn't want to have to work offshore once I was married and certainly, I would want to be at home if children were to come along.

Anyway, my plan was that I would hopefully be able to build up enough money so that I could set myself up with a nice house etc. Part of my plan was to always make sure that if for whatever reason I found I couldn't continue working offshore I would be in a position to come ashore and find a job capable of continuing to fund my outgoings. I did indeed, always regardless of income, make sure that mortgages and loans were never at a level where I couldn't service them with the sort of job I could find in Torbay or the surrounding area.

In October 1979 I completed the purchase of my first house, a nice little three-bedroom mid terraced number, on Upton Hill in Torquay opposite the coach station; I was able to use the compensation that I had been awarded following the road accident in 1977. Anyway, I put the compensation of £2,500 up as the deposit; the total cost was £14,500, goodness knows what it would be worth now! So here I was with a house, a new mortgage of £12,000 and I was about to give up my safe, secure job to embark on a course with no certainty of either passing the course and even if I did pass would I be able to get a job? I don't think my parents were impressed in fact I think they felt I had lost my mind.

So it was that just before Christmas 1979 I completed my notice period for ICI in Brixham, I had been working there for just over six years and generally I had enjoyed my time there. At the time ICI employed some fifty-odd people at the site in Brixham, we all knew one another and the place had a real family atmosphere, I made a few very good friends some of whom I am still close too and see regularly. I have to say it was with more than a little apprehension that I drove away from Brixham on Friday the twenty first of December not knowing what my future would hold.

PHOTOS FROM MY TIME WITH ICI.

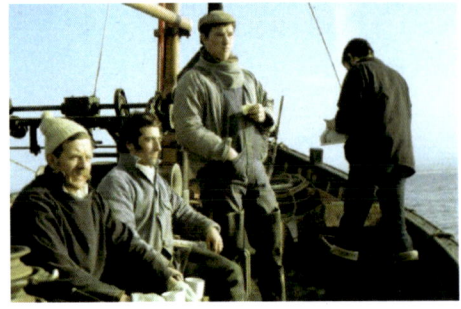

Tea break on the deck of the Achieve, all made with condensed milk!

Photo courtesy of David Taylor

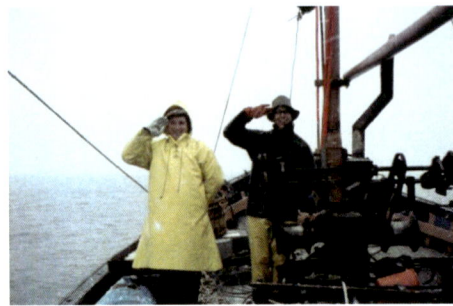

Morning parade on the Achieve.

Photo courtesy of David Taylor

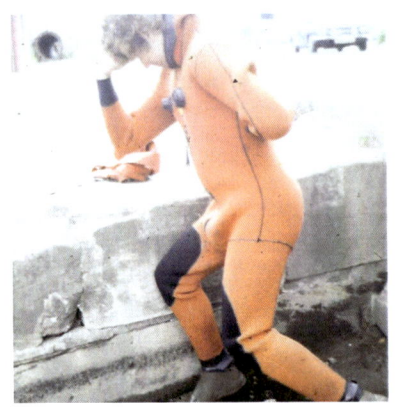

Modelling the Poseidon Unisuit, what all the best dressed divers were wearing in the 1970s.

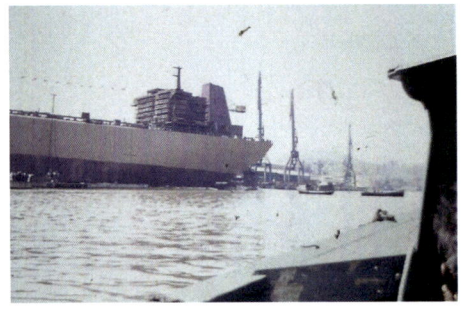

Witnessing the launch of a large bulk carrier in Bilbao in 1976.

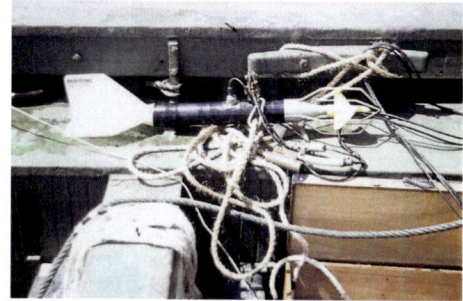

Braystoke tidal flow meter used while in Bilbao in 1976.

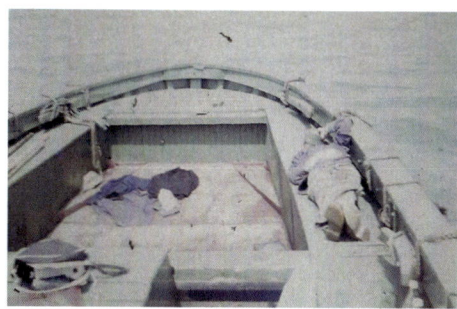

Hard at work again in Bilbao.

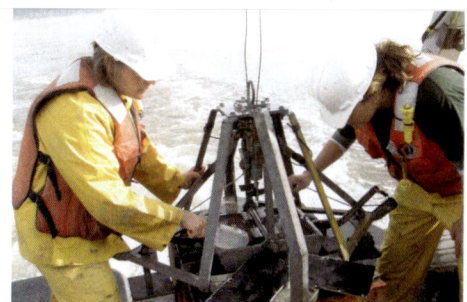

Smith Macintyre seabed sampling grab.

Photo courtesy of David Taylor

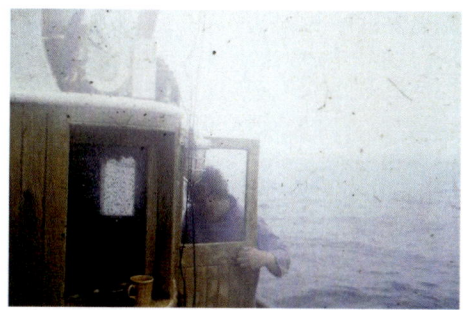

Jimmy climbing into the Achieve's wheelhouse. This was the wheelhouse that had suffered when hit by the Smith Macintyre Grab.

Photo courtesy of David Taylor

Part Two

CHAPTER EIGHT

Basic Air Diving Course (BAD 105) – January to March 1980

So, there I was on Wednesday the second of January 1980 with memories of the BBC documentary fresh in my mind I found myself on my way to Fort Bovisand Underwater Centre to commence my twelve-week Basic Air Diving (BAD) training; we had been instructed to arrive late afternoon with a view to commencing the course on the Thursday. It was a cold clear day, I was wondering what on earth was I thinking of, doubts were running rampant through my mind as to whether I would be able to complete whatever was in store for me during the next three months. I approached the Fort from the east down a roadway that only goes to Bovisand Beach and Fort Bovisand which is situated on the Eastern approach to Plymouth Sound; as I reached the car park for the beach and continued through onto the access road to the Fort, I was greeted by a stunning view across Plymouth Sound.

I was looking along the breakwater built by French prisoners of war past the Breakwater Sea Fort towards Bovisand's sister Fort Pickelcombe on the Western approach side of the Sound. In 1846 the then Prime Minister, Lord Palmerston perceived a significant threat from the French navy who were able to call on steam driven warships; he made a very pertinent remark "If your dockyards are destroyed your navy is cut up by the roots" it's a shame nobody is taking notice of this today isn't it? Anyway, within three years the first three forts forming the basis of the formidable defences around Plymouth had been completed; a quite stunning achievement even by today's standards.

In 1852 French president Napoleon III made himself Emperor Napoleon, the French enlarged their dockyard at Cherbourg and they launched the world's first armour-plated warship. Panic grew when Napoleon declared war on Austria in 1859 prompting a mammoth increase in fortifications for the Plymouth area; the Fort just inside the Breakwater was completed in 1866; things were going well. It could be said that as far as Palmerston was concerned unfortunate events took place in 1870 when the Prussian Army destroyed the French army and Napoleon took refuge in England making these massive defences completely redundant; from that day onwards, they were referred to as "Palmerston's Follies"; poor guy, he could just as easily have been labelled the saviour of England if things had gone a slightly different way.

At the time of their completion these forts were state of the art; there was nothing afloat that could touch them; they would have posed a very significant threat to any enemy ships coming within range.

As I drove my Black, Ford Escort 1,300 Sport around the access road the sea was just feet away on my left and a series of gun ports piercing the granite structure of the fort wall to my right; I parked up overlooking the harbour and got out of my car. The harbour was looking quite serene in the late afternoon light with several dark green aluminium boats lying upside down on the quayside together with ropes and other rigging equipment; this was great, I felt that this was where I belonged although I was still very apprehensive that it would prove to be beyond me. I retrieved my case from the car and made my way to our rendezvous; the letter I had received told me to walk up the hill into the fort and make my way to reception where we would be met. I of course had been here before five-years ago when I had done my original SCUBA training for ICI so knew where I was going.

Walking into the fort there was a high stone wall to my left and on my right, I was passing casemates where guns would originally have been positioned, now though they had all been closed in to form workshops, storerooms and classrooms. The road made a gradual turn to the left following the crescent of the fort, there didn't seem to be a soul about; as I climbed the hill, I found myself entering a wider area where a much more recent block building had been built on the left, I knew this was the canteen where we would be taking our meals for the next 12 weeks. Almost opposite was a large steel door standing open with a sign indicating that this was the reception I was looking for; I have to say it didn't look very welcoming but then I wasn't expecting it to be given the documentary! On entering I was confronted by a small reception desk on the left with a lady who took my name and told me to wait in the reception area until all the others arrived; I wasn't the first or evidently the last to arrive.

Reception was extremely cold, apparently the heating had been off over the Christmas period and had not yet had time to overcome the cold, I later found that although this might have been true the heating never really did overcome the cold especially in the reception area. It was all a bit foreboding as the lighting was to say the least subdued, bluntly it was dark, dank and cold! I wandered further in to find another half dozen individuals who all looked a bit like I felt, a little shell shocked, nervous and cold; we started to get to know one another, I didn't know it then but we were all to become firm friends. They became comrades in what was to be a tremendous adventure for us all.

The first to make themselves known to me were Paul Sims a motor mechanic from Dunstable and a bear of a man, Adrian Fricker a graduate from the Home Counties who over the next few weeks demonstrated the fact that he was clearly very intelligent and capable, these two already knew one another and straight off were fun to be with. Dave Pelly also from the Home Counties was also there, he was a television repair technician and a committed recreational diver; then there was a Welshman, Mark (Jack) Frost. Simon Hale was next to arrive, he was already ahead of us as he had been working as a shipwright in Portsmouth dockyard and a big part of his job involved diving already, all he had to do was pass the course and a job in the dockyard was waiting for him; lucky man. The next arrival was Craig Dickenson, a blond curly haired lad that I immediately felt was going to be a strong candidate on the course.

Next were a couple from Scotland who also already knew one another Geoff Donovan and Blair Drake, then Tom Garnett a Wiltshire lad, Trevor Glew and Tim Hancock both from Lancashire turned up.

There was not a great deal of laughter as I think we were all approaching this whole thing with varying degrees of trepidation; finally, the last three arrived, Andy Godwin representing Manchester and Henry Griffiths another one from the Home Counties and Campbell Park another Scot. There was to have been another chap but he had apparently come down with pneumonia and had to leave the course before it even started, he apparently joined the next course once he had recovered so there, we were, fifteen in total. For better or worse it had started!

When we had been checked in and had all signed the various bits of paper, we were assigned our billet or 'Grot'; we were all billeted together in one of the casemates, we were taken down and shown the room which again was very cold and displayed a complete lack of anything other than the functional. It seemed to me that Grot was a very good name for it. The room had been divided into various sections, the walls of each section extended just above head height, the walls didn't reach to the ceiling, which was a domed brick-built affair covered in sections by white paint that was flaking off. Each section did have a door so there would be a little privacy; one section at the gun port end of the room had four beds (two sets of bunk beds), this part of the room was where the gun would have been positioned, there were large iron eye bolts set into the ceiling and wall; these would have been used to rig the gun and to move it into place.

The rest of the rooms had one set of bunks so billeted two in each room, mine was the first room on the right, my room-mate was Henry Griffiths, we tossed a coin for who would take the bottom bunk and I won although I wouldn't have cared which bunk I had really. Two doors up the hill were the changing room, shower and toilet block. We were told to get settled in and to be in reception the following morning at nine o'clock ready to start the course. Breakfast would be served in the block house on the other side of the access road from seven thirty in the morning we were then left to our own devices and spent the rest of the night getting to know one another.

We all awoke early the next day; day one of the course started with us all wandering across to the canteen where we were confronted with a lovely warm canteen filled with the welcoming smells of the good old English fried breakfast. It was clear that over the next few weeks we would perhaps not be eating the healthiest of diets but it would be filling and tasty; I was sure we would be working hard enough to be able to burn off any excess calories and quite frankly at the age of twenty-four I didn't even think about this. Anyway, I was hungry and keen to get on with things.

After breakfast as instructed, we were in reception at nine o'clock ready for the day; our motley crew gathered with an assortment of pens, pads and bags looking like we were back at school although the uniform was eclectic to say the least.

We were collected at nine sharp and taken to casemate Fourteen (CM14), this was a large and airy classroom. As with all the casemates it also sported these large iron eye bolts in the ceiling and walls. We each took a seat and waited; we were apparently about to receive our domestic brief and staff introduction.

At five-past-nine in strode Alan Bax the director of the facility, I had already met him at my interview where he had quizzed me about my bringing ICIs dive logs with me to the interview, he clearly had decided that this wasn't a problem. Alan was a retired Lt Commander from the Royal Navy and Fort Bovisand was run along very military lines; he had our full attention for his introduction. He made it clear that we would not receive encouragement or be given much in the way of positive feedback, rather, we would be told if we weren't performing so, if we had not been told that we were failing then we should take that as being confirmation that we were doing okay.

There's nothing like telling it how it is, this perhaps came as a bit of a comfort but also it was chilling to know that we could expect little in the way of encouragement. Evidently, we would have to support each other, work as a team, supporting weak members as necessary; our instructors would be awarding 'day marks' to each of us every day and we had to ensure that these marks were consistently above average as below average marks would not be tolerated; there would be one warning and if we didn't pull our socks up, we would be asked to leave. There was no guarantee of a pass from the course, if we were not up to scratch then we would fail and would be asked to leave the course, he went on to describe some of the basics of the course including how we were expected to behave in the evenings and at weekends. We would have evening lectures and homework that must be completed on time, delays would not be tolerated, we would be split into groups and each group would be expected to carry out maintenance during selected Saturday mornings.

We would be expected to stay at the Fort for the complete twelve-week period, it would be frowned on if we went home for more than a couple of weekends, our behaviour would be subject to scrutiny at all times, not just during the time of instruction.

Lt Cdr Bax then proceeded to write 'DREAMS' vertically on the board; we looked at each other wondering what was coming now? Each of the letters signified a point that he wanted to highlight:

D was for Determination; many underwater tasks that could be performed quite simply in the dry become complex underwater, they could also be tedious, physically and mentally demanding and boring. A diver must have the determination to finish his or her (on my course there were no females though) allocated task.

R was Reliability; it was vital for a supervisor to know that he/she could rely on a diver to follow their instructions, so that they would not jeopardise either his own life or that of others; there were apparently old divers and bold divers but very few old and bold divers!

E was Enthusiasm; it was essential that a diver actually enjoys being underwater and feels comfortable under the water, this would enable them to concentrate on their task rather than worrying about the environment all the time. Although nothing was said at this time it became quite clear early on in our training that we were also expected to be enthusiastic when working on deck as well and our day marks would be affected by how we were perceived by the instructors at all times, not just when we were underwater.

A was Ability; a professional qualification was of considerable advantage both to the diver himself and his employer.

M was mix-ability; divers from different countries and cultures were often brought together for a project. It was essential that they were able to work as a team whatever the circumstances.

S was Stamina; to be effective in his work a diver must be physically fit and healthy.

Following this sobering speech, we were introduced to the instructors who would be taking us through the course; the chief instructors would be Ray Salmon an ex commercial diver who had worked offshore for a number of years and Bill Doughty an ex Royal Marine. They would be supported by Tony Hale, another ex-commercial diver who had worked for a number of diving companies; there was also an Australian, Monty Ham and Peter Bernardes who ran British Diver an ex Motorised Fishing Vessel (MFV) one of the vessels we would be working from.

Alan Bax then handed over to Ray Salmon and left the room, we were not given much time to think about what had been said, Ray issued each of us with a diving log book; one of the administration team took our photograph with a Polaroid instant camera, this camera took four passport sized photographs at once, we were given one of these and told to stick it into the log book in the appropriate place. Once this had been done, we were told to complete the basic information such as date of birth, address etc., I found later the admin woman was called Susie and once we had stuck our photographs into the log book, she applied a stamp across the photograph declaring my photograph to be a true likeness of me.

We were then taken en-mass to our classroom the classrooms were in the magazines below the casemates; these magazines would have been where the gunpowder and various stores would have been stored and were below ground underneath the gun rooms. Being taken downstairs to the magazines it felt like we were entering dungeons more than classrooms but classrooms were what they were to be for us, we were to be using Mag 14 as our normal base classroom.

Ray told us that each week one of us students would be assigned as Course Leader, this individual would be responsible for the security of the classroom and drying room, a place we hadn't even seen yet. The course leader would hold the keys for these rooms, he would release them as appropriate and would be responsible for cleanliness of both rooms and that the drying room had an adequate supply of bottled gas.

The course leader would also be responsible for ensuring the attendance registers were signed and returned to the admin office each Thursday morning and that all course diving logbooks and completed homework was returned to the training office by 08:30 Tuesday morning for marking. He would be responsible for the cleanliness of the dormitory and may be assigned other duties as the instructors saw fit; this sounded like a position that should be avoided at all costs! Of course, this was never going to happen and as my name starts with an 'A' I suppose it was inevitable that I had the dubious honour of being our first course leader; the course was split into two groups so as well as being course leader I would be group leader for group A with my room-mate Henry Griffiths, being group B leader I'm not sure he felt any more enamoured by this than I was.

We then had a couple of lectures about effects of pressure on the body and choice of basic equipment; mid-morning we were taken to the equipment store where we were to be issued with our basic equipment.

We followed Ray out of the door turning left heading down the dank corridor, there was minimal lighting but as we were taken down the hill we soon came to a stairwell on our right, we climbed the very steep steps which had been worn by the passage of many thousands of boots. This brought us back to the colonnade about half way between reception and the equipment store, which was situated in the casemate closest to the harbour. When my turn came, I was issued with a half mask, snorkel, fins, knife, quick release weight belt with weights (only a couple of kilos this time) and a wetsuit with a hood but no gloves! Wetsuit, in January without gloves!

Yes, it seemed that for the first week we would be going through basic drills using snorkel and occasional SCUBA so wet suits were best for this work; as for gloves; no gloves would be allowed at any time on the course not even work gloves; oh joy! We had to sign for all of this equipment and it was made clear to us that if we lost or damaged anything we would be charged for its replacement. I was quite comfortable with this phase of the course as I had already completed this on my previous course so felt that I shouldn't have any issues with this at all.

Eventually we were all standing outside the store clutching our equipment thinking, what next? Tony picked us up and took us back up the hill to the far end of the Fort where we were shown the drying room. This was another subterranean room but this one had a gas fired heater keeping the room at a good temperature, it felt dry and comfortable, clearly this was going to be an essential room for us as it would dry our kit overnight making it easier to put on in the morning, at least that was the plan. Tony said we should change into our wetsuits and leave all our dry kit in the drying room; he said that we would be expected to be on the jetty in ten minutes!

No time to lose, he left, we all rushed to get our suits on so that we were not late; I was again at a bit of an advantage here as I had been wearing wetsuits for years diving, surfing and sailing so had no problem with this deadline, some of the others were not so fortunate, anyway we all helped each other and eventually arrived on the jetty as a group to find Tony looking at his watch. "What time do you call this? I told you ten minutes and you took fifteen. This is not good enough, when you are given a deadline, you will adhere to it or will lose day marks".

I thought this was going to be difficult as there would always be times when something would get in the way of our meeting an impossibly short deadline but it was clear that missing deadlines would not be acceptable.

Bovisand had a small harbour; the walls were constructed of granite blocks with faced smooth slabs forming the top surface. There was a slipway extending down between part of a jetty on the eastern side of the harbour and the rear harbour wall, this slipway ended on a small beach only visible at low water; from the top of the slipway the main arm of the harbour wall extended due west out into the sound for some fifty metres or so; the wall was about six metres wide, the seaward side had a raised section some three metres above the deck with a walkway running along the full length with steps down to the main deck of the wall about mid-way along; anyone walking along this walkway could easily see over the wall to the sea beyond.

Mid-way along the harbour wall from the main deck there were a set of steps leading down into the harbour. At the western end of the harbour wall a jetty of about five metres width extended to the North for about thirty metres or so, this jetty had no wall or balustrade; this would be the venue for much of our shallow water training.

At the junction between the harbour wall and the jetty there was a round tower sporting a flag mast and a block house that would be the dive control when we progressed to surface supplied diving. Along both sides of the jetty wall and around the inside of the harbour there were a number of iron ladders extending from the deck all the way to the seabed; these would be used by us when we were coming back from our dives; we normally didn't use the ladders to enter the water much as we almost always had to jump from the jetty These ladders were fine to climb when the tide was in but when it was out, we would have to climb some seven to ten metres and when using some of the heavier equipment this would be very challenging. At times we would be using free flow helmets which are quite heavy in their own right and when working on the seabed we would be using a weight jacket together with lead lined boots; when we got to the top of the ladders we would be struggling for breath and would be very glad to sit down and have the hat removed.

Looking back toward the fort from the tower the fort looked just as formidable as it must have been to any marauding seafarer back in the day. The fort was again constructed with granite blocks fitting neatly together, obviously constructed by very skilled craftsmen, the gun ports were made of metal and were painted a dull red colour. I found out later that these gun ports were manufactured as a sandwich of steel, oak and lead, they were capable of absorbing tremendous energy making them almost impregnable at the time. The fort also had some additions left over from the Second World War when it had housed an anti-aircraft battery; on the roof there were two ugly block structures where the anti-aircraft guns would have been placed and where observers would have been positioned; one of these now contained the bar and the other had been converted into accommodation.

We had congregated on the harbour wall just at the top of the slipway; Tony told us to make our way to the tower. We were then briefed on what was expected of us; we were to climb onto the parapet of the tower, put on our fins, mask and snorkels and then one by one we would be required to jump into the water. Tony stood on the parapet with us and told us how to hold ourselves so that when we entered the water, we would do so in a way that would ensure we didn't hurt ourselves or lose our equipment; loss of equipment seemed to be the major concern here! We were told to place a hand over our mask, elbows were to be tucked in to our sides, the hand that wasn't holding our mask was to be placed across our chest to grasp the elbow of the other arm. We were to stand on the edge of the parapet and to look straight out (don't look down!), then step out and once in the air bring both feet together pointing our fins downwards. Sounds simple, doesn't it?

Well maybe when sitting in a nice comfortable chair reading a book but, when you are standing on the top of a tower looking down at the water (I know we weren't supposed to look down but of course, as soon as someone tells you not to look down what do you do?). Anyway, at this time the tide was about half way in so I'm sure the drop was only about twelve metres to the water but it looked a long way down from where I was standing.

Of course, they had to decide who was going first and predictably they decided we would go in alphabetical order so I was to be first! This is a cross I have had to bear all my life and indeed I was used to it, I have found that it is actually nicer not to have too long to think about things and normally people don't expect the first guy to get things as right as the last guy should, so normally it works out. So, here I was then standing on the top of the parapet looking straight ahead over a beautiful blue-green sea with Tony muttering things about how some of the last course had been hurt very badly by doing this incorrectly, this was of course a great help to me. I did what I had been told, holding my mask, gripping my elbow, tucking my elbows in I stepped off the tower; I did my best to point my fins downwards, I felt myself gaining momentum and then I hit the water.

I found myself under water in a cloud of bubbles, I let go of my mask which had miraculously stayed in place and although some water had made its way inside, I could still see. Quite quickly I came back to the surface and looked up to see a number of faces peering down at me, Tony put his thumb up and I returned this gesture as we had been told this meant we were OK, I had done it and it felt great, no injury, and I still had all my kit with me wonderful. I moved out of the way while all the others made their jump, we all managed the jump although some didn't land quite as well, some lost fins and masks but nobody had any injury and we managed to retrieve all the lost kit so no great issue.

We then swam around the end of the jetty into the harbour where we spent the rest of the day going through basic drills and exercises, learning to clear our masks of water, duck diving and other essential skills; towards the end of the afternoon all of us were cold and tired. We exited the water by swimming up the slipway and were told get dressed, have some food and be ready for an evening lecture at 19:00 in the classroom. The evening lecture covered pressure, its measurement and I have to say I found it very difficult to stay awake but luckily it was a subject that I had already covered and had a good understanding of.

We finished at 20:00 and were told that we were free for the evening but that we should report for PE first thing in the morning at 07:00. I followed everyone out of the magazine locking the door; we made our way up to our dormitory and from there up to the bar to discuss the day. The Bovisand bar was a very welcoming place accessed from reception by climbing a very steep wooden staircase; once at the top of the stairs the bar was built around one of the Second World War gun emplacements with the bar situated on the right-hand side against the back wall. The floor was arranged on two levels, the bar was on the top level, in front of this was a lower level arranged to form a circular floor area about half a metre below the upper level.

The lower level had tables and chairs arranged around picture windows giving a tremendous panoramic view of Plymouth sound and the breakwater; of course, it was dark so we were treated to flashing lights and beacons from various navigation buoys, the lighthouse on the western end of the breakwater and lights from the various boats in and around the sound.

Behind the bar was Hazel, she welcomed us with a lovely smile, we came to look forward to her smile at the end of every day; we spent the next couple of hours nursing a couple of pints, reliving our first day's experiences and getting to know one another properly it was great.

The next morning, we all congregated above the harbour in our running kit at the allotted time to be greeted by a Naval Physical Training Instructor (PTI) who was going to be taking us through our morning physical exercise. This first day we were to run to the T junction at the top of the hill and back, not too bad he said! I have never been a runner and this was not a small distance for me to run but eventually I managed it together with all the rest of the course, some of course just breezed it but most struggled up and back as did I. Anyway, we all arrived back and went to have a shower followed by breakfast, one of the high points of the day; we were beginning to get to know the girls who worked in the kitchen so more banter was forthcoming.

Day two started off at 08:30 with us seeing Doctor Maurice Cross who was undertaking some research into why some divers seemed to be more susceptible to suffering Decompression Illness (DCI) than others, it seemed he had some idea that the incidence may be related to diet and the amount of fat in the blood. As an incentive to us Dr Cross offered each of us agreeing to participate in his research an HSE offshore commercial diving medical at the end of the course free of charge so that when we left the course, we would have twelve months before having to pay for another medical. The main thrust of the research would be for us to give blood samples at the end of each week and towards the end of the course to undergo some hospital-based scans; this seemed acceptable so we all signed up.

This all took an hour or so after which we made our way to MAG14 for lectures; we then spent the rest of the day going through more drills in the harbour learning our trade, at the end of the day we were told that instead of PE in the morning we would be taking a swim in the harbour and so should be ready dressed in our wetsuits on the jetty at 07:00. It seemed that we would take it in turns, one day would be PE and the next would be a swim, I definitely preferred the idea of starting the day with a swim.

As commercial divers we were going to be 'driven' by surface crew, once we progressed to surface supplied diving equipment this would be achieved by means of voice communications but as SCUBA divers, we would be using rope signals. None of us knew any rope signals and so were all starting from scratch with this; the Royal Navy had devised a system of 'pulls' and 'bells' delivered by means of a rope to the diver. We had a lecture telling us how this system worked; the first thing to understand was the difference between a pull and a bell? It seemed a pull was a single movement with the rope being pulled steadily about a foot or so and a bell was where the rope was jerked twice in quick succession, rather like the ding-ding of a bell. There were general signals directing the diver or allowing the diver to make specific requests; there were also directional signals enabling the topside tender to direct the diver go left, right, away from or come towards the tender.

There were also more specific signals used when conducting work, this allowed the diver to request a load to be pulled up or lowered etc., anyway after a very short lecture we were presented with hand-out number 2402 detailing Rope Signals and what they were used for. We were told we would be working in pairs, to go to the store and draw ropes for each pair so that we could practice using these signals in the dry.

There we were with the whole course paired up with one of the pair holding one end of a rope and the other holding the other end; it looked like we were all going to play at skipping like kids in a playground. There was a blustery wind blowing making voice communication a little difficult but of course that wouldn't be a problem really as we had rope signals didn't, we? We were arranged along the harbour wall and surrounding area such that each pair had enough room to practice, we each had our hand-out to refer to and off we went. Just imagine all these men armed with bits of paper being blown about and tugging on lengths of rope hoping to direct operations at the other end, it was a farce!

I was acting as the diver's tender simulating being on the surface directing my diver who was Craig Dickenson, after about an hour of this we seemed to be getting the hang of it; easy! Tony then produced blacked out masks, the 'divers' would then be unable to read our crib sheets; we swapped around so that Craig became the tender and I was the diver. We did okay and although were not quick we did work well together although I did have a few doubts when I had lost my sense of direction and had to trust Craig that he wasn't sending me over the edge of the harbour wall.

Over the next few days, we continually used rope signals during our dives and became quite proficient, even when we progressed to surface supplied diving, we still used rope signals from time to time as they were a full-proof secondary form of communications.

The first week progressed with us doing basic skills and practicing with rope signals etc., I felt it was great with a good deal of light hearted banter being passed between team members and indeed with the instructors.

The second week we were issued with SCUBA gear and would be doing some real diving. Now of course I had been working with SCUBA for some five years with ICI so felt quite at home with this equipment. Our first dive using SCUBA gave me a memory which was not really that good. We were going to practice 'ditch and retrieve'; this was to simulate having a problem with SCUBA gear where the equipment had to be removed while underwater. The retrieve was where we would be required to swim back to the set we had just taken off and put it back on. We were to practice this in small pools alongside the Tinside Pool on Plymouth Hoe, by doing this in these pools we would easily be able to stand up if things went wrong, much safer.

We had already had a lecture telling us what needed to be done and how to go about it. We would start with the set on our backs sitting on the bottom of the pool; we would then loosen the shoulder straps and the waist belt before pulling the set off over our head, once over our head we would bring it down in front of us placing it on the bottom in front of us. We would then remove our mask and secure it on the set so that it wouldn't float away; once this had been completed, we would turn off the air by closing the bottle's valve (the pillar valve) and breathe down the remaining gas, as soon as we had run out of the gas in the hoses we would let go of the set and swim to the surface or in this case stand up being careful to breathe out on the way up.

Once we had achieved this, we would then reverse the process so that we retrieved the equipment until we were again sitting on the bottom breathing from the set. I had already done this a few times on my previous course and so knew what was required and how to go about it.

We loaded all our kit into the back of one of the fort's old vans and clambered into the back of another and off we went. The day was very clear and cold, it had started with a hard frost and although the sun was out, there was very little warmth in it; when we arrived at the Hoe, we unloaded the equipment taking it down to the side of the pools. Tinside Pool is a large circular art deco structure situated on the Hoe to the seaward side of the road; I had never been there and at the time it was looking quite sorry for itself, since then it has been completely refurbished and I remember thinking that it certainly needed it. There was a small changing room where we were told to get changed into our wetsuits and to be back ready to go in ten minutes; this time we made it with time to spare.

We were not going to be using the main pool but rather we were going to be using a small pool to the right-hand side of the main one; this pool seemed to be little more than a rock pool about one and a half metres deep, the sides and bottom had been painted white so it was quite bright, the water was very clear. We were all instructed to get in to the pool; when I entered the water, it was freezing! I thought this was going to be a really cold morning.

There we all were sitting in this shallow pool in early January wearing wet suits; we hadn't brought enough sets for all of us to do this at the same time and in any case the instructor had to oversee each one of us doing it to ensure we could all complete the process properly. We were all watching each other do these drills by lying on the surface with our masks and snorkels allowing us to see the action, or lack of it underwater. From time to time, I would poke my head up and try to get some heat in my limbs by working them a bit however I was getting colder and colder by the minute; this time I was one of the last to perform so by the time it came to my turn I was absolutely freezing and could barely feel my hands let alone do anything with them. I started with all the kit on sitting on the bottom of the pool; I was faced with Monty Ham who was also sitting on the bottom.

Monty gave me the thumbs up that was the signal for me to commence the drill; I managed to release the waist belt and loosen the shoulder straps quite easily, I then wiggled the set up and over my head, placing it on the bottom in front of me. So far so good, now I had to take off my mask, leaving it somewhere that I would be able to find it again, when I pulled my mask off my face burned with the freezing water, I hadn't realised just how warm my mask had been keeping my face. I immediately had a searing headache from the cold water on my face; now to close the pillar valve, I fumbled about but there was no way I could turn off the bottle, eventually I decided just to leave it and come to the surface. This was not a problem but when I went back down to the set, I found that it had been switched off by the instructor (wearing gloves) and so I had to work out a way to open the valve while holding my breath; I just couldn't do it and eventually had to give up and go back to the surface without completing the task, a failure.

I just couldn't remember ever being as cold as I was that morning, this is saying something for a motorcyclist who used his ride his bike all year round and had ridden to north Wales through freezing fog before camping without a sleeping bag, it was awful. As I was the last to attempt this test, we left the water and made our way back to the fort for lunch; I was not happy at all and neither were the other two who had not completed the task.

After lunch we were to be doing the same task again but this time, we would be doing it in the sea at a depth of 7 metres; this was the real thing, it was a task we had to complete before we could progress or we may not be staying on the course, was this to be the end for me? To say I was nervous would be an understatement; when we entered the water, I was pleasantly surprised to find that the water was a good deal warmer than it had been in the pool that morning. I was again slated to be one of the last to do the task; we were all wearing Adjustable Buoyancy Life Jackets (ABLJ) and were told to inflate the jacket and hang on to a buoy at the mouth of the harbour; this buoy was positioned in 7 metres of water so we were to go down the buoy line ditch our gear, come back to the surface free swimming; we would then need to free dive back down to the set and retrieve it as before. As the rest of the team were hanging on the buoy this pulled the buoy away from its anchor point ensuring that when we came up we were not under the buoy.

I floated on the surface trying to watch everyone complete the task although I really only saw a few bubbles rising towards me. Eventually it was my turn, by now I was very definitely nervous when Ray pointed to me for my go. We both left surface going down to the bottom, there was not a great deal of visibility, maybe a metre or so; Ray gave me the thumbs up meaning 'are you ready'? I returned the signal and started the task, all went well, I undid the quick release buckle on the waist strap being careful to make sure it was not the weight belt I had undone and loosened the shoulder straps, I pulled the set over my head and placed it on the seabed in front of me keeping the Demand Valve in my mouth; I removed my mask and put it under the set on the right-hand side so that I would be able to find it on my return.

This time my hands were functioning well and I was able to turn off the cylinder's pillar valve and breathe down the air in the hoses; I then placed the demand valve (DV) across the bottle and made my way to the surface breathing out all the way up so that the gas in my lungs was safely exhaled as it expanded with the reduction in pressure.

As a diver descends their Demand Valve (DV) will supply sufficient gas to keep the diver's lungs properly inflated so, at ten metres this would be like the balloon being completely full; if we then come back to the surface without exhaling or letting gas out of the balloon the gas will expand to twice the volume, therefore if I held my breath, I would suffer a burst lung as the air expanded. I did exhale all the way back to the surface so safely reached the surface where I took a couple of breaths before duck diving back down to retrieve my set; I came straight back down onto the set so the first worry was gone, I had found the set again. I located the pillar valve and turned it, there was the second worry gone as it turned easily; I pressed the purge button in the centre of the second stage of the DV (the part I would be putting in my mouth) to make air come out before putting it back in my mouth and starting to breathe from it again. Whew, now I could take my time, I found my mask and put it back on, of course it was full of water but this was not a problem as all I had to do was to look up towards the surface and press the top of the mask with my finger while breathing out through my nose, the mask emptied immediately and I could see clearly again.

I then placed the set in front of me with the pillar valve pointing towards me the base of the bottle away from me with the back pack and straps upward, I arranged the shoulder straps and placed my hands inside them gripping the back pack pulling it up over my head, I let it slide down my arms so that the set settled nicely onto my back with the straps lying on my shoulders, I then tightened the shoulder straps and waist belt. I then gave Ray a thumbs up which he returned and we made our way slowly back up to the surface.

That was the end of the day so we made our way back out of the water and started to strip the kit down; we returned the SCUBA kit to the store, while I was carrying my set back to the store Ray came along with me and assured me that although I hadn't achieved the task in the morning the reason was understood and the fact that I had done it correctly this afternoon would be fine and I was not to worry about it. I could have hugged him but of course I just said "thanks Ray"; I certainly was much happier than I had been at lunch time.

The end of week two was to be the end of the SCUBA section of the course, we had to pass a theoretical examination and SCUBA rescue practical; pressure was on as we were left in no two minds about the penalty of failure. The exam was programmed for Saturday; we spent Friday evening buried in our books trying to ensure we would reach the pass mark of seventy percent; the exam was to test our knowledge of all the basics of diving meaning there would be a lot of questions requiring us to work out mathematical problems using the various gas laws and Archimedes principle, the method we had been given to describe buoyancy in the water.

In all my school days I had never really revised for any exams; this was evident from my lack of achievement in this area. I was determined that as I felt I had finally found something I was good at and enjoyed that I would not let a lack of revision get in the way of my progressing. In the morning the mood at breakfast was sombre to say the least, it was something akin to the last meal of the condemned. We had been told to assemble by the chartroom (another dungeon) at nine o'clock for the theory exam; the chartroom was a room reached by the same corridor we used to get to our classroom but was on the other side of the corridor.

At nine o'clock, Tony arrived with the key to the room and in we went; the room was accessed by a couple of steps up to a much larger room than mag 14. There were ten large tables arranged as a classroom facing the back wall of the room where there was a blackboard; we had not been in this room before and it felt as though it didn't get much use at all. The room smelt damp and again was not very warm; the ceiling was the same as all the other magazines in that it was constructed of brick forming an arched ceiling, this ceiling had been painted white at one time but the paint was flaking and falling onto the tables and floor. None of this did anything to raise my mood; we were told to take a seat ensuring enough space between us so that there could be no conferring or cheating.

Tony had a hat with him and we were told that there were pieces of paper in the hat, we were to draw one each from the hat, we all did this and I found the number fifty written on mine; we were told that this number was our unique number and that in any of the exams we undertook we should not put our names on the paper, rather we should put this number at the top of the paper. This system ensured that whoever was marking the paper wouldn't know whose paper they were marking and so could not be affected by likes or dislikes of the student.

We were given one hour for the test but worryingly I had completed it in about forty-five minutes; I checked all my answers and finally got up taking my paper up to the desk at the front where Tony was reading a book. I then went to get a cup of coffee in the canteen to wait for the rest of the lads; Adrian was already there and we started to discuss the exam, it seemed that we had both found the questions relatively easy and had comfortingly come up with the same answers for the ones we could remember.

At eleven o'clock we were again assembled in our wetsuits on the jetty ready to go through our SCUBA rescue assessment, this went very well for all of us with the air full of huffing and puffing of divers carrying out expired air resuscitation (EAR) while towing their buddy to the steps. This had to be done properly and involved the rescuer placing their mouth over the casualty's nose and blowing air into his lungs. This was quite unnerving but had to be done. Once at the steps we had to shout for help when the others of our course would be allowed to come down the steps to help us lift the stricken diver to the deck of the harbour wall. If anyone actually needed help while in Bovisand harbour they would never get any as everyone would think it was just an exercise.

The rescuer then had to complete more EAR and chest compressions until the instructor told us to stop and place the rescued diver into the recovery position. Once everyone had carried out their rescue, we were lined up to be told that we had all passed the practical, there was an audible sigh from all of us; we were given half an hour in which to get changed and were then to meet in CM14 where we would be given our results from the morning's theory exam.

Again, we all assembled at the allotted time and settled in our seats to hear our fate; Tony entered with a face that indicated he was not at all happy; stress levels reached new heights; he then posted a typed piece of paper on the board and told us the results were there for us to see. He then told us where we were to be on Monday morning and left, well at least that sounded like we were all staying; there was an understandable stampede to the front of the room to see our results. We had all passed and it seemed the standard was high; my mark was ninety seven percent! I don't think I had ever passed anything with a mark even approaching that; to say we were happy would be an understatement. The instructors had gone out of their way to explain this exam was the hardest one we would be faced with as it tested all our knowledge about the basics of diving including physics and physiology; the rest of the course exams would cover equipment and procedures and should therefore be easier, well I wasn't taking any of that, I would be revising for every one as though my life depended on it.

That evening we went to the bar with high spirits, although it wasn't planned, we had a great party with various drinking games fuelling our conversations and reminiscences of the first two weeks with stories getting taller and taller as the night progressed. It was great, Hazel and Laura joined in the fun, they were to become part of the team; Hazel would eventually succumb to Simon's charms, they would marry sometime following the course; some years later Laura left Bovisand to become a professional singer at Sun City in South Africa.

Week three was the first time that we were introduced to Surface Supplied Diving Equipment (SDDE), this was of course completely new to me and I was keen to find out more about this equipment as it was how real commercial divers worked; also joy of joys we would finally be issued with dry suits, thank goodness.

Day one of week three we handed back our wetsuits and were issued with dry suits and under-suits or fleecy woolly bears instead, we were to be using a completely different type of suit to the one I had used at ICI, these were Avon suits. Instead of being made of neoprene the Avon suits were made of heavy rubber and were termed membrane suits. With a neoprene suit there was a certain amount of thermal protection provided by the neoprene material but with the membrane suit that was not the case. Thermal protection was wholly provided by the under-suit, this means that it is much more important that the suit remains dry, I was not confident of this given the fact that I had never had a dry dive yet. There was no zip; apparently, you were expected to climb in via the neck, this would be interesting and looked like hard work.

We were given a lecture on the care and maintenance of the suits and a demonstration of how to put one on, then it was our go. We again paired up as this was a two-man job, I was again paired with Craig Dickenson; firstly, we applied French chalk (talc) to the cuffs and neck seal, this would ensure that our hands and head would slide through the delicate latex without causing damage to these fragile seals. I donned my woolly bear under-suit, then sitting down I pulled the dry suit's neck over my feet and up to my hips ensuring that my feet were firmly in the suit's boots. I then stood up and pulled the neck up to my chest, next I had to stretched the neck away from my body giving space for me to push my right arm into the suits arm, I pushed my hand through the cuff such that it was nicely sealed around my wrist. Now was the point where I needed my buddy, Craig gripped the neck of the suit on the left side immediately below my left arm, he placed his foot against my left foot and leant away from me stretching the neck enough to allow me to get my left arm inside the neck and into the suits arm, once my arm was inside, he let go the suit sprung back settling around my shoulders.

Both wrist seals were now seated nicely around my wrists, all that was left now was to fit the neck seal; I pulled the metal neck ring over my head so that it rested on my shoulders, next was the latex seal, this was pulled over my head, the neck ring had a groove into which both the suit neck and the latex neck seal fitted snugly. I was now finished apart from the locking ring which was again passed over my head, I then pulled it onto the neck ring and with Craig's help fitted it nicely over the top of the neck seal and suit rubber, once in position the clamp was tightened so that the neck seal was secured to the suit firmly and wouldn't come undone.

I helped Craig with his suit in the same way and we were done; over the next few minutes the grunting and mumbled obscenities finally came to an end; we were all suited up, the suits were black and made us look like a bunch of military divers. This all took place in the road outside the store, the storemen and passers-by all had a bit of a laugh at the obvious novices getting to grips with these suits. Ray had been watching all of this and when all of us had finished he addressed us; "are you all happy?" We of course all nodded and were in fact quite pleased with ourselves; Ray went on, "well I'm not! What a shower of shit! That has just taken you fifteen minutes; you need to be able to do this in three minutes for a pair.

That's right; a pair of divers should be dressed and ready to go in three minutes". We all looked at each other and were wondering how anyone could do this in three minutes; this was going to make deadlines even more challenging. We of course practiced this remorselessly over the next few days in our own time and eventually we did conquer it to the point that we could all get a pair of divers ready in the allotted three minutes; phew again.

Over the next couple of weeks, we were taken through all the different types of equipment we were likely to come across starting with the Avon Full Face mask with its formed plastic faceplate giving very strange distortion to the edges of the diver's vision when underwater. We also covered free flow helmets and demand hats; both of which were supplied with air from the surface via an umbilical hose, this umbilical hose ran to the hat where it entered via a Non-Return Valve (NRV); this valve was an essential safety device fitted to all hats and helmets being supplied with gas from the surface.

In the past there had been instances where divers had been supplied with air via a hose from the surface but without the benefit of NRV in line, if the hose became severed during operations such as lifting or cutting, the open end of the pipe would be at a far lower pressure than the diver resulting in the diver being squeezed up the umbilical or at least into the hat; the result would be an extremely unpleasant way to die. With the inclusion of an NRV, if the umbilical became damaged the diver would not be affected other than to lose their air supply. We were taught to always check the NRV was working before attaching the hat to the umbilical.

Divers using surface supplied diving equipment are supplied with air from the surface through an umbilical, this air would be supplied from a compressor or alternatively from high pressure bottles held on the surface. Both of these meant that the diver's air supply was to all intents and purposes unlimited, which had of course been the major limitation of SCUBA where the diver had to carry all their air with them; this makes SDDE (Surface Demand Diving Equipment) preferable for working underwater where the diver may be working very hard and therefore using a tremendous amount of air. The umbilical will not only carry gas through to the diver but will normally have another smaller hose used to measure depth, this is termed a pneumofathometer or 'pneumo'; an ingeniously simple method for the supervisor on the surface to keep an eye on depth of the diver is at any time.

The pneumo hose is an open-ended hose attached to the diver at a point near to his chest i.e., close to his lungs. Whenever the supervisor wants to take a reading of the diver's depth, he will tell the diver to make sure the end of the hose is alongside his chest and will then open a valve on the surface supply panel allowing air to flow through the hose. The diver will tell the supervisor when air comes out of the end of the hose, the supervisor then closes the valve; an accurate pressure gauge attached to the pneumo hose on the surface then registers the back pressure in the hose, this can with a very simple calculation be translated to feet or metres of seawater which is how the gauge is normally calibrated. The supervisor doesn't read pressure he or she will read depth directly from the gauge. This is imperative as the supervisor can then be certain of the diver's maximum depth and can accurately calculate their decompression requirements; this again is much safer than SCUBA where the diver normally will have to look after their own decompression without help from above.

Also, included in the umbilical there will be an electrical cable allowing voice communication with the diver; all hats and helmets are fitted with speakers and microphones, there will be a diver's telephone (comms) box on the surface. The supervisor can easily communicate with the diver and vice versa; the law stated that at all times when a supervisor was not talking to the diver it must be possible to hear the diver's breathing pattern via telephone; very safe and makes divers much more useful.

Lastly the umbilical will be the diver's safety line; there will be a load member included, this was either a rope or alternatively the hoses themselves would be strong enough to lift the diver as a last resort.

At the start of day two, week three we again found ourselves in mag 14, where we were to be taken though our first surface supplied equipment; free flow hats.

Bill Doughty arrived together with Tony Hale each of them carried a helmet; Bill's was bright blue in colour, on arrival he swung his up onto the desk where it slammed down, there was an almighty crash as it landed everything else on the desk jumped and some items fell off. His first sentence introduced this as the Divex Lightweight helmet we later came to know it as the Swindell; it was clear that it was anything but lightweight! Tony's, was coloured orange and turned out to be the Aquadyne AH3 free flow helmet. Clearly, we didn't need to be treating these helmets gently as they were built to last! We all stared at these hats with some degree of trepidation; they resembled buckets with a face plate! Not at all high tech that was absolutely for sure.

Both hats had two valves, one on each side of the helmet, one was the supply valve which would be connected to the umbilical via a non-return valve and the second was the exhaust valve. Air would enter the helmet via the supply valve just like a tap; this air flowed across the diver's face and was exhausted through the valve on the other side of the helmet. Bill said that these helmets were very noisy. Indeed, the use of these helmets has since been largely outlawed as the noise levels caused the divers hearing to be damaged.

Free flow equipment such as these helmets used huge quantities of air most of which was wasted; they were only really going to be of use in relatively shallow water diving but were at the time widely used for inshore civil engineering diving.

Inside the helmet were a set of speakers and a microphone ensuring two-way communications with topside personnel; it became clear when we used these helmets that sometimes, we would have to close the supply valve to be able to hear instructions from above. There was also a very high-tech device to assist the diver to clear their ears as they descended; this was a small piece of neoprene rubber arranged as a pad beneath the face plate; the diver would hold the helmet and pushing their nose against this pad if needed. I was again very lucky in that I have never needed any devices to aid ear clearing, I could always clear my ears without any need to pinch my nose or use nose clips etc.

Other than that, there really wasn't much else to see inside the helmets. The only remaining system we had to learn about was the bail-out system. Bail-out systems were employed for all surface supplied diving equipment and were very important. In the event of gas flow from the surface being disrupted we would have an alternative supply from a cylinder on our back. If the diver lost air from the surface there would be a valve arrangement allowing the diver to switch over and breathe from the bottle on their back; they would effectively then be on SCUBA; this was known as the diver's bail-out system. All commercial divers must by law have access to a secondary air supply so that they can safely bail-out if required. In the case of free flow helmets this was supplied to the helmet via another valve arrangement only to be used in event of emergency.

We were shown how to use both of these helmets at the same time as there were a lot of similarities between them; they both had neoprene neck dams that would make a seal around our necks keeping the water out, the neoprene was clamped to a chrome plated brass ring that would in turn clamp on to the helmet; on the lower edge of the neck ring were a couple of wire 'bridles', front and back. Both of these helmets were clipped to a 'jock strap', this was a thick canvas belt which when attached to the bridle of the neck dam ring at the back was then passed between the diver's legs and back up to clip to the other bridle on the front of the neck dam; this jock strap could be tightened or loosened by the diver and would stop the helmet from floating too much.

The diver would put the neck dam over their head before attaching the jock strap front and back, then together with their tender would make sure the neoprene collar was flat against their neck; the diver would then hold the neck ring with both hands supporting it horizontally, the tender would ensure air was flowing into the helmet and would place the helmet over the diver's head lowering it down onto the neck ring. The helmet would fit snugly onto the neck ring and would then be rotated until a locking pin engaged, the helmet was then secured and the diver would be ready to enter the water.

We would be wearing weight jackets rather than weight belts these were much more comfortable than weight belts and as we would be working for up to three hours underwater this was important. We would be using these jackets whenever we used surface supplied equipment; the jackets hung loosely from our shoulders and were secured using an enormous buckle at the front. These jackets not only held our weights but also the bail-out cylinders. Weights were held in pockets all around the waist, these could be jettisoned in an emergency by pulling a couple of nylon straps that were securing the webbing under the weights; once the straps were pulled the webbing would fall away allowing the weights to also fall out of the pockets, mind your feet!

Additionally, as we were going to be working on the seabed, we would be wearing lead lined boots; we were now talking about serious weight being carried; when the diver was dressed, they would be carrying the helmet, weight jacket, bail-out bottle and heavy weight boots as well as all their basic equipment, knife, suit and any tools needed on the dive.

We were not convinced that this was going to be much fun to use but of course being a commercial diver was never going to always be fun, was it? Anyway, we all decamped to the jetty where we were shown how to lay out the dive site. Firstly umbilicals; these were stored in the hut next to the dive control: we were shown how to lay them out coiling them down in a figure of eight so that they would not become tangled as we paid them out, each umbilical included a rope load member which we tied off to one of the rings embedded in the jetty using a round turn and two half hitches knot.

We had brought down two complete sets of equipment and were going to be using the Divex helmets that afternoon; we were shown how to attach the helmets to the umbilicals correctly. The first job was to check the non-return valves were operating correctly, this was done by opening the flow valve on the helmet and then sucking on the non-return-valve; if the NRV was working then we should not be able to get any air through it and we would feel suction. Then the umbilical air hose was connected and tightened using spanners. Once this was done, we had to attached the communications cable to a couple of electrical connectors protruding out of the helmet.

We then moved into the dive control room where we connected a couple of high pressure (HP) bottles to the surface supply panel, these would be used to supply the diver in the event of failure of the primary low pressure (LP) supply. The LP supply was already connected and was supplying air from an LP compressor at the other end of the jetty along the harbour wall. We had brought a diver's telephone communication box (comms box), this was connected to the comms wire in the umbilical; when everything was connected one of us knelt down and putting their head into the helmet while another of us operated the comms box to check two-way communication was working.

When the dive site was ready, I looked along the jetty at the site, I felt wonderful, the jetty looked like a very good, tidy, well organised workplace; the sun was shining and for January it was really quite pleasant. In addition to the diver's umbilicals, helmets and other ancillary equipment there were coiled downlines for each diver and an additional workline for each diver. In short there was a lot of kit here and I could see the potential for the site becoming messy very easily if we weren't careful; I again made a mental note to make sure I kept an eye on the site and whenever I was free of other duties I would tidy up and ensure all ropes were coiled down properly and equipment stowed correctly.

After a very short time I got a reputation as a stickler for ensuring the dive sites were tidy and although some of the others took the opportunity to stand back and just let me do it others took to helping. When I returned to Bovisand sometime after my course and was chatting to the instructors who had taught me it became clear that this had not gone unnoticed and had been a factor resulting in my being awarded higher than average day marks. Throughout my whole career I have applied the same maxim to all my workplaces and indeed it has spilled over into my home life as well, 'a place for everything and everything in its place' has been quoted back at me several times!

After lunch we returned to the jetty in our dry suits ready for our first dive with free flow helmets; our task for the day would be to familiarise ourselves with the helmet carrying out drills such as bail-out operation simulating loss of air from the surface. When it was my turn to get kitted up my tender was to be Geoff Donovan, I put the neck dam over my head and Geoff made sure the seal was correctly laid against my neck. The jock strap was already clipped on at the back; I reached between my legs pulling it up in front clipping it to the wire bridle on the neck ring.

Geoff then helped me to put on the weight jacket and boots; we had been told that once we started to dress in this kit our tender must not leave us for any reason; this was because with all this weight we would never be able to stay afloat should we fall in the water. We had been supplied with a chair which I used with a certain amount of relief; the weather was not warm and, the sun had by now disappeared and a steady drizzling was falling, altogether a bit of a miserable afternoon but I was very hot already. I have to say that I had been worried about doing my course from January through to March as the weather was always likely to be colder and wetter than in the summer but, I soon came to realise that in fact, this was probably better than doing it in the summer where we could become very overheated in all this kit.

Anyway, I was excited; this was going to be my first step into the real world of commercial diving and I was going to enjoy it! I grabbed the wire bridle with both hands and held the neck dam horizontal; Geoff had applied some washing up liquid to the face plate already, this would reduce the likelihood of misting up, no more spitting in the mask for us commercial divers, he made sure air was flowing nicely into the helmet and lowered it onto my head. I felt air flowing into the helmet as it was lowered into place and after a bit of jostling Geoff managed to seat the helmet onto the neck dam properly; he rotated it until we both heard the locking pin click into place. I could now let go but as I did the helmet started to lift off my head, we had been told that this was likely to happen, it could be controlled by opening the exhaust valve a little more. It didn't take long for me to get the hang of this and I was soon ready to stand up; Geoff helped me to my feet and connected the umbilical to the weight jacket using a carabiner that had been spliced onto the umbilical.

I stood there while Geoff called out surface checks to instructor Ray who was supervising that afternoon; I carried out bail-out and comms checks as instructed by Paul Sims who was working the panel and so talking to me. Once all checks had been done, I was given the thumbs up by Geoff and moved towards the ladder; Geoff took up the slack on the umbilical and I carefully backed onto the ladder, it was really quite hard to move down the ladder given the weight I was carrying but soon I was at the surface of the water.

I told the topside crew that I was about to leave surface and they confirmed that this was OK; I took the next step down the ladder, I was now under water and what a weird feeling! The helmet had become buoyant and seemed to be trying to float free; I found that when I turned my head inside the helmet the helmet didn't automatically follow as it wasn't really attached to me other than at my neck. The jock strap was very useful as I found that tightening it really did help to make the helmet stable. I moved down the ladder until I reached the bottom where I stepped off onto the seabed; I informed the topside crew that I had made bottom.

I was told to make sure my pneumo hose was in the correct place on my chest and the topside crew opened the valve to make air flow through the hose. As soon as I felt bubbles, I confirmed this to Ray and the valve was closed on the surface, I was then told that they had my depth noted and was could move away from the ladder and to get ready to carry out a bail-out exercise; as I walked away from the ladder it felt great, I found I could move quite easily and the weight jacket was much more comfortable than a weight belt as it wasn't tight around my waist. I felt that I would be able to work quite nicely in this equipment so long as I was working on the seabed; I found that the flow into the hat was relatively easy to balance against the exhaust so that the hat was sitting on my head very lightly, it moved up and down slightly with each breath I took and didn't let much water in.

Next, I was told we were about to carry out the bail-out drill; I told them I was ready and quite soon after that the flow of air slowed down and came to a stop. It was nice that there was now no noise but of course I knew that the air in the helmet would very soon become poisoned by carbon dioxide from my exhaled breath; I opened the bail-out valve and flow resumed. In a free flow hat air flows continuously so the cylinder on my back would not last very long; if this were a real emergency, I would immediately start to make my way back to the surface but, as it was just a drill I stayed where I was. As soon as I had told topside that I was on bail-out they told me to close the valve and surface air was turned on again.

After what seemed like just a few moments I was told to "prepare to leave bottom"; I moved back to the ladder and said "ready to leave bottom"; "leave bottom" came the reply and I started to climb the ladder. All was fine until I reached the surface; as I left the water not only the weight of the equipment but also that of water trapped in the equipment came back on my shoulders, the hat slumped down; I found that I had to open the flow valve up to give me enough air.

In the time I had been underwater the tide had fallen quite a lot and so I had a bigger climb to make, as I went up the ladder hand over hand, I found that I had to stop again to open the flow valve up even more as I was finding it increasingly difficult to breathe. It was a long way up that ladder but eventually I reached the top and was greeted by Geoff who helped me to the chair; I sat down and grasped the wire bridle as we had been told. Geoff unlocked the pin in the neck dam and rotated the helmet; I was extremely glad when the helmet separated from the neck dam as I had been finding it quite difficult to breath for the last couple of moments due to the work of climbing the ladder. It was great when the helmet was lifted off, I took great gulps of fresh air; it was a great experience and I was looking forward to more of the same and working with these helmets.

Once we had all done our dives, we stripped down the dive site, stowed the umbilicals back in the hut, returned all the other gear to the store and were told to be ready for another lecture at 19:00 in mag 14; no peace for the wicked.

Over the next few days, we managed to get to grips with the heavy equipment underwater, we were to start off with air tools such as the road drill (jackhammer) and CP9, this unit was a heavy-duty concrete or stone drill that would be used to drill holes in a great number of the rocks around the harbour. Ever since we had started, I had noticed that all the rocks looked like they were making an effort at camouflage by trying to look like Swiss cheese; now I knew why they had so many holes in them. Firstly, we were focusing on the road drill or jackhammer; again, we started with a lecture telling us how to use and look after the equipment then; it was down to the jetty again to put our new found knowledge into practice.

We set up the dive site again with the addition of a road compressor that would be needed to run the tools; the tools were supplied from the compressor through large diameter 'bagging' hoses. These hoses were supplied in about ten metre lengths which were joined together using 'Chicago' fittings, these fittings pushed together and turned quarter turn to lock them together; they had a habit of undoing themselves and so we lashed the two ends of hose together with short lengths of rope. The tools would be lowered to the diver by worklines which we had brought from the store; these worklines would have their inboard (topside) ends secured to the rings set into the jetty so that we wouldn't lose them overboard.

We were then briefed that our task for the next few days was to locate a clump of rocks that were proving to be a bit of a hazard to boat movements in the harbour and to break these rocks up with the jackhammer, sounded simple enough to me.

When it was my turn to dive, I kitted up with much more certainty about what was to come, the only difference was that we were to enter the water by jumping from the jetty, we wouldn't touch the ladder until we were in the water. My tender today was Simon Hale; when I was ready Simon told me to stop at the edge of the jetty and paid out enough umbilical so that I would reach the water before it came tight; once ready he gave me the thumbs up and I stepped off the jetty. Remember I was carrying a lot of weight and wearing lead lined boots so I reached the water rather quickly; I of course found myself underwater in a great cloud of bubbles but did not plummet to the bottom as Simon had taken up the slack and pulled me back to the surface; I raised my hand with my thumb up showing that I was OK and Simon dragged me over to the ladder.

I grabbed onto the ladder and after confirming with the topside crew over the comms I left surface; very soon I was on the bottom and waiting for the jackhammer to be lowered to me. When it arrived, it had taken on a life of its own, air was spewing out seemingly from everywhere, we had been told that the tool must have air applied to it continuously when in the water otherwise water would get in and stop it from working, this was termed making the tool 'hot'; this term was applied to any tool when it was powered up and ready to work but, in this case, I had not expected air to be coming out quite so much!

I disconnected the tool from the workline and gave four pulls on the line to indicate that it could be recovered, as soon as I felt it being pulled up, I let go saying "line is clear to surface" over the comms and watched it disappear to surface. We had been briefed to take the tool across the harbour to the rock outcrop; Charlie had been the first diver that day, he had secured a line to the bottom of the ladder and run it out along the bottom to the work area so all I had to do was follow it, easy! Well, when I say easy, the tool was bulky and heavy and the air hose attached to it seemed to have a mind of its own; it was just as well

I was fitted with the weight jacket and lead boots otherwise it would have been a farce.

Eventually I managed to drag the jackhammer over to the worksite and was ready to start; I looked around the area, the viz was quite good and I could see where the other guys had been working, there was quite a lot of rubble already. I moved to start where they had left off and told the topside crew that I was ready; I pulled the tool upright and stood over it in a good stable stance and pulled the trigger. I was immediately stunned by the noise; it was absolutely deafening I knew how noisy these tools were from having seen them used on roads but that was nothing to the noise this one was making! My ears felt like they were being physically assaulted, I thought I would be deaf by the time I finished the dive.

Not only was the noise terrible but as soon as I pulled the trigger I was engulfed in a huge cloud of bubbles from the tool; this made the steady stream I had been witnessing from the tool in its dormant state pale into insignificance, there was no way I could see anything of the job site. After a few minutes I let go of the trigger and when the bubbles had cleared, I could see where I had been working; not much change seemed to have taken place yet; I pulled the trigger again and started to lean onto the tool more.

The next time I took a look I could see I was getting somewhere which was comforting; I spent the next hour or so pummelling this rock knocking bits off. I couldn't hear anything over the voice comms and so didn't know that it was time for me to stop and to come back to the surface until I felt a tug on my umbilical; I let go of the trigger, bliss, I could hear topside talking to me. "Leave the tool where it is and come back to the ladder, make ready to leave bottom", the response was "understood, coming back to the ladder" to show that I had understood the command.

That evening in the bar we were all discussing the day and how difficult the tool had been to operate; we all felt like navies working on a road, one of the lads coined the term Aquapaddies to describe us; the name stuck and in fact we used it on our plaque at the end of the course.

From time to time, we had some 'Dry' days where we would be taken through subjects that we had to have a background in but wouldn't actually be using in the water such as thermic lance and explosives. Bill and Tony gave us a demonstration of how to use a thermic lance; the day was again a very cold, drizzly day; we were all gathered on the side of the harbour on a bit of waste ground to the East of the harbour. Tony arrived dressed in a silver fireproof suit with the lance, hose and a large 'J' size oxygen bottle; we had already had the lecture telling us how this all worked but it was going to be quite something to watch. We hooked up the hose to a regulator on the oxygen bottle and when Tony was ready Bill dialled up the correct pressure on the regulator, oxygen was now flowing through the lance; this was just a 22mm diameter steel pipe about two metres long with lengths of steel wire packed inside.

Bill ignited some steel wool and Tony buried the end of the lance into it; the steel wool flared up as the oxygen fanned the flames and ultimately the lance itself began to burn; as soon as it was clear the lance was alight Tony pulled it out of what was left of the steel wool. The lance continued to burn; it was a fearsome beast spitting fire and roaring like a freight train; there was a concrete post standing upright which Tony had told us he was going to cut in half. As he approached the pillar, we started to gather around but Bill shouted for us to stand well back; this proved to be good advice as when the lance came into contact with the pillar the concrete immediately started to melt and was spitting back hitting Tony and would've hit us if we hadn't moved back.

The lance really made short work of the pillar and before long it was reduced to a smouldering heap; I was very impressed but was not at all sure how easy it would be to use underwater; in fact, I never was asked to use one underwater and I have not met anyone who has used one. We did however get to use a flexible version called Kerrie cable, this was a hose with steel wire inside and worked in just the same way as the rigid lance. We used it to cut sections of Larson Pile; thick steel plate formed into a 'U' shape, these can often be seen along the side of dock and harbour walls; I enjoyed using this, it was fun to use but it has to be said it was a fearsome beast and had to be used with extreme care for sure.

Although we did use the Kerrie cable, it was only the once each to get a feel for it. As far as the course was concerned though we had to use another derivative of the thermic lance in the form of Broco Ultrathermic cutting rods, these were miniature thermic lances about four hundred millimetres long, they work in exactly the same way, we used them to cut strips off of sections of Larson Piling as one of our tested tasks. We had to complete this cut with the rods we were given, this was not easy! If we didn't manage it there would be another black mark against our names. It was great fun and something that we would all find useful when we were out in the real world.

Another of these dry days was spent 'playing' with or I suppose I should say learning how to use explosives; we were to be using Submarine Blasting Gelatin. Ray gave us the obligatory lecture and then we all followed him to the store where he was issued with what I thought looked like quite a lot of explosives some detonator cord, safety fuse, electrical detonators and a firing box. We then clambered over the rocks to the north of the harbour until we reached one of the concrete block houses left over from the Second World War; once inside Ray demonstrated how the sticks of explosive could be moulded into shapes and how these different shapes could be made to cut metal etc., in a very precise way.

He went on to show us that this material was really quite stable and in fact was difficult to set off accidentally; he took one of the sticks and set fire to it; we exchanged glances but as he said it just burned away to nothing without the hint of an explosion, apparently it would be quite safe to set fire to it unless there were more than about five kilos stored together at which point the temperature would get to the point where an explosion could take place. We had brought a number of bits of scrap steel over with us and proceeded to apply our new found expertise to cutting and basically blowing everything to bits. We would apply the explosives to the item together with the chosen method of initiating the explosive, then we would retire to the safety of the block house, when all was ready, we would blow three times on a very loud whistle warning everyone about the forthcoming explosion and then Boom!

When it was safe, we would blow once on the whistle to indicate there would be no more explosions and when the dust had settled, we would all go and have a look at the damage inflicted; for the first couple of attempts we struggled to find anything left of the items we were interested in, they seemed to have been vaporised. We then seemed to get a bit better and found that applying even quite a small amount would be enough to cut or punch holes, it was very impressive, I learned a lot, although I never thought I would actually get to use this knowledge but I was wrong.

Before we moved into the deep phase of our course we would need to be introduced to a piece of equipment more suited to working at greater depths, Ray arrived in mag 14 with the hat we were to use for our deep diving; we would be using a hat produced in America, the Kirby Morgan Bandmask (KMB) and one produced by the French commercial diving company, Comex, this one was the Comex Pro Bandmask, these hats were favoured for use offshore and would be especially pertinent to what we would find once we finished the course, or at least that's what we all hoped. This was much more like it, the KMB had an orange frame and really looked the part to me, the Comex Pro was all black and looked quite sinister; they were both very functional in appearance I could see myself enjoying them much more than the free flow helmets.

Ray took us through the masks and how they were to be used; bandmasks were again supplied with air from the surface via the umbilical; this ran to a block on the side of the hat were it entered the hat via the obligatory NRV; the block also had the bail-out valve controlling air from the cylinder on the diver's back again for use in an emergency; In the case of bandmasks air was directed from the side block through to a demand valve second stage affixed to the front of the hat; this DV was fitted with a 'dial-a-breath' adjustment; allowing the diver to change the sensitivity of the DV allowing them to work more effectively head down or head up both of which require changes to preload on the DV valve springs. The last valve on the hat is also part of the side block, the handle protruded forwards from the block, this was the 'free flow' valve, operated by the diver it directs a high volume of air across the inside of the diver's faceplate, this could be used to clear fogging or to give the diver extra air if he has been working too hard and of course if the hat were to flood it could be used to clear the water out of the hat (more of this later on).

Bandmasks are so termed as they have a soft neoprene hood that is clamped to a fiberglass frame by a stainless-steel band. Ray opened the hood for us to see inside the hat; looking in I could see that the hood had a soft smooth neoprene section, this would be pressed against the diver's face and would form a seal between the face and the fibreglass frame. Beyond the seal I could see an oral nasal mask, inside the oral nasal was a shaped metal nose dam covered in neoprene; he told us that this would be used to help us clear our ears as again we would not be able to reach our nose to give a squeeze if we needed to. Ray then went on to demonstrate how the hat would be put on, the hood would be peeled back exposing the face seal and then the diver would put their face in so that the seal seated nicely onto the face.

The hood would then be pulled over the diver's head and a zip would be pulled down; the hat would still be relatively loose on the diver's head at this time. The hat would then be properly secured on the head by use of a rubber 'spider'; this is a rubber band with five arms, each of the arms had a number of holes these would allow adjustment depending on the size of the diver's head. The spider would be secured to the stainless-steel band by use of the five mounting studs on the band, these would be pushed through holes in the spider. First the spider was attached to the mounting stud below the side block as this was the most difficult one to get to, then the spider was pulled around the base of the diver's head and secured onto the corresponding stud on the other side of the hat.

Next were the two arms of the spider at about ear height, these were pulled tight and secured to the studs just above the side block and finally the last arm is pulled over the top of the head and secured to the stud top dead centre on the stainless-steel band.

Once this demonstration was complete Ray carried on with how the bandmask worked; air was supplied to the diver via the oral nasal mask inside of which was a microphone for the diver to use, along the side of the hat secured in pockets in the hood were speakers allowing the diver to hear what was being said to them. The shaft on the nose dam extended through a gland to a knurled knob on the outside just below the faceplate, this allowed the diver to manipulate the position of the nose dam from outside; they could push their nose onto it so allowing them to produce a pressure in their middle ear if required to clear their ears.

After the lecture we took the bandmasks down to the jetty and rigged them for diving; this time I was to be one of the first to dive and so started to kit up; we were using the weight jacket but were not using lead boots. I pressed the purge button on the front of the second stage to check air was turned on to the system, then pulled the bandmask (hat) up onto my face pushing my face onto the soft neoprene seal against the frame; I was now able to breathe from the hat and was able to talk to the topside crew; we carried out our comms check. I was able to breathe easily, it was much the same as SCUBA in that I was only supplied with air when I breathed in; this would make the hat much quieter and of course as air is only supplied when the diver needs it, they use much less air than free flow helmets.

My tender was Craig Dickenson this time, he pulled the zip down on the hood and started to fasten the spider around my head; once the spider is secured the hat is very secure on the head and unlike the free flow helmet will move wherever the diver moves their head. Once Craig had finished and had called out the surface checks to the supervisor, I completed my bail-out and comms checks then moved to the ladder; I felt much more comfortable and was easily able to climb down the ladder.

Once at the surface I again told the topside crew that I was ready to leave surface, they confirmed this was OK and off I went; as I dropped down to the next rung on the ladder, the weight of the hat came off me and I found it to be very comfortable. The hood does not keep the water out, it acts a bit like a wetsuit hood, my ears were in the water but I found I could still hear the topside crew when they spoke to me; on reaching the bottom I was told to move away and get used to the hat, I used the free flow valve which pushed a great deal of air across the face plate, this was very refreshing and would be very useful when working hard. During the dive we carried out bail-out tests and generally got used to the hat, I felt that it was much more something I would feel at home with as it seemed to be a logical step on from SCUBA. Over the next few days, we used the bandmasks to erect scaffold cubes, place concrete, work with lifting bags and numerous other tasks, it was great fun.

In week four we were carrying on with learning our trade carrying out inspections on the harbour wall, building more scaffold cubes on the seabed and cutting rings from scaffold tubes with hacksaws etc., but I remember one day when we were to carry out an endurance swim. The aim was to use SCUBA coupled to an Avon full face mask to swim as far as we could on the limited air supply we were carrying; we were provided with an inverted twinset, this is two cylinders attached to a backpack so that the pillar valves were pointing downwards, this would enable us to reach the pillar valves when we were in the water.

The method we were to use was to initially open both bottles to allow them to equalise; then we would close one of the valves so that we were breathing from just the one cylinder. When we were swimming along, we would eventually feel the demand valve start to go 'tight' indicating that the pressure in the cylinder had dropped meaning we were almost out of air, we would reach behind our back and open the closed cylinder allowing the two cylinders to again equalise. We would then close that cylinder again and carry on until again we felt the DV go 'tight'; when the first of us had equalised twice we would both make our way to the surface; this method meant that we would leave bottom with 25% of our air remaining. We were carrying surface marker buoys (SMB), these buoys were attached by a thin line to a reel that we would take down with us paying out line as we went, this would allow our instructors to keep track of where we were while allowing us to swim freely.

We loaded all our equipment into one of the aluminium assault craft, I had seen upside down on the jetty when I first arrived at the Fort. The other half of the course did the same in another boat and off we went to the north side of the breakwater (inside the sound) at the eastern end.

On arrival at the site, we all kitted up as we would all be in the water at the same time; we took a compass bearing on the breakwater sea fort; we had been briefed to head for the fort staying on the seabed. When we reached the fort (because of course none of us would miss it would we) we should turn around and start back on a reciprocal bearing, this would bring us back along the path we had approached. I thought I had a big advantage here as on my previous course in 1975 we had done the same thing and my SMB had become snagged on some pipework running from the fort to the breakwater; I was again diving with Craig and we agreed that we would aim for the gap between the breakwater and the fort, this, we felt would increase our opportunity to find the fort as if we swam between the fort and the breakwater we would catch the pipes and could just turn right until we found the fort when we got to the fort we would start back the way we had come; brilliant plan, these days it would be termed a 'cunning plan'!

So off we go, Craig and I left surface, on reaching the bottom, we organised ourselves and started off towards the fort using our compasses; the method to use with a compass underwater is to ensure the compass lubber line (the line of travel) is absolutely lined up with the diver's body and to take a point on a feature in front of you along the path you want to take and head for that, when you reach that point you again look for something ahead and head for that. Unfortunately, those of you who have dived Plymouth Sound will know that the bottom is thick mud and visibility can be very poor out by the breakwater; today was one of those days and we could see no more than about 1 or 2 metres.

Anyway, off we went swimming as fast as we could while keeping in contact with one another; we kept on swimming in to various rubbish that had found its way into the Sound. Craig was having similar problems but as we moved along the breakwater the visibility improved and we were able to make better progress.

Craig had to equalise first, once he had done that, we resumed our swim, then I had to equalise; we were doing fine, we had been going for quite some time when I began to worry that we had missed the fort. How could that be as our plan was nearly fool proof unless we had drifted off by a long way; anyway, after about seventy minutes Craig had to equalise again and we both left bottom, I took up the slack on the SMB line and we surfaced facing one another looking over each other's shoulder to ensure we weren't coming up under any objects.

When we arrived at the surface the boat was quite close to us and came to pick us up, we were not the first to be picked up, our other course mates helped us to remove our sets pulling them into the boat and we followed as quickly as we could.

It was then that we realised we had missed the fort; it seems that in the five years between my courses someone had removed the pipes between the fort and the breakwater and we had swum between the two; we had managed to get about half way between the fort and the western end of the breakwater. The instructors didn't seem too phased by our having missed the fort as it seemed all the others had as well.

During February there were a number of days when there were ferocious storms; on one of these days, we were due to jump into the harbour for our morning swim; when we arrived, the harbour was a maelstrom of foam and confused wave action. None of us were very keen to swim but the PTI was having none of it telling us not to be so pathetic; we all jumped in with the aim to swim out and around the buoy in the harbour mouth that we had used for our ditch and retrieve exercise. As soon as we got in the water it was clear that this wasn't going to happen as we were being washed this way and that; when we approached the harbour mouth huge broken waves came barrelling around the end of the jetty making it impossible for us to make much headway against such confusion. We attempted this for what seemed to be long time but was probably just half an hour or so; although we were in our dry-suits and so were protected from the cold we were though now all becoming tired, we were shouting to each other to maintain contact and we worked to come together joining hands, whenever we got close enough to grab another of us, we would.

Eventually we had all gathered into a big circle and together found that we could move towards the innermost ladder; when we reached it one of the lads, I think it was Simon held on; this was not easy at all as the waves were creating huge surge, one second, he would be almost at the bottom of the ladder and then a wave would come in making him scrabble up the ladder hand over hand; in another situation this would have looked quite comical. Simon helped the next lad to get a grip of the ladder then, when at the top of the next wave he would hang onto the ladder and as soon as the water dropped away again, he would clamber up the ladder to safety. Our circle unfurled to become a snake of very tired students. One by one we all reached the ladder and were able to climb to safety, thank goodness we were all safe and sound but had certainly learnt a lesson that even very capable people can get into serious trouble if the sea wants to take charge. We spent the rest of that day practicing our boat handling skills in the Cattwater which was sheltered from the gale some way up the Plym estuary, no diving that day.

Weekends had become great fun with the whole course and sometimes Hazel and Laura either heading off to Plymouth city centre where we would frequent the Barbican and Union Street pubs and clubs or alternatively, we would find our way up to the Bovisand bar where we would engage in various pub games such as that old favourite, climbing under a table (I know, I hadn't heard of it either). This game was one of our favourites, as we were now becoming quite fit and strong, we were increasingly being able to show this off to good effect; the game would start with two of us each lying face down on top of one of the bar's tables spaced apart by about a metre.

The referee would count down, three, two, one, go! They would then start the stopwatch; the object of the game was to climb under the table regaining the start position, the first to achieve this without touching the floor was the winner. To start with you would move your body forward bending at the hips; you would then reach under the table until you could grasp the far table legs, the tricky bit was to now pull your legs down under the table without them falling to the floor. It would inevitably mean that you would shuffle along the underside of the table until you could reach up and grasp the sides of the table back on the top surface; you would then pull your legs down and brace them against the table legs so that they didn't drop to the floor, from there it was just a matter of pulling your body back up onto the top of the table; finished.

Sounds simple but I can tell you it is anything but; we would need to ensure there were people hanging on to the table to ensure it didn't topple over. Some of us were of quite slight build but this wasn't the case with Adrian and to some extent Simon; Adrian was a big chap in all ways and Simon was tall and built like the proverbial brick outhouse, solid. Both of these guys competing in this game were great value, there would be a torrent of helpful comment and advice coming from the audience which included not only the rest of the course but also any of the other patrons of the bar; tremendous fun was had by all.

Another game was 'bottle walking'; this game involved drawing a line on the floor and with a bottle grasped in each hand you would place your feet at the line then would 'walk' the bottles as far ahead of you as you could. This resulted in supporting all your weight at full stretch; the object was to place one of the bottles as far away from the line as possible; this was not the end of the game though, to qualify as a valid placement you then had to use the one bottle still in your hands to shuffle back until you could again stand up behind the line; if you collapsed before getting back the bottle placement was void. I was particularly good at this and was able to place bottles much further than even Ray Salmon who was a good-few-inches taller than I was; small victories are worth the effort.

One weekend this all got a little out of hand; Friday and Saturday nights the bar would stay open until all of us had had enough, normally this just resulted in a good night but this particular weekend it went too far with everyone getting far too boisterous, I have no idea what time I left the bar but I was nowhere near the last to leave. I went to my bed and was just about to drop off when the main door slammed open with the rest of the lads arriving in full flow, singing and whooping it up generally. This went on for about another hour or so, it must have been about two o'clock in the morning when a very irate individual arrived at the door screaming "are you on the Ruffy Toughy course"; this received hoots of drunken laughter and Adrian who at the time was swinging from one of the large iron gun eyes set into the ceiling shouted "no we're on the Meldy Weldy course"; more laughter. Anyway, it seemed that our revelry had not gone unnoticed by some of the recreational divers who were also staying at the fort that weekend; they were not happy to say the least; once sober none of us could blame them but at the time we didn't see it that way.

There were three of them and they were given a bit of lip before we eventually settled things down; they left completely unscathed but not really much happier. We all calmed down and went to bed.

The next morning, we were woken by a very irate Lt Cdr Bax at about eight thirty; he was puce; I thought he might have a coronary. We were all told to get up and to get into the larger room towards the gun port end of the dormitory pronto! When we were all there Bax held court; we were treated to an extremely sobering monologue. It seemed the recreational divers had already been up to see him and disturbed his Sunday morning (first black mark), they had obviously told him exactly how the night had gone from their point of view which, I have to say I would probably have agreed with when in a sober state (second black mark). Evidently, he had had to promise to give them some of their money back (third black mark), and had assured them that we would be penalised for this unacceptable behaviour; this was the worrying bit. He told us that he was right on the verge of stopping the course and sacking all of us; we were to stay in the fort and not to cause any more trouble for the recreational punters; we would be told our fate at two o'clock this afternoon once he had had some time to mull over and carry out some more investigations.

Once he had left, we were all dumbstruck, what had we done, what were we thinking of! We all got dressed and went over to the café for some breakfast but I was feeling so hungover and depressed that I really didn't want anything to eat. There followed the longest morning of my life with all of us sitting in our grot commiserating about our lot, none of us blamed the others as it was clear we were all to blame. At two o'clock we were summoned to CM14 again and told to sit and be quiet; we didn't need to be told that, there was no way any of us were going to interrupt him or in any way draw attention to ourselves. There followed another very long monologue about how disappointing our behaviour had been and that if we felt this was an acceptable way to behave then we should think again.

After about thirty minutes of this he came to his conclusion as to our penalty; it seemed that he had discussed the situation with all of our instructors who must have been quite supportive of us as he had decided that we wouldn't all be sacked for this episode. We were to consider ourselves as extremely lucky and to be under notice that if there were to be any further incidence of unruly behaviour then we would be straight down the road. We all assured him that there would be no repeat; he certainly hoped not and if so, we had been warned, he then left a very shell-shocked course to our own devices.

We never did have another evening like that one until our final after course party which even then was not as raucous, I would like to be able to say I had learned a valuable lesson but unfortunately there have been several times since then when too much drink has been consumed and I have made a complete fool of myself but not while I was on the course.

Week six saw a completely unexpected development; the instructors had given us all nicknames! The first we knew of this was when we were given our programme for the week; Paul Sims was to be the course leader for the week, when he picked up the programme, he came back to our grot grinning from ear to ear. "Have a look at this you lot", they've given us nicknames and he read them out:

Paul Sims (Paul the Mod); this was probably something to do with his choice of dress.

Adrian Fricker (Bear); as I have already said Adrian was a big bearded lad and bear was a pretty fair name.

Dave Pelly (Blue Boy); Dave favoured wearing blue jeans and similar shirts but not really sure where this one came from.

Mark (Jack) Frost (Doris Loweth of the Low); again, not really sure about this one but it could be to do with accent?

Simon Hale (Dinky Doo); again, not sure about this one either, Simon was a great character but Dinky Doo?

Craig Dickenson (Harpo); this one was easy as Craig looked a little like Harpo Marx due to his hair.

Geoff Donovan (Milky Bar Kid); Geoff wore round wire rimmed glasses just like his namesake.

Alan Drake (Evil Al); don't know about this other than he was from Scotland, maybe that was enough?

Tom Garnett (Scooby Tom); again, not sure about why Tom got this one?

Trevor Glew (Marine Boy); Trevor liked to chew gum and therefore was likened to this cartoon character of the sixties by some of the instructors who kept on about Frank chewing his 'Oxygum'.

Tim Hancock (Tiny Tim); Tim was not especially small but was like me quite slight.

Andy Goodwin (Cat Balou); no idea!

Henry Griffiths (Biffer); Henry was a stocky individual with a London accent so Biffer fitted him quite well.

Campbell Park (Barnacle Bill); Campbell was even in his twenties quite weathered and so again this fitted him well.

Peter Atkey (Peter Perfect); mine came from a character in the 1960s kid's cartoon series, Wacky Racers, I really got some stick for it though.

These names really stuck though and they again helped to weld us into a fully functioning team; it was great; the end of week six marked the halfway point of the course and we were all still here, things were looking good as when I thought back to the BBC documentary, by this point a good number had already been asked to leave.

We now started to move into the deeper phase of the course where we would be working to a depth of close to fifty metres; air powered tools are really not much use when diving deeper than thirty metres, below this depth hydraulic tools are much more effective. Probably one of the most important tasks we had to master was the use of an hydraulic impact wrench to be used at a depth beyond forty metres. Before we were going to be trusted with the hydraulic wrench, we were to complete the same task using hand spanners.

We were introduced to the workpiece known affectionally as the 'pig' this was a set of eight flanges welded to short lengths of pipe, these were in turn welded to another length of six-inch steel pipe about four feet long (just over a metre); the pig was fitted with four legs so that it would stand proud of the seabed allowing access to all of the attached flanges.

We each would be allocated one of the flanges and would be given a loose flange together with a rubber gasket, nuts and bolts so that we could attach our flange to the one we had been allocated on the pig. Firstly, we would complete this task on surface and so we again found ourselves on the same piece of waste ground where we had seen the thermic lance demonstration but this time, we had the pig and were each given eight nuts and bolts, a rubber gasket and told to put the flanges together.

The tools we had were a 'podger', this was a ring spanner the handle of which tapered to a point. We were also given a 'flogging' spanner, this is a spanner that is designed to be hit with a lump hammer to tighten or loosen nuts and a lump hammer. Seems basic enough but bearing in mind that we had to work alone it is not quite as easy as it might seem, some of the guys really struggled with this. The method is that the podger is put through one of the flange bolt holes from the back, next the rubber gasket is threaded onto the podger finally the loose flange is threaded onto the podger; once all of these components have been slid together, they needed to be wiggled about until a bolt could be slid through all three and a nut fitted to the bolt, initially this nut was to be left loose.

The rest of the bolts were then threaded into the remaining holes and once they were all in place the nuts were tightened diagonally in order to ensure the gasket was evenly secured. The final tightening was to be done using the flogging spanner, the podger bar's spanner was put onto the head of the bolt behind the flange, the flogging spanner was then put onto the nut and the lump hammer was used to hit the flogging spanner to tighten fully or 'flog it up'. We all had a practice and were confident that we would be able to carry this task out at depth tomorrow.

The next day we boarded 'Deepwater' the boat we were using for the deep phase and off we went to the Victualling Yard buoy; this buoy was situated in the mouth of the Tamar River just a short distance from Mayflower marina and the Royal William Yard which used to be the Royal Navy's store where ships would be resupplied from. This buoy was sitting in about forty-five metres of water and would be the scene of all our deep-water diving for the course; when we arrived the first job was for one of us to ride to the buoy in an inflatable boat, when we arrived one of us would climb onto the buoy where we would wait for Deepwater to arrive; Deepwater was an old harbour tug; it was evidently very hard to control and was completely unable to react quickly to any developments.

Anyway, on this day I was standing on the buoy waiting patiently as the boat was edging closer and closer, Monty Ham was piloting Deepwater he was being extremely careful, the boat was headed upwind very slowly towards me; Dave Pelly was leaning over the bow with the mooring line ready for me. When Deepwater eventually arrived, I grabbed the line from Dave passed it through the eye on the buoy and back to Dave where he secured it to one of the bollards on deck; on this day the weather was fine everything was calm but on the odd occasion that it was a bit lumpy this became quite challenging as it was a bit like riding a bucking bronco while trying to gauge when the boat was going to hit the buoy; it would make a terrific theme park ride!

Once we were safely tied up, we rigged for diving, and kitted up the first two divers; we were using the Kirby Morgan Bandmask for this task, I was tending Alan Drake; once Alan was in the water and had made bottom there wasn't very much for me to do as he was not going to be moving around much. The depth was forty-five metres, I knew this from the graduations on the umbilical and could see that Alan was almost directly below me. I spent the next twenty minutes chatting to the others and appreciating the scenery; across the river on the Cornish side we could see the Cremyll arms a really nice looking riverside pub at the base of mount Edgecombe; from time to time a little passenger ferry plying between Cremyll and Admiral's Hard on the Plymouth side would pass us and although the ferry was a potential threat to divers, as we were flying the correct signals, the Alpha flag and a black ball, diamond, ball arranged vertically from Deepwater's rigging, the ferry was staying well away from us.

At the time the tide was ebbing resulting in water flowing from the river towards the Sound so the boat was facing upstream. When Alan and Geoff returned to the surface it was my turn to dive; I had already organised my kit, it took just a few moments to clean the hat, apply some more detergent to the faceplate and to make ready to dive. I was to practice the flange task, I had prepared a length of rope to take the eight nuts and bolts I would need down with me, the bolts were secured by separating the rope's weave threading the bolt through before putting the nut on the other side.

I also had the flange threaded onto my arm together with the gasket, the podger, flogging spanner and lump hammer were all attached by lanyards. Once in the water, Jack Frost who was tending me pulled me over to the shot line, I was told to leave surface and off I went; almost as soon as I left surface the visibility reduced to almost nothing. Not a problem as I knew that the pig was attached to the bottom of the shot line so I would automatically reach it once I made bottom. As I descended, I cleared my ears to compensate for the increasing pressure.

On reaching the bottom, I informed the topside crew and was told to commence my task; I spent a couple of minutes orienting myself, as I say I had landed right alongside the pig so I placed all my equipment and tools right next to the pig ready to start; I had built up a fairly good picture of the worksite in my minds-eye so I knew where everything was, there was almost no water movement now, so, perfect. I picked up the podger and slid the gasket down my arm and put my hand back to where the pig was in order to locate the first bolt hole. Hold on though where was the pig? It had gone! Where could it have gone?

I spent the next few minutes blindly searching the area but there was no doubt the bloody pig was no longer there! As part of the briefing, we had been told never to let go of the pig just in case, but of course I knew better and well, where could it go, it weighed a lot and was attached to the shot line; I mean come on, really! But after some time searching blindly around, I had to admit that it had definitely gone, I had lost it, this was a cardinal sin and would attract the anger of the instructors, I would lose day marks. Eventually I had to tell the topside crew that I had lost the pig; I was told to leave bottom, as the pig was also attached to the shot line, I had no line to follow back to the surface so I was told to climb my umbilical.

I spent a very uncomfortable half hour or so decompressing at 10 feet hanging on my umbilical wondering what wrath was awaiting me on the surface; when I made surface, Trevor was hanging over the side ready to take the flange, spanners and bolts from me, I was then pulled along to the ladder and climbed on deck. Jack helped me undress, the deck was unusually silent as the guys were all trying to keep their heads below the parapet in case, they attracted some shrapnel from the barrage I was about to receive.

When I was out of the equipment standing in my suit dripping on deck, Tony and Monty beckoned me over to speak to them in the wheelhouse; here it comes I thought. Tony started by asking me if I had understood the briefing, "yes I had." "Then why did you let go of the pig?"; of course, I had no answer for this, I apologised and said that I had learned a lesson from this. "Not bloody good enough! You were specifically told not to let go of the pig; but you still did; this was a wasted dive, if we were on a job, you would be run off for that bit of f***ing stupidity!".

This went on for a few minutes, I felt very small and extremely unhappy; when Tony told me to "get out of my sight;" I went back to the aft deck where the rest of the course members were getting ready for the next dive. It seemed that the second I let go of the pig the tide had turned, the boat had swung around the buoy coming to rest pointing downstream as the tide was now coming in; the pig must have been dragged away from me at that precise moment; of course, there would have been no sound and no indication of what was about to happen the result was that there was no way I could have found it as it had come to rest again some thirty metres away from me by the time I had realised what had happened; disaster.

Unfortunately, my bad day didn't end there though, I couldn't dive again as we were quite close to the end of the day so I would have to wait for another day when I would be given another go at this task. When everyone had finished diving, we started stripping down the dive kit as Deepwater made its way back across the Sound, I started helping Adrian to remove all the tightened bolts from the pig.

We had to use the flogging spanner as they were all very tight, I held the spanner while Adrian would hit it with the lump hammer, all went well for the first few nuts but then just as Adrian took a big swing at the flogging spanner for the next nut Deepwater hit another boats wake and rolled very suddenly Adrian lost his balance a bit and instead of hitting the flogging spanner he hit my hand. Owwie! Or words to that effect, I jumped up and holding my hand I hopped around the deck; when I stopped and looked at my hand it was looking a bit the worse for wear. The knuckle of my right hand had a big gash and was bleeding profusely, I could move everything although there was a great deal of pain when I did; I didn't think anything was broken but it was very painful; poor Adrian, he clearly felt very guilty although it wasn't his fault, he couldn't have foreseen this or done anything about it.

I was not sure how I was going to be able to work with my hand being damaged this way, would I be able to continue at all, we had been told that we could not afford to miss more than three days diving throughout the whole twelve weeks; I hadn't missed any days as yet and didn't really want to miss any now.

We were scheduled for a night dive that evening and I was determined that I would not miss it; the task was for us to make a soft eye on a piece of wire rope using 'bulldog grips'. Use of bulldog grips was a routine method of making an eye on a wire rope; the grip consisted of a U-bolt with both ends being threaded allowing nuts to wound on and tightened, there was a 'bridge' which would slide onto the U-bolt with the wire rope having been fed in between the loop of the U-bolt and the bridge.

Inside the bridge were a series of ribs that would fit snugly into the lay of the rope ensuring a secure grip, once the nuts had been tightened against the bridge the rope would be held firmly and was unlikely to slip. We had used these grips to make eyes in wire ropes a number of times already and was not a problem but I wasn't sure I could or would be able to manage it today. The team hatched a plan, when I got to the bottom with my piece of wire and grips whoever else was in at the same time would hand me one that had been completed before we went in the water.

We had all helped each other out like this in the previous nine weeks or so, it was just what we did; we had all agreed that we would feel we had all failed if any of us didn't pass the course, again it was great to feel part of such a brilliant team. The night dive was to take place from the jetty using free flow helmets, I loved night diving, we had already done a few previously on the course, the best one I remember was when we had to cut links from a chain using a lump hammer and cold chisel.

The viz was really good that evening, probably more than ten metres, it was not a particularly taxing task but it took on a completely different complexion at night; every time I hit the chisel the effect was amazing, there were a lot of minute creatures in and around all the rocks and seaweed, the concussion made them emit a flash of green light; it was like my own little light show, bang, flash, bang, flash it was great.

This evening's dive though would not be so colourful as we would not be hitting anything, when I got to the bottom Geoff quickly gave me the soft-eye he had brought down with him and then went off to complete his task. After a suitable time, I told topside that I had completed the task and went back to the surface, all well; I felt a bit bad about not having done this properly but there was just no way I could have done it that day and anyway this was not the first time we had done this task so I knew I would have been able to do it if my hand had been Okay.

Sometime after the course Ray told me he knew exactly what had gone on but as he knew I had done the same task several times before he decided to let it go; and we thought we had been so clever.

This was on Thursday and I had to stay out of the water the next day as my hand was just too painful; I decided to go back to Torquay for the weekend as I wasn't programmed for maintenance that weekend. I had a very worrying weekend but by Sunday evening I felt that I would be able to dive the following day; on the Monday I completed the flange task at depth, this cleared the way for my progressing on the course.

The final task we all had to complete was to use the hydraulic impact wrench on the flange task at a depth of at least forty metres; we were now in week eleven and could all see the end was getting very close.

Our supervisors for the day were Ray and Bill Doughty I was pleased with this as I felt they both had cool heads, we were going to be using the hydraulic impact wrench, it was painted bright yellow and looked brand new; I was the first in the water on this day and so found myself back on the bottom with the pig and this time I also had the impact wrench with me, the hydraulic hoses were very heavy and cumbersome but I didn't have to carry them anywhere so it wasn't a problem.

There was absolutely no way the pig was going to get away from me this time, I kept the shot line looped around my arm, if it was going anywhere then I was going with it. We had already practised with the impact wrench so knew exactly what to expect; I quickly got one of the bolts in and tightened loosely, the other seven bolts followed, they were all in loosely with the required gasket held in place, the podger spanner was on the head of the bolt and the impact wrench was on the front ready to tighten the nut.

I called to "make it hot" the reply came back "it's hot" meaning the tool was ready to operate, I pressed the trigger and rat,tat,tat it tightened the nut beautifully, I did the same to the other nuts in the correct order and very gratefully called "task complete". I returned to the surface again without any issues, thank goodness that was over; the rest of the team also completed the task without any problems so a good day was had by all.

All that was left to do by late afternoon was to recover the pig and the impact wrench before we could cast off and head for home; the hydraulic tool and pig were tied together, both being lifted by using Deepwater's hydraulic 'HIAB' arm, the hook was bought down to the gunwale we applied a chain stopper to the hoses and shot line, the stopper would grip the hoses and line allowing them to be lifted by the HIAB. The hook was attached to the stopper and then the HIAB started to lift, unfortunately it didn't lift very far before it became clear the shot or the hoses had become fouled around something on the seabed.

We were going to need someone to go down and clear them from the obstruction; all of us had dived so this would be a repetitive dive, not a huge problem but there would be quite a big decompression penalty. As I had been the first diver, I had been on the surface longer than all the others this meant I had a longer surface interval; I had been breathing out the accumulated nitrogen for longer and so had less dissolved nitrogen remaining in my body, this made me the obvious choice.

I was kitted up again and made my way down the shot line until I reached the bottom, I was confronted by a huge, round boulder at least two metres in diameter, the shot line was caught under one side and the hoses were caught under the opposite side. I went around the other side of the boulder where I found the pig hard up against the boulder; I called to "come down on the shot line", the topside crew started to lower the lines again; eventually I had enough slack in the shot line, I called "all stop"; I managed to pull the shot line out from under the boulder quite easily and draped it over the boulder so that both the hoses and the shot line were on the same side of the boulder.

I then worked at freeing the hoses, this was not so straightforward as they were much heavier and bulkier than the shot line and had been pulled hard under the rock; after quite a lot of heaving and grunting I managed to free the smaller 'supply' hose, I then got to work on the larger 'return' hose and found that I was able to work it out inch by inch until finally it came free. I told topside it was free and that they could come up on the pig and hoses; I made sure everything was kept clear of the boulder and once it was clear to the surface, I was told to make my way up the shot line.

I had been at one hundred and twenty feet (36.5 metres) for some twenty-two minutes. When I arrived at my first stop at twenty feet (we were using US Navy tables) I transferred over to the 'lazy shot' which was hanging at exactly the correct depth for my first decompression stop, I sat astride the scaffold pole this meant that my chest was at the correct depth and I could relax.

When the time came, I was lifted to my next stop and subsequently to the surface. This system of using a lazy shot was great, when working it was not unusual to have to carry out a fair amount of decompression and sometimes this could be in quite a fast tidal flow so hanging on to a rope by hand would be quite hard especially if the diver had been working hard and was therefore tired. Using a lazy shot the diver could effectively rest and the decompression could be easily be driven by the topside crew, much better.

Anyway, By the time I had completed my decompression the pig, impact wrench and all associated equipment was on deck and had started to be broken down; when I had removed all my kit Ray came out on deck leaving Bill to steam Deepwater back to Bovisand; in front of the whole team Ray told me that he was very impressed with my dive, he said it had been clear that the hose had been difficult to free up and I had done a good job; what a difference a day makes, I was walking on air when we got back to the harbour.

At the end of week eleven we all went in to town on the Saturday, as we had to pick up our course plaque; some of the previous courses had gone to extreme lengths to out-do previous courses. One of them had produced a papier maché head looking just like Alan Bax but we weren't that artistic and had decided to go with a brass plaque mounted on hard wood, it showed our course number BAD 105 together with all our names superimposed on top of crossed jackhammers with the title "Aquapaddies" emblazoned across it.

Suddenly it was week twelve; so soon! The best of it was that we were still fifteen students, we had done it, now all we had to do was to all pass. This was the crunch time, from Wednesday right through to Friday we were to have examinations, assessments and oral tests. Wednesday was the final theory examination we weren't to be told our marks until we sat down with Lt Cdr Bax on Friday.

We sat down at 09:00 in the chartroom again to take the theory exam, following that we started our oral tests, I finished day one of my orals with 'chamber operation' at 17:30. Thursday was day two of orals, I started this day with one testing my knowledge of compressor operation, my final one was for rigging and completed at 11:00. Following this we spent the rest of the day returning equipment and cleaning the training areas; I have to say I was exhausted at the end of the day, we all adjourned to the bar for a rather subdued couple of pints. None of us paid any attention to the wonderful view from the bar, we all sat around the tables discussing the assessments, all this did was to make us wonder whether we had done enough.

The end of the course had come so suddenly, it seemed no time at all since we had all met for the first time on that cold January afternoon but now here, we were about to complete the twelve weeks, I had done fifty-six dives with a total of two thousand two hundred and seventy-five minutes under water; it seemed to have gone in a flash, I had loved almost every second of it!

Friday the 21st March was our last day, the day started with interviews and debrief with Alan Bax; for this we were back to alphabetical order so I was again first in to see him, this didn't bother me at all as I was desperate to find out how I had got on. I was waiting in the training office outside his door trying not to look as nervous as I felt, this was *it* now, the last twelve weeks all came down to this day, had I done enough and if not, what was I going to do with myself, I had no job and very little by way of prospects having not really achieved much from my schooling. But Laura was there in the training office and it wouldn't be cool to look nervous, now, would it?

At 09:00 on the dot I was called into Bax's Office, it was a tiny affair at the far end of the training office, reached via a small sliding door; inside I was invited to sit in a chair across the desk from him. Alan was giving nothing away by his expression, he was shuffling through reams of paper until he managed to find the one he wanted; he then looked up at me, this was it! He started off by giving me a bit of a resume of the course, he covered how I had done quite well in the SCUBA exam and had performed well enough in the ensuing daily theoretical tests; it seemed I had also done okay in the practical areas.

I was beginning to relax a bit but he was being a little long winded for my liking; again, he looked up and said of course there was that little hiccough mid-course where you and all the others let the side down by making fools of yourselves didn't you? I was now quite worried as I couldn't see where this was going; then he came to the point. "Congratulations Peter, you've passed the course" I could have kissed him, it had all been worth it.

He went on to tell me that although I had done well this was just the first step and I would have to keep up with my studies to become a properly useful commercial diver; as diving was after all just the way to get to the job! Quite frankly after he told me I had passed I didn't really hear much of the rest of his speech, I was on my way into the commercial diving world. He finished off by standing, shaking my hand, we would meet again at the course presentation at 15:00, then I was out the door.

Henry Griffiths was the next in line, he looked as nervous as I had felt but was glad to be the first to congratulate me; Laura clearly already knew; she gave me a great hug telling me the result was never in doubt for Peter Perfect! what a wonderful feeling. One by one we all filed in to see Bax and one by one beaming faces came back to our grot, that is to say all but one, it seemed that Jack had failed one part of his theory tests and would be given one last attempt that afternoon. We all spent the next couple of hours drilling what he needed into him so that he would get the right result in the resit that afternoon; I felt so sorry for him, he had struggled a bit with the theory but none of us wanted anyone to fail.

Jack came back from his retest with the good news that he had also passed so he would be able to join in with the celebrations; so, we had our 100% pass rate for the course, this was the best news we could have had and it meant that we could all enjoy the party tonight; all that was left now was the presentation. At 15:00 off we all went to CM 14 where it had all begun all those weeks ago, we were now very comfortable with each other, we were a real team, we had helped each other and built very solid friendships some of which I maintain even today; it seemed a lot more like a lifetime ago we had started this and not just twelve weeks.

At 15:00 in strode Lt Cdr Bax who again took the floor with his instructors standing behind him, he again reiterated that we were just starting and needed to realise that although we had all done very well in our training it was, in every way a Basic Training course. We had all realised that while diving was what we wanted to do he again told us it really was just a method of getting to work and that there were a lot of divers out there with a lot more experience than we obviously had.

We had all signed up for a Lloyds Diver Inspector course that would be starting the following Monday the 24th March which whilst wouldn't be much, at least we would have an advanced qualification for inspection that might put us ahead of some others in the queue. He then went on to tell us our ranking on the course; I was stunned to find that I had come top of the course with Craig Dickenson coming a very close second. Alan then went on to tell us all that Oceaneering International, one of the foremost offshore diving companies at the time had agreed to take both Dave Pelly and me on as trainee commercial divers; we were to travel to Aberdeen ready to start work at their facility in the Bridge of Don on Monday 31st March; I had a job! How could it get any better?

In the programme the last sentence following the presentation was "good excuse for a booze up, hey!!" so we decided that as it was on the programme, we really should do that; back in our grot, Geoff and Alan brought out a bottle of Scotch like all good Scotsmen do, we had a couple of wee drams. The day was beautifully sunny so we all went down to the jetty to pose for group photographs; we did some of the conventional group stuff but then decided that wasn't good enough for *our* course we all ran to the tower and climbed the mast until we were all hanging off part of it.

Hazel then took a photo for posterity; the next duty was to attend the course party in the bar this evening; we arrived early and started to get stuck into the work of enjoying the evening. A disco had been laid on with some food; there were a bunch of people who it seemed had been invited, it seemed the BAD Lad discos were always memorable evenings, our instructors had all invited friends and family, it was a great crowd. I found myself getting along very well with a lovely young lady that I later found was Bill's step daughter, we were getting very friendly on the dance floor when she decided to go and powder her nose or something; I went to the bar where Bill sidled up to me, I wasn't sure how he would take my interest in his step daughter but he took one look at me and said "go on son, fill your boots" so clearly he didn't feel all that protective of her not that he needed to worry about her really; my day just couldn't get any better.

The next day started late, we all emerging around ten o'clock nursing sore heads, the canteen was still open for breakfast as they also hadn't wanted to start early having all been at the party; we got stuck in to our traditional full English, lovely. Later we all had to see Dr Cross to find out the results of our blood-letting over the past twelve weeks and to get our final medicals; these were scheduled to be done in the afternoon. When we got the results of our blood tests it seemed that the Bovisand diet of fry ups and pies had done nothing for our health as the levels of fat in our blood had all gone through the roof compared with the base levels when we arrived but none of us had suffered any kind of Decompression Illness (got bent), this clearly had done nothing to prove Dr Cross' theory. We all passed our medicals so now we had a qualification and an in-date medical; I was very nearly ready.

CHAPTER NINE

Lloyds Diver Inspector Course

Monday 24th March 1980, I was starting my first week as a qualified surface supplied commercial diver in pretty much the same position as I had spent the last twelve weeks, I was at Fort Bovisand Underwater Centre; the difference was that I was now embarking on an advanced training course. It is a little absurd to call it advanced really but this was how it was sold to us; we were about to learn a trade that would be useful to us and our potential employers when we eventually found ourselves on a diving job. The trade was inspection or Non-Destructive-Testing (NDT); I came to learn latter on that a lot of divers feel this term really means No Diving Today! But I was under no illusions about my employability and although I had a job to go too, I knew I would have to show Oceaneering quite quickly that I was useful in order to remain employed by them.

Here we were then back in CM 14 waiting for our instructor, again at spot on the allotted time Mel Bayliss and Ray Salmon strode into the room, I was pleased to see that Ray would be involved as I had got on very well with him over the last twelve weeks and, because of his offshore experience I felt he would be able to put our training into context with real world scenarios.

We were given a short introduction and then invited to follow them to our new classroom; *invited*, this was a change of emphasis from our previous experience, possibly as we were actually paying for the privilege of being on this course! Down into the bowels of the Fort we went again although this time we went straight past our old home Mag 14 and carried on up the hill to the NDT classroom Mag 16; we had been in here once before when we had a lecture on inspection but hadn't really got to grips with much of the equipment as yet. As we entered there were a lot of similarities to Mag 14, it had the same domed brick ceiling complete with flaking paint but there the similarity ended; there was seating for us all and behind these chairs were work benches loaded with large pieces of steel, lots of aerosol cans and various pieces of equipment; there was a pervading smell of paraffin.

Mel was to be taking the lecture in the morning and he led us through why inspection was required, the various methods available and which of them we would be focusing on over the next three days. I had always been interested in photography as you know; I felt this could well be a logical extension to my interest. We would be learning about Visual Inspection, Video or Closed-Circuit Television (CCTV), Photography, Ultrasonic Digital Thickness Gauges, Cathodic Protection (CP) assessment and Magnetic Particle Inspection (MPI) to find microscopic cracks in welds. We would be using these methods to identify faults and problems in and around steel structures with the aim being to identify them before they could cause the structure to fail.

We spent the whole morning running through the use of visual inspection and CCTV; by lunchtime we were all going in to overload with terms that we *'must'* remember to use properly when we undertook our Lloyd's inspection assessment on Wednesday, maybe this wasn't going to be as straightforward as I'd hoped. After another classic Bovisand lunch we found our way back to the classroom and tried to stay awake through methods of Cathodic protection and use of ultrasonic digital thickness meters.

Neither of these were riveting subjects although I did recognise their worth in terms of getting me work; Cathodic Protection was the method utilised by most steel structures to stave off corrosion in the marine environment. By electrically connecting quantities of materials that were sympathetic (less noble) to steel such as zinc, aluminium or magnesium the steel would be protected and rather than corrosion taking place on the steel the less noble material would waste away. This made some sense to me, I realised that some of the information I had been bombarded with in Physics at school might actually have some use!

Who'd have thought it; maybe if the teachers had told me how it was used, I might have paid more attention? We would be using a Bathycorrometer to assess levels of protection to the steel; this was a submersible voltmeter, we were to press the sharpened tip against clean steel and take the reading, provided the reading was greater than -0.8 V the steel would be protected and then even bare steel would not corrode. This all sounded very straightforward and certainly I felt was something I could manage without too much trouble; we then moved on to the digital thickness meter; we would be using a 'SeaProbe', this meter would send a pulse of high frequency sound into the steel, when this pulse reached the back wall of the steel it would reflect, returning to the probe, once received the meter would register the time taken from transmission to reception and would display the result in millimetres of steel.

This I felt was another machine that I would be able to handle, as it turns out the SeaProbe can be quite difficult to use when working under a ship or anywhere mid water due to the fact that you had to depress a spring loaded probe in order to activate it; easy to do when you are able to apply enough pressure but when mid-water you had to fin quite hard to be able to apply enough pressure; luckily for the exam we would be working on small test-pieces on the bottom of the harbour, we would be quite heavy so should have no problem applying enough pressure. It wasn't until I was offshore in France that I found out how hard this could be when mid-water.

We finished off the afternoon by having an introduction to MPI, again I realised that a lot of what I was being told was something I had covered in physics at school! I found myself wishing I had paid more attention but hey-ho; what's done is done; anyway, it seemed that when a magnetic field is passed through a piece of steel it will stay inside the steel unless it comes across a crack or some other defect or 'discontinuity' (a new word for me at the time!).

When the magnetic field encounters one of these it will be pushed out of the steel forming magnetic poles either side of the defect; to maximise this effect the magnetism should be made to cross the suspected defect at an angle of between ninety to forty-five degrees with ninety being the optimum. We were shown that in order to find any and all defects in the weld we needed to carry out the inspection twice at each location, for the second shot we had to apply the magnetism at ninety degrees to the first application. Doing this would ensure that no matter how a defect was situated in the weld it would show up as applying magnetism like this would mean that any defect would always be crossed by magnetism at an angle of between forty-five and ninety degrees; easy! Well, we would see about that.

This all seemed to make sense but then how could we make this useful to us? We were shown how to apply a magnetic particle ink to the surface; the particles in the ink would be drawn to these minute poles showing the location of the defect, simple! Well again, we would also see about that. To start with in the classroom, we used an ink with black particles and to make these show up we sprayed a white contrast aid paint onto the surface of the steel; this worked fine, the defects showed up as black jagged lines that were relatively easily identified. However, we couldn't apply contrast aid paint underwater so we would be using fluorescent ink, this ink didn't require contrast aid paint but would require us to carry out the inspection in the dark; once we had applied the ink, we would shine an ultraviolet (UV) lamp onto the work piece and if the particles had been drawn to a defect, we would easily see it; really?

Well in the classroom it worked fine and in fact if anything it was easier than the black ink had been; maybe it would work in the water, we would see. We spent the rest of the afternoon learning how to apply not only a permanent magnet but also two electrical methods to produce magnetic fields that would be strong enough to find defects underwater. The first of the three methods we were to use would be a permanent magnet, we all understood how the field of a horseshoe magnet looks and so this method was relatively easy. The electrical methods were though a bit more of a mystery to me in any case although some of the other lads had already trained in electricity and knew the principles, all I had was very basic understanding again from my physics lessons at school.

I did remember that electricity flowing through a cable would produce magnetism around the cable but beyond that I was lost; it seemed one of John Ambrose Fleming's laws determined how the electricity and magnetism were related. We all got the hang of this and by applying this law we could work out the direction of the magnetism produced would be running.

We were then shown the two electrical methods we would be using; the first was to use a long heavy, flexible cable, this was termed a coil, it could be wrapped around the item to be tested forming a coil, this would produce magnetism running directly through the coil. If the item was too large for us to make a coil around it then the cable could be formed into a shape resembling the element in the bottom of an old style electric kettle; effectively we would make a large coil and rather than wrap the coil around the test-piece we would lay the coil on the surface of the item and just arrange a couple of the loops one on each side of the weld to be tested, quite straightforward in the classroom where we could see everything and didn't have to hold on but in the water? Hmm!

With this method, provided the electricity was running the same way through each of the cables either side of the weld to be inspected then magnetism would run directly across the weld between the cables; I know this probably sounds tenuous but apparently it would work. As I say we all felt that again it might be possible when we were sitting on the seabed but again how would I apply this to the side of a ship or anything else mid-water? The last method we were to be using was termed 'Prods', these were a set of very heavy-duty contacts that we would be applying directly to the surface of the metal to be tested, once we had been able to make an electrical contact electricity would flow directly through the metal.

We would be carrying this out on the seabed; sounds fine until we were told that the current flowing would be something around a thousand amps! On the surface application of prods was a two-man job but underwater we were told it could be done by one diver as the prods were held in a frame enabling them to be applied with one hand, the lamp was combined with some method of applying the ink so both the ink and the lamp could be applied with our other hand; of course, this seemed plausible but I thought it would be very difficult and perhaps, dangerous?

Anyway, we were told the voltage applied would be very low (just 3 Volts) so we were quite safe; hmm, if you say so. We were told that we had to avoid any arcing at the tips of the prods as this would damage the steel being tested; OK so how do we do that then? Mel showed us, he cleaned up the surface of a test-piece so that bare metal shone, we were to be using a wire brush for this and again this was easy in the classroom but underwater on a piece of metal that had been submerged in seawater for years? Mel applied the prods to this nice clean surface and called "make it hot", Craig hit the button, the ammeter sprung up to read 1,000 amps, the current was flowing; at the tips of the prods, we could see small sparks and smoke started to rise from each of them. Hmm, it was clearly not going to be quite so easy to stop any arcing; when Mel had the current flowing, he told Dave to spray some ink onto the weld, this just made more smoke but when we shone on the UV light, we could see jagged lines which were apparently due to cracks in the metal.

When we each had a go with the prods in the classroom, we all found that no matter how much force we applied we would see a good deal of sparking and burning at the prod tips; in the water would be another matter surely, I thought that never mind using this method to find cracks I thought using prods was likely to cause more damage than might already be there!

Ultraviolet light sometimes termed 'black light', in the classroom was supplied by an appropriately black lamp about six inches in diameter, we were told not to look into the lamp as it was bad for our eyes, another reason to stay away from this whole set up. We found the permanent magnet worked very well in the classroom; it was quite strong, apparently it could lift 18 Kg; when we applied it to the work-piece it kind of took over as soon as it came within a couple of inches of the test-piece, inevitably slamming onto the metal in the wrong place!

We then had to try to slide it into the location we needed; this again was not too bad in the classroom as one of my mates could hold the test-piece while I moved the magnet, in the water when I would be on my own, I was not so sure. When we eventually got the magnet in the right place we sprayed on the fluorescent ink, turned out the white lights and viewed with the UV light, wow! The work-piece glowed bright green, in the midst of all the ink lying on the surface of the work-piece there were some brighter jagged indications; it worked; although it was clear that the cracks showed up so did a whole lot of other things caused by the shape of the weld, scratches and I'm sure some dirt and goodness knew what else was going to show up; confusing? Yes, it was, however, we were told that underwater it was much easier as none of the ink would settle on the work-piece unless there was a defect; hmm, not convinced but maybe; we would see.

Well, using the electrical methods were a lot harder, firstly the prods were quite fiery and although they could be made to work, I found them very difficult to handle, I had to apply a fair amount of pressure to get a contact and then had to apply ink while still maintaining the contact then pick up the lamp to view; it wasn't easy. We were again reassured that in the water the ink was supplied via a trigger on the lamp so we would not need three hands; not all that reassuring but it was true that the indications were easy to see using this method.

When we came to use the coil, we found that yes it did work but if we were to bring the UV lamp too close to the cable the light would 'trip' out and we would then have to wait a few minutes for it to come back on; frustrating in the classroom but much more of a problem during a timed exam on the seabed!

So, there we were, fully briefed on the methods we were to be tested on; tomorrow we would get to practice them in the water and after just one day's practice, we would be examined by the Lloyd's Inspector; no pressure then. We were given a coffee break during which we all speculated that this MPI was of course going to be impossible in the water as none of us had three hands. After coffee we all went down to the store to get our first look at the subsea-equipment we would be using tomorrow. Mel was on hand to talk us through the equipment, there was the Ultrasonic Digital Thickness Meter (DTM) together with its calibration block, which was a small steel block of known thickness 12.5mm that would be used immediately before and after we took readings on the test-piece this would confirm the meter was working properly. Similarly, the CP meter came with a lump of Zinc that was to be used as its calibration block as we knew the potential it should read.

Then we were introduced to the underwater CCTV (video) camera, this was an enormous cylinder with a handle protruding from one side, it was about two feet long and eight inches in diameter; there was a thick orange cable coming out of one end, this was clearly not going to be all that easy to use, mid-water either. We were shown the magnetised tape measures, arrows and a graduated pointer (just like the graduated pole I had used for photography with ICI); I could see this becoming a real mess in the water! How were we going to keep track of all this and make some sense of what we were looking at? Lastly, we were shown the MPI equipment, while I had been wondering how I was going to handle all of the other equipment some of the guys had been manhandling the MPI transformer outside, it was an immense lump, again, it was a black cylinder but this one was about two feet (60cm) tall and about two foot six inches (75cm) in diameter, it was very heavy and needed two to lift it.

It had a circular tubular frame running around the top and there were three terminals on top, these were where the cables would be affixed, there were large wing nuts to be used to secure the cables onto the terminals. There were short 'whips' of cable attached to each terminal and on each 'whip' there were large rubber welding connectors that could be separated underwater, this would allow us to swap between coil and prods easily. We had to make sure we used the correct terminals as the transformer could supply both AC and DC, the choice apparently was dependent on what defects we were looking for but this choice would be made for us by someone else thank goodness.

Also attached to this unit was the UV lamp and ink reservoir; there was a small pump that would continuously circulate the ink around the reservoir bag keeping it properly mixed. There was an umbilical leading away from the transformer leading to the UV lamp which was another bulky item, this was apparently the same unit as we had used in the classroom but of course it had to be contained in a water and pressure resistant housing; it was very big! On the handle we were shown a small button, just above this button was a small plastic tube extending out to a distance of about six inches, this was where the ink would be emitted when we depressed the button. I for one was a little taken aback by the amount of kit we would have to get used to but, well, it had to be possible, didn't it?

The next morning immediately after breakfast we made our way to the store where we were issued with everything we had been shown yesterday. We took all this equipment down to the jetty and started to lay out the dive site with three dive stations utilising surface demand equipment with bandmasks, Mel set up the MPI transformer for us, he attached the cables to the AC terminals he told us this was because we were looking for surface breaking defects. The transformer would be supplied with electricity via a very heavy armoured umbilical running back to the surface. Altogether this was a very unwieldy bit of kit that luckily, we would be able to sit it on the seabed for our exam, when we used this on a job site it was likely that we would not be working on the seabed so there would be a lot of rigging required in order to bring the transformer close enough to the job; I later found that rigging the site was often the greater part of the job and could take two or three times as long as the actual MPI inspection.

We rigged the transformer with a work-line so that no load would be applied to the main umbilical, and lowered it to the seabed at the base of one of the ladders. We then dressed three divers who would be the first to have a go at all this, I was not part of this first team and was left on deck running around lowering the appropriate test-pieces to whoever needed them, diver one would start off with MPI while diver two would start with UT & CP measurements while the third diver would conduct CCTV inspection of a flange that was sticking out of the wall at about five feet above the seabed; when they each completed their allotted tasks they would swap around so that they all eventually undertook all tasks.

When my turn came, I would be conducting CCTV inspection first, when I made it to the seabed, I moved across to pick up the video camera; I had thought this was going to be extremely hard as the camera was so big but in fact in the water the camera was relatively easy to handle it was almost neutrally buoyant and although it was very big (we nicknamed it the 'dustbin') I found I could manipulate it quite easily. Much harder was getting the tape measures and identification numbers to stay where I put them; both the measuring tapes and identification numbers had magnets attached to them which should have made placement relatively easy. However, although there wasn't much of a swell running with the flange being quite near the corner of the jetty there was a bit of surge, this was enough to keep pulling the tape away from the flange; eventually I did though manage to carry out some kind of an inspection with commentary.

I wasn't sure it would be what the inspector would be looking for though, I would find out at the end of the day. I then swapped to the CP and DTM; ultrasonic readings were to be taken on a step block, this was a steel block of varying thickness throughout its length, I laid on the seabed and took the calibration reading first, 12.5mm I relayed this to the surface where Jack recorded it, I then moved onto the block and gave a series of readings, I moved the probe along the block and whenever the reading changed I would give the new reading to Jack; I found a total of six variations all of which Jack recorded, then I completed the readings by another calibration check; job done.

Now I picked up the Bathycorrometer to carry out the CP readings, again I started with a calibration reading on the zinc block where I first had to make sure I found some bare metal, I applied the meter's sharp tip twisting the meter to make sure I had a good contact; when the reading stabilised it read -1.018 V, I had been told to relay this as a negative reading although the reading on the meter didn't show the minus sign. I then moved on to take readings on the various pieces of metal we had been given, one of these had a sacrificial anode attached, when I eventually managed to get a good contact, the reading was -0.86 V; I then moved on to an unprotected piece of steel where I managed to get a reading of -0.64 V; I then carried out a second reading from the zinc block as the end calibration reading. All of these were relayed to Jack again. I then put both the meters together with all the test blocks at the base of the ladder so that the next diver would easily find them.

Now I moved across to the MPI transformer, as we were to be using fluorescent ink for the MPI we had to use a 'habitat' to make the environment dark enough for us to see the defect indications; we had been told that this habitat was a purpose-built piece of kit! I could now see that it had obviously been manufactured at huge expense! In fact, it turned out to be a large steel drum with the bottom cut out, the drum was lying on its side allowing access for the diver who would effectively be lying on the bottom; earlier while I was returning from doing the CCTV, I had seen one of the others doing the MPI.

All I could see was a pair of legs sticking out of the drum, exhaled bubbles were streaming out of the top of the drum, I had thought that this looked anything but easy; cables ran from the transformer disappearing into the drum alongside the diver. As I passed the diver reversed out of the drum carrying a piece of welded steel, he turned towards me and I recognised Craig, he gave me a thumbs up and then left to get on with his next task. Anyway, now it was my turn, I moved to the drum and peered inside, I could see the prods were connected to the transformer at the time so this would be my first task; the UV lamp was also there emanating a ghostly purple glow.

I picked up the test-piece we were to use with the prods, I could see where the others had already been applying the prod tips, there were a number of burn marks on the surface; I ran the wire brush across the surface of the weld and surrounding area so that it would be clean for my inspection and took it into the 'habitat' with me.

There really wasn't much room when I got my head in as the bail-out cylinder on my back was touching the top of the drum, once I was in position it was certainly quite dark though, so maybe this would work after all. I arranged the test-piece, picked up the prods and UV lamp and called "make it hot" Jack replied "it's hot" meaning electricity was applied to the prods; I pressed the prod tips onto the metal and nothing happened! I clearly hadn't achieved an electrical contact, I pressed harder by bracing myself pushing my back against the top of the drum, I rocked the prod frame, there was a huge flash, I then felt the frame buzzing, I could see bubbles and small arcs around both of the tips so current was flowing.

I pressed the button on the UV lamp, ink flowed and I directed it onto the weld; well, that is to say so much came out that the whole place was covered in a bright green blanket of ink, I let go of the button and asked Jack to "make it cold", I dropped the prod frame and gently wafted the weld with my hand holding the lamp close enough so that I could see the weld being illuminated. Slowly the cloud of ink cleared and to my surprise Mel had been right the weld was clearly visible, there right in the middle of the weld was a bright jagged green indication, I couldn't miss it, easy; I measured its position from the edge of the plate that we had been told was the datum point for our measurements and relayed this measurement together with its length to Jack, job done!

I took the plate out of the drum together with the prods and moved over to the transformer, I unplugged the rubber welding connectors disconnecting the prods and plugged the coil's connectors in; then I pulled the coil back to the drum and went to get the test-piece we were to use for the coils. Dragging it into the drum, I managed to lay it at the end and formed the coil into the 'kettle element' shape with the cables running parallel to the weld one on each side of the weld as we had been shown.

"Make it hot", again, I could then feel the cables buzzing, I moved in to spray the ink, as I was running the plastic tube along the weld the light suddenly went out! Now what? I told topside that the lamp had gone out, Mel came on the comms and told me to sit tight and wait, the lamp would come back on in a few minutes; this was a long couple of minutes, I kept thinking if this keeps happening during the exam I could be in trouble. Eventually the lamp came back on, I could again see the fluorescence, I thought I'll just have a look at the weld before I turn on the power again, I found I could again see defect indications I measured the indication's position and dimensions and again relayed these to Jack.

All that was left for me to do now was to use the permanent magnet; by comparison this was easy although as I had thought getting the magnet in the right place was a bit tricky but by comparison to using the prods it was a doddle.

When I returned to the surface, I found that my measurements were correct and that I had found all of the defects required, my readings for the UT and CP were also OK and my video commentary had mentioned all the necessary points; it seemed I was ready for the exam, I must say I didn't feel very prepared and while chatting with the rest of the guys that evening it seemed I wasn't the only one who was a bit nervous but we would see tomorrow.

The next day the weather did nothing to help us, it was a dank and miserable day although there was very little wind so diving would not be a problem; I had not had a great deal of sleep as I was quite nervous, I was worrying about the exam as I didn't feel prepared at all. As usual we stoked up on full English breakfast and then assembled in reception to wait for the Lloyd's examiner; he arrived in reception with Mel Bayliss at eight thirty sharp they decided that we would carry out the practical assessments first as the tide was right in the morning.

We were detailed to set up the dive spread on the jetty we were told to set up three dive stations exactly as we had yesterday. Off we went to draw all the equipment from the store to set up ready for diving, we at least were confident with setting up the diving kit now but I really didn't feel the same way about the inspection equipment. Mel and Ray set up the MPI and CCTV systems and when all was ready the Lloyd's surveyor gave us a thorough brief about what he expected of us; it was nothing other than another run through as we had done yesterday except of course we had to use test-pieces he had brought with him. This time I was to start with MPI; my second task would be CP and DTM before finishing off with the CCTV.

As I took the MPI samples across to the habitat my first thought was that the exam test-pieces were much bigger than the ones we had used yesterday, this would make space in the habitat even more restricted. Anyway, this time I was to start with the permanent magnet, I had been given a flat plate as the test-piece to be used for this. I took all the equipment into the habitat and placed the magnet on to the test-piece at an angle of forty-five degrees just as we had been shown, I sprayed on the ink and inspected the weld, there was nothing to be seen between the magnet's poles but I could see a clear indication a few inches along the weld, I was a bit surprised it was so clearly visible but I thought I would report it when I got to properly inspect that part of the weld.

I then moved the magnet through ninety degrees so that it spanned the same part of the weld as we had been shown; nothing showed up but the one I had already seen further along the weld was still visible. I completed the inspection of this weld and only found the one defect; was that all I was supposed to find? I didn't know but at least I had found something.

I then set up to use the coil system, I had been given a big heavy 'T' piece for this, I had to inspect both of the welds looking for all defects; Firstly, I set the coil up in the 'kettle element' configuration with the cables running parallel with the weld, magnetism would flow across the weld allowing me to inspect for defects running along or longitudinal to the weld. I called "make it hot", "it's hot" came the response from topside, I already knew this as I could feel the cables buzzing, I moved in with the lamp to spray ink onto the weld but no sooner had I started to spray ink the lamp went out.

I had clearly got the lamp too close to the cables although I hadn't thought I was very close, it was clearly close enough; I told topside "Make it cold, the lamp has gone out", "OK just sit there and it will come back on in a short while" came the response, I was now not happy at all, I knew the lamp would come back on but I only had a short time to complete this inspection and I hadn't even started yet. After a few minutes the lamp came back on, I thought I would have a quick look at the weld before I turned the coil back on again, when I came in close enough, I could clearly see two indications, the particles must have been kept in place by residual magnetism? Anyway, I didn't really care, I reported both of the indications giving their position relative to the edge of the plate which was again the datum point for our inspection and of course I also reported their size.

I then moved the test-piece so that I could inspect the other weld; given what had happened on the other side I decided to make the coil hot and spray the ink while keeping the lamp as far away from the coil as I could hopefully this would mean I could keep the lamp far enough away from the coil that it wouldn't go out. "Make it hot", "it's hot", I sprayed ink all along the weld and waited a couple of seconds before "make it cold", "it's cold"; the lamp was still on so I went straight in to inspect the weld and again I thought I could see a small indication although it was nowhere near as easy to see as the others had been.

Was it a crack or not? I really didn't know, I decided to make a note of where it seemed to be and to see whether it came up more strongly when I applied the magnetism parallel to the weld; I wound the cable three times around the "T" piece and again "make it hot", "it's hot", I sprayed ink along the weld and made it cold again. When I came in to inspect the weld again, I could see that the indication I had not been sure about had come up much more strongly, it was running transverse to the weld and what I had seen before were some tiny branches running away from the main indication; I again reported this as an indication. There didn't appear to be any other indications on either side of the test-piece, I had completed the inspection with just a couple of minutes to spare; all that was left now were the prods.

Again, I had been given a flat plate for this inspection, I brought the plate into the habitat and then went to the transformer, where I removed the coil and connected the prods. I was quickly back in the habitat ready to go, "make it hot", "it's hot"; flash, splutter, lots of arcing and bubbles from the prod tips, I obviously had a contact, on went the ink, "make it cold". I could easily see an indication, there was no doubt this time, I reported where it was relative to the edge of the plate and gave its dimensions, again, job done; well, we would see when we were told our results.

Next, I completed the CP and DTM measurements, these all went perfectly and were reported to the surface.

Lastly, I moved over to the video camera, I had been told to carry out inspection on the same flange as I had inspected yesterday; I felt this went OK. I ran the camera around the flange's weld giving a commentary of what I saw; when complete I was told to leave the camera on the seabed and to make my way back to the surface.

Eventually we had all finished our dives, we dismantled all the equipment and took it back to the store; all we had to do now was the theory test; we were told to get changed, have a cup of tea and to be ready in the chartroom in thirty minutes. None of us wanted to be late for this one and I think we were all there ready and waiting in about twenty minutes; the Lloyds surveyor again gave us a bit of a brief about the exam, it was a multiple-choice paper and we were to make sure we read the question and all the answers properly before choosing our answer, only one answer was correct.

I found that I had clearly understood more than I realised as I didn't feel the questions were very hard, at least that was how I felt, but again we would see when the results were given. We had been told to leave quietly when we felt we were finished and to wait in reception where we would be collected when everyone had finished and the papers had been marked. There were another anxious few minutes but eventually we had all finished and were waiting in reception. The Lloyds surveyor and Mel arrived a few minutes later and we were taken into CM 14 for the results; there was no preamble at all, as soon as we were all sitting down the surveyor said "well done, you have all passed all parts of the exam"; brilliant, now we had a real skill that would help us to get a job.

That evening we all again assembled in the bar for the last time, it wasn't a huge celebration as although we were all pleased to have completed everything successfully, we realised that we were about to go out into the real world, it was scary to say the least. We had become a close-knit team and I'm sure I wasn't alone in feeling a little sorry to be leaving them all, we had already exchanged addresses and telephone numbers and assured each other that we would of course keep in touch and in any case, we would meet one another on jobs wouldn't we!

My time at Bovisand had been largely happy although there had been some trying times, it had at times seemed doubtful that I would graduate, I spent a few minutes standing on the jetty reminiscing about the course experiences with a couple of the others and then it was time for some of them to leave. I was staying one more night at the fort as I would be leaving for Aberdeen with Dave Pelly tomorrow and it didn't seem sensible to go home and then to have to come back to Plymouth in the morning.

PHOTOS FROM MY BASIC AIR DIVING (BAD) COURSE AT FORT BOVISAND

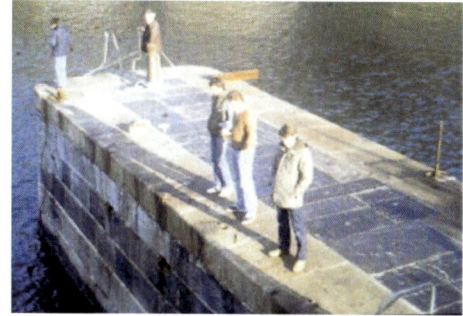

Day one of the BAD course, contemplation of the coming ordeals?

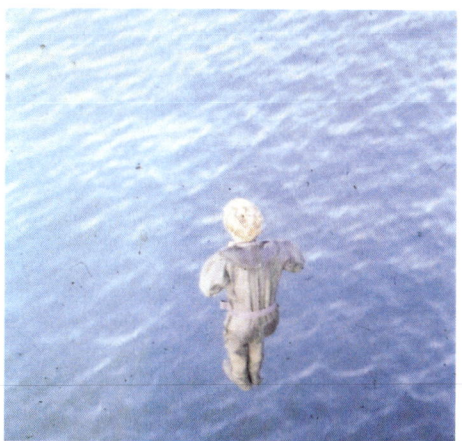

Craig was one of the first to attempt the jump from the tower, feet nicely together with arms across his chest. Perfect.

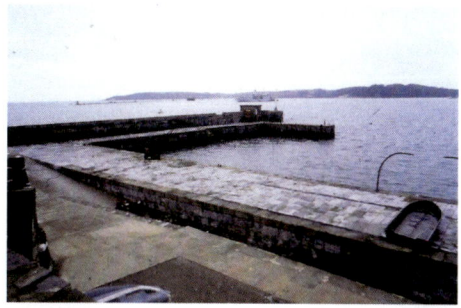

Fort Bovisand harbour on a calm day, what a lovely place to be.

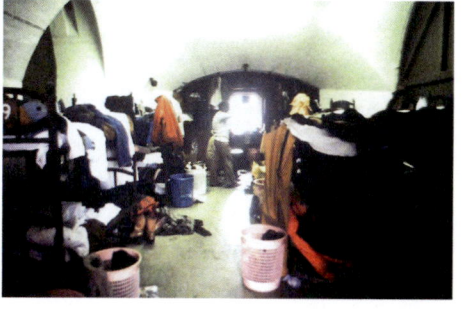

Home sweet home for some thirteen weeks. Fifteen young lads may not have been particularly good at housekeeping duties during our courses.

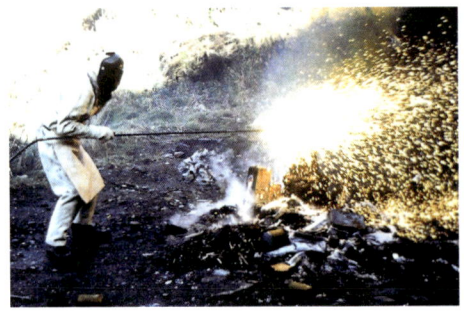

Tony Hale demonstrating the thermic lance, what a fiery beast.

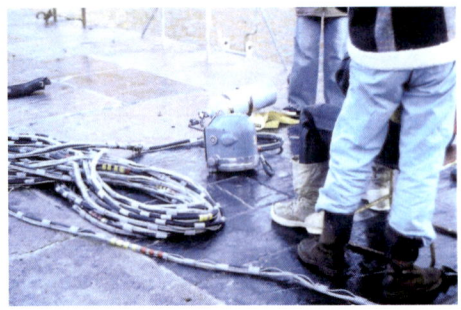

The Divex Lightweight freeflow helmet set up on the jetty attached to its umbilical prior to diving.

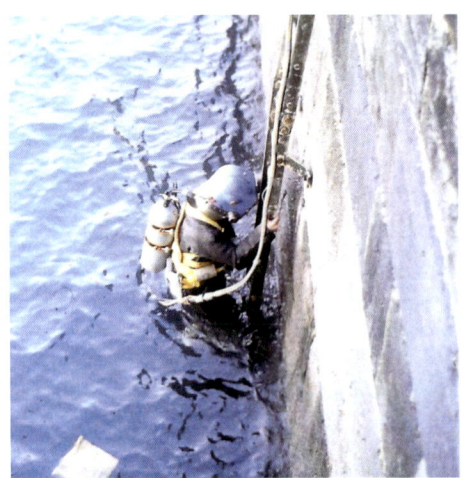

The author making his way down the ladder into the water for his first dive in the Divex freeflow helmet.

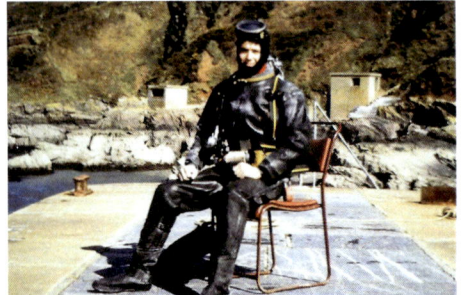

The author set up as standby diver on the Bovisand Jetty.

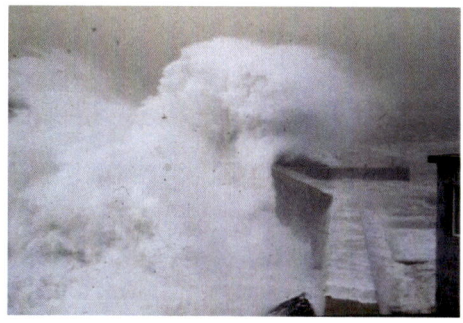

The weather in February could be challenging!

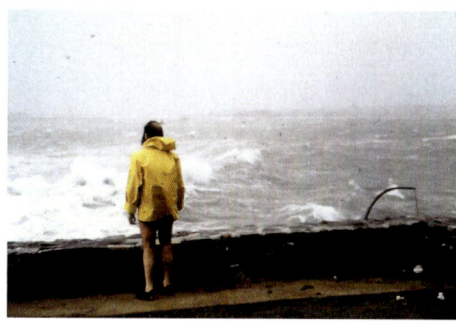

Our Aussie instructor Monty Ham contemplating where he can take us to have us blowing bubbles on this questionable day?

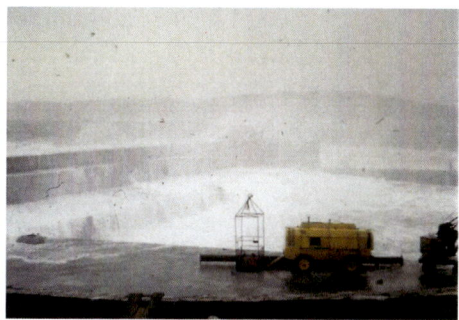

On this day we did swim in the harbour but it became a fight for survival. On the jetty in the foreground a diver's basket can be seen. This type of basket was often used to get divers into and out of the water offshore.

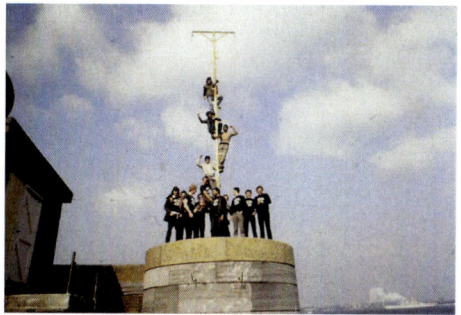

Final day of the course, we've all passed and celebrations begin. The author is second from the top on the flagpole.

Part Three

CHAPTER TEN

First Steps into the Offshore World

Finally, the day had arrived when we were to leave Plymouth, we had said all our goodbyes; I had taken all the stuff I wouldn't be needing home a couple of days before so was prepared as much as I could be. I was to be travelling with Dave Pelly as he had also been given a job with Oceaneering. We met up on the platform at Plymouth railway station and boarded the overnight sleeper to Edinburgh; this already had all the hallmarks of a great adventure as far as I was concerned; I had one suitcase which contained everything I thought I would need for my first job in the offshore diving world. We had been told to bring steel toe capped boots and some overalls; the only boots I had were totally wrong for working at sea as they were lace up, what was really needed were boots that could be kicked off if you were unfortunate enough to find yourself in the sea while still wearing them! Still, I had to go with what I had and as we were to be working in the yard at Oceaneering to begin with, I thought they should be fine for that.

We settled in to our compartment which would be our home until we reached Edinburgh at seven o'clock the following morning; we stowed our kit and headed out to find the buffet car to get something to eat and of course a couple of beers. British rail's finest sandwich and a couple of cans of Heineken were all that was available but that was fine as nothing was going to get in the way of us enjoying our first steps into the offshore world. After a very sleepless night that seemed to consist of our carriage being shunted about various sidings for most of the night, we found ourselves standing on the platform blinking in the daylight of a bright but cold morning in Edinburgh.

We finally identified the Aberdeen train and settled in to our seats for the final few hours; I was certainly a little apprehensive about what the future would hold for me, I didn't really know much about what we were going to be doing and didn't feel all that comfortable, but of course being male we didn't discuss any of this and put on a brave face. Finally, we arrived at our destination, Aberdeen; the station is imaginatively named 'Aberdeen Railway Station' and is situated alongside Union Square, although I didn't know it at the time, this was an area that I would get to know well in the coming years.

We piled into a taxi for the last few miles to our destination the Oceaneering facility which at the time was situated on Broadfold Road in the Bridge of Don part of the city. I remember standing in the car park looking at a wonderful sight, there were trucks coming and going loaded with various diving equipment all painted bright yellow and white, these being Oceaneering's colours, they looked great to me. Oceaneering's yard was behind the building so we couldn't see much from our vantage point in the car park; we decided to head in and announce our arrival, obviously they would be eagerly awaiting our arrival!

We headed into reception inside we found a lady sitting behind a desk scowling at us; at the time I felt she was not a very welcoming first impression. I later found out she was called Pamela and was renowned in the diving world as a formidable barrier to anyone wishing to access the Oceaneering site. Luckily, we had an appointment with Sam Hardy who ran the workshop; this didn't seem to make her any more welcoming but at least we were ushered through and were taken straight to Mr Hardy whose office was in a Portakabin inside the workshop.

Sam was however very welcoming he did indeed know about us and had been expecting us; we were invited to sit; we were then given an introduction to what we could expect from him and what he expected from us. Sam was very business-like; it seemed that he expected us to turn up in the morning and to work hard until the evening; simple! However, I was not sure I would be of much use to him as I certainly didn't know much about maintaining diving equipment, this it seemed was not a problem as he would be putting us alongside one of the old hands who would show us everything we needed to know; I felt a bit sorry for this chap already (this reminded me of when I had been inflicted on poor Fred at Interheat!) and we hadn't even been introduced yet!

For his part Sam assured us that provided we performed well we would be given a diving job offshore within a few weeks; this was all I needed to hear, I would do whatever he wanted so that he would recommend us for our first offshore diving job.

He then asked where we were staying, we told him that we hadn't found anywhere yet and that we would be looking as soon as we left this evening. Sam told us that we should try the Albury guest house; this apparently was where all the jobbing divers stayed, it was clean, cheap and provided a great breakfast. Well, this sounded brilliant; not only that but Sam called them and was told that they did have room for us.

Next, he called in the chap who would be looking after us in the workshop over the next few weeks; a couple of minutes later an old chap turned up and was introduced as Jimmy (I thought this was a nickname as it was common for Scottish people to have that moniker but, it seemed this was his real name! Good job I didn't say anything); he was told to look after us and to show us around. We both thanked Sam and followed Jimmy out into the workshop, he took us to the locker room where we were to leave our bags, we were told to find ourselves some coveralls which we did as there were lots of spare sets, we both put on our steel toed boots and followed him onto the workshop floor.

He had an extremely broad Scots, accent and kept referring to 'Ken' by saying "d'y Ken"; it wasn't until later that we realised that Ken wasn't a name at all, d'y ken means 'do you know'; initially neither Dave nor I knew what he was talking about for much of the time, anyway, the workshop was terrific, there was a saturation system under construction and a myriad of other diving equipment either being worked on or at least stored ready for use.

Saturation diving was the ultimate goal for divers in those days, at this time I had been trained as an air diver only, this meant that although I was qualified to dive offshore in the UK, I was limited to a maximum of fifty metres water depth. This was not really a problem other than that the average depth of the North Sea where the majority of the oil rigs were positioned was some, one hundred metres, of course this limited my usefulness. Divers who were qualified to engage in saturation diving had normally been air divers for some years and would have had further training in the necessary techniques.

Commercial air divers working in the North Sea would be supplied with air from the surface and would have to return to the surface after quite short periods, while this was useful for some tasks, it did limit their usefulness when the structures and equipment was either deeper than fifty metres or required a diver to be there for an extended period in order to complete complex tasks.

These days there are saturation systems that stay under pressure almost permanently with divers entering for a period and then decompressing in a dedicated chamber after perhaps twenty-eight days.

Anyway, back to my first day at Oceaneering, in the workshop there were various other pieces of diving equipment undergoing maintenance of one sort or another. A forklift truck was zipping around picking up pallets of hose and rope; this truck was running on propane gas and the fumes brought back memories of happy childhood holidays in caravans in Cornwall. There were a number of other men welding, painting or generally looking incredibly busy; Jimmy reassured us that we shouldn't worry about our ability as he would show us what we needed to know; at least that's what I thought he said as I say his accent was extremely broad and neither Dave nor I could really follow much of what he said! We were both pleased that he seemed very upbeat about our capability. Jimmy also confirmed that Sam would find us a job offshore within a few weeks, this was good to hear, I was again in heaven and it seemed my earlier concerns had been unfounded.

At the end of the day, we were released at about five o'clock; now all we had to do was to find our guest house; as it turned out it was situated on the other side of the city but eventually, we found it, as with all the other houses in the street and Aberdeen in general the Albury was a grey granite building, it didn't look particularly welcoming but we were there now. As we stepped inside, we were greeted by a lovely warm atmosphere and met by the owner Cecil, after welcoming us he told us to "call me Sess", he seemed a nice guy although I also found his accent a little difficult to understand as it was a lot broader Scots than I had been used to in my previous trips to Scotland with ICI.

Sess told us that we could have our own room or we could share in the 'bunk room', this was a lot cheaper and therefore the preferred option; Sess took us downstairs into the basement, he showed us the shower room and other facilities. Finally, he led us into the bunk room, told us when breakfast would be served and then left us alone; the bunk room had four sets of bunk beds arranged around the walls, two of these had guys already installed, they were reading various books or magazines.

We all exchanged pleasantries, it seemed they were both divers waiting for a job that was imminent, we of course earwigged their conversation which consisted of when and who they were last in 'Sat' with; we of course had nothing much to say to them as they would definitely not be impressed by our pedigree at this point. I chose the top bunk and put my bag on the floor in my 'area', Dave was on the bottom bunk; this all seemed OK, the place was warm, the other guys seemed friendly. Day one in Aberdeen was now complete I was officially employed by an international diving company and was on my way to working offshore, I know I keep saying this but to say I was happy would be an understatement.

I slept very well that first night as I was dog tired having not slept at all really on the 'sleeper' train last night, there were by now five others in the room including Dave and although there was a bit of snoring, I was used to that kind of living after having been effectively in a bunk room while on the course for the last three months. The next morning started at seven o'clock with breakfast which was as billed 'very good', it was indeed a very full breakfast, there was heaps of it. It was a full English although with a Scottish twist with haggis and porridge being on offer; when I finished, I felt I was ready for anything.

We said goodbye and made our way to work arriving in good time, we had plenty of time to put on our work clothes before we were due to start. Jimmy arrived and told us our task for the day was too clean and re-tape umbilicals that had returned from a job recently; when we were shown these umbilicals they were in a dreadful state, they had clearly been very well used. Originally, they had been held together by silver duct tape at intervals along their length but most of this was either peeling off or had gone altogether.

Our first job was to remove all the old tape thus separating the hoses and cables which would then be checked for damage before being put back together, Dave and I worked as a team, Jimmy disappeared and only reappeared from time to time to make sure we were still OK. Once we had cleaned off the tape from the hoses, Jimmy showed us how to check for damage and to stow the ones that had passed the check ready for the next step of the process. About ten thirty we were taken to the tea shack, another Portakabin where we were provided with coffee or tea and Jimmy lit up a cigarette, he seemed to want to chat but as I say we found him very difficult to understand, Jimmy didn't seem to notice though and after twenty minutes we finished our coffee and went back to work.

The next step of the process for the breathing hoses we were to reuse was to clean the inside of the hoses with a solvent; the solvent we were to use was 'Freon', at the time I didn't know the effect this was having on the world's ozone layer and I doubt anyone else knew either but even if they did it was commonly used. Anyway, we were given a five-gallon drum, a funnel and were told to pour a couple of pints of Freon into each of the breathing hoses then, we would hook the hose up to an airline and blow the solvent through the hose until it had all been cleared out.

We spent a good deal of the day watching the end of a hose until the air coming out was clear of any vapour; not very scientific but Jimmy said this would be fine and would have removed any nasty residues from the inside of the hoses, when complete we screwed a blank into the hose fitting either end so that the hose wouldn't become contaminated again.

At lunchtime Jimmy announced that we would be going to the pub for lunch, this seemed a bit odd but in 1980 drinking at lunchtime was not frowned on nearly as much as it would be today, anyway Jimmy was after all in charge so off the three of us went, the pub was close by so we walked there in just a few minutes. Jimmy bought himself a pint of heavy (heavy was to the Scots call what in England would be termed bitter) so Dave and I followed suit as we wanted to fit in; Jimmy quickly finished his pint and although we had hardly even touched ours, he announced it was time for another round.

We didn't need another drink yet so Jimmy went to the bar on his own; Dave and I just looked at each other and quietly wondered how we should handle the situation. We had left for our lunch break at one o'clock and by two, I was beginning to feel uncomfortable as Jimmy showed no sign of wanting to get back; in 1980 pubs in England used to close in the afternoons but in Scotland they were open all day so maybe we were in for a long afternoon. At about half past two Jimmy could see we were uneasy and announced that we would be going back just as soon as he had finished his drink (number four I think). We eventually left the pub at about quarter to three and made it back to work at a few minutes before three; Sam was waiting for us with a sour expression on his face, he took Jimmy to one side and it was clear that heated words were being exchanged; if we were nervous before we were getting much worse now.

After a few minutes Sam came back to us and it became clear that he didn't blame us as Jimmy had 'history' for this kind of behaviour, we were to make sure that if he were to suggest the pub at lunchtime, we should to tell him that we would not be going. I am not sure whether Sam felt this would deter Jimmy or not but we certainly didn't need telling twice, packed lunch would be the norm for us from now on. By the end of the day, we had managed to clean up two complete umbilicals and component parts; these had been stowed ready for final checking by a properly competent individual and then reassembly in the morning.

The next day we worked with another of the permanent staff checking the hoses and cables for nicks and other damage before getting ready to reassemble the umbilicals as we were now shown. We started by tying the load member rope to a hook in the wall and then starting to tape the hoses and comms cable together; we started by putting the breathing air hose, the smaller pneumo hose and comms cable together and whipping them to the load member rope using light rope close to the end; at this point we also whipped a lockable carabiner, this would be used to secure the umbilical to the diver's weight jacket. This would be the diver's end of the umbilical so we had to make sure there was sufficient length of hose and cable so that they would reach the connections on the hat or in the case of the pneumo that there was sufficient length allowing for the open end to be placed at the diver's chest level. We then started taping all the hoses and cable together at intervals of about thirty centimetres; this was time consuming but quite satisfying. When we reached the other end of the umbilical, we had been told to leave some ten feet of free hose and rope to allow connection on the surface; finally, we coiled the completed umbilicals in figure of eight so that when they were used, they could be paid out without becoming tangled.

At lunchtime we declined Jimmy's offer of the pub and took our packed lunches out into the sunshine in the yard. It was a beautiful day with clear blue sky, sitting in the sun was very pleasant; we spent a nice half hour watching a steady stream of helicopters carrying offshore workers out to the various rigs in the North Sea; I hoped that one day soon that would be us, we couldn't wait.

Our days were taken up with working on the various systems being readied for diving jobs; the major effort was being put into the saturation diving system that was to be going out to the 'Transworld 58' we were told that this was a Semi-Submersible drilling platform out in the Argyl field. The system was to us a fabulous 'state of the art' unit and we both loved working on it in the yard and hoped that one day we would be also working on one very like it offshore. This turned out to be sooner rather than later for Dave as he would find himself actually working as air diver support on the Transworld 58 before the end of the year.

Saturation systems would allow the divers to stay under pressure for a very much longer period than air divers could, typically they would be pressurised inside a chamber that stayed on deck, this would be termed their 'living chamber'; when the time came for them to go to work, they would transfer from the living chamber through into a diving bell. This transfer would be done under pressure termed Transfer Under Pressure 'TUP', the divers would constantly remain under pressure and would not return to atmospheric pressure for some considerable time, this could be weeks.

Once in the diving bell the divers would close doors to the living chamber and one inside the bell. As soon as these doors were properly sealed the trunking between the living chamber and the bell would be de-pressurised and the bell would be separated from the living chamber. The divers would still be at the same pressure which was normally the equivalent of about ten metres shallower than the depth at which they would be working. The diving bell would then be pressurised a little bit more so that the pressure inside would be the same as the working depth and the bell would be lowered into the water and on down to their working depth. On arrival at this depth the pressure inside the bell would be the same as the pressure outside allowing the divers to open the door at the bottom of the bell. The water would not enter the bell; the water would be level with the bottom door, rather like an upturned glass being pushed into water.

One of the divers would then don their diving kit and would be able to drop out of the bell and go to work this was termed 'locking out'. The diver's gas would be supplied via the bell, there would be a large umbilical supplying the bell with all the gas the divers would need as well as communications cables, pneumo hoses and because the divers would be breathing helium there would be another hose supplying hot water to the bell.

When divers breathe helium, they will feel cold almost immediately because helium conducts heat away from the body much more rapidly than air does; about seven times more. This means that in order for the divers to be useful for the length of time they will be in the water they need to be supplied with suit heating and in some cases the gas they breathe will also be warmed before it is supplied to the diver. The divers normally wear a hot water suit, this is a baggy neoprene suit with a connection at the waist where hot water would be introduced, this hot water then circulates around the suit via small hoses inside the suit, these hoses have small holes along their length through which the hot water is emitted. There are no seals at the collar, cuffs or ankles, hot water flows out of the ends of the suit's arms, legs and neck; the diver wears loose boots, sometimes Wellington boots and wears special gloves that allow the hot water to circulate around their hands.

The diver's umbilical has a hot water hose in addition to the other components common to diver's umbilicals we had used to date; it becomes a pretty heavy umbilical but of course in the water it can be made to be neutrally buoyant. Obviously, the bell umbilical is going to be a very heavy affair; it would run from the deck to the bell. Inside the bell there would be a distribution panel from which the diver and standby diver also known as the 'bellman' would be supplied. In the eighties there would normally be two divers inside the bell although these days there are commonly three divers in the bell.

In the case of the two diver systems one of the divers would dress ready 'lock-out' of the bell to go to work, (in a three-diver system two of the divers would simultaneously dress to go out of the bell) the diver left in the bell would become the bellman who has dual roles, he would be both the divers tender and also their standby diver. The bellman will also have dressed in diving kit except the hat, if the working diver had a problem the bellman would quickly put on his diving hat and would drop out of the bell to go and help the diver experiencing the problem.

All of this was a long way off for us or so we thought at the time although as it turns out I would be in 'Sat' within six months; I of course didn't know this at the time.

Sat systems are by necessity complex units, they have modules to supply the divers with their required gas, hot water, to maintain a liveable environment inside the living chambers and all other needs. There would be a saturation control room where there would be panels for the bell including supply for both the working diver and bellman; there would also be panels supplying the living chamber(s) (there may be more than one); there would be a separate panel for each and every part of the system that could be separated by pressure (effectively each part of the chamber system would be treated as a separate chamber). There would of course be at least one living chamber although these days it is common for there to be more than one; there would be at least one chamber that the divers would use for showering normally referred to as the 'wet pot', this would normally also contain the toilet. Often the wet pot was also the point where the diving bell would lock on to the chamber system, this then would be where the divers would leave from and return to for each dive or 'bell run'.

There would be at least one diving bell although again these days there are commonly two bells, in the eighties this would have been very rare; the bell also needed a winch and handling system enabling it to be lowered to and recovered from depth.

As you can appreciate this all would take up quite a lot of space although space is always very limited on any offshore vessel or rig; the sat system then had to be cleverly designed so that all of this equipment could be fitted into as small a space as possible.

Now clearly, we weren't qualified to do very much as far as building this system so we were restricted to painting and general duties; I spent a couple of days painting the bell and associated handling frames; I also spent quite a lot of time building the water supply system for the diver's shower inside the wet pot. I think I got this job as Sam had found out that I had spent some time as a central heating engineer although the required system bore almost no similarity to a domestic heating system and in any case, I had only spent a few months doing this and never to a very high standard.

The sat system water supply had to be fed to the chamber via a boost pump as the pressure inside the chamber would be very much higher than the normal water supply pressure; I spent a few days learning how this needed to go together and then assembling it. I have to say I was very nervous when we got to the testing phase and was very pleased when it performed as it should, phew, again!

Very soon Friday arrived; after lunch we were told to go to the boss's office, we were initially quite concerned by this but it seemed everyone was invited; when we got there, it was clear that this was a normal state of affairs. Friday afternoons were not working time, there was a large supply of beer and larger available on one of the tables, certainly enough for all of us to have several cans each. All the guys we had seen working on the various systems in the workshop were already there, they all had a can in their hands; there was a lot of raucous babble and laughter.

Dave and I grabbed a can and found a spot next to the window where we could lean against the windowsill to watch the proceedings; very soon it was clear that some of the guys were really going for it! After about an hour we were both enjoying the banter with some of the guys we had been working with when one of the other engineers decided he wasn't happy with me. He had clearly managed to throw a lot of beer down his neck and was fairly well oiled; he decided to stand about two inches from me, we were face to face and he proceeded to vent a fair amount of anger and spittle at 'us soft English twats' we apparently were coming up to Scotland where we weren't welcome and he felt he needed to tell me and most of the rest of the room how little we knew.

This was as I'm sure you will appreciate an uncomfortable time, I didn't want to make a fuss, I wanted to leave without this escalating, it seemed likely that this chap would eventually feel we should take this outside where he would be able to show me how weak and ineffectual Englishmen really were. After what seemed like an hour but was probably no more than twenty minutes, he finished his current rant and also his can and went to find another; Dave and I immediately decided to make ourselves scarce. When we saw him again on Monday nothing was said and he was actually quite friendly, I imagine he didn't remember much about it but as you can imagine Friday afternoons were something that while we always attended, but we never did stay long.

We spent three weeks working in the yard and I think towards the end we were actually becoming quite useful to them as they trusted us to swage fittings onto the ends of hoses and make up umbilicals from scratch; I actually was enjoying the work although I couldn't wait to get my chance to go offshore. This came to an abrupt end on Tuesday the 18th of April; we were summoned to Sam's office where he announced that we both would be going offshore tomorrow, for three days, the job was air diver support for one of Oceaneering's Atmospheric Diving Suit (ADS) operations.

The ADS system we would be supporting would be utilising 'JIM' suits; I had seen some pictures of these suits before but had never actually seen one yet; one of these suits later became the villain in one of the James Bond movies (the Spy Who Loved me) but more about that later. We would be tasked with hitching the 'JIM' suit to a set of guide-wires before it made its way down to the job and again when it returned, we would be unhitching it from the guide-wires; sounded like I should be able to manage that.

So, the next day Dave and I presented ourselves at Aberdeen heliport ready to go; the weather was quite good, there was something like 50% cloud cover and virtually no wind. I was really looking forward to the whole thing, one of my reasons for wanting to be a diver offshore was to experience new things and to travel to exotic places without having to pay for it. I had never been in a helicopter before but of course for everyone else queuing up to check in this was part of their normal commute; we spent a bit of time watching what the others were doing and then presented ourselves for check in.

We were going to a rig called the Nortrol that was currently drilling 'Wildcat' wells for Mobil Oil; Wildcat holes involve drilling initial wells to prove the results of geological surveys; we didn't know where this was going on but it was clear they were expecting us, we were logged in. Part of this exercise involved us being issued with a survival suit! We were told to 'get kitted up'; having never seen or worn a survival suit before we didn't really know where to start but luckily, they had a lot of similarities with dry suits so we soon worked it out. I have to say this all took me a bit by surprise, nobody had mentioned that we would need to wear a survival suit, was this really necessary?

This was in the days before compulsory survival courses that these days everyone working offshore has to do with renewal every three years; I didn't do any survival training until a few years later. When I did my first survival course it answered an awful lot of questions that were going through my mind as I put on my survival suit that morning. Anyway, when we were all kitted up, we were led out to the helicopter; it was a civilian Sikorsky H61, similar in size to the military Sea King, this one was operated by Bristow's; we were shown to our seats and were given a pair of ear defenders each. This was clearly not going to be a very comfortable trip if we needed a survival suit and some ear defenders! After a few minutes the pilot fired up the engines, the rotors started to turn, we sat there with the rotors turning for what seemed a very long time before eventually we started to roll, apparently, we would not be taking off vertically as this used a great deal more fuel.

When we reached the runway the pilot increased power and no sooner had we started to roll than we were airborne, the machine rattled and shook but I didn't care, I was flying in a helicopter and heading for my first offshore job, what could be better?

When we reached our cruising altitude the pilot set course for our destination, the Nortrol was some distance East of Shetland at the time so our first destination would be the airport on Shetland where we would be dropping some of our passengers off. After a short stop we were again on our way, this time the pilot although not taking off vertically did lift off quite steeply and when at what seemed to me to be still quite low, he tipped the nose of the helicopter forwards; all I could see out of the front windows was the ground looking very close! It seemed quite an extreme way to get moving but it was effective as we accelerated quickly and were away, we were in the air moving out across the North Sea which looked grey and a bit foreboding; several rigs came and went beneath us I loved it.

After about an hour another rig hove into view, the pilot flew around it and began to line up on the helipad. It was to me a beautiful sight; the rig was a grey painted Semi-Submersible floating in the middle of nowhere; we had been told about 'Semi-Subs' while on our course, but this was the first time I had seen one in real life. They were used for drilling operations but could also be used as production platforms as the Transworld 58 where the sat system we had been working on was destined. Nortrol had been ballasted down to a working draught and was fixed in place over the sea-bed by means of a conventional anchor pattern of between 8 to 12 anchors. As we flew towards the rig, I could see that there was a tall derrick which I knew would be where the drill pipe would be handled.

Coming in to land on the helideck, which was a very small flat area that seemed to be sticking out from the side of the rig although when we arrived I found that it was actually on the roof of the accommodation block; on the surface of the deck there was a large fluorescent H with a heavy rope net stretched across it, all around the edge of the deck there was steel wire mesh stretched horizontally across stanchions running along all of the sides of the helideck extending about three metres away from the edge of the deck. As we approached the pilot had to slow almost to a stop, we were then hovering over the helideck and descending very slowly towards it. The whole helicopter was now shaking and rattling like crazy, I was amazed that it held together at all but it did and very soon we were down on the helideck, the door was opened by one of the crew who beckoned to us telling us we were to get off.

I removed my ear defenders and placed them on my seat and made my way to the door, and down onto the helideck: as I reached the deck the wind from the rotors was blowing me about, I was beckoned to the edge of the deck by one of the rig hands; he directed me towards a set of steel steps leading down to a door into the accommodation. Once at the door I was ushered inside where my name was taken and I was told to take off the survival suit and to hand it to the attendant, once we were properly logged on board we were shown through to a hallway where we were left on our own; now what?

We had been assigned a cabin number and so made our way there wondering how we would find out what we were expected to do and where we should go after we dropped our kit off in the cabin. I needn't have worried as when we arrived at the cabin all the other divers were inside. We were met by our supervisor, Sean Harrison and the two ADS pilots, the total team was just the five of us; we spent the next few minutes chatting with all of them before the ADS guys announced that they had work to do on the suits so would see us later.

Sean then set about finding out what we knew about our task and working offshore in general, not much was the obvious conclusion; he was great though and set about the task of inducting us into the dos and don'ts of working offshore. He took us on a full tour of the rig after kitting us out in hard hat, coveralls and boots (he didn't like mine so found us some more appropriate ones which he told me to keep when I left the rig). We had a lot to learn but he helped us with where to go and where we definitely should not go; he took us to the pipe rack where he explained the process of drilling showing us some casing, drill pipe and a drill bit.

It seemed the drill bit would be threaded onto collars attached to the drill pipe which was hollow, when they were drilling a fluid would be supplied to the drill bit via this hollow tube, this liquid was termed 'mud' but was apparently a high-tech concoction of chemicals. The drill would be lowered to the seabed through a 'Marine Riser' a large pipe stretching from the drill floor all the way to the seabed where it would be attached to a 'Blow Out Preventer' or BOP; this was a set of valves that would be used to close the well if necessary and was an essential safety device. The Marine Riser effectively connected the drill floor to the seabed but of course as we were on a floating structure rising and falling with the wave action and tidal flow there was a 'slip joint' to allow for this movement, this was situated just below the drill floor; drilling mud would be fed down to the drill bit through the drill pipe and would return to the drill floor bringing the drilled bits and pieces with it thus keeping the hole clear. Once the drill had made a hole casing would be dropped into this hole, this would then be cemented in place making the well very much a sealed pipe right from the drill bit back up to the drill floor, ultimately this would allow oil to be brought to the surface without contaminating the surrounding environment.

Sean took us up onto the drill floor where we were able to see the process under-way; I looked up the inside of the derrick and saw a guy about ninety feet up standing on a small platform this was apparently termed the 'Monkey Board'. He was there to handle the lengths of drill pipe either stacking them or attaching them to the 'Draw Works'; this was used to lift and lower the drill pipe; he was working very hard slinging pipe about; it looked like a very precarious position to me. On the drill floor there were two guys (roughnecks) handling the 'tongs', these were used to tighten or loosen the drill collars attaching the lengths of drill pipe and were effectively very large 'Stillson' wrenches, they were clearly very heavy and were suspended on cables from the top of the derrick.

We watched as a new section of drill pipe was screwed on to the threaded connector, that could be seen sticking out of the drill floor. Once the connection was made the whole pipe was lifted a few feet and a wedge that had secured the pipe into the floor was removed, the driller who was in a small cubicle off to the side of the drill floor then started to lower the pipe into the hole. When the top of the new piece of pipe was almost at the drill floor the wedge was again dropped around the pipe securing it; next a square section of pipe known as the 'Kelly' was screwed on to the drill pipe. Once secure the whole lot was again lifted to allow the wedge to be removed, then, the pipe was lowered into the hole until the drill bit reached the bottom of the hole. When this was complete the Kelly had slid neatly into a square section in the drill floor this was the 'Rotary Table', the driller then started rotation of the table and Kelly thus turning the drill. Clearly this is a lightning description and just scratches the surface of what is a very complex process.

Sean then took us to the 'spider deck' this was the lowest deck situated immediately below the drill floor it ran around the main moonpool through which all the subsea drilling equipment would be lowered. We could clearly see the marine riser and its slip joint working as the rig rose and fell on the wave action; there were also four heavy duty steel rope guide-wires extending from the drill floor down into the water. These wires had to be kept at a specific tension so there was a system to compensate for the rise and fall of the floating rigs up and down movement caused by the rig riding the sea's wave action this is termed 'heave'. The wires were kept under a pre-determined load by the 'heave compensation' system; a system of winches and hydraulic rams which we could see and hear working all the time. Sean told us that these wires were attached to four 'guide-posts' on the seabed 'guide-base' at the centre of which was the 'wellhead' through which the drill was operating and of course they hoped would ultimately be used to produce oil. The guide-wires allowed the BOP and other tools to be lowered into position easily when required.

Eventually we found ourselves at the dive station; there were two white 'JIM suits' sitting on frames, apparently, they had been named after the chap (Jim) who had found the prototype in a garage in Scotland sometime in the early seventies, one of the suits had no legs on it and was clearly being worked on at the time. There was to be no diving today which suited me as I wanted to find my way around before having to go diving; the whole deck was constructed of galvanised floor plate mesh or 'Texas plate' this is made up of thick steel mesh which can often be seen making up fire escapes on buildings. This was a little unnerving as I could see through it and was looking straight down at the surface of the sea some twenty metres below me, it was lucky that I don't have a problem with heights.

We were given a quick run around the ADS system so that we knew what we would have to do when called on to dive; these suits were armoured such that when they went into the water the suit would take the water pressure; the diver inside would remain at one atmosphere. There would be no need for decompression regardless of how long they spent at depth or how deep they went. These suits were capable of diving to fifteen hundred feet (457 metres)! The main hull of the suit was made of magnesium which although extremely strong did have the disadvantage that when in seawater it would be prone to very high rates of corrosion, apparently, they would constantly need to be touched up and repaired whenever they were used. I didn't quite realise how true this was but over the next few months I would find out how bad this could get in a very short period of time.

The diver inside would be re-breathing the air in the suit so there was a system to remove the carbon dioxide from his exhaled breath and another system to replace the oxygen that he would have consumed; the suit was self-contained and did not require any gas to be supplied from the surface. The suits were fitted with a steel wire umbilical or tether which would be used to lower and raise it, this also carried conductors for communications and limited electrical power used for lighting; it was terrific, I thought it was 'state of the art', I wanted to have a go but of course was again not qualified to use them at this time.

The ADS dive station consisted of three ten-foot shipping containers arranged in a semicircle around the two JIM suits which sat on frames to one side of a 'moonpool'; a hole in the deck covered by more galvanised mesh decking. When the time came to launch the suits, this decking would be lifted to allow the suits to be lowered through into the sea. To the left of the suits was the ADS maintenance shack, to the rear was the container being used for the dive control from where the supervisor would control the diving and to the right of the suits was the dive equipment shack; this was where our equipment was stored.

Dave and I opened up our equipment store and were greeted with an Aladdin's cave; everywhere we looked there was shiny equipment and wetsuits, it all looked brand new; it certainly put the equipment at Bovisand to shame, it all looked as though none of it had ever been used. We spent the next couple of hours selecting suits that would fit us properly, at this time I was very lucky as I was a medium regular in terms of suit size; this meant that on every job I would always find a good selection of suits that were my size.

One disappointment for me was that the hats we were to use were Kirby Morgan Bandmasks, KMB18, this was great really as it was a step above the hats we had used on our course but Oceaneering was at the time famous for using the unique 'Rat Hat'. We had seen lots of these hats in the workshop and there had been a number of guys walking around with T shirts emblazoned with 'Rat Hat Diver' and I wanted to be one of those people; still, never mind hopefully next time. Eventually we had set up the equipment and were ready to go whenever required; I wandered out on deck to have a look at the rest of the system we would be using.

As I said we were some twenty metres above the water, it would be impossible to get in or out of the water by ladder; we were to be using a diving basket; this was a steel basket about eight feet high and four feet square one side was open to allow the diver access from the deck, the other three sides had steel mesh sides running about half way up to a rail that the diver could hold on to while being lifted into or out of the water. We had used one of these on our course so were quite familiar with their use; the major difference to swimming down a line was that you had no control over the rate of descent of ascent; this would be controlled by the surface crew.

Again, this is not a problem unless the diver had a problem clearing their ears; good communications were essential when using this equipment. Behind our container there was a hydraulic power pack needed to operate the winches for both the ADS and diver's basket; this proved to be a bit of a monster over the next few days as it was very difficult to start.

While we had been working with our equipment the JIM suits had been rebuilt and so everything was now ready; we closed up the containers and readied everything so that the system was safe to be left overnight. Sean told us all that we had finished for the day, so off we went in search of food; I found I was really quite hungry as we hadn't eaten much since breakfast time. We all made our way back to the accommodation block where we took off our boots and coveralls both of which we stowed in a locker, we then went back to our cabin; where we sat around for about half an hour getting to know one another before eventually getting out of our work clothes, showering and getting ready for the evening meal.

I had heard that the food was always good offshore but was not ready for the feast we were presented with: there were steaks, some kind of stew or 'gumbo', fish, salad as well as beef-burgers and a number of other things some of which I didn't even recognise. We all loaded our plates up and decamped to a vacant table, it was great, really tasty and plenty of it; what more could you want? Well pudding was mentioned and again there was plenty of choice, luckily when I was in my twenties, I could eat everything and never put-on weight so I tried to bump up my wages by eating my fill. After we had all finished eating Sean suggested watching the movie!

Apparently, every night there was a different movie screened in the lounge alongside the canteen; off we went, tonight's offering was a western or as we were informed more correctly termed a 'shit kicker', it didn't matter what it was, it passed a couple of hours which was great.

After the movie we wandered back to the cabin where four of us were sharing, Sean was in another cabin so we were sharing with the ADS operators Bill and Mike. Again, I was on a top bunk, it was very comfortable with a curtain that could be drawn along the front edge and a reading light, again, what more could a guy ask for?

The day shift started offshore at six o'clock in the morning so at five we were all up and headed to breakfast, again lots of just about anything you could want; full English with pancakes. There were of course a lot of Americans who it seemed ate strange things for breakfast such as pancakes with bacon and maple syrup! Well, when in Rome as they say so I had to try it and found it to be very tasty, even better when I found I could have a fried egg with it as well.

Sean told us that we were not programmed to dive today so we spent the day making sure everything was ready, Dave and I spent a good deal of time wandering around the deck looking at all the equipment and tools to get a better understanding of our new world.

The next day started very early, we were woken at about three o'clock in the morning and told to get ready for diving as there was some emergency work to be done on the BOP. We spent the next hour or so preparing for the dive, Dave and I changed into our wetsuits and set up the gear, we were ready, I was to be the first diver and Dave would be my tender. Bill would be diving JIM suit number seven this was identified by a large red seven painted on both sides of the body. Bill was dressed in an ordinary woolly bear, coveralls and a woolly hat, his main problem would be the cold; the dive would be at least six hours or until the job was complete, wow, I felt this would be challenging for him.

Dave and I would not be in the water for much of that time as all we had to do was to go in when the suit was launched and attach it to a set of guide-wires that would run it down to the BOP. As soon as the suit was on its way we would come back out and wait until the suit was to be recovered when we would be required to go back in and remove it from the guide-wires again.

Bill was soon ready to go, the suit was closed up; I had already kitted up and completed my checks, nobody was checking our work though which seemed a little strange at first but of course we were now in the real world and were supposed to know what we were doing, fingers crossed then. I watched the JIM suit being winched up and when the moonpool was opened the suit was lowered carefully though it; as soon as it was in the water Sean signalled for me to get ready; I put the bandmask on, Dave zipped it up and pulled the spider around my head securing it as we had been taught; I gave him a thumbs up to indicate I was ready.

I walked over to the basket and climbed aboard; I turned around so that I was facing the entry side and watched Dave put the safety chain across; The basket had rails along the sides which were inside the frame so that when I held them my hands would still be protected by the basket's frame. I established comms with Sean and he gave the order for me to be lowered into the sea; this was it my very first offshore dive was about to commence and it was to be a night dive, I was so excited. I was lowered through the moonpool and suddenly was under the deck, I felt very alone but not in a bad way, I could see for miles out past the legs of the rig, I was still some ten metres above the water which was coming towards me slowly. The sea looked very black, I was going to enjoy this for sure; very soon my feet touched the water, the basket continued down, I could feel water entering the suit, it was cold but not too bad.

As the water rose up my body, I felt myself become light and buoyant; I could keep my feet on the bottom of the basket only by holding on firmly. As my head came level with the surface, I remember thinking "this is it", I called "left surface" and then I was under water; the basket was still descending as it was supposed to but I found I couldn't breathe; when I tried to take a breath all I got was a steady stream of sprayed seawater. I called "All stop" and the basket immediately stopped, Sean called what's the problem? I tried to tell him but there was just too much water coming into the hat, I really didn't want to abort my first offshore dive but what could I do?

I decided to turn on the free flow valve and quickly found that this worked, the water stopped coming into the hat, I could breathe; great this would be OK, I would do the dive using the hat on free flow, no problem. I told Sean all was well and that I was OK to proceed to depth; the basket started dropping again; my buoyancy was perfect, I was almost perfectly neutral which had been another worry so that one was gone, if buoyancy hadn't been right, I could have been bobbing around at the top of the basket or unable to swim across to the JIM suit; I was desperate that nothing would get in the way of my completing this my first offshore job. I now had time to look around and what I saw was fabulous; the visibility was excellent, maybe 30 metres or so!

I really couldn't remember being in better vis; even though it was night time I could still see a great deal as there was a lot of illumination from the moon and from the lights of the rig above me, to my left I could see a massive pontoon looking like a submarine sitting just under the rig, the rigs legs running down to it, I could see anchor chains disappearing away into the distance. Off to my right was the JIM suit and beyond that the white painted

Marine Riser and in the distance the other pontoon; when I was level with the JIM suit, I called "all stop" again and the basket stopped.

I told Sean that I was ready to leave the basket and was told "fine, off you go"; I left the basket swimming out through the side of the basket so that my umbilical would run from the surface through the basket and out to me, this meant that if the current was strong, I would always be able to get back to the basket by pulling myself back along my umbilical.

There was virtually no current though and I quickly reached the JIM suit; the suit had a tag line clasped in both its pincers at the ends of its arms, the line dangled about three feet either side of the suit's pincers; at either end there was an eye containing a shackle. I grabbed one end of the line and pulled the suit over to one of the guide-wires which I could see were just a few feet away; when I got there, I hooked one arm around the wire and started to undo the shackle, I removed the pin, I could see nothing below me except black water, I knew the depth was about three hundred and fifty feet so if I dropped the shackle or pin, I would be in trouble! I pulled the shackle over and fitted the guide-wire into it, then refitted the pin and finally turned the shackle around so that the pin was held inside the tag line's eye; I had been told to do this as otherwise the pin could undo itself when rubbing on the guide-wire either on descent or at the end of the dive when the suit was coming back to the surface.

OK that's one done; I moved over to the other end of the tag line and fixed the shackle to the other guide-wire, I also managed that one without dropping anything, I finished this off by turning the shackle around in the same way. All that remained for me to do was to remove the safety line from the ring on top of the suit; this line was attached for the suits launch and recovery so that when it went through the splash zone if the main lift wire parted the suit would only fall as far as the end of the safety line. I undid the safety line shackle, replaced the pin, didn't drop anything again, gave four pulls on the safety line and watched it being recovered to the surface I told Sean "Safety line clear to the surface".

I then went around to the JIM suit's ports and gave Bill a thumbs up which he returned and told Sean "Suits all secured to the guide-wires and ready to go", Sean responded with "OK make your way back to the basket". I saw the suit start its descent and made my way back to the basket; making sure I entered the same way I had come out and made myself secure inside the basket ready to be recovered; I told Sean "In the basket and ready to leave bottom", the basket started to ascend, I said "left bottom," when I broke surface told Sean "Arrived surface". As the basket continued to rise out of the water, I felt the full weight of the diving kit come on my shoulders again and the water that had entered my suit pooled in the legs of the suit; when I got back on deck I called "on deck"; Sean said "well done, good dive". I was really chuffed, my first offshore dive was now complete and I hadn't made a complete hash of it, brilliant!

Dave helped me undress and we both went into dive control, Sean gave me a cup of tea and asked me what had happened when I initially left surface; I told him the story and said that I would go and check out the hat to see if I could find the reason, he seemed happy with that. Dave and I went to the dive store and swapped the hat for another one so that we would be ready whenever the JIM suit came back to the surface Dave would be ready to go and do his bit; I then sat down with the hat I had used and started to take the second stage apart as I was almost certain this would be where the problem was.

I expected to find the exhaust mushroom valve was either missing or had become inverted, either of these would have allowed water to come into the hat. However, when I removed the front plate containing the purge button it became immediately obvious that the problem was the diaphragm; it had not been fitted properly, it was not seated in the groove so when I had inhaled it came away allowing water to flow uncontrolled into the hat. It was very easy to fix and didn't even need a new diaphragm, brilliant, not only had I overcome the problem in the water but had now been able to fix the hat. I went back to Sean and told him of my findings, he seemed happy with this and went back to supervising the JIM suit dive.

My first dive of the day, I left surface at four forty-six in the morning, the dive had lasted a total of thirteen minutes; Dave and I took it in turns with Dave doing the recoveries and me doing the launch dives; we both did a total of four dives that day with my final one completing at twenty-one twenty-five after a ten-minute dive, I was clearly getting quicker. Our day finished at about two o'clock in the morning when we finally were able to get to bed; it had been a very long day but I loved it, towards the end of the last JIM dive we were in dive control still in our wetsuits with the American client whose favourite line was; "When I say jump the divers all I want to hear is splash", this uttered in a broad Texan drawl! We all had to laugh at this no matter how often he said it; this for me was a good introduction to Texan humour.

The job wasn't complete though, we were back ready to dive again by about ten thirty in the morning, I left surface at five past eleven for the first of my four dives. Diving during the day was even better, I could see for what seemed like miles and although I had seen the pontoons during the night, they were much clearer and more impressive during the day; they were covered in marine growth and had lots of fish swimming around them although as the dives were so short, I really didn't get a lot of time to look at them.

The twenty eighth of April was my birthday, I was twenty-four, obviously there were no celebrations as nobody knew the significance of the date. This was a non-diving day so we spent the day making sure all the equipment was ready and carrying out maintenance as required. We were able to help with maintenance of the ADS suits which I enjoyed and again I learned a lot that would become of use to me over the coming years.

Over the next week or so we dived almost every day supporting the JIM suits and learned a great deal about offshore life; on the thirtieth of April the weather took a turn for the worse. We would not be able to dive so we stowed all the kit and retired to the accommodation to wait the storm out; over the next four days there was really nothing much for us to do as the weather was dreadful. The rig was very stable but the waves were so large that we were being pitched up and down quite dramatically.

We spent our days watching movies and eating four times a day, it just had to be done and was of course all part of the wages. Eventually the weather finally settled down enough for us to get back to work on the fifth of May. On the eighth of May we had finally finished the job and could return to the beach, I must say I wasn't really very happy about this as I was enjoying being offshore, I liked the work and of course when we arrived on shore again, we would have to go back to buying our own food and accommodation.

Still, I suppose as we had been told initially that we would be offshore for three days having actually got twenty-one days and during that time I had completed eighteen dives I certainly couldn't complain; I supposed all good things come to an end and hopefully it wouldn't be too long before I was given another job. The helicopter flight back to Aberdeen was entirely uneventful which of course is how the majority of them are and I must say when we landed and returned our survival suits, I was quite happy to be ashore again.

Dave and I made our way back to the Albury where we were met again by Sess who asked us "now you're offshore divers would you like to move out of the bunk room?" Although we had earned a fair amount of money, we didn't know how long it would need to last us so we both decided to remain in the bunk room for the foreseeable future. In the morning, we made our way back to the yard where we were put to work again helping to maintain equipment, this was not anything like as good but beggars can't be choosers and I felt it was much more likely that I would get offshore again if I stayed working in the yard.

That evening we were wandering along the road going in to town for something to eat and I noticed that as we passed gardens full of flowers, I was especially aware of their scent. I doubt I would have noticed them before but it seemed that being at sea for even quite a short period where smells are definitely not fragrant in the way that flowers are I had become more sensitive to these lovely fragrances. Although this hypersensitivity wouldn't last very long it was something I always appreciated whenever I returned from a trip offshore.

I didn't have to wait long working in the yard as, I was sent offshore again on the twentieth of May; this time I would not be going with Dave. The job was to travel out to the Beryl field where the Transworld 58 would eventually be located, at this time the rig was still being refitted part of which was to have the saturation system we had been working on before fitted. As I say the rig wasn't there when we got there but this didn't matter as our job was to check the mooring chains of the large buoy that would be used to export produced oil to waiting tankers.

We travelled out to the job on the Stirling Ash supply boat, the dive spread had been loaded on board the previous day so while we were steaming out to the field, we were busy putting everything together so that when we arrived, we would be ready to dive. We were on site the next morning and transferred all our kit into an inflatable rubber boat to take it across to the buoy as the Stirling Ash had other work to be going on with; we loaded all our kit onto the buoy which was about twenty feet (6.5 metres) across and really quite stable.

My first job was to check the angle of the six anchor chains and to check the sacrificial anodes to make sure they were working properly, checking the chain angles would tell the engineers whether the buoy had been pulled away from its proper position; my Lloyds Diver Inspector qualification was already coming in useful, maybe it had been worth if after all. We were to use an inclinometer to check the angles, this consisted of a straight edge which was to be pushed up against the chain link, there was a pendulum attached to the top edge which would of course hang vertically, the angle could then be read from a scale, it was actually very easy to do. The hardest part was cleaning marine growth off the link and holding the edge against the link; I had to gauge when the wave action would allow the pendulum to stabilise to give an accurate reading. This felt like real work and together with the Cathodic potential readings I really felt a sense of achievement when I had finished; this was again a very short job and I was back ashore again on the twenty-second of May.

Dave and I spent our evenings visiting the various hostelries in the town centre, normally this would be just a couple of pints and some pub grub but I remember one evening, the twenty-fourth of May when Scotland were at home to England in the home championships the football match was being played at Hampden Park in Glasgow. The evening started very well and was all quite good natured but when it became evident that England were getting the better of the match which England eventually won by two goals to nothing it became clear that the two English Sassenachs were very definitely not welcome and we decided discretion was the better part of valour and left before the end of the match.

Up to this point all my work for Oceaneering had been in the UK sector of the North Sea but Oceaneering at this time was probably the world leading diving company; they had ongoing worksites throughout the world. My next job was to be in Norway on another Semi-Submersible; this one was the West Venture; she was positioned some distance off Bergen. At the time I didn't know it but the West Venture was of the same design as the Alexander L Kielland, the Kielland had been utilised as an accommodation platform working alongside a platform in the Ekofisk field until in March 1980 during a storm it suddenly capsized killing 123 people.

As soon as this disaster happened the West Venture had been taken into the safety of a Norwegian fjord for safety checks but when I travelled out on the twenty-sixth of May it had been relocated back over its original wellhead and was going back to work. I was again going to be working as one of the air divers supporting ADS suits; this time one of the suits was a free swimming 'Wasp' suit number five, another first for me, this suit was supported by a JIM suit number nine. I duly arrived onboard just after lunch on the twenty-sixth minus my bag which had apparently gone on holiday to Barcelona without me! I was very glad to see my bag when it eventually turned up on the twenty-ninth as my clothes definitely needing to be changed by then!

When I arrived on the twenty-sixth, I was again met by Bill Hayes so at least I knew someone as Dave had not come along with me again this time; the other ADS pilot was Wayne Horton who eventually went on to star as the baddy pilot of a JIM suit in the James Bond film.

The next day we were scrambled to repair a broken guide-wire, again my job was to attach or detach the suit's tag line and safety line in much the same way as I had done with the JIM suits previously; the one thing that soon became clear was that there was no limit to working hours in Norway at this time. My shift started at six o'clock in the morning of twenty-seventh with my first dive being at eight twenty-five in the morning, we worked continuously through until my fifth and final dive ended at four fourteen in the morning of the twenty-eighth!

I was absolutely knackered and very hungry; as soon as I was showered, I went to see if I could get a sandwich, I found the galley and although it was not a meal time the guys were very nice to me and made me a cheese sandwich; I thanked them and made my way to my bunk. We had some seven hours off before we were again woken to carry on as the job was still not complete, we had to manufacture some parts to help the suit with its job of replacing the guide-wire, although this would be a very easy job for a diver the suit had very little power and could not stab the bayonet into the guidepost on the seabed so we had to work out a method that would allow the suit to do the job.

We couldn't send a diver as the depth was over one thousand feet! As soon as I arrived in dive control, I was taken to one side by the supervisor, Danny King who informed me that the galley crew had complained about my behaviour last night, apparently, they felt I shouldn't have been in 'demanding' food between meal times. I explained my side of things and although I think he believed me he made it quite clear that this was unacceptable and that I should not repeat this.

I went to meet the 'camp boss' who was in charge of the galley and apologised to him, he was very nice about it and seemed to me to realise that this had been blown out of all proportion; another lesson learned!

Anyway, we again worked right through until my last dive (again dive 5) completed at one forty-five in the morning of the twenty-ninth, there didn't seem to be any fixed shifts and as there was only one set of divers the client wanted us to work until the job was complete. During May at these latitudes, it never really gets dark so I found myself not knowing whether it was three o'clock in the morning or afternoon, I was completely disoriented and towards the end found myself falling asleep while I was sitting as standby diver! Not at all safe, but this was the way things were done offshore in Norway in those days.

Things carried on like that until there were a couple of very high-profile accidents that were put down to human error; this forced the Norwegian Government to impose very tight restrictions on offshore companies. Today in Norway workers have to be given the same work benefits and practices as their shore-based counterparts and the hours we were working would never be allowed now; but, in 1980 we were stuck with it and the job carried on in the same vein until I left on the second of June.

I returned to Aberdeen where I met with the operations director who informed me that I was up for a two-year job in Brunei, I didn't really know where this was but a two-year job; this would be great and it was going to be real work not just ADS support. I told him that I was definitely up for it but had to go home first to organise things for my being away for this length of time; he agreed and told me to be back in Aberdeen ready to go in two weeks. I bade farewell to Dave and boarded the milk train to travel overnight back to Devon via London, this was probably the worst journey I have ever had as the train travelled at snail's pace stopping at every station, it was however very cheap which was the reason I was on it.

I had a couple of great weeks at home getting ready for my extended trip; I spent a lot of time with my old mates hanging out at bars such as the Yacht on Torquay's harbourside, this was a great bar situated immediately adjacent to the inner harbour in Torquay. There was usually a DJ playing great songs such as Geno by Dexy's Midnight Runners and Freebird by Leonard Skynyrd.

In those days Oceaneering would contact me via telegram; these would normally be delivered by a young chap who arrived on an old BSA Bantam (125cc) motorbike; in fact, I got to know all the delivery guys quite well as they were often delivering to me, this got to the point that they knew my local pub was the Upton Vale and would sometimes deliver the telegram to me there, great service.

Anyway, towards the end of the second week I was contacted to be told that the Brunei job was not going to happen, I was gutted; what now? Well, there was nothing about for me at the moment apparently, so, I was out of work, not good, I didn't know when or even if I would be offered any more work. I spent the next week or so mooching about until a telegram from Oceaneering arrived telling me that if I wanted, I could come back and work in the yard until something came along; I was on the next train and worked the next month in the yard, I'm sure I really was becoming quite useful to them towards the end of this month but I was getting fed up with not really going anywhere especially as I heard that Dave had been taken on to the Transworld 58 as an air diver on contract, a steady job! I was pleased for him but couldn't wait to be offered something better than working in the yard.

Towards the end of July, I was offered another three day's work on another ADS support job in Spain, I wasn't very happy that it was so short and only another ADS job but I had to take it. On the twenty-fourth I joined the rest of the crew at Heathrow airport, we were due to fly out to Barcelona, not just my bag this time we would both be going, at least I hoped my bag would come along for the ride!

We both did arrive in Barcelona, in those days getting into Spain could be a little challenging but this was by no means as difficult as it had been to get in to Bilbao the last time I had been to Spain as Barcelona was not in the Basque area so we were not treated with the same level of suspicion. Eventually we were all standing at a taxi rank where our supervisor Chris Lane flagged down a cab to take the five of us down the coast to Sant Carles de la Ràpita. I think this would have been a small fishing town but was beginning to be taken over by tourists who brought some very expensive looking yachts with them; we arrived quite late on in the evening and as soon as we were installed in our hotel Chris informed us that we would be going for a meal "down in the town".

I don't know if he had ever been there before but I was not about to give any opinions and just followed; we found a nice and very noisy hostelry where we all had that very Spanish meal of steak and chips, apparently that was what all good Spanish people enjoyed according to Chris! I didn't like to say that the other tables seemed to be proving him to be a bit wide of the mark but hey I enjoyed the meal and a good-few-beers; we left the bar at about ten o'clock only to find that the real party was going on outside. The street had been cordoned off and the crowd were massed at a barricade, what was going on?

We found ourselves at the barricade sticking our heads through to see what was happening; I was faced with a young bull looking around frantically the poor thing was being taunted by the crowd one of which would run up to him but as soon as the bull started to run after him another bloke would run in and taunt him so he kept stopping and getting more frustrated and angrier. Well, being in my early twenties and with a bunch of other fit, healthy young men we all decided to get involved. We climbed over the barricade and went to join the fun I use the term loosely as I'm sure the bull wasn't enjoying himself; we spent the next hour or so running to and fro in front of the bulls; there wasn't just the one.

Eventually it seemed the Spanish organisers felt that the original bull had been too timid and so some bright spark came up with the jolly jape of tying flaming torches to the bull's horns. This had the effect of turning an already angry beast into a real raging bull, he became frantic, we left at about eleven as we had an early start and I for one was completely knackered by then, we made our way back to the hotel just stopping a couple of times on the way for another couple of beers.

The next day at breakfast we were told that the evening had got even more frantic after we had left; one of the bulls had broken through the door to some poor blokes flat where the bull caught him minding his own business watching TV; the bull proceeded to gore the poor chap but the waitress said it wasn't a problem as he wasn't badly hurt! I think I would have felt a bit miffed if that had happened to me but it seemed to be just one of those things for the Spanish.

After breakfast we all went down to the harbour where we had to be weighed with all our luggage so that they could work out the loadings for the helicopter for our journey out to the vessel tomorrow. It was a beautiful day and once we had finished, we had nothing to do for the rest of the day. Beach, bar and restaurant was the rest of the day until the evening when we graduated to a make shift bull ring that had been set up in the town centre where we watched bull fighting although it wasn't the full-on fight as none of the bulls were hurt other than the torment of being taunted by people waving capes at them and goading them, it was a spectacle for sure. After another great evening we made our way back to the hotel it really was hell this working offshore lark.

The next day we made our way out to the job using an ancient helicopter, it was an early model Sikorsky H58 which had been in service since the mid-1950s; if I had thought the H61 flying out of Aberdeen had shaken a bit I was soon to find it was nothing by comparison to this one! We climbed aboard together with a bunch of Spanish crew none of us had survival suits but nobody seemed to think we needed one? I had been told we were going out to the 'Delta Platform' but this meant nothing to me; we couldn't really see out of the helicopter as we were seated on a bench running along the side of the fuselage, I was facing one of the Spanish crew who didn't seem to speak any English but of course as soon as the engines were running there was no possibility of conversation anyway. There were no ear defenders issued this time either!

After a very short flight we were deposited on a helideck, I quickly moved to the steps at the edge of the helideck and down onto the main deck of a huge tanker; the Delta Platform was in fact a Floating Production, Storage and Offloading (FPSO) Platform. No sooner had we all reached the deck than the chopper took off and headed back to the beach; the helideck was right at the bow of the vessel; I was looking aft towards the rear of the ship where there was a huge white superstructure this was where the accommodation was situated. Leading from where I was standing, I could see masses of pipes extending the whole length of the deck; an FPSO is a floating platform, it was essentially a ship this one was an old tanker that had been modified for its current role. The vessel was anchored to the seabed via a large frame attached to the bow, this frame was hinged to a static tubular steel structure that was standing on the seabed and extending to a few metres above the surface of the sea.

The structure supported a marine riser through which oil made its way up from the well on the seabed this oil was then fed into the tanker's storage tanks. When oil was flowing the tanker would fill over a couple of weeks. When the time came another tanker would be brought alongside, the oil would then be transferred to this vessel and would be taken off to the refinery. When oil was being produced the FPSO would be free to rotate around the structure attached to its bow and because of the hinge arrangement the ship could rise and fall with the sea's wave action. At the moment there was no production going on as we were there to do some work on the wellhead so the well had been closed; the stern of the ship had also been anchored so the ship was fixed over the well to make it safer for us to work.

We were taken to the accommodation and shown our cabins, I was to share with Bill the ADS pilot I had worked with on the Nortrol and the West Venture; our cabin was directly over the engine room, it was very noisy and extremely hot! Obviously, Spain in late July was going to be warm but our cabin's proximity to the engine room meant that it was going to be very difficult to get comfortable. Air conditioning had not reached this part of the marine world yet, we did have a porthole but even with this fully open there was so little air flow that the cabin felt more like an oven than a place of refuge.

We dumped our bags and made our way back to the deck to start setting up the dive spread; the day was hot and there was really nowhere to shelter from the sun, I was at the time a bit of a sun worshiper so this was OK for me but even I was finding it a bit too hot. I was tasked with setting up the air diving system, we had a very nice little two-man dive panel, a couple of brand-new umbilicals, some lovely new KMB 18 Bandmasks and all the other equipment I needed.

After an hour or so I had finished setting up and testing the kit, I then looked at how I was going to get into and out of the water; I looked over the side of the tanker, to find that there was a bosun's ladder running down to the water. I couldn't see a cage or basket anywhere I asked Chris what his plan was; he told me that I was to use the bosun's ladder! I was not at all sure this was going to be safe, the ladder extended from a strong point on the deck down to a couple of metres below the surface of the sea.

The Delta was a fairly large tanker; it wasn't fully loaded, meaning the deck was some ten metres above the surface of the sea; memories of those ladders on Bovisand's jetty wall came back to me but at least I would only be wearing a very thin wet suit as the water was warm and I would only be in for a very short time so I wouldn't have to carry much weight. On the other hand, climbing a bosun's ladder was not as easy as a fixed ladder; the rungs laid against the ship's side and although the planks were quite wide, I would be climbing on the balls of my feet rather than with the rung of the ladder being in the arch of the foot.

Oh well I was sure I would cope; the other air diver Simon also didn't look wildly happy about this situation either but there was really nothing we could do about it and, in any case, I wasn't going to refuse to use the ladder. Sometime later after the job had finished and I was safely offshore in France I pondered the situation of the bosun's ladder. I came to the conclusion it might just about be acceptable for a diver to enter and exit the water that way but there had clearly been no thought given to use of the standby diver.

How would an injured diver have been recovered? Anyway, this was another lesson learned it reminded me that I had to look after myself as I couldn't rely on anyone else to do it for me! I resolved to refuse to dive if I was put in this type of situation again.

I then went off to help with setting up the ADS system, we would be using wasp number five again for the majority of the dives; soon it was lunchtime. We made our way to the mess room; when we got there, I was stunned to find there were bottles of wine on the table. This was completely foreign to me as although I hadn't much experience of offshore,

I knew that ships and rigs in the UK were 'dry' in that they didn't allow any alcohol and that had certainly been my experience to date. Anyway, clearly that was not the case in Spain, we all sat down and were served a very nice concoction, not at all sure what it was but it tasted good, I took some wine and watered it down with mineral water in the same way that I saw some of the Spaniards doing.

This seemed to be very civilised to me; I was going to like it here; when we finished our meal, we all went straight back out to the dive spread but we weren't joined by the locals for about an hour as they all had a bit of a siesta, again not something I was used to. By the end of the day, we were ready to dive and again I fully expected the client to insist we at least start, but no, we were to start diving tomorrow. At six o'clock in the evening the helicopter turned up again and most of the Spaniards boarded to be taken back to the beach, apparently, they didn't stay on the ship overnight; I can't say I blamed them if the accommodation available was anything like ours! They would be back in the morning; we finished up so that we were completely ready for the morning and then made our way to the accommodation.

I decided to shower and change before dinner, the showers were along the corridor from my cabin; none of them had a shower rose and I found they were tepid at best still this wasn't a huge problem as in fact it was quite nice to cool off.

Dinner was again nice food that I couldn't name but tasted good; the wine was again there and nobody seemed the least bit concerned when we finished that bottle as another one turned up! Weird. After dinner I went out on deck to relax a bit, we were only a couple of miles offshore so I could clearly see the coast and looking down into the water I could see lots of large fish, Simon said they were 'Jacks' they were extremely fast and looked to be about two or three feet long. On the horizon I could see a more conventional semi-submersible platform much like the Nortrol, I didn't know at the time but this was the Afortunada on which I would be spending the Christmas of 1981.

The next day we started diving, my first dive commenced at eleven forty in the morning; the job was to attach a large magnetic hydrophone to the hull of the ship, this would be used to track progress over the next few days, already the job had extended from the three days I had been promised to two weeks; OK with me. I made my way down the bosun's ladder, this was by no means easy as the ladder moved quite a lot but eventually, I was in the water, I left surface and again the visibility was great, at least twenty metres.

The sea was a beautiful deep blue and nice and warm; I didn't see any of the Jacks which was a bit of a disappointment, I made my way down the side of the ship, it was quite a long way down, my depth was forty-six feet (just over fourteen metres) but as the sea was so clear there was still plenty of light even at that depth. I then had to make my way under the ship, the first thing I encountered was the bilge keel, it extended away as far as I could see both ways towards the bow and stern. I made my way under the keel and wow what a difference, it got really quite dark but soon my eyes adjusted to the gloom and I could see enough. I had to give a bit of a marine growth assessment; once I had completed this. I cleaned off a small area where the hydrophone would be positioned; when I had done this, I went back out to the side of the ship and collected the hydrophone, that had been lowered on a line and was ready for me.

I took the hydrophone back under the ship positioning it as I had been told, I then had to back off and wait while it was tested; I spent the time looking around, it was amazing, the ship had a flat bottom and extended off as far as I could see in all directions other than towards the side of the ship where I could see my umbilical going back under the bilge keel towards the side of the ship. While on our course we had been told that people diving on large ships like this using SCUBA without lines to the surface had been known to get lost and find it difficult to find their way back out from under the ship; I could see how this could really be a possibility particularly if the visibility wasn't good.

We spent the next week supporting the wasp and generally enjoying diving in the Mediterranean Sea, the fish did turn up from time to time which was really nice to see; they were so fast, they would come and go in a flash, they never bothered me, in fact they didn't even seem to notice me. After five days of this we were stood down while the oil company did some tests of the well, there was nothing much for us to do for two days; we were not allowed to go ashore so we just set about topping up our tans. As I said the Delta was an old tanker, on top of the accommodation just behind the bridge there was swimming pool! Yes, a pool, it was empty when we first saw it but as there was nothing much to do the client had it filled, this was not a big job as it was already plumbed to be filled with seawater and only took about half an hour to fill.

The client was a keen sport diver and was very eager to try one of the bandmasks so Chris tasked us to set one up using a bail-out bottle so that he could use the KMB on SCUBA; he had a great time wandering around on the bottom of the pool. In the evening after dinner, I was up on the bridge wing with Bill and Steve and as is common with bored young men dares started to be bandied about; I was dared to jump off the bridge wing into the sea. Of course, there was no way I could back down, so I climbed up onto the rail. There I was looking down what seemed a very long way, I don't know exactly how far it was but it looked much further than I was comfortable with, I think it would have been about twenty-five metres at least.

I stepped off the rail, no going back now, I remember thinking oops it's taking a long time to get to the water but of course no sooner had I got this thought done with than I hit the water. We had been told how to jump from height into the water and so I had my ankles firmly together and an arm across my chest with my hand covering my nose but I really wasn't ready for the impact, I was only wearing a swimsuit that gave me no protection at all, it certainly hurt, my left arm had been outstretched to keep balance this slapped the surface, ow! I came back to the surface with no real damage just a little bit bruised, now I just had to find my way to the ladder and climb back on deck; this was another lesson learned, I never did another jump like that although there were times when I was tempted,

I always remembered this moment in time.

The second week went by much like the first and very soon we were getting ready to leave; Chris came towards me from the accommodation with a big grin on his face. "You've got another job", I didn't know what he was on about but he went on "you're not coming back to the UK with us, you're going to a job in France instead". I didn't quite know what to say so I just gabbled something about how was I going to get there; he just laughed, "there will be tickets waiting for you at Barcelona airport, we'll find out more when we get ashore".

Over the next few years, I came to find that this kind of thing was not unusual, I would often go directly from one job to another; I was quite excited at this prospect. These days there would be a great deal more communication between the diver and the office but, in those days, communication was very much more difficult and so was minimal and often just via the supervisor. This would lead to my often being given minimal information about a destination or how to get there, leading to some very interesting episodes as you will see.

When we got ashore there was a telegram waiting for me detailing the travel arrangements; I was to fly to Bordeaux and from there I was to take a train to Biarritz; the contract was a twelve-month job doing rig support on a rig in the Bay of Biscay. Seemed good to me, this of course meant that I wouldn't have the worry of finding a job for a full year; I said goodbye to the guys at Barcelona airport and made my way to my flight.

A couple of hours later I found myself going through passport control at Bordeaux airport, again, in those days you still got a stamp in your passport even going into France so I was gathering quite a collection already. When I exited into the arrivals lounge, I looked for the signs to direct me to the railway station; you could say that I had studied French at school but in fact I had given it up as soon as I could, this happened at the age of thirteen and I had really been no good at it even then!

Still as nobody seemed to speak English, I had to try to make myself understood, I went to airport information and in my extremely pigeon French asked "ou et la Gare", which I was sure meant where is the railway station. It seemed to work as I was directed out of the terminal and told to board a particular bus that would take me into town to the station; I boarded the bus and again was faced with having to ask a Frenchman for a ticket to the station, he looked at me and I said "une billet pour la Gare, sil vous plait" again it worked although his answer was lost on me but I thought he must be telling me how much the ticket was.

I presented a fist full of French Francs, he took some and gave me a ticket, I went and sat down; maybe I had learned more than I thought; well in truth I wasn't sure, I had to sit and wait to see whether I did actually get taken to the train station.

Off we went with me enjoying the trip, Bordeaux is a lovely city that I had never been to before so I was very glad to be seeing a bit of it from the bus. Eventually I saw the train station come into view, success; when the bus stopped just outside the main entrance, I picked up my bag and went to find the ticket booth so that I could buy my ticket to Biarritz. As I had been able to buy the ticket for the bus without too much problem, I thought the train ticket would be a breeze; well, not quite so easy as it turned out. I waited in line at the ticket booth, when it was my turn, I thought it was worth asking if they spoke English only to be told "non!" Oh well it had been worth a try, nothing else for it then I trotted out my best schoolboy French again "je voudrez une billet pour Biarritz sil vous plait"; I was fairly sure this meant I would like a ticket to Biarritz please.

Unfortunately, this time it didn't have the desired effect as he just sat back and looked at me with a puzzled expression, I tried again with the same result; hmm, what now? He just looked around and talked to some of his co-workers this seemed to be a great joke as they all started laughing, at my expense, I think. Well, I didn't know what to do now; meanwhile the line behind me was beginning to show signs of mutiny with a lot of people talking over my head to the ticket booth, a woman standing in the line about three back from me decided to come to my aid. She spoke some English and asked me what I wanted, with a good deal of gratitude I told her that I had to get to Biarritz; she nodded and turned to the ticket seller, she proceeded to speak in very rapid French to the man and although I can't be certain, it sounded as though she said exactly the same words as I had but for her it had the desired effect, I got my ticket!

I later found out that the reason I wasn't understood was because of my pronunciation, well never mind, I had the ticket; I thanked the woman and made my way to the train that was just about to leave.

The train journey was completely uneventful, we travelled very slowly through some lovely countryside until finally arriving in Biarritz at about five in the afternoon. I disembarked climbing down beside the tracks as there was no platform, I had been told I would be met by one of the other divers so I put my bag down and looked around. I saw a big guy wearing a bright yellow T shirt, when he turned around, I saw the cartoon of a Rat carrying a diver's helmet, this was the Rat Hat T shirt I had seen while working in the yard in Aberdeen, ah I thought this must be my contact. I caught up with him and introduced myself, he presented me with a huge grin and a hearty handshake, he introduced himself as Doug, I later found out his full name was Doug Rank, he was a larger-than-life character and made me feel very welcome.

He grabbed my bag and told me to follow him, we went out through a very dusty station building to his car; I climbed into the passenger seat and off we went. Over the next few minutes Doug and I swapped information about ourselves, he was a Canadian from Toronto and his sister was visiting him at this time so we were going out to their villa where we would get a bite to eat. This sounded like a great plan to me; on the way I told him that I had only been qualified for some five months which he seemed to already know, he said not to worry as the job would give me lots of opportunity to learn my trade. I asked him about the job and it seemed we would be working on another semi-submersible, the

Glomar Semi 1; this one was some half-hour offshore by helicopter.

The rig was sitting in some five hundred feet of water and I would be part of the team that would be maintaining everything from the surface all the way to the seabed! I was stunned, I told him that I wasn't qualified to work at those depths he seemed completely unfazed by this, he said that this didn't apply in France and that I would get into sat if I proved myself as capable to the supervisor; wow again.

Doug then told me that we would be going offshore in a couple of days as there was an inspection contract to be carried out, the whole team would be offshore for about ten days. This was apparently unusual as normally the team which consisted of five divers one of which was the lead diver or assistant supervisor and a supervisor. The team was split into pairs with each pair normally spending two weeks on the rig followed by four weeks on the beach. Anyway, it seemed over the next couple of weeks I had to prove I was up to the job so that I would be trusted to carry out the full duties including going into sat!

When we arrived at the villa that was some five miles out of town in the middle of some lovely rural countryside, I met another two of the team, Paul Latham the assistant supervisor and Bill Latham, the others were offshore at the moment; we had a nice meal and then Doug took me in to the centre of Biarritz to a bar where a room had been reserved for me.

The bar was in a very atmospheric little street, Rue Mazgran, this was right in the centre of the town. He parked up and we made our way into the bar where he introduced me to the landlady who was very pleased to find that I was at least trying to answer her in French although it must have been clear that I was very limited in this respect. I came to know my landlady quite well, she was a lovely woman, she was probably in her fifties and clearly had decided that I needed mothering. She became my French mum while I was working in Biarritz and made my stay there more comfortable as she welcomed me into her family even to the point of inviting me to her house on special occasions.

Anyway, I was shown to my room which was fine, it was above the bar with a single bed, a desk, chair and small wardrobe. The room was all I needed and it was cheap, not only was it OK but they would keep it for me when I went offshore so I didn't need to cart all my kit out to the rig with me each time, not that I had much stuff with me. But of course, if I was going to be here for a year, I would very likely accumulate some stuff that would be hard to drag offshore each time I had to go. I decided to get my head down as it had been a long day and Doug wanted to get back to his sister to say goodbye to her, we arranged to meet up in the morning when he would show me around the town.

I slept well and was woken by the sun coming through the window at about nine o'clock in the morning: I went down to the bar for breakfast which consisted of some lovely croissant and café au lait served in an enormous cup, it was more like a soup bowl. As I was finishing up, Doug turned up on his motorbike, it was a nice little Honda 125 dirt bike; he said they had all bought bikes when they arrived so that they would be mobile. Apparently as they would be taking them home with them at the end of the job in effect exporting them from France, they had been able to buy them tax free. I hopped on the pillion seat and we headed off, in France there was no need for helmets at that time, so off we went.

We headed out to look at Biarritz; Biarritz is a lovely little town right at the south-western corner of France, it nestles in the corner of the Bay of Biscay only a few miles from the Spanish border. There are some great beaches most of which are very good for surfing which suited me down to the ground as surfing was one of my favourite pursuits.

Just around the corner from my hotel was a great little colonnade of shops and bars, the bar that became our local La Tireuse was in this colonnade, it looked out over the harbour area; we all spent a lot of time in that bar whenever we were ashore.

In the evening, we met up with another couple of guys who had been drafted in to help with the inspection of the rig, the inspection controller was Matt Isbitt and another NDT qualified diver Nobby Clarke would be helping out with the work underwater. We met them at their hotel and had a nice meal with a few beers before heading back to our respective lodgings having arranged to meet up in the morning to go to the airport together. The next day we arrived at Biarritz airport; a small provincial airport that seemed to be asleep when we arrived; Spud led the way to one of the check-in desks where we were all weighed together with our bags. There was very little administration required, nothing like Aberdeen, without delay we were led out to the waiting helicopter.

This was another Sikorsky H58 and I was told by Bill that this one had actually seen service in the Korean war! Of course, I have no way of knowing whether this was true or not but it certainly looked pretty beat up; anyway, we climbed aboard, there again was no requirement for survival suits or any kind of briefing. One of the ground crew slid the door closed and the engines started, it was extremely noisy and didn't really sound very well. After only a couple of minutes, the rotors picked up speed and we started to lift off, as we took to the air the chopper lurched worryingly to the right which although I thought was a bit upsetting nobody else seemed to bat an eye; I later found that this was normal, it seemed level flight wasn't really something this helicopter aspired to!

Off we went and very soon were crossing the coast heading eastward, although I couldn't really see much as we didn't have windows in the cabin other than a small one in the door which was not really much use at all. After about half an hour we arrived at the rig, the pilot made a couple of circuits and then came into make a reasonable landing although again this thing really did seem to be about to shake itself to bits but we made it, the door was opened from outside and slid along the fuselage. Out we got and headed to the edge of the helideck then down into the accommodation to be logged onto the rig, this didn't take long so very soon we were heading down to the diver's cabin.

On arrival at the cabin, I met the other crew members, there was the supervisor a Scotsman

Ian Little, Ian would become pivotal in my offshore career as he would leave Biaritz to become Oceaneering's Operations Manager just a couple of months after I arrived. As Ops Manager he was in a position to offer work which he did for me whenever I wanted it. I also met the other diver, a South African Phil Lloyd, so the team was complete; after the traditional half hour chat during which everyone learned about each other and their experiences I was taken for a look around the dive system by Doug.

It was another new experience for me as I had never been on a dive site with a sat system, this one was actually a very small system it consisted of just one living chamber in which two divers would live, sleep, eat and generally exist for the time they were under pressure, there was a second lock this was the transfer lock or 'wet lock'. The wet lock was where the divers would get dressed into and out of their diving suits, there was also a shower and toilet in this lock; once the divers were dressed, they would lock through from the wet pot into the diving bell via a short 'trunking'; this would all be done under pressure when the divers were in sat so that they would only decompress once at the very end of the job.

I was awed by this as although it was nothing like the Transworld 58 system, I had helped with in Aberdeen this one was certainly capable of short sat dives and if Doug was to be believed I would eventually get to use it, I couldn't wait.

As I say the rig was another semi-submersible, this one was operated by Global Marine, a Texan company and was working for Elf Oil, they were also drilling wildcat wells although Doug said that this hadn't been going well as the present hole had taken some eleven months to drill already and kept causing problems. Continuing with my tour we soon came to the breathing gas storage area, there were what seemed like hundreds of 'quads', metal frames holding some twelve to sixteen bottles containing helium oxygen mixtures that we would be breathing when in sat. The water depth was about four hundred and sixty feet, so we would be using a breathing mixture containing ninety seven percent helium and only three percent oxygen. If we were to breathe this mixture on deck it would not provide us with enough oxygen to survive but at depth because the pressure was some fifteen times greater than at the surface this mixture would keep us alive beautifully.

Next, I was shown the diesel fuelled hot water machine, this would pump hot water down to the divers to keep them warm by being circulated around their hot water suits. Eventually we made our way to the equipment store where I found a few medium regular hot water suits that would fit me just fine but perhaps the best find was Rat Hats. There were four of them and it was clear that these were the hats we would be using not only during sat dives but also during the air dives over the next few days for the platform inspection; this was great, at last I would officially be a Rat Hat diver.

We then went to meet the rest of the team, the client's rep and barge master (captain of the semi-submersible) to discuss the inspection job; Matt took the lead, I just sat and listened. It seemed that we were not going to be inspecting the whole rig, apparently this was normal, we would be doing one quarter, the idea was that this would be done every year so that after four years the whole structure would have been inspected. Matt laid out the plan showing which part of the rig we would be concentrating on this was going to be the starboard aft corner; OK but I didn't know which was the front or the back of the vessel! Again, Doug came to my rescue and showed me how to tell the difference; it seemed that I was continually learning new things; once the basic plan had been outlined to the whole team Ian told Doug, Phil, Bill and me to go out on deck to assemble the diving kit so that we would be ready to dive in the morning.

Matt and Nobby went to sort out the various Non-Destructive Testing (NDT) kit; we would be carrying out MPI using prods, Digital Ultrasonic Thickness (DTM), Cathodic Potential (CP) meters and photography. We met up again towards the end of the day when it became clear that the chap who was supposed to be the photographer had not arrived, this presented a bit of a problem as none of the others knew how to develop the film which was a requirement for the contract. I stuck my hand up to offer my services as I had done some developing before, it was very simple and straightforward as we were using slide (transparency) film.

The process for developing this type of film was the E6 process, very easy although I might not have mentioned that it was so easy. So, yes, you've guessed it, I got the job, I was now the official photo technician for the contract, I then started to worry that I had bitten off more than I could chew; but too late now.

There was no dark room but luckily, I didn't need one as I could transfer the film from its cassette into the developing tank by using a lightproof black bag, I had not used one of these before and although it was fiddly it was quite straightforward. But where would I be able to set up the equipment? The barge master offered the bridge as this was not in use while the rig was at anchor for drilling; this turned out to be fine, there was fresh water, a sink and power so I had everything I needed. The camera I would be using was another Nikonos camera although this one was a Nikonos IV; it was fitted with electronic strobe so very similar to the system I had used at ICI, but being the most up to date model had much improved metering which should make things easier for me, simple!

Of course, to begin with there was nothing to photograph other than a few shots to show the accumulations of marine growth which I could do whenever as we weren't going to be cleaning the whole rig so there would always be something representative that I could photograph. No, the first thing was to clean some of the welds, we were to be using a high-pressure water jet with grit entrainment; another thing I had never used.

The equipment was supplied by another company who were also supplying an operator so we wouldn't have anything to do with the topside equipment, he would do it all. I was given a briefing to tell me how the diver's gun worked and what I would need to do in order to keep myself and the other divers safe. The gun was an evil looking piece of kit, it had a pistol grip with a trigger and trigger guard; the high-pressure hose entered at the rear of the trigger assembly just above the hose carrying the grit, there was no lock on the trigger so I would need to keep the trigger depressed all the time which seemed simple enough.

There was a short barrel about a foot (30cm) long (this would be too short these days as now the minimum length is sixty centimetres for safety's sake). This was where the high-pressure water would be coming out, just before the end there was a fitting onto which the grit hose was connected; it seemed that the grit would be fed down this line entrained in air, as it arrived at the gun it would be drawn into the HP water with the resulting mixture of high-pressure water, air and grit being fired out towards the weld or anything else it was aimed at!

I was made very aware of the damage it would cause if I were to shoot myself or anyone else with it, this thing could kill or at least maim someone. The last thing to mention was the retro jet, this was a second water jet that exited backwards and was enclosed in a large diameter tube about two inches (50mm) in diameter, this tube was to be tucked under the diver's arm so that the retro jet would exit behind them; why did the gun need this? You probably all know that when you hold a garden hose you can feel it trying to push you backwards, this is fine when you are standing on firm ground but underwater this would result in the diver being pushed away from the job all the time, the retro jet counters this and if it has been set up properly there is absolutely no force either pushing the diver off or onto the job; it all seemed simple enough but tomorrow we would see as this was to be my first real job.

The next day our task was to clean one of the very large welds running around one of the main support legs where it connected to the horizontal pontoon at a depth of about fifty feet. I wasn't the first diver so when my turn came at about eleven o'clock the job site had been set up with a down line leading to the job and the water jet gun already on the job. I started to get kitted up, this was for me another momentous day as it would be my first dive in a Rat Hat, I was really looking forward to this as I had heard so much about them, they were supposedly the best hat available at the time.

The hat was a demand hat with an optional free flow that could be used to clear a flooded hat or to demist the face plate, if necessary, the free flow valve was on the right-hand side outside the hat; just below this on the same side was a very small 'duckbill' water purge valve. This valve would pass air or water out of the hat if the hat was slightly over pressured and could be used for clearing water out of the hat; on the other side of the hat there was the main exhaust valve that would exhaust exhaled gas from the hat. Inside the hat there were communications speakers and a microphone all held in place by spring clips and on the left-hand side was a small diameter rubber hose leading from the back of the hat forward to the second stage.

This was a new one for me, I had never seen a hat where the second stage regulator was inside the hat; it would of course function in exactly the same way as it would if it were outside the hat but it seemed a bit strange to me, the regulator nestled into a recess in the side of the helmet's shell and was held in place by a springy length of rubber. There was no traditional mouthpiece such as you would see on a SCUBA demand valve, instead there was a breathing tube that extended to a point at the bottom of the face plate; at the end of the breathing tube was a mouthpiece although this was not designed to be put wholly into the mouth, there were no lugs to bite on; the Rat Hat mouthpiece was designed for the diver to just make a seal with their lips. On top of the breathing tube was a shaped piece of plastic for the diver to press their nose on to help with ear clearing, luckily again, I never needed this.

First, I put on the neck dam, this was very similar to the neck dams I had used on my course, it consisted of a chrome plated brass ring that would be passed over my head, the seal was a latex job as opposed to the thick neoprene ones I was used to. The latex seal was very thin and I was a bit worried that it would tear as it was made of the same kind of material used for the Avon dry suit cuff seals, I had used on my course these had been prone to tearing if we weren't very careful. I passed my head through the latex seal and neck dam and pulled it over my head, the seal seated nicely against my neck, so far so good, the water was quite warm so we were just using thin wet suits. This meant that there would be no problem with the neck dam seal being covered by a dry suit seal which could sometimes lead to air being allowed to pass into the dry suit. If this were to occur the dry suit could inflate causing the diver to lose control of his buoyancy.

The neck dam had wire bridles at the front and back onto which a 'jock strap' was clipped, just the same as the free flow hats we had used on the course, Doug who was acting as my tender for this dive hooked the strap onto the bridle at the back of the neck dam he then passed the end of the strap between my legs; I pulled the other end up and hooked it onto the bridle at the front of the neck dam, there was a buckle that would allow me to tighten or loosen the strap to suit my work position.

Next Doug helped me to put the bailout cylinder on my back, the bottle was held upside down in a backpack; making the bottle's pillar valve accessible to me if I needed it while in the water. The hat had no dedicated bailout valve, so, if I needed to utilise the bailout supply, I would need to reach behind me and turn on the bottle's pillar valve. The bottle's supply hose would be attached to the hat via a quick disconnect fitting just before the hat was put on my head. As we were only using wet suits there was no need for a weight belt as the hat was a negative buoyancy hat, this meant the only other weight I had to carry were a couple of very small ankle weights, I was a little sceptical that this would be enough but Doug assured me that everything would be fine.

I put on a pair of fins and the mandatory diver's dagger then was ready for the hat, I had already selected the correct size padded liner, again I was a medium so the black one was my size. Doug had already applied a smear of liquid soap onto the inside of the hat's faceplate to stop it from misting up and had also fitted the liner into the hat, it was secured firmly into the hat. I stood up and Doug handed me the hat, he then attached the umbilical to my harness using the carabiner and threaded the pneumo hose across my chest. He lifted the hat over my head, I had to slightly twist my head to one side so that my nose cleared the breathing tube and nestled my head into the liner, I was holding the neck dam bridle so that the neck dam was horizontal. There was a small tongue on the front of the neck dam that Doug slotted into the corresponding slot on the front of helmet's ring then he settled the hat onto the neck dam making a seal and I felt him latching the two handles fixing the helmet and neck dam together.

We then carried out a comms and bail out check and I was ready to go, I stepped into the diver's cage and was very soon on my way, it was a nice day although there had been a bit of a blow over the past couple of days so I could see that the water was not going to be very clear. When I reached the water, the cage kept on descending, I called "left surface" Iain responded with "roger that". I found I could easily breathe, the hat was dry and seemed very comfortable, I had been told that if I removed my lips from the mouthpiece while I was inhaling the demand valve would free flow, this was a safety feature allowing the diver to get a great deal of air without any effort, to stop it free-flowing all I had to do was to put my lips back onto the mouthpiece it really was a lovely hat.

I had a couple of practices just to get the hang of how the free flow feature worked, it was simply great. Very soon I was at the right depth, the cage halted and I prepared to go out to the job. I was pleased to find that Doug was right my buoyancy was perfect, I found I could hang midwater without any effort at all. I followed the line, making my way to the job, the visibility was poor, just a couple of feet (0.5m) at most, this was much more the conditions that I was used to from my days with ICI and on the course in Plymouth. However, I could see the gun and the weld to be cleaned so no problem; I set myself up to carry on cleaning where the previous diver had finished.

I spent the next couple of minutes setting myself up, there was a constant flow of air coming out of the gun, I had been warned this would be the case as air had to be kept flowing to keep the inside of the hose dry, if it were to flood then the grit would not flow properly and would block the hose. Soon I was ready, I called "make it hot" the gun came alive and when I pressed the trigger the jet of water really built up, the level of noise was horrendous, I would never be able to hear the comms while the gun was active. Anyway, very soon I could see that grit arrived as the water jet changed colour to a dark grey, I could start cleaning, I moved the gun close to the weld and all the marine growth was blasted away with very little effort on my part; a huge amount of grit was being blasted onto the weld before just falling away.

Although when I was below the weld the grit fell onto me and the hat, with the Rat Hat's second stage being inside the hat it was protected, if I had been using any of the Kirby Morgan hats the second stage diaphragm would be at risk for sure as grit would get into the water side of the second stage which could then wear the diaphragm. I really started to enjoy myself although my hand quite soon became fatigued by having to hold the trigger depressed all the time, the hat though was really comfortable it sat very nicely, it wasn't always floating up as I could adjust the jock strap to keep it exactly where I wanted it to be.

After what seemed like a very short time the water jet lost power and Iain told me that my dive time was up so I should prepare to leave bottom, I hung the gun up so that the next diver could easily find it and made my way back to the cage. My first dive in a Rat Hat had been great, I loved it, it was definitely the best hat, I had ever used.

Over the next few days, I dived every day jetting more welds, inspecting and photographing everything we found to be out of the ordinary; during this time, we found a very large dent in the top of one of the horizontal braces. The dent was about three metres long, half a metre wide and about twenty centimetres deep, this had to be photographed but photographing dents can be challenging, how could I demonstrate the size properly; I knew dents tended to be flattened out in photographs?

On the day I was to photograph the dent luckily the visibility had greatly improved and was good at about eight metres and there was a lot of sun giving very good conditions for photography. I had decided to use the 'taut wire' method; this involves stretching a thin wire along the brace so that it runs along the axis of the brace directly over the dent at its worst point, the wire was graduated at ten-centimetre increments allowing measurements to be taken. There was nowhere convenient to attach the wire so I placed a couple of horseshoe magnets one either side of the dent making sure that they were both at the same orientation on the brace so that the wire would run parallel to the brace.

I measured the position of the magnets relative to the welds at the end of the brace and ensured the magnets were far enough along the brace so that they were both on undamaged steel. When I had finished setting up the wire it was nicely positioned running parallel to undamaged brace; I had magnetic identification tags that I stuck to the brace alongside the taut wire these would be clear in the photograph showing which brace we were on. I took some photographs of the identification and then a general shot of the taut wire spanning the dent. I then called for another diver to help me with the measurements; Bill was also in the water at the time so Iain directed him to come over to help me. I had already discussed what I was going to need him to do. As soon as he arrived, he started by placing a ruler perpendicular to the wire pressing down into the dent this showed the depth of the dent at a fixed known location.

I then proceeded to take photographs showing each vertical measurement at all the graduations along the taut wire, this information would then allow us to build up a profile of the dent. These measurements would allow engineers to assess its effect on structural integrity. When I had finished photographing and recording these measurements, we repositioned the wire so that it ran along the side of the brace and repeated measurements, this showed that the brace had been squeezed outward by the impact, another factor the engineers would be interested in.

At the end of the sixth day, we had found a number of cracks in the welds inspected including one in an anchor chain fairlead as well as the dent, it was clear the rig had suffered a lot more damage than had been expected; bearing in mind that the job was supposed to be completed in nine days this needed to be discussed with the client. Of course, I was still a very junior diver at this point so was not involved in these discussions but, at the end of the day's shift we were all called together to be told that it had been decided to extend the inspection to the whole rig!

Clearly this would now take a lot longer; a revised plan was set out for us to clean and inspect all the welds; in the end this took us ninety-three days, I was quite happy with this as while I was offshore, I didn't need to pay for food or accommodation and of course I would be doing what I liked which was working underwater.

One morning I was given the task of rigging the MPI equipment close to a particular weld so that it could be inspected that afternoon; the weld was some distance away from where the MPI transformer could be lowered into the sea. I waited in the basket until I could see it coming down, again the viz was wonderful, while I waited, I was treated to a show being put on by jellyfish; there were some enormous ones accompanied by some much smaller ones. They all looked very colourful and exotic; there were always a lot of them around the rig in Biscay, they never bothered me until when I was using a hot water suit. A jellyfish must have been sucked into the seawater intake of the hot water machine, its body must have then been mashed up inside the machine and then directed down my umbilical where it was injected into my suit: Ow!

I didn't know what was going on but when I took off my suit later, it was clear that I had been stung over large areas of my body. We could see tracks of where the suit's hoses had been. Oh, well it didn't put me off using hot water as it was generally so comfortable.

Anyway, back to the dive where I was rigging the MPI unit, for this dive I was wearing a normal wet suit so there was no issue with the jellyfish; I waited until the transformer was level with me, I told topside "All stop on the transformer". I swum out to the transformer and then started to fin with it across to the node where the weld we were to inspect was; I had to push hard I found I was not winning. I could get to within about a metre of the brace but no closer, I was knackered, I stopped finning and of course the transformer swung back to where it had started. I then sat on top of the transformer while I had a rethink; it was then that one of the most annoying things about diving particularly in helmets and hats was concerned happened.

I had been working hard and the water was relatively warm meaning that I was sweating buckets, sweating works very well to regulate our body temperature when we are in air but, when we are in water it doesn't work at all! It works in air because the sweat evaporates from our skin but in water no evaporation can take place, we can overheat if we are not careful.

Now, this was not going to happen to me here as the water was certainly cool enough, all I had to do was to pull the zip down on my wet suit and I started to cool off. The annoying part though was that a couple of drips of sweat trickled down from my forehead, they travelled down my nose itching all the way! Itches are incredibly annoying as you can't scratch them, I was pushing the hat onto my nose and using the ear clearing device to try to get to the itch but neither of these worked very well. It's annoying but in the great scheme of things it's no big deal really, amazing how annoying these things can be though isn't it?

After I had cooled down and got my breath back, I had come up with a plan, there were some shortish lengths of rope attached to the transformer. I made a longer length which I tied to the transformer and then swum off to the brace holding the other end; then sitting on the brace I just pulled the transformer over to me this was much easier and within a few minutes I was able to start rigging it securely in location. I was of course still learning how to work effectively; I have never been particularly strong so always had to think of ways to overcome my lack of strength; I often had to work smart, not hard; rigging and the use of blocks and tackle were my friends.

When we had completed the inspection of the rig, we had identified nine cracks in various welds around the rig but none of them were deemed to be in need of immediate repair; the engineers decided that we would dot punch the ends of each of the cracks and would inspect them on a weekly basis. We would be able to see if any of the cracks had visibly grown beyond the dot punched points; the engineers would then re-evaluate the rigs capability but at this time the rig was cleared to stay on location drilling for oil.

As we had all been offshore now for over three months it was decided that most of us would be sent ashore for a week's R & R; Iain and Paul were the only ones who had to stay on the rig as there had to be two of the team on-board at all times to ensure the dive system was ready should it be needed.

On arrival ashore again I went to my room above the bar to drop off my bag and to get changed then we all hit the town for a well-earned beer or three! I had come to realise already that the first night ashore could be a dangerous affair as there was always more beer consumed than was anything like sensible, this often resulted in one of the crew suffering some kind of injury.

As I've said communications in the early eighties were much more difficult than they are today, when I last saw my parents, I was under the illusion that I was just going to be in Spain for a few days but had been there for over two weeks and then had been sent directly from there to France to start this job. Spain and France both were not places where you could call overseas from a call box so I hadn't been able to keep my parents informed of the change of plan. When I arrived in France my feet didn't really touch the ground and I was very quickly back offshore so no chance to call anyone again. I'm ashamed to say that it was some three and a half months after I had left home that I first had a chance to contact people at home. Anyway, I was now intent on making a call to them to hopefully put their minds at rest if nothing more.

In those days in France if you wanted to make an overseas call you had to go to the main post office and arrange with them to make the call for you; you would then be directed to a booth where the call could be taken once they had established a connection with whoever it was you were trying to contact. This being the case, the first day I was free I went to the main post office in the centre of Biarritz and placed the call, I was directed to a little booth where I waited. After about ten minutes the phone rang; I picked it up to find my dad was on the other end obviously a little confused as to why a French lady who spoke very little English was contacting him!

Well once he realised it was me, he was clearly quite relieved to hear from me and was very keen to chat about what had been going on with me; he was amazed that I was on a job that should last for a year but was happy that I was at least gainfully employed. I promised that I would write to give more details and then our time was up so I had to hang up. I was really not a good son my parents must have been extremely worried for all the time I was out of contact but I'm afraid I hadn't given it much thought. I went straight back to my room and wrote a long letter to them detailing all that had gone on and sent it off to them the same day; I would like to be able to say my communications with them improved but, I'm afraid they probably didn't very much. Oh well, they were certainly keen to speak whenever I did manage to call.

Luckily nobody suffered any injury that first night ashore after the NDT job but over the coming months the team did suffer somewhat from this phenomenon. As I said we had to dive every week to keep an eye on the indications we had found to ensure they were not growing, there were always two of us rig sitting so each week an extra two of us would need to be flown out to the rig as the minimum dive team was four. Doug and Phil were programmed to do the first dive; they would fly out to join Iain and Paul. The day before they were due to go out, as I was effectively off-duty I went out with some of the locals, this turned into quite a long night! I rolled in to bed at about three in the morning very much the worse for wear, as soon as my head hit the pillow I was out like a light; after what seemed like a few minutes I was woken by someone hammering on the door.

Eventually I managed to crank open an eye and made my way to the door; my head was banging (that last beer again must have been off!), when I opened the door Bill was there looking very red faced, in fact, he was looking very much how I felt. He was very agitated and pushed his way into the room, "I can't find Doug or Phil, they must have got pissed last night!" This didn't make much sense to me as they had both told us they were going home early to be fresh when they got to the heliport this morning, we had waved them off at about eleven last night. Now, if they couldn't be found things changed for Bill and I, he said; "We're going to have to go and do the dive", this was very bad news on a number of levels as both of us had definitely had far too much to drink last night and this very definitely should disqualify us from diving today. Unfortunately, neither Iain nor Paul had been briefed on the specifics of the defects we were to be keeping an eye on this duty had been assigned to Doug and I as the qualified NDT divers. As Doug and I were on opposite teams that would mean there was always one diver who knew what to do available for the weekly dive.

There was no way we could refuse to go out as Iain had made it very clear that not being available was not an option, I would have to go and dive! I didn't need much kit as the plan was for us to fly out to the rig do the dive and then after a couple of hours when it was safe to fly in the helicopter again, we would be flown back to shore, we wouldn't be staying overnight.

We hightailed it out to the airport, both of us looking white as a sheet, we must have been a real sight; when we arrived, we could see the helicopter already had its rotors turning ready for take-off. We were rushed out and jumped on-board; as soon as we were seated the pilot lifted off, as usual the chopper took on its list to starboard which had initially been of a concern to me but I now knew wasn't a problem so didn't really take much notice. After about ten minutes I began to feel very queasy; I looked across at one of the Maltese deck crew who were flying out with us, he looked very concerned.

I must have looked a state but I didn't care about what he thought, I had other things on my mind. After another couple of minutes of normal flight in this chopper which was anything but smooth at the best of times, I knew that I was going to throw up, I looked around for something to use but, this being a very rudimentary helicopter there was nothing like a sick bag available. I remembered that my boots were in a plastic carrier bag in my rucksack at the front of the cabin; I got up staggering to my bag, rooted around in my rucksack and eventually found the carrier bag; I pulled my boots out and made my unsteady way back to my seat. No sooner had I sat down than the inevitable happened but not before I had been able to open the carrier bag; I heaved the contents of my stomach into the bag only to find that in my haste to remove my boots I must have also removed the bottom of the bag! Everything went straight through the bag onto the deck!

As soon as I had finished, I felt a bit better but I don't think the same could be said for any of the guys on the bench facing me, they all looked like they would follow suit, when I looked across at them, they were all looking at my feet or rather at the rather unsavoury pile between them. Luckily, we soon arrived at the rig and were deposited on the helideck, the chopper was shut down to wait for me to finish the inspection dive, I tried to apologise to the rest of the passengers but they were definitely not listening; as soon as the door opened there was a stampede, I was left sitting on my own. Can't say I blamed them!

I made my way to the galley to get some water and coffee, no sooner had I sat down than Iain came in looking like thunder; "what the hell are you doing here?" I explained the situation to him but he really didn't look any happier when I had finished. "Well, you're going to have to dive so get your arse in gear and get ready". I had no option; quarter of an hour later I was standing on deck in my wetsuit kitting up ready to get in the water; the indications were spread all around the rig so I was going to have to swim a full circuit but I thought I could do this relatively quickly. I was dropped into the water via the basket and made my way to the first defect, all I had to do was to look at the dot punch mark at each end of the indication, assessing whether there had been any visual extension beyond these punch marks, it was very easy to find the location and took just a couple of minutes to identify that the indication hadn't extended.

I made my way around the rest of the defects none of which had visibly extended, this information would be relayed to Det Norske Veritas (DNV) the rig's insurer so that they knew the status of the rig; the whole dive took me just forty-seven minutes with a maximum depth of fifty-eight feet well within the 'no stop' time limit meaning that I didn't need any decompression stops. When I arrived back on deck, I was extremely glad it was over although in truth the dive would have been very pleasant in other circumstances as the visibility was excellent and the sun was shining. I went and had a relatively cool shower, dressed and met the others in the galley for a bite to eat before we could return to the beach; Iain was keen to find out more about what had gone on last night. Neither Bill nor I could shed much light on the circumstances which didn't please him but he made it quite clear that he would get to the bottom of it when he got ashore at the end of the week.

After I had been on surface two hours, we made our way back to the helicopter for our flight back to the beach, I was ready to get down on my hands and knees to clear up my mess but someone had already done that for me thank goodness. The flight back was completely uneventful thankfully; when I got back to my digs, I found Doug and Phil having a cup of coffee sitting at one of the sidewalk tables; it seemed that they had met up with some friends the previous night, one thing led to another and neither of them woke up until midday, at one of the local's houses; oops! It could have been worse for sure but, I wasn't quite so sure Iain would see it like that when he got ashore but there wasn't much I could to about that.

We settled into what was supposedly the 'normal' routine, this meant that we were paired up and each of the pairs would be spending two weeks offshore with the others being ashore for four weeks on a four hour call out in case of a dive being required. I was normally paired with Doug whenever we were offshore with no diving planned our days were taken up with maintenance of the diving kit and ensuring everything was kept clean and tidy. In truth we spent a lot of time eating, reading and sleeping. This situation didn't actually last very long though as very soon after settling in to this routine I was in the client's office overlooking the moonpool when one of the guide-wires snapped; this wasn't a huge problem for the rig as drilling could continue but the guide-wire would need to be replace with some urgency.

This meant sending divers down to the wellhead at a depth of four hundred and sixty feet; Doug and I were the team offshore at the time and apparently this meant that I was in line for the dive! I couldn't believe this was happening to me as I had just finished my basic air diving course and shouldn't be anywhere near going into a dive like this, but this was the way Oceaneering worked at that time. The client set about calling the rest of the team out to the rig. Doug and I started readying the dive system, well I say Doug and I but in truth I didn't really know what I was doing so Doug led me through what needed to be done.

We had checklists to follow which made the job that much easier, quite quickly I got the hang of things, between the two of us we had the system ready for when the rest of the crew arrived. The others turned up after about six hours, Iain and Paul spent an hour or so discussing what the client wanted us to do and then they came to the rest of us to explain the plan; it seemed that although the guide-wire would need replacing the client was more interested in seeing whether the BOP had been damaged by the wire when it let go.

The plan was that Doug and I would go down to the BOP but would not pressurise the bell as the client wanted us to observe the BOP looking for leaks; once we had done this a decision would be made about what we needed to do.

We prepped the diving bell for the dive, we set up a Rat Hat for the diver and a KMB for the standby diver who would also be the bellman; I thought I would be told to be the bellman with Doug going out to actually do the work but this was not the case. Iain briefed us telling us that Doug would be bellman, his job was to stay in the bell, helping me to dress and when I dropped out of the bell ('locked out') Doug would act as my tender. In the event of an emergency Doug would also be my standby diver; although I didn't properly understand at the time, the diver locking out to do the job was by far the easiest and less skilled part of the process so this situation made perfect sense under the circumstances.

While I would be well qualified and able to dress Doug and carry out the tending duties, if I had to lock out to recover Doug I wouldn't have known where to start in terms of recovering him into the bell as I hadn't had this training at the time. Over the next few weeks, I was given the necessary training but at this time this hadn't been done. Even though the plan was that we would not be diving during this bell run, Doug and I kitted up as though we were going to dive just in case. I had already picked out my hot water suit some time before so off we went to get kitted up. Eventually we were ready for the observation dive, we were sitting inside the bell, Doug established communications with Iain in dive control and we closed the bell's bottom door, the bell had two doors, one was termed the 'top door' this one would be closed when the bell was to be pressurised above ambient pressure, this would be used when we were carrying out a dive where one of us had to leave the bell.

In this case the bell would be kept at ambient pressure 'one atmosphere'; at depth the pressure outside the bell would be much greater, this would keep the bottom door firmly closed. Very soon we were ready, it was five in the afternoon, the date was the twentieth of September and considering my basic air course had finished on the eighteenth of March I had only been a qualified offshore diver for six months, fabulous!

We were lifted off the deck and although I couldn't see what was happening, I knew the crew outside would be attaching the bell's drop weight to the hooks on the side of the bell, the drop weight made the bell negatively buoyant, without it the bell would float. The hooks were part of the bell's emergency system and even when the bell was under pressure the divers inside would be able to jettison the weight if necessary. When the drop weight was jettisoned, the bell would float back up to the surface theoretically taking the divers inside to safety although I don't think this was something anyone would want to test. As soon as the drop weight had been attached the bell's moonpool door was opened providing access to the water some sixty feet (18m metres) below us; the crew outside then attached the bell to two guide-wires, the bell would slide down these wires taking us down until we were alongside the BOP.

When all was ready Iain told us that we were about to be lowered into the sea, Doug gave me a thumbs up which I returned, I was ready! The bell was lowered through the moonpool, we were being lowered on a steel wire rope running from a winch on deck; I looked out of one of the ports. I could see the sea coming towards us. As soon as we came into contact with the water I could see some water coming in around a gap between the bottom door and the bell trunking but very soon this stopped, the door had sealed, we continued to descend, I could see bright blue water through the lower port and very soon I saw water covering the port on the top of the bell; there was not much swell but what little there was pushed the bell about, it was a bit uncomfortable but as soon as we were completely submerged the ride became much smoother.

Doug told Iain that we had a seal and were clear to commence our descent proper to the job, off we went; it took about fifteen to twenty minutes before I saw the BOP come into view through the port, there was very little light coming from the surface at this depth but we had lights on the outside of the bell and these illuminated the BOP well enough so we could see it sufficiently for our purposes. When we were at the right depth Doug told Iain "All stop", we spent the next couple of hours observing the BOP through the port looking for leaks as the drilling crew carried out a number of tests. All I had to do was to check the oxygen monitor from time to time to make sure we replenished the oxygen we were breathing; the carbon dioxide we were breathing out was being 'scrubbed' from the atmosphere by a scrubber with a fan pushing the bell atmosphere through a cannister filled with soda-lime; both of these kept the atmosphere in the bell breathable for us.

We had no way of manoeuvring the bell at all so only had a very limited view, we could only see one side of the BOP and really in truth couldn't see much of anything; after we had been there for two hours, we were told to make ready to leave bottom. There was absolutely nothing for us to do to make ready to leave bottom so we just sat and waited to be lifted back to the deck, the journey back to the surface was uneventful although it was nice to see daylight through the port when we reached the surface again. As soon as we were back on deck with the moonpool closed Iain told Doug to open the bottom door, there was a rope attached to the centre of the door which I held while Doug undid 'undogged' the latch, I then lowered the door until it was hanging on its hinge. As soon as it was open Bill's grinning face appeared and he said "enjoy the ride?" I had indeed enjoyed the ride, the only thing that would have made my day better would have been to have actually pressurised and locked out but that would be for another day.

The next day following discussions between the client rep and Iain it was decided that the guide wire did indeed need to be replaced! We were actually going to be doing it! I was so excited; Iain brought the whole team together for a full brief. The plan was that we would go down to the bottom in the bell but with the bell being kept at one atmosphere, when we were at depth, I was to kit up with all my equipment ready to leave the bell. The bell would then be pressurised as quickly as possible then as soon as the bottom door opened, I would lock out and move straight to the job. This was termed a bounce dive, it seemed that ideally, I would complete the replacement of the guide wire and be back in the bell within twenty minutes! If I was able to do this then we would be able to decompress fairly rapidly but if the bottom time went over twenty minutes, we would have to carry out a full saturation decompression, over a much longer period.

The plan was that the BOP would be separated from the wellhead and lifted some distance above the bottom so that it was safe for me to work below it. The end of a new guide wire would be dropped to the sea bed, I would pass this end into the top of the guide post, then, make a soft eye secured with bulldog grips just as we had done a number of times on my diving course although the wire was a good deal thicker than we had used then. Once I had completed this the guide wire would be tensioned up, the eye with the bulldog grips would jam inside the top of the wellhead's guidepost thus securing the wire effecting the repair; this was apparently a proven method of repair.

Doug and I made ready for the dive, we put all our personal equipment into the chamber so that we had all we would need such as soap, tooth brush, books etc., we then kitted up again in our hot water suits and made ready to dive the bell in exactly the same way as yesterday. The only difference would be that this time we would be pressuring the bell with Helium/Oxygen and I would be locking out to go to work; I was nervous but excited as I'm sure you can imagine. We went through the same routine as yesterday and very soon were beside the BOP, we carried on down past the BOP until we were about fifteen feet (5 metres) above the seabed.

With Doug's help I put on all the dive equipment and seated myself alongside the bell trunking with my feet on the bottom door, I had hot water running through my suit and the hat was ready for me to don as soon as we were at depth. Doug confirmed with Al that we were ready; we received the response that all was good to go for pressurisation, Doug asked me if I was ready, I gave him a thumbs up and he said if I wanted to stop just to hold my hand up in a fist as we would not be able to hear any spoken words, another, thumbs up.

Doug opened the blow down valve fully and we were off, I was very glad again that my ears cleared without any problem, in fact, it was Doug who had to stop a couple of times but generally all went well and quite soon the bottom door fell open meaning the pressure inside the bell was exactly the same as that outside, we had arrived at 460 feet (140 metres).

One of the main things I felt was the increase in temperature, we had pressurised from one bar absolute to fifteen bar absolute in a very short time the result was the temperature inside the bell increased significantly. In 1808 a French physicist Gay-Lussac noticed that whenever gas was compressed there was a corresponding rise in temperature. So, as we had increased the pressure in a fixed volume (the bell) the temperature had risen.

The other thing I noticed immediately was that of course my voice had changed! As we were now breathing Helium and Oxygen at a high pressure my vocal cords vibrated differently and I sounded like Donald Duck. This made me chuckle and Doug clearly was amused by my reaction as well. This effect does make voice communication somewhat more difficult but in fact after a short time you get used to it and it is not much of a problem. It was of course all new to me, I loved it. Doug helped me with my hat and very soon I was dropping out of the bell, I stopped just below the bell sitting on the drop weight so that Doug could check to see all was well and then I was off to the job, the date was the twenty-first of September 1980 just six months after I completed my air diving course!

I made my way over to the job, but not before I had looked around at a wonderful vista, the bell's lights lit the wellhead and I could see everything, the viz was at least thirty metres, brilliant! I felt great, breathing was easy, I was warm; life couldn't get any better. My right hip felt a little strange, it felt a bit loose but wasn't painful, other than that all was well. The wellhead was some fifteen feet (5 metres) below me and off to my left, I could see the hole in the centre which was the actual well, this was a thirty-six-inch diameter hole raised some three feet above the guide base. The sealing face of this I had been instructed needed to be checked for damage as this was the point at which the BOP would seal and was vitally important. Before that though I had to get the guidewire fixed.

I could see there were four guide posts, one at each corner of the guide base, the one I was to be working on was helpfully the one closest to me. I was not wearing fins but found it very easy to drift down to the seabed which was soft and silty but was easy to walk on; as I approached the guide base, I was able to look around at this area of the world that I was confident had been seen by probably fewer people than had been to the moon! The seabed was flat with no rocks or boulders to be seen, there were a few fish swimming around the guide base, all was so tranquil, it was wonderful. I made my way over to have a look at the damage, the old guide wire was nowhere to be seen and I could see that the hole into which I had to put the new wire was clear, so far so good. I asked topside to send down the new guide wire, Paul was on my comms and told me the new wire was already on the bottom; I looked around and saw that it was coiling down just off to my right, I told them to all stop as there was already enough wire on the bottom.

In fact, the wire had made a large coil on the bottom and right in the middle of the coil I could see there was an enormous Monk Fish (Angler Fish); I had seen a number of these before but never one this big! These fish have an enormous mouth and look truly ugly! But they taste good, I told Paul about the fish and his response was "great, go and stick your knife in it, we'll have it for tea". Well, there was absolutely no way I was doing that especially as I was here to do a job and, I had very limited time available to do it. Anyway,

I wasn't sure who would win that battle, I would leave that for another day.

I moved over to the coil and finding the end of the wire I pulled it across to the guide base ensuring that it would not tangle when the wire was tensioned up. I then climbed up the guidepost which was about two metres tall and clinging on to the top I fed the end of the wire which had been burned with a cutting torch so that it came to a nice point and would not fray; I found it easy to feed the wire down through the hole at the top. There was a slot about forty centimetres down the guidepost and I could see the end of the wire in the slot, I was easily able to hook the end of the wire out of the slot and pull it down to the seabed with me. After pulling a couple of metres of wire through I had enough to make the eye. I set to work; I was then told I had already had half my allotted time so the pressure was on!

When we had made soft eyes in wire rope at Bovisand the wire was quite small, about half an inch diameter and so would bend easily. The guide wire was more than twice as thick and was coated in thick grease, this was not going to be easy. I made the eye fairly easily and started to put the first bulldog grip on to secure the eye, holding both wires together while pushing the threaded ends of the U-bolt through the body of the grip's saddle; I threaded the nuts on securing the grip. Once this had been done, I was able to pull the wire through so that there was an eye of the right size, once the eye was good and the wires were properly in line, I tightened the nuts. Once finished I sat back to survey my handiwork, I had managed to make the eye, I remember thinking 'well, that's the hard part done', I then had to apply the other two bulldog grips keeping the short end of the wire held against the main part of the wire. As I was just tightening the second grip, Paul told me I had just five minutes left, well, there was no way I was going to complete this in the time available.

I still had to have the slack taken up and the wire seated in the guidepost in five minutes and then of course I had to inspect the wellhead and get back to the bell where we should be leaving bottom before the twenty minutes had elapsed. No way! I tried to explain this but as I was breathing helium my voice was very distorted and I couldn't make myself understood, anyway I tried.

Once the eye was complete and all the bulldog grips were tightened, I told Paul that I was ready for them to start taking up the slack; quite soon I could see the coiled wire being taken up, eventually the wire started to come under tension. I was very relieved to see that there were no knots in the wire so I had got that right, meanwhile I had managed to force the wire eye complete with bulldog grips into the guidepost slot, I then stood back to watch; I have to tell you my fingers and toes were all crossed that it would hold! As the tension in the wire increased, I could see the wire eye being pulled into the guidepost, the eye was deforming and I could see the first bulldog grip being pulled up hard against the top of the slot, I was anxious that this would work but at the moment I could see there was still movement.

After a few more minutes Paul came over the comms and gave me the great news that the wire was at the correct tension, he asked me to go and have a look to see whether I could see any problems. This was in the days before CCTV was commonplace so the only eyes on the job were mine; I had a good look and could see that the eye was scrunched up tightly in the slot but there didn't appear to be any movement so I reported that and was told, good job.

The last thing I had to do was to inspect the wellhead sealing face (my Lloyds diver inspector qualification coming in useful again). I went across to the wellhead and started to look at the smooth sealing face, I had been told to look for any scratches or impact marks as these could cause a leak which would be something of a disaster. I must admit that I found the thirty-six-inch black hole in the centre of the wellhead a little unnerving as I knew that it led down to the bottom of the well which at that time was some three-thousand-five-hundred metres below me. After a few minutes of looking very closely using the lights from the bell I reported that the sealing face looked to be undamaged. Paul then told me that was great and that I should make my way back to the bell, I have to say it was with some reluctance that I returned to the bell, I had really enjoyed my first Heliox dive and couldn't wait for more. At that depth everything was so still, the visibility was great and with hot water being fed to me I could have stayed there all day quite happily.

Anyway, it was not to be, I made my way back to the bell and with Doug's help climbed back into the bell; Doug sat me down on one of the seats and removed my hat, he turned off the hot water and now that I was safe and secure, he turned his attention to the doors of the bell. Doug told me that I had been outside the bell for some fifty-five minutes so we were in sat meaning we would have several days of decompression to look forward to. Firstly, he stowed my umbilical securely on the horns inside the bell then he pulled up the bottom door with the aid of the rope attached to the handle and dogged it in place once this was secure, we spent a bit of time tying the umbilicals in place and clearing the other ropes etc., away from the top door sealing face.

Once all was clear he lowered the door down onto the seal, there were no dogs to secure this door as it would be kept closed by pressure inside the bell being greater than that outside. Once the top door was closed Doug informed Iain that the top door was closed, Iain then told Doug to increase the pressure inside the bell by thirty feet, this would be above the pressure at the seabed so that if the bell did for any reason fall to the seabed the door would not open thus keeping us safe.

The topside crew then started to winch us back to the surface, meanwhile we started to break down all the diving gear and stow it securely. The bell was tiny by today's standards and was in fact something less than, six feet diameter inside and given that inside there were two men, two lengths of umbilical of some fifteen and seventeen metres respectively (the bellman's umbilical being two metres longer than the diver's so that he would always be able to reach the diver in the event of emergency). There was also one rat hat, one Kirby Morgan Bandmask, two weight jackets and all ancillary equipment (fins, knives etc.) it was true to say that it was somewhat snug in there!

When we got back to the surface the deck crew replaced the moonpool cover and then lowered the bell so that the drop weight could be disconnected. While this was being done Doug was told to start venting the bell to bring the pressure in the bell closer to the pressure inside the living chamber which was some thirty-three feet (10 metres) shallower than the seabed depth, this was termed the 'storage depth'. Now the system we were using was built by an American company, Perry Engineering, it was designed as a bounce diving system but was equipped for short duration saturation dives just as we were carrying out now. As I said before space was very limited on-board rigs and for that reason Perry had designed this system to have a very small footprint (it took up very little space).

In modern diving systems there would normally be two doors in a bell, the bottom door as we had and a side door which would be utilised to lock on to the main system. Or there would have been the facility to lift the bell onto the top of the wet pot so you could again use the same door in the bottom of the bell, but we didn't have either capability. We just had the one door and couldn't lift the bell onto the top of the system; this meant that the bell had to be rotated through ninety degrees allowing the bell trunking to be secured to the wet pot of the main system. This seemed to be no problem but as the bell started to rotate, we of course had to move around at the same time, this became very disorientating to say the least especially given that I had only been in the bell twice I was completely lost as to where the various valves were positioned.

It seems I was not the only one, Doug fell and I heard him gasp, at the time I didn't know what was going on but it seems that he had fallen onto the open-ended valve through which the bell pressure was being vented! His hand made a seal over the valve and he was being sucked onto the valve, he was luckily able to prise himself off the valve but even though he had only been stuck there for just a few seconds his hand at the base of his thumb had been sucked into the tube and a big blood blister was the result, very painful but ultimately not life threatening.

Those of you who know about pressure systems will be saying how could this happen? Whenever there is a tube that has the capacity to remove gas from a chamber or bell there should be a device fitted to stop this kind of problem from occurring, this is normally achieved simply by fitting a 'T' piece to the open-ended pipe; once this is fitted it is very much more difficult to inadvertently make a seal. As soon as the bell was back on the surface, we ensured there was a 'T' fitted I can tell you.

Anyway, when the bell had completed its rotation, it was pulled hard up against the wet pot trunking being clamped on to form a gas tight seal. The trunking was then pressurised and following a leak check was brought up to the same pressure as the storage depth inside the main system. We then continued to decompress the bell until we could open the top door. This is the most dangerous time for divers who are transferring under pressure (TUP) the integrity of the system is reliant on the clamp holding the bell onto the system, if this were to fail the whole system would decompress explosively.

Clearly nobody wanted this and so once the doors were open, we were encouraged to move through from the bell into the wet pot as fast as we could, we did this and closed the chamber door, the bell was then decompressed some thirty-three feet shallower and was left there as it was our lifeboat in the event of an emergency. We were now safe and secure inside the deck system, happy days.

As I had been in the water Doug suggested that I shower first, this was nice of him but first we checked to see whether there was anything we could do for his hand but it seemed that he felt there was nothing to be done and that it would be fine. I then started to take my hot water suit off. I noticed that lifting my arms was quite painful, it seemed both of my shoulders were affected? I didn't know what was going on, it couldn't be decompression illness (DCI) as we were still at almost the same depth and had not commenced decompression yet, the pain was not great and in fact if I didn't lift my arms up there was almost no pain.

Bearing in mind this was my first deep dive I was very reticent to report this and indeed I didn't tell anyone at the time after all I was only twenty-four and therefore still immortal! Some time, later I discovered that I was suffering from Compression Arthralgia, this affects some divers who are compressed to depth too quickly as we had done as they wanted us to bounce if possible. It seems that during the compression the synovial fluid inside the joints is displaced and the diver feels as though his joints are arthritic; painful but no real problem and indeed after a couple of days at depth it resolves itself. In my case it resolved during the decompression quite rapidly and although I did other similar dives following this, I never experienced it again this is one of the reasons that deep bounce diving was discontinued not long after my first deep dive and these days would probably not be undertaken at all.

Saturation decompression from that depth using the Oceaneering Saturation decompression tables that were in turn a derivative of the US Navy tables took just over three days during which there was really not much to do. In those days there was no video inside the chamber so we couldn't watch movies or TV really all we could do was eat, sleep and read books; I found it not too bad if a little tedious. During our decompression I was told that nobody had thought there was any way that I would be able to complete what needed to be done in the twenty-minute window so it was OK and indeed Iain and Paul, both told me that I had done a good job, fabulous, I was chuffed to say the least.

Clearly, we were going to be in the chamber system for some three and a half days or so; we needed to be able to satisfy our basic needs, such as use a shower, use a toilet and of course be fed. The wet pot chamber was equipped with a hyperbaric toilet for our use, we would use this as normal whenever necessary but there was no conventional flush system. In order to remove the offending materials from the toilet, a system of valves needed to be operated in a very well controlled manner so that the pressure inside the chamber could be utilised to push the materials out of the chamber to be ejected overboard. This kept us safe, also our food and drinks would be brought into the chamber via an equipment or medical lock; this is a large diameter tube that penetrates the hull of the chamber there is a door inside the chamber which will be kept closed by the pressure in the chamber.

Outside there is another door which will be kept closed by some kind of clamp arrangement there are some very safe systems available now but, in the eighties, there were some significant issues with some of the systems and they had to be operated using good and well controlled procedures. When the inner door of the lock is open the chamber, occupants are again at risk of explosive decompression so everyone takes this procedure very seriously. Food is of course always important but perhaps more so when you have nothing much to do! When under pressure food still tastes the same but there can be some change in the texture of some food making things seem a bit stodgier but of course it is still nice to be fed.

Finally, after the decompression was completed and the door opened, I have to say it was nice to be out of the chamber although I was hopeful that I would not have to wait too long before I was again inside. We had to wait close to the chamber for twenty-four hours just in case either of us suffered an episode of DCI but thankfully neither of us did and Doug's hand healed nicely.

When working offshore most days are very similar in the case of divers when there is no planned diving taking place the day revolved around maintenance of the equipment. This could be chipping and painting of the heavy plant such as lifting frames etc., or perhaps routine maintenance of the actual diving equipment, checking bottled gas pressures and cleaning inside of the chamber and suits. In the case of a rig support contract such as the ones I undertook in France, Italy or Spain, the maintenance days are fairly low key so there is no rush normally and as I say one day looks pretty much like any other; weekends don't exist for example.

During December of 1980 I was again offshore in the Bay of Biscay, it was my first Christmas as a commercial diver and I was quite happy to spend it offshore, however, on Christmas day the client decided that there was a dive that absolutely couldn't wait! It seemed that the rig had a towing bridle that had become damaged during the last rig move and as the rig was due to be moved again as soon as the current hole had been completed this bridle needed to be removed for repair.

My dive took seventy-four minutes, I was quite glad to get back on deck and de-rig all the kit, when this was completed, I showered and changed then we all went to the galley to find a festive environment with everyone seemingly enjoying a really good spread albeit without any alcohol. It was a nice day and definitely a different way to spend Christmas.

Guidewires were a bit of a perennial problem on rigs in those days and another dive to repair them brought me a memory that I could probably have lived without! Again, I was in saturation, this time I was accompanied by Bill Latham, it seemed that on this occasion not only had the guidewire broken but this had taken place when the BOP had not been on the bottom. When the BOP had been put back down so that drilling could recommence the BOP could not be seated properly onto the guide base and had apparently bent at least one guide post. This meant that the BOP had to be lifted back above the guide base and was hanging mid-water. We were to go down and remove the damaged guidepost completely; the guidewire would then be fixed to a convenient padeye on the guide base which it was thought should be a good enough fix. For this dive I was initially to be bellman for Bill, when we arrived, we could see that not only had one of the guideposts been bent but in fact all four of them were damaged. When this was noted, we were told to sit tight in the bell until discussions had taken place with the client. This was not a problem for us as being under saturation conditions there was no issue with us staying at depth for an extended period if necessary.

After some twenty minutes or so we were told that all of the guideposts were to be removed with the guidewires to be re-attached to the corresponding padeyes on the guide base. OK so now we could get on with the job; I dressed Bill ready for him to lock-out; he left the bell and after we had carried out the required safety checks with him sitting on the bell drop weight just below the trunking, he moved off to start removing the first guidepost. He carried on working to remove guideposts and transfer the guidewires to the Padeyes on the guide base for about four hours, he was then told to come back to the bell and I would take over to complete the job.

As I locked out following the changeover, I could see that Bill had done a great job, he had in fact managed to complete removal and transfer of three guideposts and guidewires so there was just one left for me to do. I moved over to the guide base and started work, the guidewire had been slackened off and was hanging in a loop so that the rise and fall of the rig floating above me would not affect my work. The guidepost was attached to the guide base by four large nuts and bolts, I got to work removing them, the top two were going to be quite straightforward but the lower two were buried beneath silt and grout; I would need to dig around them to gain access. This took me a few minutes, I then started to undo the nuts on the bottom bolts, they were not too tight and actually came off very easily.

I then moved on to complete removal of the top bolts and again they didn't prove to be too difficult so quite quickly the post was free and was lying on the seabed beside the guide base. I put the bolts back through the holes in the guide-base so that they would be recovered together with the guide-base. I then moved to the issue of removing the guidewire and moving it to the padeye on the guide-base; again, no problem, the whole job took me about an hour, I was then told to make my way back to the bell.

When we were both back in the bell and settled, we asked our supervisor what he wanted us to do next. It seemed there had been some discussion taking place on deck and the client wanted us to observe as the guidewires were tensioned up and once this was complete, they would try to lower the BOP onto the wellhead and hydraulically latch it. The client wanted all of this to be observed by a diver in the water; as Bill was by far the most experienced of the two of us it was decided that he would be the one to observe, he would lock-out and sit on the bell drop weight from where he could see everything easily. I dressed Bill again he locked-out and was again sitting on the drop weight, all was ready.

Now the BOP was an enormous set of valves and equipment it was some ten metres from top to bottom and about three or four metres square, it weighed some two hundred tonnes or so; a big bit of kit! The client gave the order for the drill floor to commence lowering the BOP; we watched, Bill from his seat on the drop weight and me through a port; they were lowering the BOP very slowly but as you may already know the Bay of Biscay is a very exposed area and it was certainly not unusual for there to be a fairly large ground swell which on this day resulted in the floating rig above us rising and falling by several metres. Of course, the people on the rig really did not have much perception of this movement but we could see it quite clearly. As the BOP was lowered the last few centimetres onto the wellhead the rig must have been at the top of one of the swells above.

This being the case when the BOP touched the wellhead but without the guideposts for support and even though we told them to stop lowering, this didn't happen although I was later told they had stopped lowering on our command but, the BOP continued to come down because the rig was slipping down into the trough between swells. The BOP at first seemed to be sitting quite nicely but as the rig kept coming down it started to topple, as soon as it was out of vertical gravity took over. Things started happening very quickly then. I kept my eye on the situation through my port and saw the white painted BOP coming towards me very rapidly, this enormous metal contraption then came into contact with the bell, there was an almighty crash resonating inside the bell which knocked us sideways.

Inside the bell I was knocked over and lost my footing, my left foot fell through the trunking and the bell tilted dramatically to an angle of some 45 degrees or so, gas started to escape from the bell trunking, I worried that the bell might flip over! However, the rig then started to rise onto the crest of the next swell, the bell righted itself, the BOP returned to vertical. Bill must have told the supervisor what was going on and I assume he informed the drill floor as I could see the BOP rising away from the wellhead, it was raised to a safe distance so that it would not impact on the wellhead again. Bill didn't wait to be asked, he immediately climbed back into the bell; we quickly lowered the top door and pressurised the bell making a seal, having done this we were for the time being safe. I don't mind telling you that we were quite shaken by the whole incident, bearing in mind we were at a depth of some one hundred and forty metres water depth and didn't know whether the bell or lift wire had suffered any appreciable damage from the impact!

After a few minutes the supervisor came back on the comms and told us that the client wanted us to check that the wellhead had not been damaged! This news was not very well received in the bell I can tell you, however we had already decided that one of us had to go back outside to have a look at the bell to see whether we could identify any damage that might affect us being able to get back to the surface. We decided that as Bill was already virtually ready to lock out again that he should do the dive, it was with some reticence that we decompressed the bell to allow us to reopen the top door but all went well and before long Bill was ready to lock-out again.

I again fed his umbilical out and could see him moving up the side of the bell checking whether anything had been damaged or knocked off, he also went up to the top of the bell and took a good long look at the lift wire and fixings. It seemed like the majority of the impact had been taken by the heavy steel tubes around the bell that were designed to keep the pressure hull safe were there to be any impact such as the one we had just experienced. As far as he could tell everything looked OK so hopefully all was well for us to be recovered to the surface, but, before that would take place Bill had to go and look at the wellhead sealing face.

Off he went with me paying out his umbilical carefully so that in the event of any unexpected event I could pull him back quickly; Bill's inspection of the wellhead was carried out without any issues; he could not see any damage, he returned to the bell and we again made ready to leave bottom.

Once we had sealed the bell again and were ready, we were safely recovered back to the surface, I think we were both quite worried that there may have been some damage Bill hadn't been able to identify but as it turned out nothing went wrong and we very soon had transferred back into the living chamber on deck. After we had both showered and had some food, we were told that the rig crew would make another attempt to latch the BOP while we were asleep so we should get our heads down for the night; we were both happy to do this and I certainly had a good night's sleep wondering if I had used another of my nine lives?

When we awoke the next day, we were told that the BOP had been successfully latched but that during the following test procedure there had been a failure; we would be required to go back down to see whether we could identify the problem and of course fix it. We were given our breakfast and then locked through into the bell again, all was well and we were quite soon on our way back down to the seabed. It was my turn to dive, so as we were descending, I started to put my kit on and by the time we were at depth and the top door was again open I was ready to go.

As I dropped onto the bell drop weight waiting for Bill to signal that I had no leaks and was good to proceed to the job I had a good look around; the job site was just as we had left it with no evidence of yesterday's drama. I moved off towards the BOP again wondering at this terrific spectacle. As I had thought before I again felt how lucky I was to be doing this job, I really couldn't believe it was great.

I arrived at the BOP and was directed to where they thought the problem would be found; the BOP is a complex piece of kit with hydraulically activated valves to close the well were there to be a problem. There were rams that could be used to temporarily close the well by clamping the drill pipe and I'm sure lots of other functions that I was not aware of. But the issue today was to do with the method that the BOP used to clamp on to the wellhead and I was directed to a series of hoses that were all attached towards the base of the BOP, sure enough I could see that one of the hoses was flapping about, it was only attached at one end. I found that the fitting that should have been threaded into the metal at the base of the BOP had sheared off, all I could see of it was the broken end of the fitting attached to the loose hose end. The subsea engineer who was in dive control confirmed that this would cause the issues they were experiencing so it seemed I had found the problem, now, what to do about it? They could of course take the BOP back to the surface and fix it on deck but, given the issues they had with seating it back on the wellhead they didn't want to do that if possible. Could we fix it on the seabed? It was decided that we could indeed carry out the fix and as I was already on the job it was down to me.

So, now I had to fix it, I had spanners etc., so I could easily remove the broken part of the fitting from the hose end, this took just a few minutes. The other end of the fitting was a different story though, it was not clear where the hose should be attached; I grabbed the end of the hose and used it to see where it would easily stretch to and in that area, I started to look for the other end of the sheared fitting. Eventually I found a hole with what looked like a broken piece of threaded pipe protruding from it, this was the correct size. I used the part of the broken fitting I had removed from the hose which seemed to fit nicely onto the protruding stub; I described this to the topside crew who confirmed with the engineer that this was the right fitting.

There was of course no hexagonal head on which to fit a spanner and there was not enough of the fitting standing proud for me to be able to get a pipe wrench onto it; there is though, a tool called an 'Easy-Out'. This is a tapered tool; with a thread running along the taper this thread is arranged such that it tightens as it is turned anti-clockwise therefore as the tool is screwed into a damaged fitting such as this one, as the tool tightened the broken fitting would unscrew. It's an ingenious tool that makes for a very simple fix when removing broken fittings, the problem was that I didn't have one with me.

I explained what I needed to the engineer and he told me he had a set of these tools and would get one sent down to me, great! The comms were handed back to the supervisor who told me to go back to the bell and sit tight there to wait for the tool to be sent down the guidewire on the port side of the bell. No problem, I swam back to the bell and took up a position next to the main lift wire; I looped my arm around the lift wire and settled in to wait for the tool to be sent down. In this location I would be out of the way but would be able to see when the tool arrived. Well, I didn't know how long it was going to take for them to get the tool down to me so I all I could do was sit and wait.

I was in a nice comfortable position, I had lovely hot water flowing around my suit, it felt like I was diving in a bath, the hat was very comfortable and I had lots of gas to breathe; in short, I was quite relaxed! It seems I nodded off, the next thing I knew was the supervisor calling repeatedly to find out whether I was alright? Bill later told me that the tool had arrived some ten minutes before but evidently the topside crew couldn't get any response from me, they were just about to get him to come out to see whether I was OK; oops, oh well no real harm done. I quickly moved over to the guidewire where I found the tool together with the correct spanner and a replacement fitting. I took these back to the job and started work, it took only a few minutes to remove the broken part and to then replace it with the new fitting.

Once the new fitting was installed and tight all I had to do was to refit the hose being careful to route it correctly as described by the engineer and then the job was complete. Once I had told them it was complete, they asked me to stand off a short distance and to observe while they pressure tested the line; I moved away far enough so that if the fitting should break, I would not be in range of the loose hose and again sat and waited. I couldn't see anything happening but there was quite a loud rushing sound that I assumed was them carrying out the test; after about an hour I was told all was well and that I could return to the bell. We were recovered to the deck chamber again and later that evening started our decompression.

A few weeks later I was again in sat with Bill and this time our first dive was to commence at a shallow level of just forty feet (12 metres), we were to carry out a visual check of the marine riser all the way down to the bottom. This would involve one of us swimming across to the riser where the diver would circle around the riser checking all the joints etc., as we would be working mid-water, we would this time be wearing fins. When the bell reached twelve metres the topside crew stopped lowering us; the bell was still at one atmosphere at this time, Bill who was to be locking out for the first stint sat on the bell trunking where I helped him dress ready for the dive, as soon as he had his hat on and all the checks had been carried out, I told Iain who was our supervisor today that we were ready and was told to begin the blow down. I put my right hand up to the red handle of the main inlet or blow down valve, this was a large bore quarter turn valve, I cracked the valve (opened it slightly) and gas started to enter the bell. Very soon we had equalised the pressure inside and outside the bell, this was indicated again by the bottom door falling open.

Bill gave me the thumbs up and dropped through the trunking, after his leak test just below the bell, I told Iain he was good to go and he swam away from the bell. Iain came onto the comms and told me that he would not be able to talk to me while Bill was out of the bell as he could only listen to either the diver or the bell not both at the same time so I should expect to be left alone. These days this would not be acceptable as there would need to be a more complex comms system able to speak to all personnel under pressure at all times, but, not so in those days and being young and probably a little stupid it didn't bother me at all!

I now had very little to do as my main job was to tend Bill's umbilical which as he was staying the same distance from the bell did not need much input from me. I spent the time checking the bell's internal equipment, this included for the first time two brand new subsea flashlights, these were sealed beam units with a diving depth rating of we had been told of two hundred metres. I picked one of these up and inspected it closely, it had a white painted aluminium body with a red circular flange, this was secured with four small wing nuts, this flange held the sealed beam unit into the main body of the housing where the battery was located. There was a handle extending below the lamp with a light lanyard attached, it looked exactly the same as the lights we used when I was with ICI but of course it couldn't be as they were only rated to fifty metres water depth.

As soon as Bill had completed his inspection at this level, he started dropping down the riser inspecting as he went, the topside crew commenced lowering the bell alongside him so I was also getting deeper as he progressed down the riser. Moving deeper, I noticed that the water level in the trunking was rising and soon was level with the door seal. This was not an issue as knowing Boyles law I was expecting this to happen as the bell was lowered, the ambient pressure would increase, compressing the gas inside the bell allowing the water to encroach into the bell.

As we descended though the water continued to rise and before long it was getting worryingly close to the bottom of the CO_2 scrubber. The scrubber we had in the bell consisted of a small twelve Volt electric motor powering a fan that drew the bell's atmosphere continuously through a canister containing the soda-lime. By now the water was just a couple of inches from the base of the scrubber, I knew what I had to do to reverse this issue, I just had to open the blow down valve to let more gas into the bell but, there was a problem. During the dive briefing I had been told that if the blow down valve was opened while a diver was outside the bell it would starve the diver of gas. Clearly, this was not a good thing but what could I do?

If I did nothing the water would damage the scrubber and that would lead to us having to terminate the dive early, so not an option. I had no comms with the supervisor so couldn't talk to them, I quite quickly came to the conclusion that the only realistic option I had was to open the blow down valve for a couple of short bursts. This would help the situation by letting more gas into the bell but would also be heard in sat control and they would then likely realise I needed to talk to them; if I did this in short bursts Bill would lose his gas but only for a very short time and I knew he would be OK with that.

Decision made I grabbed the blow down valve handle and turned it through the complete quarter turn, after just two seconds I closed it again, I repeated this a second time and then waited, Iain's voice came over the comms asking what the hell I thought I was playing at? I explained the situation as clearly as I could and was told they would tell Bill to expect loss of gas for a short time while I was sorting out the ingress of water into the bell; within a minute they came back telling me to go ahead. I opened the valve again and this time kept it open until the water had been pushed all the way back down the trunking, with the valve closed again I confirmed that all was now well.

Iain then told me to do the same again if I needed to repeat the process, with that he went back to talking to Bill and I was alone again, the bell again being lowered. I had to do this again a few times before we reached the seabed but without any real issues.

However, as I was descending, I watched the caisson gauge (depth gauge) showing the pressure inside the bell; I watched our depth increasing, at a depth of ninety-two metres there was a sharp and very load **Crack**! This made me jump and I started to look for the source of this unwelcome development, what had broken? I knew it would be very unlikely to be anything to do with the bell's pressure hull as the pressure inside the bell was exactly the same as the ambient pressure outside. I started to look around the inside of the bell, soon I found a lot of shards of glass some with silvered appearance scattered around the top door sealing O-ring and the bottom of the bell, it didn't take me long to find that one of the flashlight sealed units had failed, it had imploded!

While I was not injured at all by this it did give me a couple of potential problems, firstly I had another flashlight still in-tact at the moment but for how long? I decided that I didn't want it to implode inside the bell so I carefully picked it up tied its lanyard onto a longer piece of rope and dropped it through the trunking so that it was hanging some two metres below the bell. This wouldn't stop it from imploding if it was going to but at least it wasn't inside the bell any more.

The second problem was much more significant to both Bill and me, as I say there was a lot of broken glass sitting on and around the bell's top door sealing face; I was not sure whether this could have damaged the seal potentially causing it to fail when we were being lifted back to the surface. I spent the next ten minutes or so clearing up the mess and making sure the seal had not been damaged; I used my hot water hose to flush the glass out of the bell. I then inspected the seal and good news, the seal looked fine so fingers crossed all would be well. I knew the seal was made from a very hard neoprene material and so was unlikely to have been significantly damaged. As I was just finishing cleaning up there was another **Crack**, this one was not as loud as the first one had been and was accompanied by a bubble of gas surfacing inside the trunking, the second flashlight had failed but was not in the bell, the depth was now just ninety-seven metres; I thought I was right in my thinking that these flashlights were the same as the ones we used at ICI and were certainly not rated for two-hundred metres!

The rest of the descent went without further issue, we completed the tasks required, when we were both back inside the bell and had closed the top door there was a bit of an anxious time when we over-pressured the bell before leaving bottom. We waited for fifteen minutes watching the bell's caisson gauge and when the pressure was clearly holding, I told Iain that all appeared to be OK and we started our trip back to the surface; indeed, all was well and continued to be fine for the rest of our repeated dives during that saturation period but I have to say it went down as another memorable compression in a bell.

When not offshore on the rig we would spend our time in or around Biarritz we had to be within four hours as we were always on call-out but, this meant that we had some lovely times on the beach as we called it. There were usually four of us on the beach and two on the rig, we would spend two weeks on the rig and then four on the beach although often our month on the beach would be punctuated by visits to the rig for dives when all of us would be needed to be on the rig. We spent a fair amount of time on the beach and had managed to get to know some of the locals quite well, to the point that we were invited to some of their parties; it was a very nice laid-back time.

One time I was on the beach with Bill Latham who had a very old, bright green, Mk one Ford Escort which he used whenever the weather was not looking good or for longer trips when his Yamaha dirt bike was not appropriate. Unfortunately, the engine had stopped charging the battery and rather than get this fixed he thought we should buy a battery charger and just charge the battery whenever it needed it. I decided that as he was always ferrying me around that I would buy the charger for him. So, the normal procedure was that every night the battery was removed from the car and put on charge, all good.

Anyway, one day we had been on the beach for a week and were getting a little bored, we decided to take the car and make a trip to Lourdes; this was not far away it was some way up into the Pyrenees. Early in the day we dug out the appropriate map and making sure the battery had a full charge, off we went. The route took us via Pau. After that we headed up into the mountains and eventually found our way to Lourdes, unfortunately it had now started to snow quite heavily but hey what could possibly go wrong?

Lourdes is a really beautiful town with a famous church, it is rumoured that a vision of the Virgin Mary sometimes can be seen, people suffering illnesses and disabilities have been known to experience a revelation while there resulting in them being cured! There was a small grotto on the side of the church near the river where there was a small statue of the Virgin Mary and alongside this there were old crutches, walking sticks and even wheelchairs supposedly abandoned by the lucky individuals who had been cured; it was quite moving.

We spent a few hours taking this in and looking at the church before deciding we should head back; making our way back to the car we started back to Biarritz. Now the time was getting on and being late November, the sun was setting, it was getting dark, quite soon headlights would be needed, more electricity needed! Well, to cut a long story short as we were still some eight miles from home the car started to misfire and the lights were becoming very dim. Luckily, we just made it back before the poor battery gave up completely, truth was that we were very lucky indeed that we weren't called out that day!

With respect to first night ashore incidents, one time when I was offshore, I had relieved Phil who together with the others tied one on during their first night ashore, he though would live to regret it as he ended up in intensive care in a coma, it was touch and go for a week or so but eventually he did pull through. The result was that Phil had to go home to complete his recovery in South Africa, this left a vacancy in the team; this was filled by one of Doug's Canadian buddies who joined us for the last few weeks of my trip. In early February I was called back to the UK as Iain Little had arranged for me to go on a course to become an Atmospheric Diving Suit (ADS) pilot/operator and technician. While I loved diving and particularly saturation diving, I was very keen to experience all aspects of diving and being an ADS pilot would I thought be another string to my bow.

I arrived home to my little house in Torquay with a nice bit of money stashed in my bank account and determined to enjoy myself. Anyway, I arrived home sporting a nasty gash just under my left eye. During one of my recent dives, I had been transferring from the wet pot through into the bell while under pressure; unfortunately, we couldn't get a seal on the wet pot door; I wedged a spanner into a threaded hole in the door and was pulling with all my might while topside were pressurising the wet pot. As the door sealed the spanner slipped out of the hole, I was still pulling for all I was worth and the ring end of the spanner hit me in the face causing a cut below my eye. Another war wound don't you know!

Anyway, when I arrived home, there was a beautiful vision awaiting me in the form of Chrissie, she was visiting my lodger; I of course didn't know it at the time but she would later become my wife (definitely punching above my weight!). Over the next couple of weeks, we had a great time, frequenting the pub just across the way from the house and generally having fun. One of the main things I wanted to do while I was home was to get another motorbike and so John and I went to Portsmouth where I purchased a Honda CB900FA a wonderful bike, christened Harry by Chrissie!

PHOTOS FROM MY TIME WITH OCEANEERING INTERNATIONAL

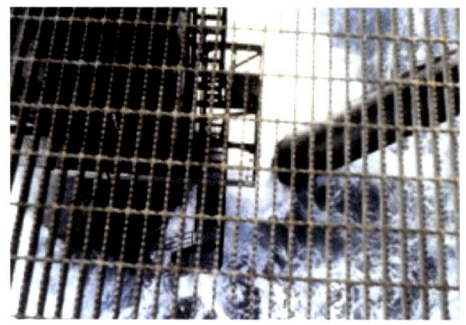

My first offshore job on the Nortrol semi-submersible drilling rig. Looking down through the deck 'Texas' plate at the wave action.

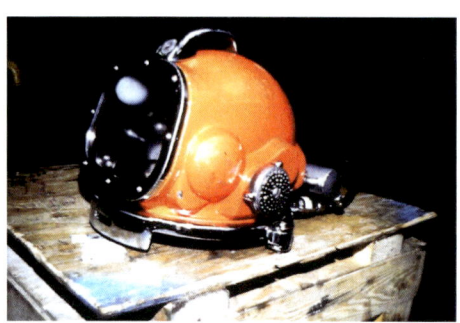

The fabled 'Rat-Hat' what a lovely working helmet!

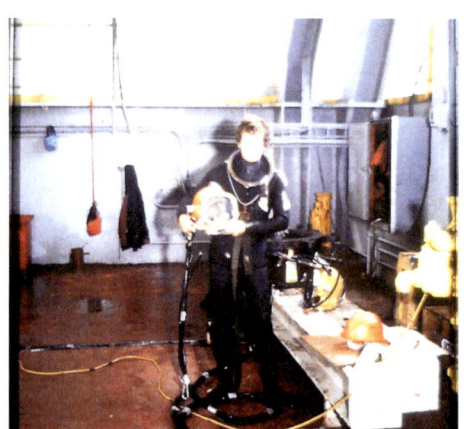

The author in France on the Global Semi One dressed for a surface-oriented dive using the Rat-Hat.

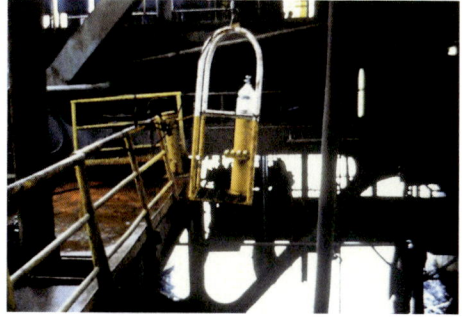

Diver's basket waiting for me to be lowered through the moonpool. Backup air bottle can also be seen inside the basket.

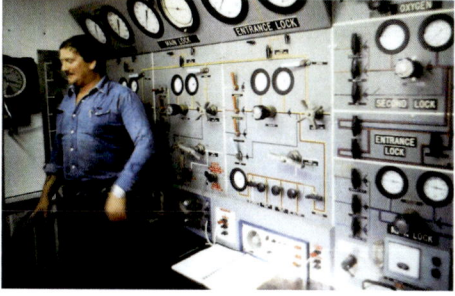

Iain Little in Saturation Dive control on the Glomar Semi One.

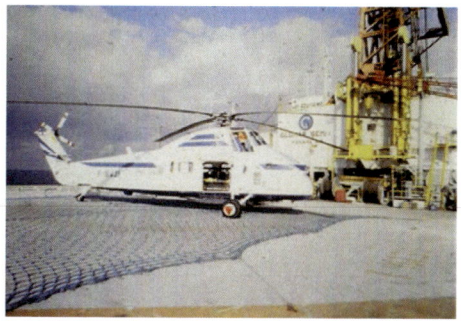

Sikorsky H58, our transport while in France.

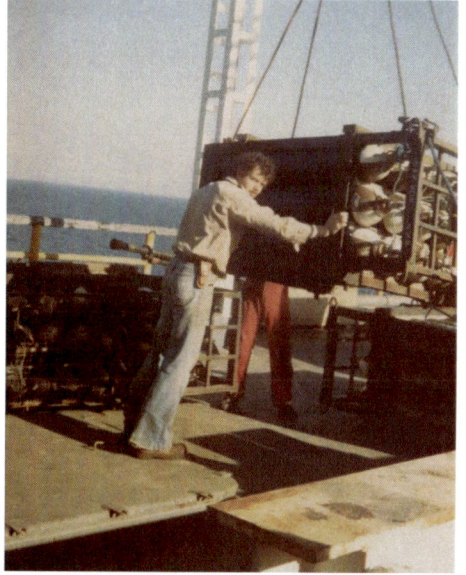

The author handling a Heliox gas quad on the Afortunada in Spain.

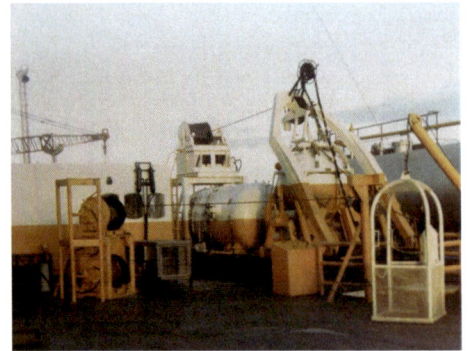

Perry 'Roll-Over' deep bounce/saturation system. This one was in Spain on the Afortunada. But it was almost identical to the one the author used in France for his first saturation dive.

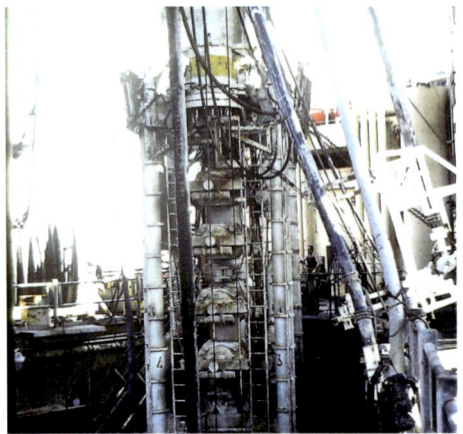

Blow Out Preventor (BOP) similar to the one that was dropped onto the saturation diving bell the author was inside in France.

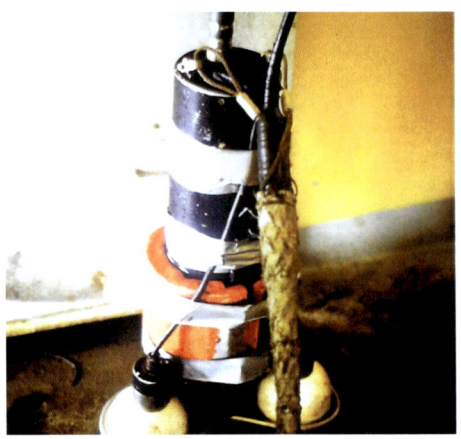

'State of the art' subsea CCTV system or '*dustbin*' as we labelled it!

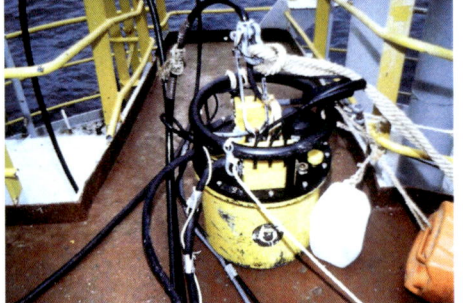

Magnetic Particle Inspection (MPI) subsea transformer.

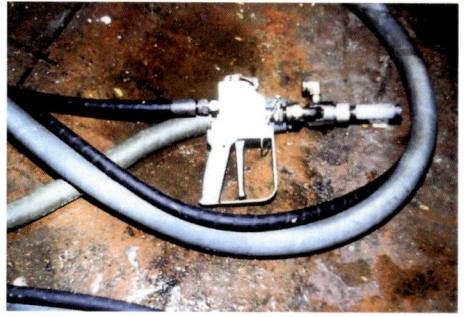

High pressure water jet with dry grit entrainment, this was the system employed by the author in France in 1980.

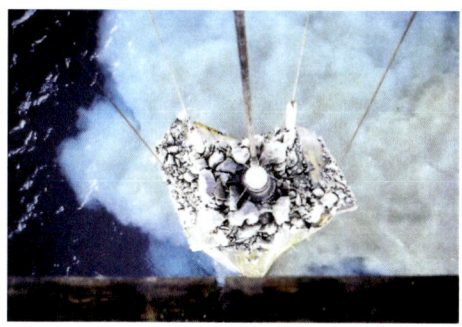

Subsea wellhead and guide base similar to the one the author worked on in France. This one was in Sicily on the Scarabeo four.

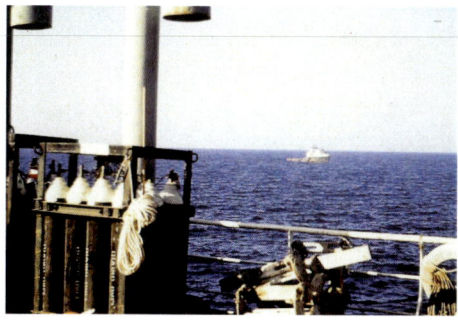

Twelve bottle oxygen 'quad'.

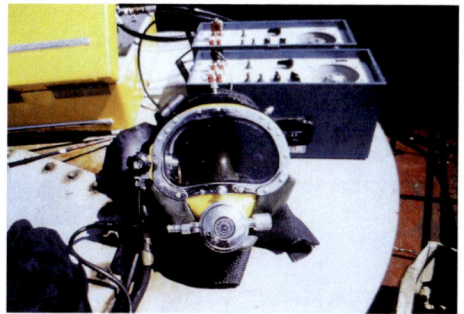

Kirby Morgan Bandmask KMB18. Also in shot are two diver's communications boxes.

CHAPTER ELEVEN

Atmospheric Diving Suits (ADS) 1981

On Sunday the fifteenth of February 1981 I made my way by train up to Alton in Hampshire to join my ADS course starting the next day at Oceaneering's subsidiary DHB Construction, this company operated and maintained all of Oceaneering's ADS operations. The course was to be carried out over a four-week period and covered use of both JIM and Wasp suits, I was really looking forward to it. This was nothing like the BAD course at Bovisand, I was being paid offshore rates to be there by Oceaneering and we were put up in a nice hotel right next door to DHB's facility, the rest of the guys on the course were from all over the world, some from the USA, one from South Africa and of course others from the UK. Both the Wasp and JIM suits were armoured, when a pilot was inside them, he/she could go to their deepest depth for hours and come back to the surface without any decompression being required as the pilot never breathed gas under increased pressure.

The JIM suit was an armoured bi-ped suit, capable of diving to fifteen hundred feet (457 metres) it had two articulated arms and legs, at the end of the arms there were fairly rudimentary pincers which allowed the operator to grip and manipulate items, they were clumsy at best and it took a lot of time and patience to achieve even the simplest of tasks.

The suit was designed to walk on a solid seabed and could not at that time work midwater although there was sometime later a version termed Jet-JIM that was fitted with thrusters and could work midwater. At the time I was using them the suits were mostly used for rig support and so would be working on BOPs such as I had done in sat while in France. In order for the JIM suit to be able to work on a BOP stack there needed to be walkways constructed around the stack; there would normally be two sets of walkways, one near the seabed at guide base level and one further up near the top of the stack. The suit would be sent down on guidewires so that it landed on the appropriate walkway and would carry out its work while being able to walk around on the walkway.

The Wasp on the other hand was a swimming suit capable of diving to two thousand feet (609 metres), it could work midwater, it consisted of a fibre glass tube in which the pilot would stand and an aluminium torso (no more magnesium so corrosion was much less of a problem for Wasps) from which two articulated arms just like JIM's extended; finally, there was an hemispherical plastic dome that closed over the pilot's head. This seemed to me to be a great improvement to the JIM suits four small ports through which the pilot had to peer; this was true but the optical distortion caused by the dome and the water when we were in the water meant that everything outside the suit seemed small and far away, this took some getting used to. The wasp was fitted with thrusters allowing the pilot to fly the suit up and down, rotate left and right, fly forward or backwards; these thrusters were operated by the pilot dancing on a set of switches on the floor of the tube. The switch sequences were a little complex, the pilot had to learn a series of sequential operations whereby these four switches could make the suit move in all directions. We all spent hours learning these sequences but it was not until we actually got into the suits and had to make them move that we learned them properly, initially we had a crib sheet taped to the inside of the suit's dome to help us remember!

On the first day of the course, we assembled at DHB's unit in Alton, this was alongside the hotel, we were immediately into the workings of the suits, we spent the first three days of the course classroom based; we were learning how the suits worked and how they would keep us alive. We spent a lot of time pulling the suits apart so that we could learn how to properly maintain them. The main advantage Oceaneering's suits had was the type of fluid supported flexible joints they employed in both the arms and legs of the JIM suit and the arms of the wasp. These joints would allow us to go down to two thousand feet and still be able to carry out tasks by moving the arms and pincer claws; this is true but it must be said that while everything may be able to be done, it all takes a long time! But the time taken would be the same at eight feet or eight hundred feet; this meant the suits only really became truly viable at great depth.

Anyway, we had to learn how to strip these joints and put them back together as when they were being used offshore this would need to be done with monotonous regularity. We also had to learn how to repair the JIM suit's hull which as I had learned when working as their air diver support; being made of magnesium would corrode very rapidly: this was to be brought home to me very firmly on my first offshore job as an ADS pilot! Repair of JIM's hull was carried out by using Araldite the two-part epoxy glue, some of the experienced guys told us that some of the older suits may have more Araldite than magnesium! The practical part of the course for JIM suits was carried out in their twelve-foot-deep tank inside the unit, nice and warm and completely controlled, great; no cold-water swims on this course.

My first dive in a JIM suit was to be in JIM 3, we were all weighed as the suit would only have sufficient buoyancy to lift with a pilot who weighs no more than twelve stone (76 Kg) in an emergency. This being the case we were all of a similar size and shape but, of course we were quite different heights, apparently, the majority of difference in height tends to be in the lower leg so we all were measured up and leg spacers were chosen so that we would be able to operate the suits properly. All done and the correct spacers fitted I was briefed on my first dive; the main point of this dive was to go to the bottom where I would be told to unscrew and jettison the large lead weights installed front and back of the suit. This was an important skill to master as this would be our main safety action in the event that we needed to bail out from a dive.

I would be installed in the suit where I would be wearing an oral nasal mask so that my exhaled breath would be taken to and pushed through cannisters holding soda-lime, to remove the carbon-dioxide from my breath in just the same way that scrubbers in the saturation systems had done for me. Meanwhile the suit was fitted with systems that would automatically replenish the oxygen that I consumed we had been told that there was enough life support carried on the suit that we could survive quite happily for forty-eight hours. Not sure I would have been happy after forty-eight hours though! This dive was also being witnessed by surveyors from Lloyds Register as the suit had just been refurbished and they needed to witness the suit coming back to the surface after dropping its weights.

OK so here we go, I climbed into the suit dropping my legs into the suit's legs, my feet fitted into the boots nicely, I had a pair of wet suit booties on; I was comfortable. I found that I could sit on the section between the suit's legs and could fold my arms and rest them in the arm holes; we had been told not to put our arms into the suit's arms until the suit was submerged. The reason for this was because if the suit dropped uncontrolled into the water the arms would be forced upwards and could break our arms, OK that was enough for me! Once I was sitting comfortably and had established communications with the supervisor the dome could be closed, my Canadian friend Tom Gilchrist pushed the dome up and it closed above my head, there were two levers on the inside of the suit just above my head, these were used to secure the dome. I turned these levers and gave a thumbs up to Tom, all was well and I was ready to go.

I had been told that when the suit first entered the water it was common for there to be a small amount of water to come in around the dome, this would seal almost as soon as the suit entered the water and was not a problem. The suit was winched up and across the tank and started to be lowered, as I was lowered into the water, I felt that I could use the legs quite easily, the water came up and started to cover the lower of the four ports in the dome; as the water rose to cover the other ports a fair amount of water came into the suit soaking my head and face. I had been told that if a lot of water came in, we would just need to adjust the eccentric hinge bolt for the next dive.

This was all well and good but the Lloyds surveyor would not want to see a very soggy pilot at the end of this dive; I didn't have a towel or anything else to dry myself and had quite long hair then but hey, ho! The dome did seal quite quickly and by the time I was on the bottom of the tank water had stopped flowing; from then on, no water came in so all was good; the water depth was only twelve feet (3.6 metres) so it wasn't long before I was standing on the bottom.

All good, inside the suit I had a depth gauge and an altimeter, the altimeter would keep me informed about the status of the suit atmosphere if it went up then this meant that either there was too much oxygen coming in or there was carbon-dioxide building up in the suit. If the altimeter dropped then it would mean that there was not enough oxygen being fed in to the suit and I would need to manually top it up.

All was well and I was told to go ahead and jettison the weights, I started to unscrew the front weight, it is a little strange to do this as the weight was positioned just above the suit's feet and would fall right onto the foot. It was a very big weight but of course the suit was armoured and so when the weight fell it didn't hurt at all, still, it felt a bit odd to intentionally drop a big weight onto my foot. Once the front weight was gone the suit's attitude changed, it tipped backwards, I then started to unscrew the rear weights; as soon as they had gone the suit took off for the surface, job done; I was bobbing around on the surface with the suit lying face down. I was then winched back out of the tank and the suit was again placed into its support frame I was told to release the dome which was opened by Tom again.

I was faced by the Lloyds surveyor who took one look at my wet hair and said, "well it leaked then did it?" I told him it was just a small amount when the suit first entered the water and although he didn't seem convinced, he clearly didn't feel anything needed to be done as he passed the suit as fit for use.

When the work was done for the day, we would normally adjourn en-mass to the Barley Mow a pub just across the road, it was a very welcoming little local pub. We very soon made good friends with the locals and inevitably after a few days some pub games were necessary between us and the local lads. We set up the same games as I had on the BAD course such as bottle walking etc., but also the more traditional pub games of darts and skittles; the locals seemed to take to us immediately. It was great and I had a wonderful time with another group of new friends. During one of the weekends, I was asked by Tom and one of the Americans Simon if I would take them up to London and show them around. I was very happy to do this and indeed while I showed them all the sites, they introduced me to the McDonald's Big Mac, McDonald's had only made it to London at that time, it had not found its way to Devon as yet so this was a treat for me.

We spent the next two weeks diving the suits in the tank learning how to carry out rudimentary tasks such as attaching shackles, walking the suit up and down steps and replacing guidewires in a guidepost attached to the side of the tank. It was a lot of fun but very hard work; we were also learning how to put the systems together so that we could mobilise a system offshore without needing people from base to help us.

During this time, we continued to work learning how to maintain the suits and it was clear that we would spend a great deal of time pulling them apart and replacing parts as well as combating corrosion whenever we were offshore. We learned that the old salts who had been working with JIM suits for years termed them the Alka-Seltzer, this was because as soon as they were immersed, they would start to fizz!

Just prior to our course Oceaneering had supplied a JIM suit and another type of ADS the Mantis, to feature in the James Bond film 'For Your Eyes Only'; the JIM suit and the Mantis were part of the villain's arsenal in the film and so ultimately, they both came to a sticky end in the film, the pilot of the JIM suit for the filming was Wayne Horton a friend of mine who I had worked with on the West Venture in Norway. The Mantis was piloted by the designer of the Wasp and Mantis, Walter Downing. In the film the JIM suit came to a sticky end by James Bond affixing a limpet mine to the back of the suit, this then exploded and destroyed the suit! This was all well and good but, the model that had been used and subsequently destroyed had silver joints on the legs whereas the real suit had green anodised joints.

It had of course previous to the filming been decided that both the real suit and the model had to look the same and one of them would therefore need their joints to be painted. I would have thought that the best solution for this would have been for the model to have its joints painted green; but of course, that is not what happened, the real suit had its joints painted with silver paint! The part of the joint that had been painted was a part that needed to slide and rotate and would not operate properly with a layer of paint on the joint, so, you've guessed it I was given the task of cleaning all the paint off the joint. This took hours as I had to be very careful to get all the tiniest flakes off as they could damage the small O-ring seals that kept the joint working and water tight.

During the third week of the course, we were to start using the Wasp, the tank in Alton was not big enough for us to do this so, we had to decamp to Stoney Cove; Stoney Cove was an old gravel quarry pit in Leicestershire where there would be space for us to really get to grips with the suit. Stoney Cove had a maximum depth of thirty-five metres (115 feet) and had a variety of sunken objects for recreational divers to explore. The suits we were to be using were Wasps eight and nine, they were loaded onto a big truck for the trip up to Stoney Cove overnight, we would follow in a Mini bus. Our trip took a couple of hours and during this time we listened to the radio featuring tunes like 'kids in America' by Kim Wilde and 'Breaking Glass' by Hazel O'Connor and other similar eighties classics.

When we arrived, we were immediately put to work offloading the truck and setting the equipment up, this was a very important lesson for us as it was a practice of mobilisation of equipment such as we would be required to do on any job in the future. Luckily, a lot of thought had been put into this and although there were a large number of hydraulic hoses and various pieces of kit that had to be connected all of the fittings were unique which meant that each end of a hose would only fit onto the correct piece of kit, brilliant! This made the set up very easy and quite quick to achieve; by the time we had finished there was time for a brief about the tasks we would be expected to carry out and then it was time for our first dives.

Again, having a surname starting with 'A' meant that I would be in the water first, this was fine by me as I was very keen to have a go. When all was ready, I was told to get suited up, this was a lot easier than having to dress for regular diving as I just had to put on a set of coveralls and a warm jumper with a pair of wetsuit booties; I was ready. I climbed in to Wasp eight and settled my feet on to the switches that I would be using to operate the thrusters, we carried out the pre-dive checks and I was ready; the Wasp differed from the JIM suits in that there was no need to me to wear an oral-nasal mask as the Wasp had a powered 'scrubber'; the system would draw the suit's atmosphere through a soda-lime cannister thus 'scrubbing' the carbon-dioxide out of the air.

The Wasp held enough soda-lime and bottled oxygen to give a maximum endurance of seventy-two hours! When all was ready the plastic dome was lowered over my head and latched, now I was isolated from the outside world, it was very quiet inside the suit, all I could hear in my little cocoon was a small whirring of the scrubber motor and random noises from dive control; this was new. Previously all my diving using spoken communications had been with a 'press to talk' system; arranged so that the comms were continuously open from the diver to the topside control room but I could only hear them when they pressed the switch to talk to me. This is sometimes referred to as a two-wire system; the Wasp though used a four-wire system, this meant that it was more like a conventional telephone in that I could hear the topside crew all the time and they also could hear me all the time. It was a bit of a novelty to hear all the banter in dive control while I was underwater, very different.

I was lifted from the frame by a crane and swung out over the water, then was lowered into the water, as the suit entered the water it started to float although when completely immersed it should be neutrally buoyant, this would allow me to be able to 'fly' it via the thrusters. The suit had a small air bottle that I could access from inside the suit via an electronic circuit, this bottle could be used to blow a small ballast tank on the back of the Wasp, allowing me to trim the buoyancy of the suit while at depth. Anyway, when I was first on the surface, I had to press a switch that would vent the ballast tank thus allowing water in making the suit slightly negatively buoyant.

This done, I started to descend, as the water came up above the dome again a small amount of water dribbled into the suit around the dome seal but, it was really a tiny amount and nothing like the previous drenching I received from the JIM suit on my first dive. The task for my first Wasp dive was to go down to the bottom and to get used to operating the thrusters, I was to move away into the centre of the quarry; it was fun to work out how to make the suit move by dancing on the foot switches, I found I could easily make the suit go up and down, rotate left and right as well as go forward and backwards. I started making my way into the deeper part of the quarry and eventually managed to get to one hundred and six feet (32 metres) at this depth I came across an old car that had been submerged in the quarry to give recreational divers something to look at. I later found that there had been all sorts of stuff, lobbed into the quarry for the divers to play with including a small aeroplane!

I found that while I recognised the car for what it was the dimensions seemed wrong, this was due to the refraction of the dome and as I had been told would be the case the car looked smaller and further away than it actually was; this would take some getting used too. I was given two hours to play with the suit but this seemed like just a few minutes to me, I was then recovered and brought back to the suit's handling frame without any need for decompression, it was fun.

We spent the next four days working with the suits and trying to achieve meaningful tasks, the culmination of this was that we had to show we could complete some rudimentary tasks in a given timeframe such as doing up a shackle! The main task that we all had to complete in order to pass the course though was to connect an hydraulic quick disconnect hose. This is a very straightforward task for a human but, not so much when this is being done with a couple of manipulators, it involved having to hold the collar of the fitting up with one pincer while pushing down on the fitting with the other. We had to do this midwater using the thrusters to keep us in place and indeed to try to apply some downward thrust to latch the fitting.

While the arms do not need much effort to move, they do require some and I found that when I was holding the fitting effectively at full stretch applying pressure to slide the collar up while pushing down on the fitting was very hard work. Overall, it was hard to achieve and took a great deal of practice and patience to complete; luckily, we did all manage this eventually which was great news, job done again.

Once we had all completed the tasks with the Wasp's we were taken back to Alton to finish our course. There was of course the perennial written exam and practical assessment in the tank, this would be a timed assessment of a series of tasks. We were given a list of tasks that had to be completed and were told that we would be given no longer than one hour to complete them all! This might seem like a long time but let me tell you achieving anything with a JIM suit could be very time consuming, anyway, with a certain amount of trepidation I was readied for my turn, I was the last in the queue this time which was of course something of a novelty for me.

Anyway, I had been sitting on surface watching everyone else complete the tasks with varying degrees of rapidity, they had all done well enough though, now it was my turn. At seven minutes past five in the afternoon I entered the water in JIM ten and started the tasks, all went very well and after just thirty-two minutes I was back on surface having completed all tasks satisfactorily, great. This was the twenty-fifth of March, I was now a fully qualified JIM and Wasp operator/technician, what next? Well before I left to travel home one of the staff members told me to call Iain Little in the office in Aberdeen, OK, now what? Well, Iain was very pleased to hear that I had passed the course and told me that I had my first job using JIM suits, I was to travel to Sicily for a six-month contract, great here we go again. I hitched a lift to Bristol with one of the other course members and stayed with him overnight then made my way by train back to Torquay the next day.

I had two weeks off before the Sicily job, I spent the time playing with my new motorbike and my friends, I had a great couple of weeks with no real worries as I knew I would be back at work very soon. Before I was to travel to Sicily and bearing in mind, I was going to be there for six months I was debating with myself whether I should take my new bike with me. This would be a great road trip albeit on my own but that didn't bother me and when I got there, I would have transport as the job was another where I would be living on the beach four weeks out of six so this seemed quite attractive to me. I spent time debating this with myself but eventually came to the conclusion that even though it would be nice to have the bike down there with me. There were a lot of unknowns such as where would I store it when I was offshore but for me the major one was, I had already been sent somewhere for a fixed period for plans to change in a second and the bike could then be left in Sicily with me in some other part of the world. I decided that although it would be great, there were too many unknowns for it to be sensible.

Therefore a few days before I was due to travel to Sicily, I got in touch with Iain's secretary a lovely lady by the name of Diane, I had got to know Diane quite well when I was working in the yard in Aberdeen, she had always been extremely helpful to me. I did get to know her well but purely platonically, it was an extremely bad move to date the operations manager's secretary as all would be fine when things were going well but if the relationship didn't last then this would likely lead to problems; so, although I liked Diane and I think she liked me we were just good friends. Diane was my normal contact with respect to travel and directions but it has to be said the directions part of things sometimes left a bit to be desired to say the least! So, my comprehensive instructions and directions were as follows: "There will be a ticket left at the Alitalia desk at Heathrow for you, you will be travelling to Catania via Rome.

When you arrive in Catania make your way to Gela on the south coast of the island. Where you are booked into a hotel for the night". She then gave me the hotel address. I said OK, so what do I do in the morning, where do I have to go? She said "It's no problem, just take a taxi and ask them to take you to the heliport". What could possibly go wrong?

On Thursday the ninth of April I made my way to Heathrow airport finding the ticket was indeed waiting for me, so far so good. Checking the time between arriving in Rome and leaving again I could see that it was going to be tight! I saw that I had to change terminals, hmm, there really was not a lot of time. As I was supposed to be away for six months, I had decided to take a fair amount of clothing etc., unusually for me I had a carry-on bag and one bag to be put in the hold; again in 1981 it was unusual to be able to check bags all the way through to a final destination so I would need to pick the hold bag up in Rome and carry it to the next check-in desk.

The flight to Rome went without a hitch we arrived spot on time, I hurried through to passport control and joined the queue, this was before seamless travel in Europe; looks like we might be returning to something similar now what with UK leaving the EU doesn't it! I didn't have long to wait and very soon was heading to the baggage reclaim, my bag eventually turned up which in itself was a relief as I would never make my connection if I had to chase lost luggage. Now I took off to get to the other terminal as quickly as I could, I had just over twenty-five minutes; in those days I was fit and so ran all the way dodging around other passengers making myself quite unpopular with some. I made the connecting flight with just minutes to spare and indeed I had to take all my bags on board with me as there was no time to get anything into the hold.

This was again something that was allowed in those days despite the fact that I had a couple of knives and a rigging kit in my bag, nobody was the least bit concerned by this all I had to do was to give the offending items to the pilot who looked after them, when we arrived in Catania, he gave them back to me! Different times. As we were coming in to land at Catania airport, it was a beautifully clear afternoon; I had a very good view of Mount Etna Sicily's active volcano, there was a plume of smoke rising from the crater but apparently that was the norm and not a problem. I was impressed to see this as I had never seen an active volcano before, I made up my mind to make the effort to visit while I was in Sicily if at all possible.

Once on the ground I made my way into the terminal after collecting my knives and rigging kit from the pilot, the time was a little after two in the afternoon so I had lots of time. The issue I was now facing was much the same as when I had arrived in France heading for Biarritz in that nobody here spoke English, the difference was perhaps that even though my French had been very limited at least I had a bit. As far as Italian was concerned, I had none! There was of course nothing like Google maps, Trip Advisor or any other electronic help as this was still some thirty years before all that came about.

I started by looking to see whether I could find a map of the island looking to see whether I could get a train or other options that might be available for me. In those days there really was a lot more printed help than there is today and I soon found a very helpful map on a wall in the arrival's hall, it showed rail lines and roads. It was clear that there was no rail link between Catania and Gela. OK then so a bus was to be found, again bus timetables were very easy to locate and I soon found one that showed I could get a bus from Catania airport to Gela and they ran quite frequently, great. I had no problem finding the bus station and as I arrived there a bus showing that it was going to Gela was waiting for me; I had changed some English Pounds into Italian Lire before I left London so no problem with having money although I wasn't sure how much the trip would cost.

I approached the ticket office and having learned from my experience in France I had a map ready and with a mix of hand gestures and pointing at the map I managed to get my point across. A ticket was duly passed across and I was told I needed to part with three thousand five hundred Lire, sounds like a King's ransom doesn't it but this related to about one Pound forty and as the trip was about one hundred Kilometres, I thought that was not at all bad.

My bus was plush and had air conditioning! It was a nice trip although a little slow, it took about three hours to make it to Gela but, this was very nice as the island is beautiful and it was a lovely day. I arrived in Gela at about six thirty, the bus station was busy and there were a lot of people around so I thought I would try to find someone who might be able to direct me to the hotel. Not a chance, I didn't seem to be able to get anyone to even want to look at the address I had let alone tell me how to get there, after about half an hour of this I decided to just get in a taxi. This was easy and luckily the taxi driver seemed to know exactly where the hotel was, well, in any case he nodded and as soon as I was in the car he took off.

I was not quite prepared for the fact that all Italian drivers seemed to feel they were born racing drivers, they all compete for every square inch of road and traffic lights were treated like grid starting lights. It was with some level of relief that I was eventually deposited at the door of the hotel in a big cloud of dust and fumes from a very hot engine; as soon as I had paid and was safely out of the car, he took off in another cloud of tire smoke and exhaust fumes clearly, he had just made a pit stop and was back to join the race.

The hotel was fine, there was a room reserved for me, thanks Diane, I was shown up to the room without any further delay, it was a nice room with en-suite which in those days was something of a rarity. I dropped my bags and decided to head out and find something to eat, on the way I stopped at reception and found another rarity, an Italian who spoke a bit of English. I enquired about taxi to the heliport the next day, he said there would be no problem, it was not far and should take no more than fifteen minutes, I thought that given the speed taxi drivers seemed to travel in Italy meant it could be as much as fifteen miles away but said nothing! Heading out of the hotel I turned left to find several very nice eateries almost next door, I settled in and had a lovely pizza and a couple of beers, I felt very happy and comfortable.

The next morning, I didn't have a very early start as I didn't have to be at the heliport until ten thirty so I had a leisurely breakfast and at ten o'clock I was checked out of the hotel and waiting for the taxi. The same hotel clerk was on duty and agreed to come outside with me to make sure the taxi driver knew where to take me, what a helpful chap, I thanked him and climbed into the taxi. Off we went and again I was treated to a master class of competitive driving. It did indeed take about fifteen minutes before we arrived at the heliport. In fact, this turned out to be a field with absolutely nothing in it at all! In my best Englishman abroad gesticulating I asked the taxi driver whether he was sure this was the heliport, the response was "Si, Si Senor, helicoptro inchinari".

Apparently, this meant that the helicopter would be arriving soon, unconvinced I decided that I had very little option other than to get out and to wait in the field. I spent the next hour and a half kicking my heels in the field completely on my own, I was though getting quite worried that I had been taken to the wrong place. I knew that I was going to be working on a rig that was drilling for the Italian oil company Agip and I could see a large building with an Agip logo on its side about half a mile away so I decided I would go and see if I could get any joy by asking someone there. I set off to walk there as there was no traffic at all, I continually kept looking and listening for the helicopter but nothing was moving at all, where was I?

I eventually rocked up in the reception area of the Agip office building, here I was faced with a nice lady who clearly didn't speak or understand any English. After about five minutes of me again trying to explain about helicopter and asking if there was anyone who spoke English a penny seemed to drop and she picked up her phone, there was a relatively short conversation in very quick Italian, then she hung up and just looked at me. I thought, what now? She didn't make any attempt to engage me at all so I sat down on a chair and decided to wait a bit. After a couple of minutes, an harassed looking man turned up, he proceeded to berate me in very broken English accompanied with a lot of exaggerated gestures (I was soon to learn that Italian's usually accompany any spoken words with exaggerated gestures). Anyway, it seems I was an idiot and that the helicopter was due within minutes and it would indeed be landing in the field where I had been waiting.

Oh, right, I had better get back there then, evidently, he didn't think I had time to walk and decided he would take me in his car, very decent of him I thought. Almost without delay, I was again deposited in the field where there was still nobody else? He just said that I was to wait and the helicopter would arrive, OK, so I will stay here then. He jumped back in his car and left in another cloud of tire smoke and dust, so there I was then on my own again. After about another hour a bus turned up in the field and a bunch of men got out, they milled about smoking, chatting and seemingly enjoying the afternoon.

They all seemed to waiting for something, I took this as a good sign; there was hope, after about another half an hour a very small helicopter turned up and set down in the field. There was no way we were all going to get on this chopper? Four of the men opened the doors to the helicopter and flung their bags into the door at the back, again no sign of survival suits at all. They climbed in and off they went, the helicopter took off and disappeared away to the south, the rest of them all looked content so I thought maybe this was expected. After a few minutes the helicopter returned and landed, four men jumped out and retrieved their bags from the back of the chopper, they then wandered over to the bus and boarded. Four more men boarded the chopper and off they went; this was repeated until there were just two men and me waiting, sure enough the chopper came back and when the returning crew had made their way to the bus we boarded and off we went.

I knew the rig had to be close but I wasn't prepared for just how close, as we rose up out of the field, we cleared a small row of sand dunes and there less than half a mile offshore was the rig. The Scarabeo 4, it was yet another semi-submersible, this one was operated by Saipem and was drilling for the Italian oil company Agip, it had a bit of an odd design or at least one I hadn't seen before, it had just three legs, it looked great to me though, it would be home for me for most of the summer. The chopper landed on the helipad and we all got out, the final three men waiting for the chopper including the chap I was replacing took our places and off the chopper went with them.

I followed the others off the helipad and entered the accommodation where I was greeted by someone who spoke reasonable English, I was logged on board and told my cabin number. I soon found my cabin and the rest of our crew who were already there, there followed the usual chat where everyone finds out about the others, the first to greet me was the Italian supervisor Matteo Romano, luckily Matteo spoke good English but he turned out to be a bit of an odd individual, my first impressions of him were that he looked ill, he looked anaemic and was extremely thin. When I got to know him properly, I came to the conclusion that this was due in no small part to his diet; in my view it was letting him down'. He was macrobiotic, this seemed to involve him eating not much and what he did eat consisted of beans, pulses, nuts and not much else, it didn't seem to have much goodness to it!

The other ADS pilot was Adrian Morris, Adrian was an ex Royal Navy clearance diver who had been part of the deep trials unit and so had been involved with both saturation diving and atmospheric diving suits in the navy, it seemed that Adrian had arrived just a day or two before me. And lastly the two air divers were an Englishman Keith Lewis who was a newly qualified air diver, he was in much the same position as I had been on my first trip offshore. And lastly an Italian, Guido. Guido was a real character, it turned out that he had previously made a lot of money diving for red coral; this involved him using scuba equipment with the bottles being filled with Heliox that he had mixed himself.

He would routinely dive to over one hundred metres on his own with only a boat on the surface following his bubbles, he would collect coral which he would put in a bag and when ready to leave bottom he would send up a small line attached to a small lift bag that he would inflate on the bottom. He was relying on the boat on the surface having been able to follow him and to locate the small lift bag, they would pick this up together with the attached line, they would then send a thicker line down to Guido which he would use to ascend. The surface crew would have lowered more bottles to the depth at which he would complete his first decompression stop, this was necessary for two reasons, one, he would not have enough gas to complete the necessary decompression and two, he needed to breathe a different percentage of oxygen during his decompression.

This all seemed very hit and miss to me but it seemed that he had been doing this for years and had made a very good living at it. After about half an hour Matteo told us that he had to go and see the client and directed the team to show me around. It didn't take long, there were two JIM suits (numbers 4 and 12), Oceaneering always sent two suits on any job, one would be used as the working suit and the second was a standby just in case of problems. The suits were positioned above their own dedicated moonpool together with all the required equipment to winch them into and out of the water as well as all the ancillaries; the main issue seemed to be that the position of the moonpool and therefore the suits being just below the drill floor meant that they were constantly being drenched with drilling mud! This was not good as drilling mud was quite corrosive, I was told that whenever the suits were not being used, we had to make sure they were covered with tarpaulin to protect them.

It was a nice little set up and the guys were all helpful, in addition to the ADS suits there were a lot of Heliox quads; it seemed that we were also geared up for surface oriented mixed gas bounce diving. This was music to my ears as I was keen to keep diving as well as using the ADS systems; after we had finished the tour, we headed to the galley for a bite to eat as it was by now nearly six o'clock.

The galley was very familiar as it looked just like the ones I had seen before; the food being made available though was not what I was expecting, it seemed that there was really just one main course and tonight that was tripe! My mum used to boil tripe as food for our dogs and my enduring memory of it was the smell, it was rank! I decided that maybe I would be living off bread and fruit if this was going to be the kind of fare produced on a daily basis, still things could be worse. Matteo turned up again and informed us that we should finish up our meal and then make ready to dive as there was a problem that we needed to go and sort out.

As I had just arrived it was quickly decided that I should be the diver as the others knew their way around the system, this made perfect sense and was fine by me. We made our way out on deck and started to prepare the suit for the dive, I was to be using JIM 4, I started by topping up the cannisters with fresh soda-lime while Adrian made sure the oxygen bottles were full, I also made sure the calf spacers were the correct length for someone of my height. Very soon all was ready and we stood by for the briefing from Matteo; when he arrived with the client who was of course Italian, Matteo told us that there had been an issue when they were grouting the thirty-six inch well casing resulting in a large quantity of grout (cement) being deposited over the whole of the guide base, it was thought that there was so much there that the BOP may not be able to latch and of course that would mean there couldn't be any drilling. My job was to go and have a look at the guide base to make an assessment of what could be done, great, let's get going.

Keith was to be my air diver support; he went off with Guido to dress for his dive. Meanwhile Adrian and I continued to prepare the JIM suit for me to use, within another twenty minutes or so we were all ready to dive; I was excited but this was tempered with a little apprehension as this was to be my first real ADS dive after completing my training and I didn't want anything to go wrong.

I climbed into the suit donning the oral-nasal mask, I carried out comms checks with Matteo and gave him the required readings of gas pressures etc. Adrian had readied the tag line which would be used to attach the suit to its guidewires for the descent, I put my arms into the suit's arms and grabbed the right-hand manipulator, inside the hand area globe the operator had a 'D' which when gripped could be used to rotate the pincer; inside this I was able to locate the 'T' bar that I knew could be used to open and close the pincer. If I closed my fingers around the bar and pulled it the pincer would close and if I pushed it away the pincer would open. The 'T' bar was on a threaded bar that extended through to the pincer, so, by rotating the 'T' bar clockwise I could screw the pincer closed; so, I wouldn't have to keep pulling on the bar to keep the pincer closed.

Adrian put the tag line through the right-hand pincer and I rotated the bar until it was tight; we then did the same with the left-hand pincer now the tag line was held firmly in both pincers. When all was ready, I gave a thumbs up Adrian closed the dome, there was a soft thump as the dome closed, I rotated the locking levers and gave another, thumbs up to Adrian. Meanwhile Guido and Keith had made ready for Keith's dive, we were all ready, let's go. Adrian moved across to the winch controls and I felt the suit being lifted; as soon as the suit was clear of its frame Adrian stopped the lift and moved across to open the moonpool, he then moved back to the winch controls and I started to be lowered through the moonpool. I always found this to be a wonderful time on any dive, it was the first time that you were all on your own, inside the JIM suit was extremely quiet as there were no fans or anything else to make noise, I was effectively isolated from the world outside.

I looked around at the underside of the rig, I could see the rig's legs and the sun which was setting, the time was nineteen twenty-seven on the eleventh of April. I suddenly remembered that we had been told to keep our arms out of the suit's arms during our transition through the air water interface just in case, so I pulled my arms out crossing them resting my elbows in the arm holes. Very soon the suit reached the water and as I entered the water I duly reported "left surface" to Matteo, when I was at thirty feet, I told Matteo to stop the descent. I had to wait a few moments for Keith to reach me, once he arrived, he had a quick look around the suit to make sure there were no bubbles coming out of it; he gave me a thumbs up grabbed the tag line and started to drag me across to the guidewires which were only a few feet away. Once he reached the first guidewire, he attached the first shackle, then, he moved over to the other end of the tag line and again attached the second shackle to the other guidewire, good job. Keith then gave me a thumbs up before making his way back to the basket so that he could be recovered. I had been talking to Matteo and had told him all was ready for me to start the descent; he clearly passed this on to Adrian as I started to be lowered.

As I descended, I remembered that we had been told to keep the joints moving as we descended so I started to kick my legs and put both arms into the suit's arms and started to operate them. This would keep the joints free we had been told that if we didn't do this the joints could become seized as the pressure outside increased. As I descended past about one hundred and thirty feet there was a loud crack! This was a little off putting but we had also been told to expect this as it was the ports seating and was nothing to worry about, I continued to be lowered and expected another three cracks as the remaining ports seated. Very soon I saw the guide base come into view, the water was so clear in this part of the Mediterranean that even at depth I had a fair amount of visibility and could see some fifteen metres.

I told Matteo that I had reached the bottom and read off the depth from my depth gauge, I was at a depth of three hundred and thirty-three-feet (101 metres), well within the suit's fifteen-hundred-foot depth limit. I could feel that my feet were on the seabed but, I would not be walking anywhere as there was a huge amount of cement grout all over the guide base; we had agreed prior to the dive that there would be no need for me to let go of the tag line as it would be enough for me to give an assessment from where I was standing alongside the guide base. I spent the next ninety minutes observing as the driller sent down the drill string and tried to break up the cement; all of this was illuminated by a CCTV camera's light that had been lowered on the BOP's guide wires and was sitting some five metres above me. It was by then clear that I was no longer needed and I must admit I was somewhat concerned that this very large and heavy pipe was being raised and dropped just in front of me; I could see the potential for this to go somewhat wrong for me, so, the decision was taken to recover me to the surface. Once I was back on deck, we spent another hour or so stripping the suit down to make sure it had not been damaged in any way and washing the sea water off to try to reduce corrosion.

The next time I dived the suit was not so straightforward, we were just carrying out a practice dive to ensure all was working and to allow me to have a go at walking the suit around the BOP walkways as I had never had this experience as yet. The dive went to plan to begin with, I had been on the seabed for about half an hour when I felt my lower chest on the right side was getting wet!

This was definitely not in the script I took my arms out of the suit's arms and immediately saw that there was a small jet of water coming into the suit just below the right arm. I told Matteo that I had water coming into the suit and he told me that I should make ready to leave bottom; all I had to do was to pick up the tag line again so that I would be brought up the guidewires, this didn't take long so quite soon I told him I was ready. The suit started to rise I could see the guide base receding into the murk; the water was still coming into the suit but as the outside pressure eased the jet became less forced. Very soon we were back to thirty-feet and Keith was there to release me from the guidewires, as soon as that had been done, I was winched back on deck I saw Adrian close the moonpool and place the suit's support stand under the suit. He went back to the winch controls and lowered the suit gently onto the support stand, then he came over to the suit and stood ready for me to open the dome.

I glanced at the altimeter in the suit and could see that the pressure in the suit had increased due to the water coming in so when I undid the locking levers I did it slowly ensuring the pressure would be released gradually; as soon as the dome seal was broken, I heard hissing and then Adrian was easing the dome away from me settling it onto its support. As I started to climb out of the suit it was clear that quite a lot of water had come in as my whole right side below my arm was drenched and there was a lot of water in the right boot.

We started to break the kit down as there would be no more diving until we had fixed the problem, Matteo was not as unhappy as I expected him to be as he felt that the dive had not been a complete loss. When I had changed into some dry clothes Adrian and I started to remove the suit's right arm so that we could locate the leak; what we found stunned me! The suit's arms and legs were threaded into aluminium inserts which were in turn bolted to the main magnesium pressure hull, what we found was that corrosion had been acting unchecked for some considerable time and had actually corroded the hull completely through.

At this point the suit's hull should have been some fifty millimetres thick corrosion had been going on for some considerable time although it has to be remembered that magnesium and seawater are not a good mix, plus, bolting more noble metals onto it in the form of aluminium or stainless-steel only makes matters worse.

It seemed that I had been lucky that the leak had not been much worse! Over the next few days, we did a lot of work on repairing the suit and did get it back to a dive-able state but it was decided to replace it so that it could be fully refurbished properly back at base. We were to be sent a Wasp to replace it, that made perfect sense to me, I was looking forward to seeing the change.

Normal service was soon resumed, as far as we divers were concerned rig support on a drilling rig consisted of quite long periods of not much to do other than a bit of maintenance followed by short periods of feverish activity when the drilling hit a snag as this would need to be sorted in very short order. So, a few days after we had fixed the suit it was decided that Matteo, Adrian and Guido would go ashore and Keith and I would stay for our stint offshore. This was OK with me as I wanted to really get to grips with the suit maintenance and to spend a bit of time learning about atmospheric suits in the offshore real world.

After a few days of this I was happy that I knew the status of the suits and was looking for something to keep me occupied; working offshore in the early eighties would have me reading a lot of books and doing a lot of sleeping and as we were in Sicily a good deal of sunbathing on the helideck. Soon our two weeks were up, we were due to be relieved by Adrian and Guido, Keith and I were ready and waiting as the same helicopter started to ferry the crew off bringing the replacement crew back. We were told to wait until the very end as the helicopter would take us back to its home base which was in Syracusa a town on the east coast of Sicily, this was also where I would be making my home for the time being.

When our turn came, we climbed aboard and off we went, it was great, we were the only two passengers and I was allowed to sit in the co-pilot's seat which put me up in the plexiglass bubble at the front of the chopper, great view. The pilot did speak a little English and just told me not to touch anything! Message received and understood. It was a nice trip taking about half an hour, we flew over beautiful coastline, olive groves and small villages all bathed in wonderful sunshine. We landed at a very sleepy little airfield, there didn't seem to be any administration the pilot just waved us goodbye and off we went to find a taxi into town. Keith had been on the job for a few weeks before I arrived and knew his way around; the taxi took us to the old town on the Isola di Ortigia and dropped us right by the harbour, it was lovely and very picturesque.

Keith was at the time living in a small hotel right on the harbourside and luckily, they had another room for me, as soon as I had dropped my bag in the room Keith suggested we head into town for something to eat, this sounded good to me so off we went. The hotel was very close to the town centre so we didn't have far to go, Keith had a favourite Trattoria (restaurant to you and me) where they sold wonderful Pizza and of course nice cold beers, terrific. We had a lovely relaxed evening, I resolved to explore the old town properly the next day.

The next day Keith agreed to come with me, we left the hotel at about nine o'clock, the hotel was on the harbour front with just a quite road between the two; it was a beautiful morning with almost no wind and was very warm for April. After we had wandered along the harbourside with Keith pointing out the ferry terminal serving ferries to Malta. Keith was into guns having represented the RAF at Bisley where he had won several trophies; he was very keen to show me points where he said there was evidence of gun-shot damage on the buildings from when the Allies had fought the Germans and Italians during the war. We spent a couple of hours wandering along the harbourside and generally around the Isola so that I could get my bearings, Keith took me to a lovely little square called Largo Aretusa, in the centre was a legendary spring and fountain powered naturally from an Artesian well, Keith told me this fountain was very significant for the ancient Greeks?

According to Greek mythology, the fresh water fountain is the place where the nymph Arethusa, the patron figure of ancient Syracusa, returned to earth's surface after escaping from her undersea home in Arcadia. The whole place certainly had a wonderful atmosphere, we approached the spring across cobbled streets with the sea to our right tiny streets leading off to the left, the buildings were clearly very old, the Greek inventor and mathematician Archimedes had lived in Syracusa and it was through these very streets that he reputedly ran naked screaming Eureka! Meaning 'I've found it' apparently, he was so happy because he had just worked out how he could prove whether the king's crown was made out of gold or some other cheaper metal; I expect his neighbours probably stopped what they were doing when this was going on, shrugged their shoulders and muttered something along the lines of "It's just that nutter next door again!" Just around the corner from this square was the Via Capodieci where we found another little bar that became my local while I was living in Syracusa, all was well with my world.

Over the next few weeks, we managed to find a much more suitable two-bedroom flat in a complex just a couple of miles away from the old town; I had discussed transport with Adrian and it was decided that we would buy a cheap car between us, we only needed one as either Adrian or I would be on the rig at any time so the other would have use of the car. Eventually and with Matteo's help we purchased a Simca 1000 LS; this was a truly awful car but as we only needed a cheap run around it served the purpose admirably. We spent a lot of time in this car visiting areas of interest including Mount Etna and lots of Roman and Greek ruins so it did us proud; after I had left, I met up with Adrian who told me that the Carabinieri had confiscated the car as evidently, we weren't authorised to own a car in Italy?

After our two weeks on the beach Keith and I made our way back to the rig to relieve Adrian and Guido again, it was clear that Adrian had been on top of all the maintenance so there was very little for me to do, I was bored!

Working offshore on an Italian rig with a largely Italian crew had a few oddities the first of which came to light not long after I had arrived, Keith and I were the only divers on the rig with Adrian, Guido and Matteo having gone ashore. In the morning, I left the accommodation to check out the dive system and carry out the daily checks, but, as I walked out on deck there was a weird silence. Normally there would be engines running and a lot of noise from the drill floor above our dive station; this morning though there didn't seem to be anything going on? This was very strange, I decided to check it out but couldn't find any of the deck crew to ask, even the bosun was absent and this was unheard of!

Eventually I decided to head for the galley and sure enough everyone seemed to be there; I saw the bosun who was a good friend by then and knowing he spoke English should be able to clue me in on what was going on. I sat at his table with a cup of coffee and asked the question; he laughed and told me the crew were all on strike! I had never heard of anyone offshore going on strike and indeed the very idea would not have been contemplated in the North Sea in those days anyway. He told me that Saipem operated the rig to the same standards as onshore facilities and this meant that they were heavily unionised; evidently the onshore facilities were on strike for some reason and the offshore crew had come out in sympathy.

Nobody seemed to be the least bit phased by this at all, there must have been negotiations happening somewhere and by the end of the day everyone was back at work, very odd. I later learned that the offshore crew were paid at a similar rate to the onshore personnel and seemed to feel that it was their right to strike fairly regularly; indeed, they did this a few times in the four months I was there.

There were other times when work on the rig would come to a halt, for instance, I was again offshore over Easter, Easter Sunday that year was April 19th, around lunchtime we were made aware that our presence was required in the galley. When we got there, we were seated amongst virtually the whole day crew and the Camp Boss paraded a huge cake around; he then proceeded to cut the cake and distribute a chunk to everyone there. We were each treated to a very large tot of Whiskey and a great deal of Bon Homie; it was a nice day but I don't think a lot of work was done after lunch certainly not by the divers!

Something that really brought home to us how religious Italy was happened in May 1981 I was again offshore with Keith when everything again came to a standstill; Pope John Paul II had been shot! He had been hit twice and a couple of bystanders had also been hit. The Pope was taken to hospital where he underwent a five-hour operation, it was touch and go for a while; the rig was at a standstill with most of the crew sitting in front of the TV until the Pope was deemed to be out of danger.

Again, I was offshore on the twenty-ninth of July 1981 when Prince Charles married Lady Diana Spencer. It seemed that the Italians had a great fondness for all things Royal, this again was to me odd as they had done away with their royal family by referendum when they became a republic in 1946 ending King Umberto's 34-day reign as king. Umberto at first refused to accept what he called "the outrageous illegality" of the referendum, and took his deposition badly. Can't say I blame him. Anyway, on the day of the wedding again, I went out on deck to do the daily checks to again find everything silent. I just thought the crew had gone out on strike again but when I went for a cup of coffee Keith caught me and told me to come along to the TV room with him. When we arrived, the room was packed with Italian crew all watching the wedding on TV, I was stunned that this had been allowed to halt work on the rig but when in Rome and all that, we settled down to watch.

Sunday afternoons were often quite quiet especially when Ferrari were racing in the Formula One World Championship, a lot of the crew would down tools to watch the race and indeed a lot of them would also stop to watch Moto GP (in the guise it was in those days).

Soon Keith and I were back on the beach again, and I was looking for something to do, I saw that there were a lot of people windsurfing in the large enclosed bay on the south side of Syracusa and so I set about looking for somewhere that I could learn to windsurf. Given I now had access to our wonderful staff car, I headed out on the Via Elorina the coast road running alongside the beach to the south of the town.

I soon saw a sign with a windsurfer image on the left side of the road, there was an arrow pointing along a small unmetalled track. This track obviously did not carry much traffic and was in a poor state of repair. There were a lot of potholes and random rocks strewn about, the Simca was not an especially luxurious vehicle and I think it would be fair to say the suspension had seen better days, I went along the track at little more than walking pace, eventually I came across another sign signifying that I had reached the school. I parked up in what looked like it might be an area meant for cars just to the right-hand side of a one-story building. I got out of the car and started to look for someone that, might be working there, the building had been constructed from concrete blocks covered in white painted render although it has to be said the decoration had clearly been done some time ago and the place looked to be due for another coat of paint! The roof consisted to rusty corrugated iron with no gutters at all.

Built along the side of the building there was a wire mesh construction secured with a padlock, this was being used to house a number of windsurfers and their sails. The building had a couple of small windows with a door in the middle of the wall facing the car park; I wandered over and knocked on the door; there was no immediate answer so I walked around the building. As I walked past the cage containing the windsurfers, I came to a wonderful beach, looking left and right I could see that it ran for about a mile in either direction. The beach was bordered by wooded areas I was impressed, there was nobody on the beach at all, I turned left and walked along the beach front of the school's building where there was another door; this door was open, inside I could see an athletic looking man.

I tentatively approached, once he noticed me, he stopped what he was doing and came out onto the beach with me; I went through the normal, do you speak English with predictable results so we had to converse with gestures and signs. He was quite good at this I had the feeling this might not be his first time of being approached by an English idiot who didn't speak any Italian. Anyway, I was able to take him around the building to the windsurfer cage where I was able to get through to him that I was interested in learning how to windsurf; eventually it became clear that he was in fact one of the school's instructors and he was game to take me on. He helped me to choose an appropriate windsurfer and rig (mast, boom and sail), he then showed me how to rig it, I spent the next hour or so with Carlo (we had been able to swap names by this time) he showed me how to stand on the board and what to do to make it move.

It was now time to take the windsurfer and my new knowledge into the sea, the beach was perfect for this, it was very shallow shelving very gently, the wind was enough but not too much, it was coming off the beach which meant there were very few waves, we spent the next couple of hours with me trying to pull the mast up and to then bring the boom around so that I could move forward. Despite my surfing background I found this quite difficult but soon realised it was because I was working against the wind and not using it properly, the instructor was very good and patient and despite not speaking English he soon got me sailing. My main memory of this was Carlo standing in the shallows with the water up to his knees bellowing inoltrare (forward) when I needed to push the mast forward, this would push the bow of the board down wind and Indeitro (backward) when I needed to pull the mast backward, this would bring the bow of the board back up into the wind.

He was brilliant and after a couple of lessons I was given a key so that I could come and go as I pleased and borrow the windsurfer whenever I wanted, I used to go and practice with the boards whenever I could and over the next few weeks became quite proficient.

The next couple of months came and went with me rotating offshore where I spent most of my time carrying out daily checks on the JIM suits, servicing legs and arms as necessary, when I was ashore, I spent a lot of time windsurfing, in the main I had a great summer. During one of my stints offshore with Keith and Matteo the client asked us to go and have a look at the tide gauges on the rig legs, this would just involve one of us swimming over and taking a couple of readings, the gauges were at a depth of some ten feet so this would be a simple little job. Keith was up for doing the dive and I would be his tender/standby diver; we would be lowered through the rig's main moonpool using the dive basket.

The plan was for me to stay in the basket, Keith would swim away from the basket, to go and do the job. Initially the basket would be lowered into the water so that we were immersed up to our chests, then Keith would leave the basket and Matteo would raise the basket out of the water so that I was just a couple of feet above the water while Keith was off doing the job. All went fine to begin with, Keith who was using a KMB 18 hat, left the basket, I was lifted to a couple of feet above the sea, it was a bright sunny, flat calm day so all was good. After no more than twenty minutes Keith was back at the basket and indicated to me that he was ready to get back in the basket; I had a walkie talkie with which to contact Matteo but, I couldn't get any response.

I told Keith to try talking to Matteo via the diver's communications, Keith clearly did this but he could not get any response from dive control either? After about fifteen minutes of trying to raise Matteo without success I managed to attract the attention of one of the rig's deck crew who was peering over the edge of the moonpool and got him to drop the basket enough so that Keith could climb back in. We were then lifted back to deck level and were able to transfer from the basket onto the deck, I thanked the crewman and started to undress Keith. Once this was done, I left Keith to break down the diving equipment and went to look for Matteo; I was not in a very good mood; this wasn't improved when it became clear that there was nobody at the dive control at all? After another few minutes I was able to locate Matteo, he had apparently abandoned us to go to the radio room! We had words as I didn't think it was appropriate to leave divers in the water swanning off to the radio room, he made some lame excuse but realised that I was not impressed at all. Good job we didn't have an emergency!

Eventually we were told the planned suit change was going to take place, as I said it was not going to be like for like, as Oceaneering had convinced AGIP that a Wasp would be more appropriate for the type of work required. This was fine and before long we were told that the replacement suit had arrived in Catania. This was great news but it was not plain sailing at all, it seemed that there was some doubt about what was in the crate. At this time Matteo was on leave and so was not available to help sort out the issue; this meant that the suit could not pass-through customs until he came back! After a couple of weeks Matteo returned and got to grips with negotiating release of the suit; he was able to resolve the issues very quickly, not sure how? When he arrived on board with the Wasp, he told us that the customs officers had opened the crate and seeing a large yellow painted cylinder they thought it was a bomb!

In July a Self-Elevating platform (normally known as Jack-Up rig) took up residence about a mile away to the east of us; Jack up drilling rigs were used principally for shallow water work but could work in water depths of up to about 250 feet. They differ from the semi-submersible rigs in that although they were floated onto location, once there they lowered legs onto the seabed, then the legs would be jacked up raising the hull out of the water. Once this had been done the rig would give a stable platform from which drilling operations would be carried out. The legs would not be anchored to the seabed in any way other than by gravity. Because of this there was a danger of the legs being undermined by scour (seabed removal). For this reason, Jack up Drilling rigs must have the legs carefully inspected looking for scour, it is quite common for divers to be employed to go and look at the base of the legs. The diver assessing scour would normally lie on the seabed alongside any depression near the leg, topside would then take the depth using the diver's pneumo; the diver would then move to the bottom of the scoured depression next to the leg where their depth would again be checked using the pneumo. This would give the depth of the scour around the leg and can be used to assess the rigs continued stability.

The rig alongside us was called 'Black Dog' and had no divers of their own, Matteo told us that we would be transferring our equipment onto the jack up and would be carrying out scour checks for them. We had the capability to do this as we had Heliox and all the necessary equipment, the main issue was that the team had not actually done any wet diving together so, it was decided we should carry out a 'work up' dive prior to moving the equipment. This would allow us to practice the required procedures and would help with making sure that when we moved to the Black Dog the dives would go without a hitch. I was to be the diver and the plan was to use this dive to check the Scarabeo 4's marine riser during the dive, all's good, I dressed in and was quite soon ready for the dive, I was using a Rat Hat and would be breathing Heliox for the deeper part of the dive, the dive was due to be to a maximum depth of one hundred and fifty feet, the plan was for me to carry out surface decompression.

Well, all went to plan when I entered the water, at forty feet I was paused in the basket while my gas was changed from air to Heliox for the main part of the dive. I told Adrian that I was ready for the gas changeover he then informed me I was on Heliox, I opened the free flow valve to flush the air out of the umbilical. Quite soon I heard a change in the sound of gas entering the hat which signified that air had gone and had now been replaced by Heliox the change was due to the density differences between air and Heliox. Once this had taken place, I told topside that I had Heliox, I was then authorised to carry on with the dive, I left the basket and made my way down the marine riser checking that all looked as it should, this went without a hitch and quite soon I was on my way back up. I completed all my in-water decompression as required and was subsequently brought to the surface in the basket, when I arrived on deck the crew didn't seem in any hurry to help me get my equipment off, I was being left to do it by myself.

I said to Adrian, "Come on mate, I've got to get in the chamber". He said "Why, are you doing surface decompression?" "Yes, I am", Adrian, and the others then jumped to it and I did get into the chamber and down to depth within the allotted surface interval time so all ended well. When I eventually managed to talk to Adrian, he told me that Matteo had not told the crew that Surface Decompression was being done, good old Matteo. I decided that following this and the previous issue where Keith and I had been left hanging in the moonpool the next time I was ashore I would call Ian Little to express my concerns.

The next day we transferred ourselves and all our equipment onto the waiting supply boat, we were taken to the Black Dog where we set up our dive spread ready to carry out scour checks in the morning. We settled into our accommodation and set off to find the galley; when we found it, I was amazed to find there was a pool table there, I was not expecting that but then thinking about it we were not afloat and as the rig would not move a pool table was a logical recreational piece of kit I suppose. Eventually, having had our supper and relaxed all evening I found my way to my bunk, I then proceeded to have the worst night I think I have ever had I don't think I got any sleep at all. The air conditioning in the accommodation did not seem to be working at all and with the mattresses being covered in black PVC, these two facts led to us all sweating profusely and not being able to settle; as I say it was possibly the most uncomfortable night I've experienced; I remember thinking, I hope we're not on here long.

The next morning, we were ready to start scour checks on the Black Dog's legs, my turn came around at about half past four in the afternoon. The depth of the dive was to be around two hundred and thirty feet (70 metres), this was too deep for air so I would again be breathing Heliox with an oxygen percentage of ten percent (ninety percent helium).

We had worked out that ten percent oxygen would provide a partial pressure of oxygen of 0.8 Bar Absolute (BA) when on the seabed at the working depth, this would be absolutely fine. However, as before if I were to breathe ten percent oxygen on deck the partial pressure, I would be breathing would be just 0.1 BA. Not enough oxygen and I would lose consciousness.

So as before, I would start the dive breathing air, would be lowered to forty feet (12 metres) on air, halt the descent where my breathing gas would be changed over to the ten percent Heliox mix. At forty feet the ambient pressure being higher the ten percent mix would provide a PpO$_2$ of 0.22 BA which is of course fine. We would be carrying out surface decompression using oxygen as we did before. I had been involved in the brief and everyone knew the process and their duties, all good.

I was now ready to dive, I had dressed and was again using a Rat Hat, I had carried out all my surface checks and was given the go ahead to enter the basket. As soon as I was in the basket Matteo confirmed that I would be leaving deck level and off I went. The day was again beautiful with bright sunshine, the sea was flat calm, as I was lowered to the surface of the water, I again had a good view of the underside of the rig and the three legs disappearing into the water. As I reached the water, I told Matteo "Leaving surface", I continued to drop down in the basket until the topside crew measured my depth as forty feet, the basket stopped and I was told that they were changing over the gases. I opened the free flow valve to drain my umbilical of air, as before I was listening to the flow of gas and quite soon heard the expected change in pitch of the sound made by the gas entering the hat, I took a couple of breaths and then spoke to confirm I was breathing Heliox and once confirmed I told topside I was ready to continue the descent.

The basket started its descent again, it was very pleasant as the water was very clear and I could see lots of fish that seemed to be keeping pace with me. Quite soon the bottom hove into view and while I was still some five metres above the seabed, I told topside to halt the basket, I left the basket through the side so that I wouldn't lose my way back and made my way across to the leg; I could see that there had indeed been significant scour. Matteo told me to lay on the seabed at the top of the scour for them to take the first measurement. As I lay on the seabed topside put gas through my pneumo hose, as soon as I felt bubbles coming out, I said, "I have bubbles" after a couple of minutes I was told that they had the depth and was asked to go down into the deepest part of the scour pit and lie next to the leg at the bottom of the pit. I wandered over and down into the scour pit where there was soft mud resulting in all the visibility disappearing, I laid down at the bottom of the pit right next to the metal leg where we repeated the pneumo process allowing topside to measure the depth at the bottom of the scour pit; once these readings had been taken the depth of scour was known allowing the engineers to assess the rigs stability, I was told to move back to the basket and make ready to leave bottom.

When I had confirmed I was in the basket and ready to leave bottom the visibility was again wonderful, I was in deep blue water with a number of small fish shoaling around. I felt the basket start to rise and watched as the seabed fell away from me, as I was rising through the water column, I was accompanied by a huge shoal of sardines that seemed intent of staying with me. The shoal looked great, as each fish turned sunlight would reflect off its scales so there were thousands of tiny flashes of light all around me, it was lovely and kept me amused all the way up to my last in-water stop at forty feet.

The basket stopped and I was told I had some forty minutes at this stop; this was normal and for me it was no issue, I was in a wet suit in fairly warm water, I had lots of gas to breathe so I just had to sit back and relax. The first thing I had to do was flush my umbilical again as I had now been switched back to air, this went smoothly and I confirmed I was back on air as soon as I had heard the change of pitch.

Normal practice when undertaking surface decompression with the diver being recovered in a basket like this was for the diver to remove the majority of their equipment while they were at their last water stop waiting to be recovered. The first items I took off were my fins which I hung on a lanyard provided for this purpose, the lanyard was attached to the top frame of the basket on my right with a carabiner at the loose end. I passed the lanyard through each of the fin straps clipping it back on itself leaving the fins to dangle from the lanyard just to the right of my head, I continued to take off as much of my equipment as I could until all I had left on was the hat, bail-out bottle and of course my wet suit.

There were still about twenty minutes to wait at the stop so I sat back and contented myself with watching the sardines, there really were thousands of them all milling around just in front of me. The visibility was now magnificent at about thirty or forty metres so I could see all of the Black Dog's legs, where I could see some larger fish swimming around the legs, it was a lovely vista and very reminiscent of the Jacques Cousteau programmes of old. Suddenly the whole sardine shoal seemed to polarise such that they were all facing in the same direction, then they shot off leaving me on my own. Now, as I may have said before we are blessed with a wonderful brain which has the ability to add two and two together and come up with five! Well, my imagination went into overdrive; what had spooked that shoal? At that moment an enormous black fin drifted across my field of view!

I took a sharp intake of breath and "Oh…shit!" came out of my mouth as I recoiled into the back of the basket; I then saw that this big black fin was in fact my own fin swinging to and fro on the lanyard! To say the least I felt extremely foolish especially as the topside crew had heard my exclamation and were now asking "What's wrong!" I just said nothing was wrong but I often wonder what they thought. After my stop had been completed, I was brought back to the surface and transferred into the chamber to complete my decompression without any further drama. I would like to say that there was no repeat of anything like this but I'm afraid that from time to time my imagination has got the better of me a couple of times since then.

With the job complete on the Black Dog we transferred all our equipment back to the Scarabeo 4 and life returned to normal. I thought I would call Ian Little to discuss my concerns about Matteo. Oceaneering had access to an agent in Syracusa, I turned up there to make my phone call, eventually I got through to Iain and said "Hi Iain, I just wanted to talk to you about Matteo…" he cut in then and said "yeah, great guy isn't he!" I was taken aback by this response and it was clear he wasn't going to hear anything bad said about Matteo. The phone call achieved nothing, oh well I tried, Adrian and I had already agreed that we had to look after ourselves and the others on the team.

I received a letter from my mum, this was not all that unusual as we were conversing by mail fairly routinely by now but, this letter was very definitely not good; it seemed that my dad had suffered his first heart attack and was recovering in hospital. I hot footed it back to our agent to get access to the phone again and called mum; we had what for us was quite a long call, maybe five minutes. It seemed that dad was recovering well, I asked whether she felt I should come home to see him; she thought that would send the wrong signal to him and that he might feel that I had been told he was about to die, she felt I should stay in Sicily. I was not happy about this as I wanted to see him or talk to him, in those days there was no option to call someone who was in hospital so, I couldn't do anything other than send some flowers and a card; this seemed totally inadequate to me but was all I did. I felt very dismayed when I left the agent's building.

The Scarabeo 4 had completed drilling the hole off Gela and was due to be towed to a new location near Palermo, all the dive team had to be on board when the rig was under tow so off we went. When a semi-submersible rig is drilling it is ballasted down so that the pontoons are at a depth of seventy feet or so, this gives a very stable platform from which to carry out drilling. However, when it is to be towed it is ballasted to raise the rig so that the pontoons are all that is left in the water, this reduces drag and makes the rig easier to tow.

I had not seen this process done before so was interested to see the supply boats moving off to handle the anchors as they of course all needed to be recovered, the Scarabeo 4 had three anchors on each leg, nine in total. Raising these took the best part of a full day, while they were being raised one of the supply boats took up position with a towing line attached to the rig.

Matteo arrived on board to tell me that I would be leaving the job the following week as I was needed in Angola! This took me by surprise as I still had two months to run on my contract but, I was not displeased as I was looking forward to visiting another country and this time also a new continent, Africa, great.

I travelled home directly from the rig which meant that I could not get back to Syracusa to pick up some photos I had in for development but this wasn't a huge problem; just as well I hadn't brought my bike with me to Sicily though wasn't it! I did have all my clothes etc., so didn't really need to go back there, and anyway I was pleased that I would finally be able to see my dad. The trip back went without any issues, I landed in Heathrow in early August to be greeted with a dull dreary day with a fine drizzle falling. Normally this would not be something that was memorable but having been in Sicily for four months, during which time having seen no rain at all it was actually quite nice to see rain again; this feeling wore off quite quickly though!

PHOTOS FROM MY TIME WORKING WITH ATMOSPHERIC DIVING SUITS (ADS)

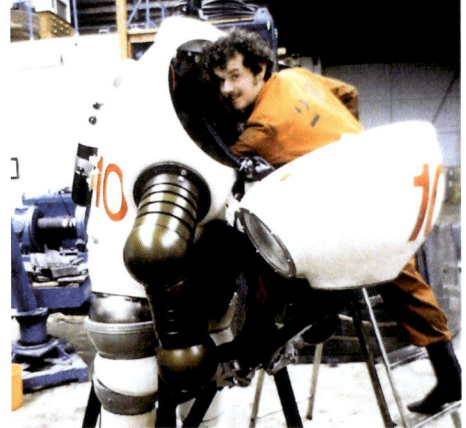

The author climbing into Jim 10 during his atmospheric diving suit (ADS) training course.

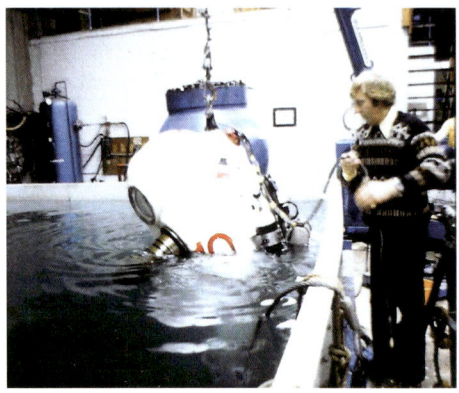

The author being lowered into the training tank at DHB in Alton.

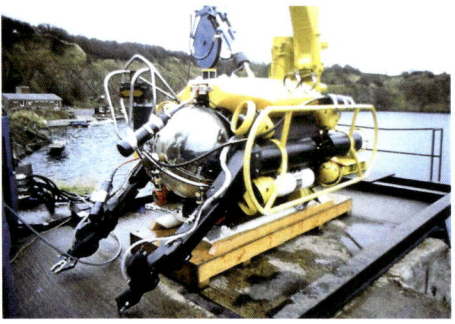

Mantis ADS at Stoney Cove.

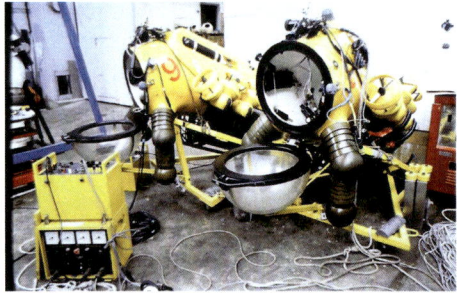

Mk 2 WASPs at DHB in Alton.

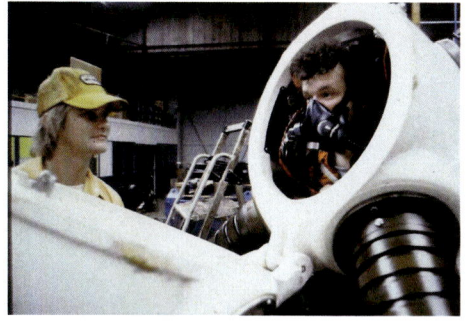

The author in Jim 10 carrying out pre-dive checks.

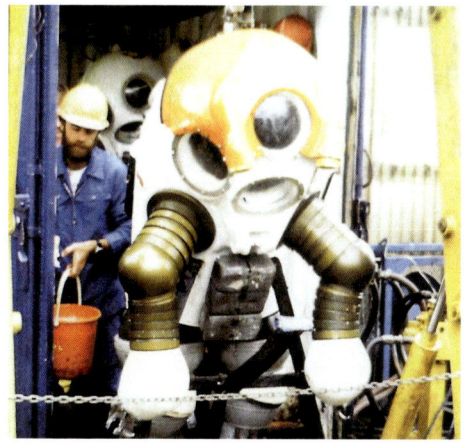

Bill Hayes maintaining the Jim suit on the Nortrol during the author's first offshore trip.

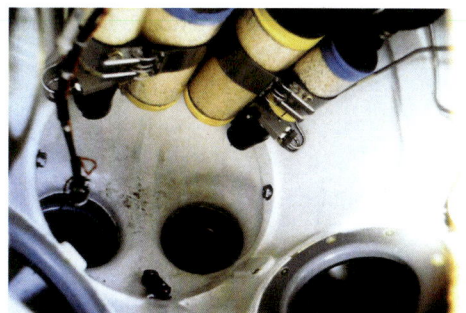

Inside the Jim suit showing canisters of soda lime used to 'scrub' CO_2 out of the diver's breath.

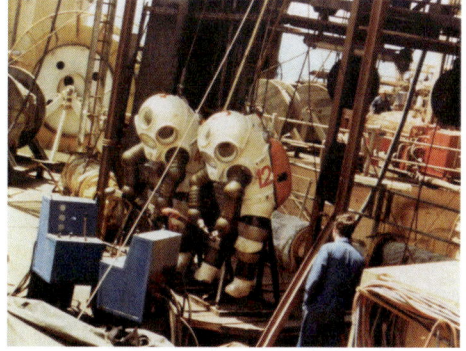

Jim suit dive station on the Scarabeo 4 just off the south coast of Sicily.

CHAPTER TWELVE

First Trip to Africa – 1981

On arrival home in Torquay, I took up where I had left off four months ago, I had one week before I was due to fly out to Angola, I put this time to good use. The first thing I did was to go out to see my dad; I was relieved to find him in very good spirits and in fact he was looking very well. Hopefully, this was just a little blip and he would be fine, he had an appointment with surgeons to discuss him being given a heart valve replacement, it all sounded very positive.

A few days before I was due to leave for Angola, I called Diane to find out my travel details; I was told that my ticket would be left for me at airport information in Heathrow terminal two, I was due to fly to Paris Charles de Gaulle where I would transfer to a UTA flight to Libreville in Gabon (I have to say that at this time I don't think I had heard of Gabon let alone Libreville!). On arrival in Libreville, I would be met and directed where to go for my onward journey; as before this was all suitably vague but I wasn't overly concerned as I was sure I would find my way.

I had a few things to do before I left, I needed a couple of jabs, the first was easy as it was Typhoid and Cholera, in those days I would normally get these jabs at the airport before leaving. I needed anti-malarial tablets for the whole six-week trip, these were available from my GP. The main problem was that I also needed a smallpox vaccination, this was not required for either Gabon or Angola but was a requirement for entry into Zaire (now the Democratic Republic of Congo), I had already applied for and been granted a visa for Zaire while I was in Italy but I was a little confused as I wasn't due to go to Zaire, was I? Diane explained that I would need the ability to travel to Zaire as, apparently, I would from time to time need to go to Kinshasa in Zaire, this would be for the purposes of visa renewal and indeed as Angola was engaged in a civil war at that time Zaire was a safe haven should we need to evacuate quickly!

This now was beginning to feel a little more uncertain but as I was in my mid-twenties, I was sure, I would cope with whatever was thrown at me I just chose to ignore any concerns as again, what could possibly go wrong? Well, it seemed that the Smallpox vaccine was not available locally so I would need to travel to Hampshire to get it, not only would I need to travel there but I would need proof of my need as the world health organisation had officially branded Smallpox as eradicated, it was just that nobody had told Zaire and they still had this down as a requirement before entry would be allowed!

Given that emails and indeed faxes were still not even being dreamt of it was decided that the vaccination centre would accept a telegram from Oceaneering. Diane told me that this was not a problem and would be provided the following day. I travelled up to Hampshire on my bike and was sitting in the waiting room of a fairly non-descript health centre, it didn't look anything special but I had been told was one of the very few places in the UK still authorised to offer Smallpox vaccinations.

The doctor asked me a number of questions about my health and previous vaccination history all of which seemed to satisfy him and so he gave me the shot; I was told not to get the injection site wet for at least a week this could be tricky given my job but I told him I would do my best. He then decided that as I hadn't had a Polio immunisation since I was a kid that I should have another one of these too. When I had been given the Polio vaccine before, it had been given to me on a sugar cube but of course now being an adult, I was given the vaccine directly dripped onto my tongue, Yuk!

So, it was on the eighth of August I said goodbye to Torquay again and travelled by rail up to Heathrow airport, I went immediately to the medical centre where I was provided with the Cholera and Typhoid vaccination, I was told to avoid alcohol for a day! I then found my way to airport information where my ticket was available, all good although it was a one-way ticket, I had been told that this would be the case and was not a problem as the return ticket would be purchased when it was clear which route, I would be taking for my journey home; hmm, OK?

My flight to Paris was via British Airways and on arrival I saw that I had plenty of time to find the UTA desk for check in. I had no bags to check in as again I had been told that when travelling in Africa it was best to travel light; this turned out to be very good advice. Quite soon I was settled into my seat on an UTA McDonnel Douglas DC-10 for the flight to Libreville. It was a very nice flight and the French cabin crew looked after me very well although in those days the in-flight meals were not as good as they are now and as for entertainment well, that didn't exist really so I settled in with my book and off we went. The flight time was about seven and a half hours and was overnight, we arrived early in the morning; I must say I was quite excited I was looking forward to my first glimpse of Africa.

As is the norm with any flight everyone stood up immediately the flight came to a standstill which I never do, it seems crazy to me to be standing in the aisle for sometimes fifteen or twenty minutes before the doors are opened, but that is what the majority of people seemed to want to do and still do today don't they?

Eventually the doors were opened and we started filing out of the plane, as I emerged from the door at the top of the steps I was assaulted by a sudden hit of high humidity and heat; it was still dark, nevertheless it was stifling; there was a wonderful smell of damp vegetation, it was unlike anything I had experience before; wonderful I loved it.

The plane was positioned some hundred metres from the terminal building; in Africa in those days there would be no such thing as busses to ferry passengers to the terminal we would all be expected to walk to the terminal. I made my way down the steps; I was now starting to wonder what I should do next Diane's directions had again been vague to say the least telling me I would be met, but where? After looking around for a few minutes to see whether there was anyone waving a board or something, I decided that as I couldn't see anyone I should follow the rest of the passengers to passport control, I was in the midst of the passengers so I had to wait in line for a good twenty minutes although there were a lot of people behind me. When I arrived at passport control the African guard took my passport and spent a few minutes looking through all the pages, I was not really concerned at this point and started to look around.

The arrivals hall was as you would expect, a large, mainly featureless room painted in a non-descript light grey with lots of extensive spider's webs in the corners, eventually the border guard seemed to come to a decision. He kept my passport and pointed to me indicating that I should stand to one side while he dealt with the other passengers. Hmm, this didn't seem so good; I was left standing there until all the other passengers had been processed, then the guard looked around and beckoned another uniformed individual over, this chap was enormous, he was dressed as a soldier carrying a sinister looking rifle. It became clear that I should follow him although this was all done by gesture, they didn't seem to feel they wanted to converse with me not that I thought I would understand their language even if they did want to chat.

The three of us left the arrival's hall with the official keeping my passport, I was shown into a small, windowless room that smelt of body odour and other nasty odours. In the centre of the room was a table that had been bolted to the floor, the only other furniture were two chairs, the original border guard gestured for me to sit, he then had a short conversation with the soldier who spent most of that time looking at me in a bored manner. The border guard then left; with the soldier standing guard just inside the door; I sat on one of the chairs facing the door putting my bag on the floor beside me; I settled in to spend time contemplating my situation.

Clearly this hadn't gone well, I had done something wrong although at the time I had no idea what that was. The soldier clearly was not going to enter into any dialogue with me although even if he had wanted to, I doubted we had a common language anyway; I settled back to wait, I had a bottle of water so was reasonably comfortable although very hot and more than a little concerned. I was left like this for some three hours with the only break in the monotony being when the soldier was relieved by another equally big and well-armed individual.

I was of course by now very apprehensive as to what fate was awaiting me; eventually the door opened and in stepped an harassed looking individual. I was relieved to see he was a white man and hoped he would speak at least some English he was wearing a creased white, sweat soaked shirt with the UTA logo above the left breast. He took the seat opposite me and started with. "What the hell are you doing here?" I thought this was a strange opener as I would have thought he would know what I was doing there, but, still, never mind at least he spoke English. I explained my story which seemed to make him angrier, apparently, I should not have gone through passport control as my onward journey was supposed to involve me transferring to another smaller plane on the tarmac without going anywhere near the terminal! I should have been told that I was to wait on the tarmac at the bottom of the planes steps where someone would have come to get me to take me to the other plane.

He told me that the other plane had left already and so I was stranded here and not only that but had attempted to gain entry to Gabon without the necessary visa! Ah, well that would be the problem then! This did nothing to reassure me though, I was becoming very worried as to what he would tell me next. When he paused for breath, I asked him what was going to happen to me; he rolled his eyes and in a matter-of-fact way he proceeded to tell me that I would be arrested and would be deported on the next available flight. I thought that meant that I would be sent back to France but no, apparently, I would have to wait a few days until there was another flight to Angola.

He stood up and had a brief conversation with the soldier, then turning back to me he told me to follow him, all three of us walked out into the arrivals hall where we were joined by another soldier. I was almost frogmarched out of the terminal building where there was a waiting police car, I was roughly shoved into the back seat where I sat with my bag on my lap, I was sandwiched between soldiers either side of me and the UTA guy got in the front seat.

We then left the airport, nobody seemed at all interested in telling me where I was being taken and I must confess to feeling more than a little worried at this time; the level of body odour in the back of that car was overpowering; as we drove out of the airport, at the first roundabout we headed left towards the town which was signposted albeit in French although I now had enough French to be able to make out that we were heading for Centre Ville. I was expecting the car to drive to the nearest police station or some other jail where I would be incarcerated for the necessary few days, I was not over confident that this would be any fun at all. After about half an hour we were travelling along a small road next to a beach with coconut palms between the road and the sea; in other circumstances it would have been idyllic.

The UTA guy then tapped the driver on the shoulder and pointed to a hotel on the left, the driver turned into the hotel parking area and pulled up beneath a portico. Mr UTA got out of the car and so did the soldier to my right, I was invited to also get out, the three of us then entered the hotel, approaching the reception desk Mr UTA spoke to the receptionist and after a few moments he handed me a room key; he told me that I was under house arrest and should under no circumstances leave the hotel.

As soon as he finished telling me this, he turned on his heal and left together with the guard, I was stunned, after what had been a stressful day, here I was standing in the foyer of a fairly nice hotel in a country where apparently, I was illegally and I had been left with a room to use? I was then taken to the room by a bell boy, I had no money so couldn't give him a tip but then I had virtually no luggage so all he had to do was bring me to the door I suppose. This was Sunday early evening and I was not feeling at all well either as was often the case following Typhoid and Cholera vaccination particularly when I had partaken of some alcoholic beverages on the flight despite being advised against taking alcohol, I just got my head down and fell asleep.

The next day, I was up bright and breezy for breakfast which was a lovely buffet served in an open area that looked out over beautiful gardens, and swimming pool. I had to pinch myself to check I wasn't dreaming! When the bill came, I had been told to sign everything to the room; I wasn't worried about this as I had a credit card that I could use to settle the bill at the end of the stay. I decided that I needed to try to let Oceaneering know that I was OK and to try to find out whether I still had a job; I went to reception and found someone who spoke passable English, he told me that the hotel had a Telex machine and he would be able to send a Telex for me. I thanked him and sat in the foyer composing my apologetic telex to be sent; I gave this to the receptionist and he assured me that it would be sent that day.

I spent the rest of the day relaxing by the pool with a couple of beers followed by a nice lunch and a nap it was really like being on holiday other than the worry I had as to what Oceaneering would make of it all. I was worried that effectively from their point of view I just hadn't turned up on the job and I felt this could never be a good thing; still, I was under arrest and could do nothing about it. The day was rounded off with a nice meal of roasted antelope (another first for me) and a couple more local beers, all in all a bit of a result.

Tuesday dawned and I thought I should try to find out what was happening; I decided I would walk into town and try to find Oceaneering's agent. As it turned out Oceaneering didn't have anyone in Gabon at the time but the Gulf oil company that were running the oilfield in Angola did. I was conscious of the fact that I had been told not to leave the hotel but nobody seemed to be keeping tabs on me so I just walked out; I had a small tourist map from the hotel, it showed clearly that I was only a couple of miles from the centre of Libreville. I walked back to the road that we had come in on from the airport where I turned left which I thought would take me into town; It was a lovely day, although the sky was overcast, I later came to realise that this was normal for this part of the world but, it was very warm.

I was walking along the road, the sea was off to my right and looked serene although there seemed to be a fairly large swell running, between me and the sea there was a narrow fine sandy/gravelly beach and a stand of coconut palms, it was lovely. To my left there was nothing much, probably now there would be a lot more hotels but at the time there was just what looked to me like virgin forest with lots of colourful birds none of which I could identify other than I thought they looked like parrots and were pretty. After about half an hour walking, I found myself on the outskirts of town, it had the feel of a frontier town with just a few cars and dusty pavements running intermittently along the sides of the roads. There didn't seem to be many shops as far as I could see but there was a market where people were grouping buying food, clothes and almost everything else; it was for me a real eye opener and a great introduction to Africa.

I had been given an address by the hotel receptionist who had marked the location on my map, the map I had was actually not at all bad and led me straight to the building I was looking for. I entered and found a list of companies on the wall, this told me where the office for Gulf Oil could be found, I climbed the stairs to the first floor where I knocked on a door sporting a Gulf Oil sticker.

I was invited to enter where I was greeted by a local lady receptionist who, luckily spoke English, she told me to take a seat and went to find someone who could answer my questions. After about five minutes she returned and told me to sit and wait; after another fifteen minutes or so I was told to go upstairs where I should knock on the first door on the right. After my first, timid knock I heard someone inside but didn't hear an invitation to enter so I decided to knock a little harder. This worked and I heard a gruff voice with an American accent call me in, I poked my head around the door and was told to come in and sit down.

I didn't get the chaps name but it seemed that he was in contact with the office in Angola and knew my story; he reiterated that I should have waited on the tarmac and should not have tried to enter Gabon, he didn't seem overly angry about the situation but was concerned that I had not been given information by Oceaneering. I asked what he wanted me to do and he said that there was another flight leaving at midday on Wednesday and I should make every effort to be on that; I asked him where the flight would take me and was told that it would take me to Malongo in Angola which was the nearest airfield to Cabinda where the oilfield was situated that Oceaneering was looking after. I thanked him and was dismissed; I walked back to the hotel where I found a note from UTA informing me that somebody would be at the hotel at ten o'clock the following morning and I should be ready to leave with them; this sounded positive but meant that not only did I still have a job but I also had another day at the hotel, I concentrated on relaxing with a few more beers and lunch by the pool.

The next day I was in the hotel foyer at the allotted time, I had tried to settle the bill but the receptionist told me that the bill had been taken care of already? To this day I have no idea who picked up the tab for my stay but, I am very grateful. Mr UTA turned up at ten o'clock on the dot, he was alone and without any preamble presented me with my passport, I was loaded into his car and taken back to the airport where I was quickly ushered through passport control and out onto the tarmac to find a small executive jet waiting. There were other people already seated in a very small cabin, I couldn't even stand upright but there was a seat waiting for me, as soon as I was seated the door closed and we were off.

The plane was very comfortable but the flight was short, only about forty-five minutes in the air I think; very soon we were coming in to land; I could see a great number of small tripod structures; with a few larger structures these structures are commonly termed 'jackets' as they surround at least one oil well. These jackets were out to sea just south of the airport, on our final approach to the airport, we flew over a fair-sized town.

Once on the ground the door was opened and everyone got off, we all walked over to a very dilapidated terminal building, here we had to go through passport control where we were all required to surrender our passports. Now I was in an African country in the midst of a civil war and I didn't even have my passport, to say I was nervous would be an understatement; I was assured by the Americans who were arriving with me who had clearly been through this process dozens of times before that all was well and we would be given our passports back two weeks before we were due to leave. During my next leave period I applied for and was issued with a Seaman's card, this was an alternative to a passport and at the time could be used as a substitute, at least I would be ready if things went pear shaped in the future. Anyway, as I was due to do a six-week trip I thought that maybe this would be OK, we would see.

Once passports had been collected, we were all herded through to another very dilapidated room where there were several trestle tables arranged in a line, behind which there were four guards/officials who were clearly waiting for us. I watched the others to see what was expected of me and it seemed that the officials wanted to look in our bags; OK that wouldn't be a problem for me at all. As I reached the table, I swung my bag up and plonked it down, I pulled the zip across revealing the contents; as you know I was a keen photographer and had a nice camera with me, it was a Canon A-1. As the zip opened the camera was there right on top. The guard looked delighted and grabbed it, just as he was hauling it out of the bag an arm came over my shoulder brandishing a pack of twenty Marlborough cigarettes which were waved under the guard's nose, the promise of twenty American cigarettes was clearly an attractive proposition for the guard and a much better prospect than a camera so he went to grab the packet. A short tug of war ensued between the guard and the owner of the pack of Marlborough's, it was clear that neither was going to let go.

The American who had offered the cigarettes pointed to my camera. the guard nodded and gave my camera to the American behind me who then released the pack of cigarettes; the guard looked chuffed with himself and waved my bag away. The guy who now had my camera gave it straight back to me and told me that whenever I came through any sort of official bag search area that I should ensure there were at least one or two packs of Marlborough cigarettes on top, all would then go well as once the guards had their cigarettes, they would be happy to let the bag go unmolested. Well, another lesson learned and while I didn't smoke, I resolved to get hold of some packs so that I could pack properly. Soon everyone had passed through the bag check and the guards retired with their booty to smoke themselves to death, although, I later learned that an unopened pack of Marlborough was really currency and was worth a lot to them.

We were ushered through the terminal which was tiny and little more than a couple of large rooms with a series of stations set up inside for passport and bag checks. When we were all through, we congregated on a forecourt outside where there was an orange painted American school bus parked, all my travelling companions who clearly knew the drill started boarding the bus and I followed; I found a seat next to the guy who had helped me with the bag check. He turned out to be a very helpful and friendly chap who was one of the oil company's crew, they were working four weeks on and four off. As the bus pulled away, we chatted and he told me that American cigarettes were almost legal tender in Angola, it seemed you could buy almost anything with them.

The local currency was the Kwanza but evidently, it was not worth the paper it was printed on; he told me that I could buy a pack of two hundred Marlborough at the bar on the camp, this would be sold to me tax free so that it would cost me just a couple of UK Pounds, I could then sell them to any of the locals for a thousand Kwanzas these could then be used to purchase beers in the camp bar and would be enough to last a whole six-week trip! I resolved to do this at the first opportunity and in fact I purchased four hundred so that I had some for seeding my bag on the journey home as well.

The airfield was some distance from the Gulf compound at Cabinda so I settled back to see what Angola was like, Malongo was bordered to the north by Gabon and Zaire to the east and south; Malongo was in fact a very small enclave separated from the main part of Angola off to the south, by a narrow band of land running along the banks of the Congo River, this land was part of Zaire, giving Zaire access to the sea which was of course very important. The town of Malongo turned out to be quite large it had been built by the Portuguese when Angola was one of their colonies.

It seemed that pre-independence Malongo had been a great tourist destination for the Portuguese, how life changes? There were certainly no tourists now, as we were driven through the town, we drove down nice wide tree lined boulevards, I saw great arcades of shops all empty with smashed windows, lovely town squares, piazzas with dry fountains and even a beautiful open air swimming pool that looked like it could have been Olympic size complete with diving boards and heaps of broken sun loungers piled both alongside and in the bottom of the pool. The pool itself was empty of water and was overgrown with creepers and jungle plants, clearly the whole place had been ransacked and neglected to the point where nature was reclaiming the town, it seemed such a shame but, as I would learn over the coming years this was a common theme to most African states that had been colonised by any of the European countries once independence was won.

The road finally brought us to the beach where the road turned right to run parallel to the sea on our left, quite soon we arrived at the gate to the Cabinda compound, there were armed guards on the gate, I later learned that these guards were supplied by the Cuban government as Angola was at this time a communist regime supported by the Soviet Union and their allies. Angola had been fighting a civil war since 1975, this war started just after Angola secured independence from Portugal continuing, until 2002. The war was a power struggle between two former anti-colonial guerrilla movements, the communist People's Movement for the Liberation of Angola (MPLA) and the anti-communist National Union for the Total Independence of Angola (UNITA). The war was used as a surrogate battleground for the Cold War by rival states such as the Soviet Union, Cuba, South Africa and the United States.

History lesson over our bus was waved straight through the gate without any checks at all; the landscape changed immediately to that of a regimented almost military compound, it could have been somewhere in the USA, there were American pick-up trucks everywhere being driven by men wearing Stetsons with their arms hanging out of the windows looking very relaxed. The road was dark brown and looked somewhat sticky to me, I had never seen anything like it; my new friend who was Kyle informed me that the road was constructed by crude oil being sprayed directly on the dirt and left to dry, it seems that once dry the surface while not as good as tarmac, was perfectly adequate for the purpose of carrying the traffic of the camp although he told me whenever it rained the surface became treacherous.

The bus drove on up a hill away from the sea, where there were various collections of buildings, Kyle pointed out the administration block, engineering area, accommodation blocks and finally the mess hall. This was to be our final destination, the bus pulled up to the main entrance and we all disembarked; I was glad to be here but was apprehensive as to what my reception would be given that I was some four days late!

Looking around I could see that the mess hall was on a large flat area of grass which was brown and clearly had not seen water for some time, I had arrived in the middle of the dry season and rain was not expected for some time yet. There were a number of large trees providing shade for the mess hall as well as a roost for hundreds of huge, black fruit bats; everyone was lining up at the entrance where we were to be logged in, the camp needed to keep track of everyone who arrived or left for obvious reasons.

After being logged in I was told the number of my billet and directed towards how to find it; my accommodation and that of the other divers was in the same block as the mess hall (convenient I thought), I quickly found my room and went in. I was confronted by another individual who introduced himself as Bart, he was the lead diver, he told me that the team was not diving at the moment as their boat had been taken away for a few days, it had been seconded to help with some anchor handling apparently. This meant that my absence may not have caused any issues as there was not much going on at this time other than a bit of maintenance, he reassured me that nobody was the least bit miffed by my late arrival as they were used to issues like this; in his words it was described as 'WAWA' standing for

West Arica Wins Again! Bart showed me my bunk area where I had a nice clean bed and a personal locker, at the time the team consisted of four and had two adjoining rooms with a bathroom between them, it looked great to me and I was very pleased with it, I thought I could rough it like this for six-weeks no problem.

Once I had put my bag on the bed Bart told me to put my coveralls and boots on, he would then take me to meet the rest of the team. I followed Bart out to a parking lot adjacent to the accommodation block, he pointed out a blue pick-up truck which I later found out was a Chevrolet Silverado. We climbed aboard, Bart fired up the obligatory V8 and off we went, Bart told me that the pick-up was Oceaneering's and we had sole use of it; he told me the compound had a perimeter of about six point five miles and inside there was the 'Malongo Country Club' this consisted of a small golf course, a softball field and other recreational facilities. He told me that the Country Club sometimes organised events such as barbecues etc., he told me that Sundays in the camp were half days for everyone he said these Sundays were always very laid back with soft ball matches with lots of free beer supplied, golf and in the evening barbecued steaks; it sounded great.

Bart continued my tour around the camp heading towards the engineering compound that Kyle had pointed out from the bus, he pulled up in front of a single story white painted unit that was in a row of some eight similar lock-ups. We both got out of the car, Bart led me into the unit, inside were two other men, the first to greet me was the supervisor Richard (Rick) Newman, the other was another diver he was a stocky individual with multiple tattoos called Billie.

Rick filled me in with how things operated in Cabinda, it seemed that normally the dive team was assigned a supply boat and would board the vessel at six in the morning, we would then be taken to an agreed location where we would carry out the required oilfield maintenance for the day returning to port at around six in the evening. I was really looking forward to getting involved with proper oilfield maintenance as opposed to the drill support, I had been working with up to now. It seemed that the Cabinda field had been looked after by Russian companies previously but that it was clear that the ageing field was falling to bits meaning there was plenty for us to do. Rick then disappeared to go and see the client to find out how long it would be until we were able to get our boat back, the rest of us set about seeing what needed to be done to maintain our equipment.

We had a small air diving system consisting of compressors, dive shack containing a two-diver panel, two umbilicals and a couple of Rat Hats all looked good to me and it all seemed to be in a pretty good state of repair. Bart decided that we should take a trip around the camp to show me the layout so that I could begin to find my way around. Firstly, we took a right outside the unit's door and walked to a low fence about fifty metres away, when we arrived there, a panoramic view of the working facility opened up below us. We were at the top of a hill about fifty metres above sea level; below me and to the left was the camp's entrance, directly in front of me was the harbour; this consisted of a solid pier extending about eighty metres straight out from the beach, at the end there was a second arm at right angles to the right of the main pier this resulted in a small sheltered area where supply boats could tie up for loading and unloading. Bart told me that this was where we would board the boat in the mornings. To my right along the beach there were some buildings that Bart told me were the harbour administration buildings, further along there was a heliport.

As I looked on there were a steady stream of helicopters that seemed to be on a circuit landing, dropping people off and picking others up before taking off and heading out across the sea towards the oilfield. The helicopters were operated by Petroleum Helicopters Incorporated (PHI) on this job they were operating a fairly large number of Bell 206 Jet Rangers, small helicopters that could seat the pilot co-pilot and four others, Bart told me the majority of the work was done by these small helicopters but there was a bigger Huey (UH-1 Iroquis) that was used for longer trips, apparently, most of the pilots were ex Vietnam US military. He went on telling me that these helicopters were used pretty much like city dwellers would use taxis and we would from time to time be hitching a ride on them. As I looked out to sea, I could see the small tripod structures I had seen from the air, each of them had a small helipad on the top with pipework dropping down into the sea. I was looking forward to getting up close to find out more about the work I would be doing.

We spent the rest of the afternoon touring the camp and around six in the evening we knocked off, showered and changed before meeting up again to go to the mess hall for our meal. The mess hall was a real slice of America, and the food reflected that, there were huge steaks with French Fries (not chips!), pizzas, tacos, gumbo and other American fair. The portions were massive, and were accompanied with all the condiments that Americans love, there was of course ketchup, blue cheese and ranch dressing and French's mustard; I certainly would not go hungry on this trip.

After our meal we all adjourned to the bar where I was told we could have four cans per person per night, the only beers on offer were American favourites such as Coors, Miller, Budweiser etc., well maybe these were not my usual choice but I was sure I would manage. Rick decided to take me under his wing a bit, he took me up to the bar where he told me to buy two packs of two hundred Marlborough but not to open them. I duly did this paying with US dollars which I always used to carry as they seemed to be the universal currency, Rick then purchased eight cans of beer using Kwanzas, four were for himself and four for me; we sat down to enjoy them.

He told me to bring one of the packs of Marlborough with me in the morning where we would sell them to one of the locals, he confirmed what I had been told by Kyle on the bus that this sale would be enough so that I could buy beers for the whole trip. Apparently, I would get some ten thousand Kwanzas which he said seemed like a lot of money but he told me that all the locals were paid in Kwanzas but that they were pretty much worthless as there was nothing for them to buy with them whereas Marlborough cigarettes could be used to purchase almost anything; it's a funny old world isn't it? We had a nice evening talking about people we all knew and polishing off our beers, we were all ready to hit the sack by nine o'clock though as we were going to be up for breakfast at five in the morning.

We didn't get our boat back until five days later, we then spent the first few hours loading our equipment back on to the rear deck of a supply boat called the Tropic Service, this was the boat that the team normally were assigned and for them it was like a bit of a homecoming. The Tropic had a dark blue hull with the accommodation towards the bow painted white, although it was plainly still these colours, they had been applied some years previously and now were streaked with rust, dirt and more than a few dings; while it was scruffy it looked to be very serviceable. The deck crew were all locals and didn't really interact with us, the officers and chef were however were very helpful, it was a happy ship, the chef was Portuguese and used to spoil us with great Portuguese dishes served for lunch, more food!

As soon as the gear had been loaded onboard, we cast off, Rick had been briefed by the client earlier; we headed out to one of the tripod structures where we were to remove a couple of risers that needed replacing. Risers in Cabinda carried the well's produced oil to the beach where it would be stored in large holding tanks. At intervals tankers would arrive to take this oil for export; a tanker would tie up to a Single Buoy Mooring (SBM) to load this oil, the SBM was part of our remit and we would visit it to carry out inspection and maintenance from time to time.

As we headed out to the dive site, I worked with the rest of the team setting up the diving equipment so that it would be ready for the dive as soon as we arrived on site. On reaching the site we moved out of the way while the deck crew tied up the vessel to the jacket. The deck crew then clambered onto the jacket and started rigging the two risers we were to be removing; once the first one was supported on the Tropic's crane they commenced cutting. Meanwhile I spent some time familiarising myself with the jacket and pipework it supported; up close I could see that the vertical legs were not truly vertical they were all slightly leaning in towards the centre of the jacket; this gradient was termed the batter, apparently the fact that they were not actually vertical made the structure stronger. The well was producing oil via a thirty-six-inch pipe held in the centre of the jacket, the 'conductor', it was bringing oil from the well on the seabed to the surface.

At the surface the conductor continued up for about another six or eight metres where it ran through a horizontal deck; just above the deck there were a series of valves terminating the conductor, these were the wellhead valves sometimes called the 'Christmas Tree'. From these valves the oil was diverted into the various risers that would take the oil to the beach for storage, I could now see clearly how the risers all ran down the outside of the jacket where they were held by large bolted clamps.

The ship was tied up stern-on to the jacket laying off just a few metres this would mean that when we entered the water, we would not have a very long way to swim to get to the job. We were ready to dive at about midday, I had been looking at the water and was a little concerned, there seemed to be a lot of movement and the water looked to be very murky. I was chatting to Bart as I was getting him ready for the first dive, he said that the surface of the water was always quite murky and tended to move quite fast; this was due to the fact that we were just north of the river Congo. The Congo was of course a very large river, Bart told me that the water I could see was mostly fresh water from the river carrying a good deal of river silt; this water ran along the surface above the seawater, he said that the sea water was about ten feet below and would be clear and still; Hmm, we would see.

Bart's first task was to establish a down line, this was a light line he would attach to the jacket close to where we would be working. While he was getting ready Billie with the help of a couple of the deck crew manhandled the recovery ladder over the stern of the ship. As soon as Bart had completed his surface checks and was ready for the water, he was handed the down line and stepped to the edge of the deck, he then leapt off into the water, I had his umbilical and pulled him back to the surface, he gave me a thumbs up and immediately left surface. I paid out his umbilical and Billie tended the down line; quite soon Rick told me that Bart had reached the job and was establishing the down line, within minutes the line was secured and Bart got to work on one of the risers that needed to be removed. After about forty-five minutes the riser was ready to be recovered on deck, Bart needed to be recovered first and when he was safely on deck the deck crew hauled the riser up onto the rear deck.

Once it was on deck, I was able to have a good look, it was a six-inch pipe that had clearly been in the water for years, it was covered in a thick layer of marine growth including huge oysters, mussels, clams and loads of other growth that I hadn't seen before.

Now it was my turn, Billie was going to be my tender and helped me to dress ready for the water; my job was to remove another of the six-inch risers, this would involve me cutting the riser using a large three-wheel pipe cutter. I had used pipe cutters a lot when I was working as a plumber's apprentice with Interheat all those years ago so I knew how they worked and how to use them but, I had never seen one this big before. The pipe cutter had a threaded 'T'-bar that could be used to wind the cutter open and closed; there was a cutting wheel that would run against the pipe on the side of the pipe to be cut and just beneath the T-bar there were a couple of rollers that would run around the pipe. When I was at the work site, I would roughly clean the surface of the pipe then open the pipe cutter and fit it around the pipe.

OK, so here I go I jumped into the water, Billie brought me back to the surface and pulled me over to the down line, as soon as I had the line, I told Rick I was ready to leave surface and he told me to go ahead. More or less as soon as my head left surface my world went dark, I couldn't see anything much, the visibility was thirty centimetres at most. I started to make my way down the line when I had gone just a few feet suddenly I dropped through from the murky surface water and, what I saw took my breath away, the water visibility had improved immeasurably, it was gin clear! I felt like I was flying! I could now see the whole three leg jacket including the well's conductor pipe rising vertically in the middle of the jacket, it was awesome, I could see that Bart had tied the line to one of the horizontal braces and the riser he had cut was just to the left of the jacket's leg.

Very quickly I made my way to the jacket, I confirmed with Rick that I was on the job site, he told me to wait there while he took my depth; I checked that the pneumo hose was across my chest and when I felt bubbles coming out of the hose, I confirmed I had bubbles. I was then told "you are at forty-two feet". I now needed to confirm which pipe I had to cut as there were four pipes to my left plus the one that Bart had already cut; Rick told me that the one I needed to cut was the second pipe in from the left. I set myself up and again confirmed that I was on the right riser and also where I was supposed to cut, all confirmed I started to clean off an area to allow access for the pipe cutter around the pipe.

This took me about ten minutes, I then fitted the pipe cutter around the pipe, once the cutter was wound in so that the cutting wheel and the two sets of rollers were nicely in contact with the pipe all was ready. I pulled the T-bar so that the cutter wound around the pipe, after a full rotation I checked and could see that the cutting wheel had indeed made a line all around the pipe. I wound the T-bar in so that there was again pressure on the cutting wheel, then pulled the cutter around the pipe again, I found that I needed to wind the cutter around the pipe twice and then wind the T-bar in to again increase the pressure on the cutting wheel. I continued to wind the cutter around the riser winding the T-bar in until finally the pipe jerked a little and I could see that the cut was complete; all I had to do now was to remove the face plate from a clamp holding the riser onto the jacket. This was a simple matter of cutting the bolts with a hacksaw, the bolts were quite corroded so this didn't take long at all, my job was then complete, I told Rick all was done. I was then recovered to the surface; I was very pleased that my first job with this new team had gone well.

When I was back on the surface and had removed my kit, I watched as the riser I had cut was brought on deck alongside the one Bart had done earlier, the deck crew moved both of the risers across to the edge of the deck on the starboard side and then one of them grabbed a broom and started to sweep all the marine growth that had been knocked off the risers over the stern into the sea. I saw that there was another broom so I thought I would give him a hand, but as soon he saw that I had started to sweep he dropped his broom and disappeared back towards their tea shack. Bart was in fits, he said that the deck crew would be very happy for me to do all their work, they would be very happy to watch! I clearly needed to learn quickly, I stopped sweeping and a couple of the deck crew came back and finished the job; clearly it was not the done thing to help them.

Actually, I was quite glad that I had to stop as I had an awful headache, it seemed that in my desperation to show that I would do a good job quickly I had been working too hard and was suffering from a carbon dioxide (CO_2) build up in the hat. I should have taken a breather more regularly and used the hat's free flow facility to flush out the CO_2 from the hat, this was a lesson learned again, I never suffered a repeat of this problem; this was no big issue really and after a couple of hours my headache went away so all was well.

As the resident dive team, we not only looked after the oilfield but also, we were often asked to carry out work on the numerous supply boats and tugs. One morning we were asked to go and have a look at the rudders on another supply boat, the Nordic Service, when we arrived the deck crews moored both ships together so that both ships sterns were alongside each other. The Nordic's engineer came on board and briefed us; it seemed that the skipper had noted his ship was not responding to the helm properly and it was thought there may be a problem with the rudder system. The Nordic had two rudders; my job was to go and take a look at them and to report any problems I found. We were moored with the Nordic in a quiet location so I would not need to contend with much tidal flow, it should be an easy job; I was soon ready for the water, jumped over the stern and made my way to the Nordic's stern, once there I left surface and went looking for the rudders. The draft of supply boats was not great, just about ten feet or so, it didn't take me long to get to the location, when I arrived at the position where I should find the starboard rudder all I found was a flange with four bolt holes I thought this flange was the rudder stock, the rudder stock was at the base of the shaft protruding through the hull, it would rotate and move the rudder as required. However, there was no rudder at all!

I knew I was in the right place as I could see the propellor just a few feet forward of the flange. I turned left and went in search of the port rudder, I soon found it well, at least it was there however, of the four bolts that should be attaching the rudder to the rudder stock, one was missing all together and the others were very loose so the rudder was just hanging loosely and would be less effective than normal. I certainly was not surprised the ship was not responding properly to the helm. I was recovered to deck and reported to Rick and the ship's engineer; we were in favour of tightening the bolts on the rudder and replacing the missing one but the engineer felt it wasn't worth doing this as they would have to go to South Africa for a replacement rudder anyway. I was very surprised by this but we were effectively dismissed and the Nordic Service left to steam south straight away; I heard later that the port rudder fell off before they arrived in South Africa so maybe they regretted not letting us do the work.

The majority of our work was carried out on the jackets but from time to time we had to follow and repair flowlines on the seabed. This was a different prospect completely, midwater there was excellent visibility but near the surface the viz was not so good as I've already said, however, that was nothing compared to the viz near the bottom. The first time I was required to follow a flow line we had been asked to place buoys along the line as a jack up rig was going to come alongside the jacket to carry out some work. The jack up would come in alongside the jacket; when in position it would jack down its legs to the seabed, our buoys would ensure that the jack up did not place its legs onto the flowlines.

This dive was quite an eye opener for me, as I dropped down the riser all was great until I arrived at about eight feet from the seabed, at this point visibility was suddenly reduced to zero, I literally couldn't see a hand in front of my face. Well, I continued down until I felt the riser bending away to the left, this meant I had reached the tube-turn where the riser turned from a vertical pipe to run along the seabed. I had been provided with a light line running up to the surface where it was attached to a small buoy, the plan was for me to swim along the flowline until it either became buried too deeply for me to be able to continue or alternatively I was told to stop; whichever was the case I was then to tie the line to the flowline, simple. Well as I've said before our imagination can go into overdrive when underwater and that was especially true for me when in black water in the tropics.

As I started out along the flow-line all was well, I had a thin pair of white polka dot work gloves on and I could feel the pipe together with its marine growth quite easily, I progressed along the pipe by touch constantly expecting to come across a Moray Eel or some other sea monster that would bite or sting me. Of course, neither events occurred but it was a little unnerving and I never did get completely comfortable with it and following discussions with the others I found I was not alone. There were enough horror stories and folklore to keep us all a little on edge; however, in all the years I was doing this work I never did get bitten or stung by anything so it really was all in my mind.

Sometimes we had to follow flowlines along their whole length looking for damage or foreign objects, this would normally be much too far for one dive, in this case when the first diver came to the end of their dive, they would tie the buoy line in such a way that the next diver would know which way would be the correct direction for them to continue along the pipe. This was achieved by swimming along the line until told to prepare to leave bottom, at this point the diver would pass the buoy line under the pipe ensuring the line to the surface was on the right of the flowline, quite often this would involve digging. The line would be passed under the pipe so that the line wound clockwise twice around the pipe, the next diver down would then know which way they had to go to continue along the line and not retrace backwards.

A common problem was items being dropped overboard, we would often be called upon to carry out searches to locate and recover these items. Of course, these searches would always be carried out at the bottom which in the case of Angola meant the visibility was always zero so, the search would be done by touch alone. One instance that comes to mind was being called to the harbour area where we were told that a down hole tool had been lost while being loaded onto one of the supply boats. Apparently, the tool was about a metre and a half long and seven centimetres in diameter, it was made of stainless steel; the tool had been loaded on a pallet and while it was being lifted onto the boat the tool rolled off and dropped into the water.

The harbour was only about twenty feet deep (6 metres) the deck crew were pointing to the point where they had apparently seen the tool enter the water, this should be no problem I thought. I was going to be carrying out a circular search just like I used to do when looking for paint panels in Brixham harbour, the difference was that the viz would be zero so again I would need to be doing this by touch. Having done a number of these searches now I had found that it was significantly easier if I didn't wear gloves as I could differentiate between what I was looking for from other items on the seabed.

We put a shot line down, I took a workline with me to tie around the tool when I found it, as well as another line to use as a distance line, a compass would be useless as I would be unable to see it and being in the harbour there was likely to be a lot of metallic junk on the seabed which would cause the compass to be useless. My circuits would be observed by my tender on the surface following my bubbles, this would be tricky when I was close in to the shot line but as soon as I was a little further out it should be easier.

On arriving at the seabed, I located the shot weight which was again a fifty-six-pound (25 Kg) weight, this weight had a handle on which the down line had been attached and there was plenty of room for me to tie my distance line to the same handle. Once this was done, I told the supervisor I was ready to start searching and off I went, the first thing I found was that the seabed was covered with what felt like slimy plastic bags so not only did I have to search the top of these but also, I needed to dig under them just in case the tool had rolled or slipped underneath. As I progressed around the first circuit, I had to keep stopping to feel under the plastic bags, there was a lot of junk on the bottom and each circuit took me a long time.

On my third circuit I put my hand onto something that was very slimy which was expected but this thing, whatever it was decided it didn't like my hand on it and so squirmed off and disappeared away from me, it must be said that all sea creatures have to be careful as they are constantly aware of predators and divers must look pretty big and scary to them. It is true to say that in the main they are much more scared of us than we are of them. Continuing my search, I was told I had completed another circuit and should move out and go back the other way again. I was moving out about a metre at a time as with no viz at all I had to search everything by touch. Now I was on my fourth circuit some four metres away from the shot.

I was somewhat surprised that I had not found anything yet, I knew I hadn't missed it as fingertip searches are extremely successful normally and it was not that we were looking for a tiny item. I carried on and completed my fourth circuit, I had been looking for about an hour and it was decided that this was enough, I was told to come back in to the shot and leave bottom. This was disappointing but there you go, these things happen I suppose; when I was back on deck, Bart was supervising at this time as Rick had gone home on leave, so, Bart came out of the dive shack and climbed up on to the pier to talk to the client. He came back a few minutes later to inform us that it was no wonder we hadn't found anything as in his words "They've found the bloody tool on the pier!" It seems that it had never been loaded onto the pallet at all so I don't know what they all saw fall of the pallet? Maybe they were telling Porkies?

Most of our days consisted of travelling out to one of the jackets and either removing a riser or two with us returning the following day with newly fabricated replacements to be refitted. We would each normally carry out two dives per day, this meant that at lunchtime it would not be unusual for us to have downtime while we were breathing out the accumulated nitrogen from the first dive. This was particularly true when we were diving on one of the deeper structures where we may be needing a couple of hours between dives. During these surface intervals there was almost nothing for us to do other than eat one of the Portuguese chef's wonderful lunches. It became the custom for us to play scrabble to pass the time; this had been the norm before I arrived and so consequently, Rick and Bart were particularly good at the game and tended to win by some margin although my game improved over the time I spent working there.

Very soon my six weeks were up and I was due to fly home, there was a bit of a tradition for people going on leave from Cabinda. This was that they would all take crayfish home with them. All the structures in the field were home to hundreds of lovely big, fat crayfish, routinely we used to catch some whenever we completed our work some of these would be given to our Portuguese chef who would cook them up for us for lunch; wonderful. Well, a few days before we were due to fly home, we would go on a crayfish hunt, in my case I would catch four or five, these would then be frozen ready for us to take home. On the day we were due to leave the crays would be wrapped carefully and secreted in our bags, the journey home would take about twelve hours so by the time we got home the crays would be nicely defrosted and ready to be eaten.

As promised my passport had been returned to me a couple of weeks before I was due to leave; I was all set although I was a little worried about my journey as I knew I was not welcome in Gabon. I'm not sure whether Oceaneering took this into account but my homeward journey was to be via Luanda the capital of Angola where I would catch another UTA flight directly back to France. On the day of departure, I packed up my crayfish tails and made ready to leave, I was the only diver leaving that day but was accompanied by another seven others; our transit from the camp to Malongo airport would be via the Huey helicopter. We all assembled at the mess hall for the departure paperwork to be completed then walked over to the main heliport which was quite near the mess hall. I found my seat, placed my bag on the floor at my feet, with very little preamble we were up and away, it was nice to be flying over the oilfield knowing that I was not going back to work for a while, I was definitely ready for home.

When we arrived at Malongo we were directed to the terminal building again, this time the passport control and administration was very lax, we were then directed to a small waiting area to wait to be called for the flight. There were some locals who it seemed were also going to be flying with us, the males were almost all dressed in cut-off jeans, T shirts and flip flops, none of them seemed to have much in the way of baggage. The women on the other hand were all dressed in flowing brightly coloured dresses with extravagant head ware, these looked to be a cross between a hat and a turban, all very colourful.

Departure time had come and gone but nobody seemed the least bit concerned, I could see the plane on the tarmac about a hundred yards from me and there were steps all ready for us. We had not been issued with boarding cards and there didn't seem to be much by way of officialdom in evidence; suddenly a uniformed guard appeared outside the terminal, he started to unlock the sliding doors that seemed to be the departure gate. As soon as the doors were slid open there was a stampede, everyone picked up any bags or babies they had and just took off at speed! Luckily, I was in those days quite fit and as I only had my carry-on bag I also took off; it was clearly a free for all, the fittest arrived at the aircraft steps first and without any hesitation started to board.

I was not far behind and was probably one of the first dozen on board everyone then just found a seat and that was that; the flight crew were clearly expecting this and stayed well out of the way until the feeding frenzy had calmed down. The doors were then closed and the engines started, if I was expecting a safety brief, I was to be disappointed, one of the flight crew stood at the front and using the local language started to berate those who were still standing at least that's what I assumed was being said. Eventually the attendant sat down and the flight took off, now we were in the air I had a look around the aircraft, firstly under my seat where the life jacket was according to the sign on the seat in front of me but, no, there was nothing there. Oh well, at least we weren't going to be flying over water very much, the seat belt seemed to be fine and I could see the emergency exits were properly labelled, I just hoped that the aircraft's maintenance was up to date!

The flight time from Malongo to Luanda was about an hour so there wasn't much by way of catering although they did give me a beer, which I thought was very civilised. As we approached Luanda, we did a circuit giving me the chance to have a look at this capital city; from the air it looked a little ramshackle, it was spread over a large area, it was right by the sea and looked to have nice beaches. Once we had landed the plane taxied to a point quite close to the terminals, again when the steps had been brought up to the plane and the doors were opened, we all just took off; everyone piled out of the plane down the steps and started walking/running towards the terminal building. The terminal was large, it had clearly been a significant international airport in the past, however, now it was sadly very dilapidated, there were tiles missing from the outside face of the building and it looked in need of a good coat of paint.

Inside was no better, a lot of the lights were damaged or were missing, the suspended ceilings had holes in them and again everything needed cleaning and a good coat of paint. There was an all-pervading smell of unwashed bodies with a hint of spicy food although I couldn't see where that was coming from; I later realised that it was from some of the other passengers who had brought their own food with them, some of these being pots of curry with rice and nice-looking bread. They clearly knew that there was to be nothing available at the airport, oh well, another lesson learned. As ours was an internal flight there was no requirement for passport control or it seemed any other administration; we were all directed to a large area where a lot of people were congregated, they were all milling around and shouting, the noise level was immense.

I looked around for something official for UTA and saw over in the left-hand corner what looked to be the UTA check-in desk, I made my way over to find a sort of queue although people didn't seem to understand how queues operated and were jumping the queue all the time. I thought, when in Rome and pushed my way to the front of the queue, again, I know it shouldn't make any difference but it seemed that as I was the only white face in the queue and had managed to get to the desk the UTA operative behind the desk immediately started to handle my query. It seemed that I was indeed at the check-in desk and that there was a valid ticket in my name for the flight that would be leaving in a couple of hours, she checked me in and gave me a boarding pass; that's more like it I thought.

She told me where to go and when to be ready to board, it seemed there would be no announcements as there was no PA system, fine. I left the desk and found a seat close to the point where I had been told the departure gate was, I pulled out my book, I was halfway through Shōgun a great novel by James Clavell, I started to read. After about an hour and a half I could see UTA personnel getting ready at the desk by the gate and so made my way up to them. I was efficiently dealt with and was told to walk through the gate and go to the plane; I walked through the gate and found another McDonnel Douglas DC-10 ready and waiting, I made my way up the steps and was directed to my seat, all very civilised.

The flight continued to be very civilised with proper food and even wine being served although there was still no in-flight entertainment, the flight time was eight hours which brought us to Marseilles in France. I spent a bit of time thinking back over my first trip to Africa and all that had happened, it was certainly eventful and not at all dull. Even forgetting the issues, I had just getting to Angola, the job had been varied. I had put a lot of the skills I learnt on my BAD course into action; using hacksaws, spanners, hydraulic impact wrenches, oxy-arc cutting, heaps of rigging exercises and of course a number of inspection tasks; I had loved all of it.

In the early eighties all flights from Angola had to clear customs at Marseilles so we landed and everyone had to leave the plane to go through French passport control and customs procedures. After about an hour we were herded back onto the same plane for the short hop back to Charles de Gaulle airport in Paris, having cleared customs in Marseille I just had to find my way to the British Airways transfer desk where I checked onto the next flight to London. After another uneventful flight and a subsequent re-entry into Britain I caught the 'rail-air' link to Reading; once at Reading station I purchased my rail ticket for the next train to the south-west which was due in fifty minutes.

PHOTOS FROM MY TIME IN AFRICA

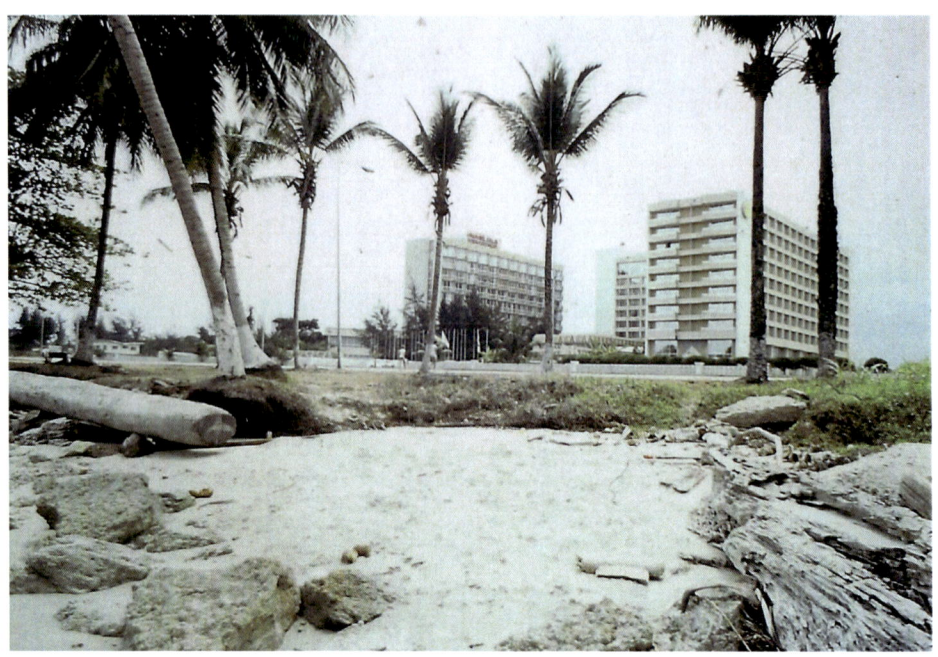

The hotel where I was under 'house arrest' in Gabon (Awful!).

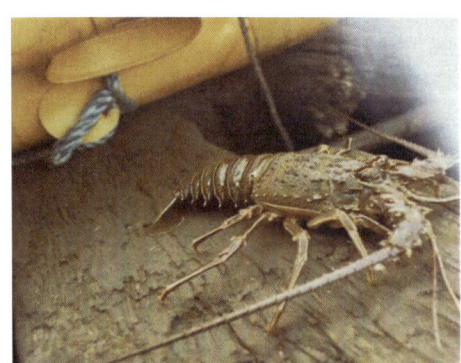

Crayfish almost ready to make his way back to Torbay.

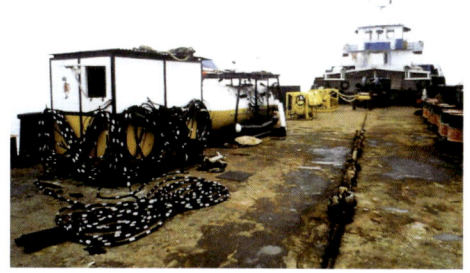

Air diving system set up on the aft deck of the Tropic Service our usual supply boat. Note the umbilicals coiled up on the side of the 'dive shack' in the foreground and the small chamber right behind.

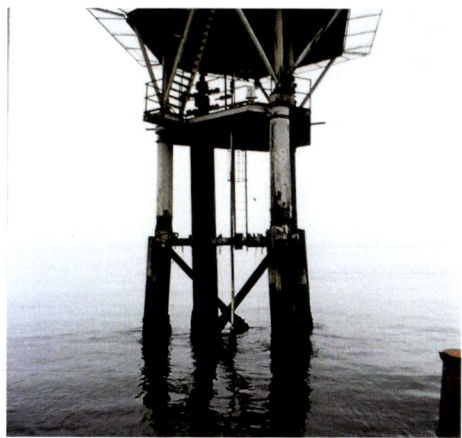

Typical tripod structure in the Cabinda oilfield in the early 1980s.

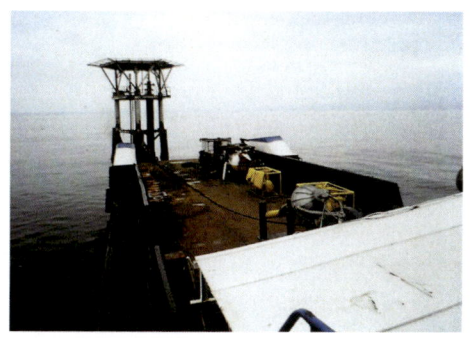

View from the bridge wing on the Tropic Service supply boat looking out across the after deck towards the tripod structure that we were to be working on.

Part Four

CHAPTER THIRTEEN

Late 1981

Following my return from Angola I took a couple of weeks off I had been expecting to be home for a month but after just a couple of weeks I received a telegram from Oceaneering delivered by my old friend on his BSA bantam, the telegram was asking me to call Diane. I made the call from the phone box just across the road from my house later that morning, Diane told me that I was to travel back to Sicily for a short job, it would be just a couple of days. As was now the norm, I had to pick up my ticket at the airport the next day and find my way to Catania in Sicily; apparently, I would be met at the airport by one of the team and we would make our way across to Trapani near Palermo by road the following day.

The journey to Catania was a carbon copy of my previous trip and although the transfer in Rome was again very tight, I arrived in Catania on time. As I went through the airport into the arrival's hall, I was met by a chap holding a sign with my name; I went straight across to him and we introduced ourselves, he was a Brit who introduced himself as Joe O'Neil he was the supervisor of the job Matteo had apparently gone; I was very glad to hear this.

We made our way out of the airport to the car park where Joe had left his car, he told me that we would be staying the night at his flat in Syracusa; it took us about forty-five minutes to reach his flat, which was on the first floor of the building. The rest of the crew were already there, we settled in for a meal with a few beers before we bedded down for the night. The next day we had to drive across pretty much the whole width of Sicily, it was some three hundred and fifty kilometres and would take at least five hours. We had to be at the heliport by two o'clock in the afternoon so didn't have to leave at silly o'clock, after a nice breakfast we loaded up the car and off we went, leaving at just after seven o'clock.

As we drove Joe brought the team up to date about the job; it seemed that we would be going out to a rig situated just off Trapani, this rig had a resident dive team from an Italian company who it seemed were refusing to dive. The reasons for their refusal were apparently contractual and not issues with safety; we would be using their equipment so would be staying offshore for at least one night or as long as it took for us to become confident and happy with the equipment. It was clear that the client was very unhappy with the dive team they had on board and would be sending them all ashore so we wouldn't have to deal with any antagonism from them which was I thought a good plan.

Joe told me that the job was to fit a corrosion cap to the wellhead as the rig was moving off to drill another well but would be returning to this well at a later date. This procedure was not unusual and indeed was common for rigs drilling 'wildcat' wells; so, while the well was being left dormant it needed to be protected from corrosion, the well would be filled with a corrosion inhibitor and a cap would then be fitted to the wellhead to temporarily seal it. Joe wanted me to do the dive as I was by then the most experienced member of the team, this was great as far as I was concerned; the diving depth was to be three hundred feet (92 metres) and would be a surface-oriented dive. I would be taken to depth in a basket with gas being supplied from the surface via my umbilical as there was no diving bell available; I would be using surface decompression again.

The trip across Sicily went according to plan, we arrived at the heliport in good time; Joe found a spot to leave the car and we all piled out to make our way to the terminal however, before we reached the terminal we were met by Guido, it was really nice to see his smiling face again. He had news though, it seemed that when the Italian diving company heard that we were coming to do the job that they had so far refused to undertake they had a bit of a rethink and decided they would do the job after all! Guido told us that the job had been completed that morning, oh well never mind; the client thanked us but as we were no longer required; we turned around and made our way back to Syracusa. There were no flights the next day so I had to wait in Syracusa for a couple of days, what a hardship! I was being paid and had nothing to do; I spent a nice couple of days revisiting my old haunts, it was again sheer hell!

After a few days at home, I was asked to travel up to Aberdeen to help with some work on ADS systems in the yard for a few days. By this time Oceaneering had moved to a new facility on the Pitmedden Industrial Estate, in Dyce, Aberdeen, this was a brand-new building with a lot more space for Oceaneering's expanding requirements. This meant that the yard in the Bridge of Don where Dave and I had started our careers had been closed with everything being moved to the new facility, DHB also moved from Alton in Hampshire (where I had done my ADS course) up to Aberdeen; everything was now centralised in one place.

I arrived on an early morning flight and went straight to the facility, it was impressive, much more corporate than the old Bridge of Don facility had been, Pamela was still the gate keeper but as she now knew me, I was admitted without much of an issue. As I walked through the facility I was stunned by its size and the variety of equipment being stored and worked on; I saw Sam Hardy and said hello, he seemed pleased to see me but it seemed that Jimmy was no longer employed with Oceaneering.

Sam directed me towards where the ADS systems were stored and maintained and I set off through the workshop, along the way I walked past an 'Arms Bell', this was a diving bell that had been fitted with a very sophisticated (for the early eighties anyway) hydraulic arm. The operator of the Arms Bell would operate the arm from inside the bell which would not be pressurised, they would remain at one atmosphere with the bell taking the pressure of the water much like the atmospheric diving suits I had used. The Arms Bell was another of Oceaneering's high-tech solutions to deep diving work and indeed I had been on a job with an Arms Bell on the West Venture in Norway some time ago but I never actually used one or even saw one used as the West Venture's bell was out of action while I was there, indeed that was the principle, reason I had been sent out there with the Wasps.

I eventually found the DHB compound in the far corner of the workshop, here I found Terry and Bill both of whom I knew from previous jobs. I was given a tour of the facility and saw a number of JIM suits, Wasps and one Sam suit, all of these were in the process of being maintained. Bill took me to see their new diving tank, the tank was outside the building, it was much bigger than the tank we had used in Alton, he told me that they had already used it for some much more demanding trials with more planned which I hoped I might become involved with. The tour finished back at the compound where I was detailed off to start working on one of the JIM suit's life support systems, I spent the rest of the afternoon working on this until at half past five, Bill told me it was time to knock off. He also let me know that now I was an Oceaneering regular I qualified to stay at their staff house; he told me he would drop me off at the guest house on his way home.

When we arrived, I was faced with a classically solid Aberdeen house constructed from granite, the boarding house was called the Allen Guest House. Oceaneering maintained rooms here which were made available to visiting divers and staff, it was very nice, I was assigned a single room and told Breakfast was at seven thirty in the morning.

There was no evening meal supplied but, by chance just across the road was the Inn at the Park pub where they did very good pub fare and of course sold beer so fitted the bill very nicely; I wandered downstairs where I came face to face with Dave Pelly who was also staying the night. We decided to make our way across the road to the pub where we spent a very agreeable evening catching up with each other's experiences. Towards the end of the evening, I remembered that I had agreed to call Chrissie my girlfriend, so, at about ten o'clock I found the pub's payphone (mobile phones were still a long way off). I dialled her number and when she answered it was clear that all was not well; Chrissie was not enjoying my being away so often and had apparently stopped on her way home from work to get some essential shopping.

This sounded like a very normal thing for her to do but it seemed that she had only bought a litre of vanilla ice cream and a bottle of Bailey's Irish Cream! Again, no issue there but, it seemed that when she got home, she had proceeded to pour the bottle of Bailey's over the ice cream and had eaten the lot! By the time I called she was clearly not feeling well and of course all of this was my fault for leaving her on her own; we chatted for a while and she thawed a bit in every way so that we parted on good terms when I ran out of change for the phone. The joys of working away in the eighties, these days of course there would be photos of the event uploaded to various social media platforms which I would have been able to trot out whenever I felt like making her feel embarrassed for years to come.

I spent about a week working at Oceaneering's yard doing a number of interesting and some boring jobs, the work was quite varied though ranging from painting of winches through to cutting up some syntactic foam. Syntactic foam is a class of material created using pre-formed hollow spheres (commonly made of glass, ceramic, polymer or even metal) bound together with a polymer. The "syntactic" portion refers to the ordered structure provided by the hollow spheres. The "foam" term relates to the cellular nature of the material. Syntactic foam was used offshore to provide deep water buoyancy for whatever equipment required; the foam can be used at great depth without losing its buoyancy. My first job with the foam was to cut it to a specific size and shape using a chain saw, the aim was to make a buoyancy aid for use with an High Pressure (HP) water jet making it possible for the water jet to be used by a Wasp.

I was taken out into the yard and was pointed to a large piece of foam with the helpful instruction of 'There it is, let me know when you're done'. This piece of foam had clearly been designed to fit around a sub-sea hose, it was about five metres long and one metre in diameter, the surface of the foam was shiny and smooth. Well, I marked out where I needed to make cuts using a permanent marker, picked up my safety PPE consisting of clear visor and a pair of gloves; all ready, I started the chain saw, I had never used a chain saw before and the total training I had received was from the guy in the hire company who told me how to start and stop it! I felt totally prepared of course being a young man, what could possibly go wrong?

It must be said that although I enjoyed this job it did not go well, the foam was far too hard, whenever I applied the chain to the surface it just skittered about and refused to cut the foam; it soon became obvious that a chain saw was just the wrong tool for the job, I eventually reverted to using a cutting disk but even then, the resulting chunk of foam turned out to be useless. We finally abandoned the foam and ended up using a plastic buoy attached to the water jet by a rope, this actually turned out to be a very good buoyancy aid allowing the suit to manipulate the water jet fairly easily. We were due to go back to Stoney Cove and carry out some trials with the Wasp to see whether we could use an HP water jet to clean some welds.

After about a week of working in the yard we packed up all the equipment and watched it disappear down the road on trucks on its way to Stoney Cove, the team followed to start the trial. We had been put up in a nice little hotel in Stoney Stanton about half a mile from Stoney Cove, we all assembled in the bar, had a nice meal and a couple of beers. The next morning, we all travelled the short distance to Stoney Cove to set up for the trial; when we arrived, the familiar bright yellow suits had already been offloaded and were sitting ready and waiting for us. Alongside the Wasp was another type of atmospheric diving suit made by Offshore Submersible Electronics Ltd (OSEL), this suit was called the Mantis (As had been used in the Spy Who Loved Me) it was however quite different from anything I had seen before the operator lay flat inside the suit and operated its thrusters by fingertip controllers, their feet did nothing.

I felt that this would make flying the machine and operating its arms at the same time very difficult. Mantis arms were also completely different, they were powered by seawater hydraulics which would give them a lot more power than the Wasp and JIM suits arms but they suffered with limited dexterity making them hard to use apparently. The dive control container was off to my right, this was a permanent fixture and had been there when I had last visited. To the left of dive control there was a walkway leading down to a floating pontoon where the suits and equipment would be launched from. Alongside the dive control there was a second container which was fitted out as an on-site workshop and a quad of oxygen; there were the required hydraulic power pack and winches for launching and recovering the suits as well as a high-pressure jetting system capable of supplying pressure of upwards of one thousand bar to the water jet!

We started prepping for diving, my job was to prepare the suits, I wandered over to the container alongside dive control, the door was already open and I could see there was nobody inside. I went in and located the plastic carboys of soda-lime (CO_2 absorbent) and cans of Castrol R which was the oil used inside the arm joints there was a small work bench and tool box that had all the tools we would require to maintain the suits. I turned around and went back out to the suits, where I started to prepare Wasp six by opening the dome and leaning inside, all looked to be as it should be, I dropped back to the ground and opened up both on board oxygen bottles then stuck my head back inside the suit to check the contents of the bottles indicated by readings on the suit's gauges.

All was well, the bottles were full, I then removed the CO_2 absorbent container, took it into the workshop container where I filled it with fresh soda-lime before refitting it in the suit. When I had completed the suit checks I left the suits and wandered into dive control where I was introduced to Edward Patrick, Edward was a world-renowned underwater photographer who was there to make a record of the trial as well as to take some promotional shots.

Once all was ready the team assembled outside for a briefing on how the trial was to be conducted; there were two aspects, first was to work out if and how a Wasp could be used for HP water jetting, for this a six-hundred-gallon oil tank had been placed in the water.

We were to clean the welds on the tank to SA 3; this was the term applied to a bright shiny finish; all of the paint must be removed but this should be no problem when using the water jet. The second part of the trial involved the Mantis, at the time OSEL were in the process of converting some of their fleet of Mantis subs from manned to unmanned Remotely Operated Vehicles (ROVs).

These units would effectively be 'flown' by topside personnel situated in dive control; at this time the vehicle had been rigged for remote operation but evidently this being the first time it had been used in open water confidence was not high. So, for the trial there was to be a pilot inside the suit whenever it was launched; if necessary, the pilot could take control of the suit in the normal way.

My first dive was to be a target for the Mantis, I was briefed that I should take the Wasp away from the pontoon and 'hide', the Mantis would then come and find me using its sonar systems, effectively my job was just to sit there and wait to be found. Soon I was ready inside the Wasp, I was dropped through the pontoon's moonpool and started to find somewhere to hide; now as you know I had spent a bit of time playing with the suit in Stoney Cove while I was on my course and so remembered that there was a car on the bottom some distance away, I thought I would go and sit next to this car and see how long it took to be found.

The visibility was very good so I had no problem locating the car and nestling up against it, I adjusted the suit's buoyancy so that it was nicely negative and settled onto the bottom. I had come prepared for a long wait and had brought a book and some sandwiches; I was very happy just sitting there; over the next couple of hours, I sat and watched a number of fish gambolling around the car and from time to time I would see the Mantis come past. For the trial the Mantis' CCTV cameras had been disabled and the pilot in dive control on the surface was relying on the sonar only, each time the Mantis came past I would wave to the operator inside and he would respond. After a couple of hours of this cat and mouse game my supervisor came over the comms and asked whether I had seen the Mantis at all? I told them that I had seen it several times and indeed at that moment it was sitting mid-water just in front of me facing away from me, this information was relayed to the Mantis crew and they rotated the vehicle, switched on the vehicle's cameras and immediately saw me; apparently, I was not playing fair by sitting next to the car!

Stoney Cove was and still is a Mecca for recreational scuba divers, during the week there would be a steady stream of cars bringing people to dive either for recreation or maybe training, there was a shop and café so they could recharge their sets on-site it was a very nice setup. At the weekend though things became a little more hectic with hundreds of divers arriving to engage in their hobby, it was amazing, I had never seen anything like it! When Saturday arrived, we were due to start the trial with the water jet, this gave us a bit of a headache as the recreational divers were showing a lot of interest in us and especially the suits. The issue would be if any of them were to come too close while we were operating the water jet, being shot with a water jet can cause tremendous injury and so we needed to find a way of keeping everyone away from the area where we were going to be working.

We put signs up in the shop, the café and a number of large signs alongside the access to the pontoon, we asked all Stoney Cove's staff to reinforce that all should stay well clear of us as it was very dangerous. We were assured that this would not be a problem as they had good control of the diving taking place at their site! I was not convinced but between us we decided we would go ahead with the trial and post lookouts to keep an eye on bubbles approaching our site.

My turn came around at about two o'clock in the afternoon and just before I closed the Wasp's dome, I saw that a large number of individuals were getting ready for the water just off to the left of our site. I completed my pre-dive checks and very soon was ready to go, the water jet was already affixed to the manipulator pincers, all I had to do was find my way across to the tank to get started. When I left surface, I had to rotate the suit ninety degrees to the right before heading out to the tank, this highlighted the first problem, I knew from previous dives that the Wasp was underpowered but now it seemed this was going to be a real problem.

The water jet was supplied with HP water via a heavy hose and the suit just wasn't powerful enough to allow me to rotate as I needed too; I found though that as I descended and more hose was paid out by the surface crew that I was able to power forward and after motoring just a few feet forward I found I could start to turn. This was more about me learning how to make best use of the suit and after a few minutes I seemed to be getting the hang of it; eventually I reached the work site, Bill had already started to clean one of the welds and my brief was to carry on to completely clean this weld.

The weld was running horizontally mid-way down the side of the tank; I could see that Bill had not found it easy to follow the weld as there were jetting marks running away from the weld both above and below the weld. Oh well, we would see how we got on; I lined myself up on the weld as best I could, this involved me constantly adjusting the power to the thrusters by dancing on the foot pedals, this was to say the least, challenging. The jetting gun was fitted with the float (buoy) that we had worked on in Aberdeen, it was attached to the gun by a short length of rope and was doing a good job of supporting the weight of the gun perfectly. This meant that I could move the gun around with the thrusters and also to a limited extent by moving the arms, as I was lining the gun up on the tank I was suddenly engulfed in a huge cloud of bubbles; I didn't know what had gone wrong but all seemed OK in the suit, I wasn't getting wet and the gauges showed that oxygen pressures were still good so where was the gas coming from?

Suddenly a face appeared in my eyeline, a diver was coming up from below me just in front and to my right, the gas had come from his exhalation while he was still below me. I told topside what had happened and they told me to stand off from the tank while they decided what to do. After a couple of minutes, I was told that the diver had been recalled and moved away, evidently, he was carrying a surface marker buoy (SMB) and the Cove's safety boat had managed to signal to him to surface. I was told I was clear to move back on location and to start cleaning, without much delay I was back and ready to start, I called 'make it hot', I knew there would be a few minutes before water pressure was supplied to the gun but, soon I saw the hose shift as they do when pressure builds inside them. The suit could not depress the gun's trigger so the trigger had been replaced with a solenoid that I could control from inside the suit, I was told all was ready for me to start.

Again, I checked I was in the right place with the nozzle of the gun close up against the weld, I pressed the button to activate the solenoid; immediately I saw HP water coming out of the gun and hitting the weld surface, luckily the retro-jet equalising the forces was working very well and I was able to stay in position quite easily. I found visibility poor when the jet was active as it was creating a lot of turbulence around the end of the nozzle; when I had carried out jetting as a diver before I had found it relatively easy to gently move the nozzle across the weld to clean the area as required. Using a water jet from a Wasp was not so easy, I found that to move the nozzle across the weld I had to physically fly the suit a little up and down; not easy but, after a little time I found that I could do this in the still water of Stoney Cove, whether it would be possible in the sea with tide and wave action would be another thing entirely!

Well, as I moved along the weld, I could see that the jet was doing the job very nicely and the weld was being cleaned to the required standard with very little effort from me. I had cleaned about a metre of weld and was approaching the edge of the tank, when the nozzle was no more than a hundred and fifty millimetres from the edge, I could see the wash from the jet pushing bits of removed paint clearly around the edge of the tank when suddenly I had a big shock! Without warning a diver's head appeared around the edge of the tank right in line with the end of the weld his half mask was already being buffeted by the wash from the nozzle, I immediately let go of the button and the water jet shut off, making it safe. The diver was clearly unaware of how close he came to disaster as he held his hand up making the classic 'O' with his forefinger and thumb as I'm sure he had been taught to signify he was OK. He might be ok but I can tell you my heart was going like the clappers knowing that I had come within a whisker of blowing his head off! It was decided to call it a day after this and I was recovered with the gun, I can't say I was unhappy to be finished with this trial.

When everything was tidied away again, we had a debrief and although the trial had been prematurely terminated, we had proven that it was possible to carry out HP water jetting with the Wasp although its lack of power would be an issue. Sometime later Oceaneering upgraded the Wasp with larger more powerful thrusters, the suit would then be termed a Hornet and although I never used one, I was told it was a much-improved vehicle.

Following the end of the trial I arrived home at about midday and started making plans for the evening, all was going well until six in the evening when I received another telegram; I was required to go to Sicily again and had to leave immediately to catch the flight!

As you can imagine this didn't go down very well but it was the way things worked for a day rate diver in the eighties, you just couldn't turn work down as the unspoken threat was that if you did maybe they wouldn't call again. So, it was I returned to Sicily in mid-November; the journey was again via Rome and Catania to Syracusa where I again met up with Joe O'Neil and the others on the team. The next day we were taken back to the Black Dog jack-up rig; the rig was still situated just south of Gela; in fact, it had not changed location since the last time I was on board.

When we arrived on board, we were briefed by the client who told us that a down-hole logging tool had been lost overboard and we were to search for it; I don't know how much these tools cost but it must be a lot! Mobilising a dive spread with all the required equipment for surface-oriented bounce diving to two hundred plus feet together with the team of divers would not have been cheap. Our first day on board was spent setting up and testing the equipment, day two was diving, I was to be the first diver and duly dressed into the equipment, we were again using Rat Hats and would be breathing Heliox for the majority of the dive. Once I was ready my tender helped me to put the hat on and I carried out the necessary checks of comms, bailout etc., as before I would be breathing air for the first part of the dive, when Joe confirmed that all was ready for me, I stepped into the basket and was winched over the side of the rig.

The weather was again playing ball, it was a beautiful bright sunny day with almost no wind, the sea was flat calm; as I entered the water, I gave the 'left surface' report and could feel bubbles coming from my pneumo hose as topside checked my depth. When I reached forty feet the basket stopped and we carried out the drill for changing from air to Heliox. I reported, I have Heliox with my Donald Duck voice and was told OK we're lowering you to the seabed, as before I was accompanied by a shoal of sardines almost all the way to the seabed.

The visibility was again excellent and even as I neared the seabed, I still had enough light from above to be able to tell topside to 'all stop on the basket'; the basket was some ten feet above the seabed which was fine. I had been supplied with an underwater metal detector to use during the search, I was to use the circular search technique again with the basket acting as the centre of the circle, I left the basket through the side and swam down to the seabed. As soon as I was on the seabed, I called for topside to check my depth, topside confirmed they had my depth (two hundred and nineteen feet, 67 metres). At this depth I had very limited time, my bottom time had to be kept to less than twenty-five minutes. I switched on the metal detector and held it just above the seabed, and started finning in a clockwise circle listening for the tell-tale sound that would signify a metallic contact.

There was nothing on the first circuit, I moved out a further few of metres and retraced my circuit going anticlockwise, again nothing found; I carried out four circuits before I was told to get ready to leave bottom. I moved back to the basket where I tied off the work line, I had been given to tie onto the tool in the event I had found it, my umbilical was being tended from the surface and I could see that it was pretty much straight up and down so

I called, 'ready to leave bottom', the basket started to rise and I said 'left bottom'. I was brought up in the basket stopping at the required 'stops' until I reached my last in-water stop at forty feet; again, here my gas was changed back air.

I again had a long stop at forty-feet with nothing much to do but blow bubbles, I was due to undertake surface decompression so had removed most of my equipment that I had hung in and around the basket. There was no repeat of my mistaking my fin for something more sinister this time; after about half an hour at the stop somebody came over the comms telling me that a present was on its way down to me? I looked up and saw a weighted line approaching, a small plastic bag had been attached to it, I could see there was something inside the bag but, it was not until the bag came level with me that I realised the bag contained a nice big slice of pizza! Very thoughtful, they were all apparently having pizza on the surface and thought I shouldn't be left out; as I say very thoughtful but as I had no way to get the pizza from the bag to my mouth it just sat there taunting me until I left the decompression stop.

My decompression was completed without issue, we spent the next couple of days searching along the side of the rig where the tool had been dropped but never got any kind of response from the metal detector so it was all for nothing. As soon as the client decided enough was enough, I was sent home; when there was a resident team on a job, the clients never wanted day rate personnel to stay on board any longer than necessary as we were too expensive so, I was sent home in the afternoon of the fifth day. Owing to my afternoon departure from the rig I didn't get to Rome until too late to get a connecting flight to London so had to spend a night in Rome. I stayed in a fairly nice airport hotel, my one regret was that I didn't get to see any of Rome as there was no time, so, now I had been to Rome six times but had never had time to do anything but sleep one night and never did see any of the sights. It would be some years before I was able to spend enough time in Rome to see the sights, this would be when I became a board member of the European Baromedical Association (EBAss) much more about this later.

I was only at home for one day before I was called back to Aberdeen; the job was to get ready for a promotional shoot with the Wasp, this was due to take place in that old favourite location, Stony Cove. In the early eighties Oceaneering spent a huge amount of money promoting their high-tech diving operations and it seemed I was going to be involved in the next effort, I spent a week in the workshop making the suits we were to be using look perfect and of course making sure they worked properly. The suits would once again make their way to Stoney Cove via road but, Bill and I flew to Birmingham airport where we picked up a hire car before heading to the same hotel as before in Stoney Stanton.

When we arrived, we met the rest of the team one of whom was Edward Patrick, again he would be the photographer recording everything for posterity, the job was to make the Wasp look good and in order to do this we had some props. There was a Rubik's cube, this puzzle toy that was at the time taking the world by storm; the plan was to show that the Wasp could complete this puzzle while underwater.

Following discussion, it was decided that it would be good to also photograph the Wasp playing poker with a diver with the Wasp of course holding all the aces. This sounded like we would be having a fun couple of days playing with the suits while being paid offshore wages, sounded good to me.

The next day when we arrived at Stoney Cove the suits were again there ready and waiting for us, the suits looked great; they were pristine. The Wasp we were to be using was suspended inside a frame with a large spool holding its umbilical/tether, this was Oceaneering's first attempt at fitting the Wasp system with a Tether Management System (TMS). This was new to me I had heard about TMS but had not actually seen one before. As I've already said, one of the major limitations of the Wasp was its lack of power; the Wasp had a very good depth rating of two thousand feet (609 metres), when diving at depths like this with the suit's lift wire stretching all the way back up to the surface the whole length of the wire would have tide and water currents acting against it, the effect of this was that the suit often couldn't make way towards the worksite.

The idea of a TMS was that the frame in which the Wasp was held would be lowered to depth on a heavy wire; once the TMS and suit were at working depth alongside the worksite the suit would be released on a much lighter excursion tether. Given that the excursion tether would never have to lift the suit in air it could be much lighter and in fact the tether utilised was neutrally buoyant; the suit was latched in the TMS frame for launch and recovery, when at depth the suit would be unlatched and would 'swim' to the job. The TMS winch would pay out and recover the excursion tether as required, the TMS winch was operated from the surface. The suit would only have to pull this light tether along with it, this made the suit's operating footprint much improved, it was a great idea and in fact has been very widely and successfully adopted by Remotely Operated Vehicles (ROVs) worldwide.

I started prepping the suit for the dives while the others went looking for more props. We had decided that it would look good if a poker game was being carried out on a table so the guys were off looking for something we could use. After half an hour or so they returned with a metal patio table 'borrowed' from outside the café and also a Martini parasol, this was great and would make things look much more atmospheric. The first day was to be the Wasp playing cards with a traditional diver with Edward taking photos showing how much better the Wasp was.

First job was to set up the table and parasol on the bottom; this took a bit of organisation as initially when the parasol was up it caught the divers exhaled gas and took off for the surface. We recovered the parasol I went over to the café and asked them whether they had an old parasol that they wouldn't mind us putting some holes in. I was told I needed to talk to the boss, he turned out to be a really sound individual who was very happy for us to make holes in the parasol we already had and not only that, he also had a nice heavy parasol weight that he was happy for us to take into the water with us. I also picked up an empty wine bottle and a couple of glasses, more atmosphere.

I took all this back to the rest of the crew with the good news; we spent an hour or so cutting slots in the parasol so that any air would not be trapped and working out a way of rigging the weight onto the bottom of the parasol. One of our air divers, Doug was given the task of rigging up the site and Edward was drafted in to help so that he could set up the shot the way he wanted, this took an hour but by two o'clock we were once again ready for the shot, the pack of cards had been stuck to the table together with the bottle of wine and glasses; we also had some gambling chips, the result was very effective, it looked great. The Wasp was being piloted by Bill and as he was settling into the suit, we organised his poker hand with all the aces as agreed, the diver would of course have a random useless poker hand full of haphazard low cards.

When all was ready, we launched the suit with Bill; when the suit was submerged and Bill reported all was well, we unlatched the suit from the TMS; Bill applied gentle downward thrust to swim below the skirt of the TMS frame. He then motored over to the table he of course already had the hand full of aces firmly gripped in his manipulator. Edward made his way to the table ready for the shot, Doug was by then also in position together with his useless poker hand, all was ready. Edward took a great number of photographs of this spectacle none of which I ever saw used in advertisements but maybe they turned up in promotional presentations, who knows. When Edward had completed his pictures and had taken some promotional video, he came back to the surface; we had decided to leave the table, parasol and weights on the bottom overnight so that, if necessary, Edward could take some more shots in the morning. Bill motored back to the TMS while his tether was wound back in by the topside operator, the suit was drawn back into the TMS where it was again latched successfully enabling us to recover the suit.

The next day was to be our final day, I would be travelling home as soon as we had finished diving. I had arranged for Chrissie, my girlfriend to come to pick me up in her car; she would be bringing her sixteen-year-old brother Mike with her; they arrived mid-morning when we were just finishing off the last photographs of the card scenario. The next dive was to be the Wasp completing the Rubik's cube; now, as none of us knew how to complete the Rubik's cube the plan was that the Wasp would go down with the cube in a perfect, pristine condition with all the faces one colour, once photographs had been taken with the Wasp pilot looking very smug the diver would take the cube out of the Wasp's pincer and mess it up before putting it back in the Wasp's manipulator. This would then be photographed with the pilot looking suitably pained, when the photographs were shown in reverse order it would look like the Wasp had completed the cube, great plan!

Bill was again the Wasp pilot and Edward completed the photos over the next hour so all was well again. As I say the dives went very well with Edward getting some great shots showing how superior the Wasp was, again I am not sure any of these pictures were ever used, I certainly never saw them.

Before we packed up Bill suggested that perhaps Chrissie would like to have a dive in the Wasp; Edward was keen as he felt some pictures of a pretty girl in the suit would go down very well. Chrissie however was not looking quite so sure; she is not a diver by any stretch of the imagination and was really not showing any signs of wanting to have a go at all! However, she was still in the period when she wanted to impress me so allowed herself to be persuaded to go ahead and have a go. Eventually she was installed in the Wasp, I was on the comms and spent a good deal of time reassuring her that all would be well. Bill closed the dome and came back into dive control chuckling to himself; the crane driver was given the signal to lift the suit and to swing it out over the water. Edward had already taken a few pictures of her climbing into the suit and some with her smiling as the dome was closed.

To say Chrissie was apprehensive at this point would be an understatement, at the time I didn't know but she doesn't like heights or going underwater, but she didn't tell me that she wanted to stop. I was chatting away to her trying to take her mind off things as the crane driver started to lower the suit into the water, as the suit started to be immersed it started to float up a bit; Chrissie was doing her best to remain calm but it was clear she was not really enjoying this experience. As the suit left surface a small amount of water leaked in through the dome's seal and fell on her head, she definitely was not happy with this situation but, I was able to reassure her that all really was OK. I had already told her to expect a small amount of water as the suit left surface, she did calm down when she realised that the water had stopped coming into the suit. To her credit she didn't freak out and actually spent fifteen minutes underwater before we brought her back to the surface.

The only time she showed any signs of freaking was when Bill said that we were about to let her go! That didn't go down well at all; when the suit was back on the surface and the dome was opened, she was full of beaming smiles having survived her plunge to the depths, more photos. She was a great sport for doing it at all; I think her brother was a bit miffed that he was not offered a dive though. We spent a couple of hours getting the system ready to be taken back to base before we left for our journey home, I had enjoyed the few days and I think Chrissie had enjoyed herself if only a tiny little bit. As far as the TMS trial was concerned it was declared an emphatic success and was employed on Wasp systems in the future.

I had been at home for a couple of days when on the morning of the second of December, I was carrying out some work on my bike when there was a knock at my front door; on opening the door, I was faced with a policeman standing on the doorstep looking a little uncomfortable. He introduced himself and asked my name, he then asked if he could come in, I showed him into the front room, he then proceeded to tell me that my dad had suffered a heart attack and had died. Understandably I was stunned, apparently, dad had been in court in Teignmouth supporting his neighbours who were applying for a licence to open an off-licence in Buckfastleigh when he had been taken ill.

I was told that the magistrate presiding was a doctor who had tried to resuscitate him but there was nothing that could be done, he had been pronounced dead at the scene, I thanked the policeman and he left. I went straight down to the phone box and called my mum, my brother-in-law Bob answered the phone and confirmed what I had been told; I said that I would put my bike back together and would come over as soon as I could. When I arrived in Buckfastleigh an hour later obviously mum was in bits, dad had been ill for some time and had had a previous heart attack when I was in Sicily but, was on the list for a replacement heart valve. We had been led to believe that he would be fine once he received this; clearly that was not going to happen now. After I had spent a couple of hours with mum, I went next door to see Tim and Sharon Patterson who were the ones that dad had been supporting in their application; they of course also were dreadfully upset as you can imagine. I did my best to reassure them that dad would have never wanted them to beat themselves up about what had happened which I know to be true but of course they were still very upset; they were however awarded their licence so my dad's last act was at least successful.

I was just glad that I was at home when it happened so that I could be there to support my mum and sister. I was able to stay at home for two more weeks which meant I was able to help organise and attend dad's funeral, it was a horrible time as these things always are but especially so as dad was just fifty-seven when he died far too soon! Dad had always been there for me and although I'm sure I had tried his patience many a time, he never washed his hands of me (I would not have been surprised if he had). He had a great sense of humour and even when he was ill, he never lost his ability to make us all laugh.

A couple of days later I had to go to the police station in Teignmouth to pick up dad's personal effects which didn't amount to much, there was just his wallet, watch, glasses, signet ring and clothes; I found this to be quite upsetting but someone had to do it. I took everything back to mum who was staying with my sister in Ashburton, when I got there, mum wanted to go through the bag with me, understandably she found this very difficult.

So it was that two weeks later I had to go back to work, I was sent to Spain to a rig called the Afortunada, the job was to cover a diver who was to go home for Christmas; It seemed the job was a carbon copy of the one I had been on in Biarritz, France the previous year. There was a crew of six living on the beach in Salou rotating offshore as and when needed. Oceaneering had another small saturation system on board. Diane had told me that I should make my way to Salou however I could, Salou is some one hundred kilometres south-west of Barcelona; in the early eighties Salou was not the tourist destination it is now. In fact, it proved to be quite difficult to reach, I arrived in Barcelona on a dry and reasonably warm December Monday afternoon, I changed some money at the airport and armed with what I thought would be plenty of Pesetas I started to look at how I could get to Salou.

I again had no Spanish so had to rely on gestures and pointing at maps to make myself understood. I eventually found another trusty wall map showing Barcelona and surrounding area, there didn't seem to be a direct rail link between Barcelona and Salou and it seemed that even if I could get a train, it would take upwards of four hours. I then tried to find a bus but again could not find any bus going to Salou until the following morning, I had to be at the heliport by ten o'clock in the morning so really had to get to Salou that evening. With limited options available I decided to take a taxi, as I walked outside the terminal there was a taxi rank immediately in front of me with several yellow taxi cabs available. I had bought a map and was able to show the taxi driver where I needed to go, he seemed very happy with a fare of this distance, I threw my bag on the taxi's back seat and the driver offered for me to take the passenger front seat which I did. We headed out of the airport and onto a dual carriageway road heading west, the scenery was nice if a little like a desert, as we drove, I saw some rugged hills off to the left sporting interesting advertising hoardings in the shape of a huge black bull.

After a couple of hours, we arrived in Salou, the time was now mid evening. Diane had given me the address of an hotel which I showed the driver; it was clear that he didn't know where the hotel was and in the days before sat-nav he had to resort to stopping at a bar to get directions, it seemed that going into a bar just for directions was not an option in Spain. The driver had to have a drink, I suppose after a couple of hours driving, I should have expected that, eventually, he came back to the car armed with a bit of paper on which were scrawled directions and we were off again.

The hotel finally hove into view, it was quite a modern affair and looked fine to me, I have to say that I was ready for food, beer and bed by then so pretty much anywhere would have been fine by me. The foyer of the hotel was reached via a revolving door, and was all marble and hardwood, looking very posh, the reception desk was off to the right and was manned by a pretty young lady who I very quickly found spoke no English.

She looked crestfallen when it was clear that I didn't speak Spanish so she told me to wait by hand gestures; she disappeared through a door behind reception and was gone some ten minutes, when she returned, she was accompanied by a man armed with a beaming smile and the most horrendous comb over hair do! He didn't have much English either but we eventually were able to make sense of my requirements and it seemed there was indeed a room I could have; great. The next fifteen minutes or so involved me filling in forms (luckily the questions were in both Spanish and English) however it seemed Spain still had not really got to grips with mass tourism and wanted to know everything short of my inside leg measurement.

Eventually all was finished, it then became clear that I had to pay in advance, I thought this was a little strange but hey-ho, never mind; I put my credit card down on the counter as the taxi had taken almost all my cash. The two staff members exchanged looks and then looked at me with an apologetic look, it soon became clear that the hotel only dealt in cash and did not accept credit cards! Oh dear, I certainly didn't have enough cash and there was no such thing as a cashpoint in those days, I tried to show them English money and US dollars but, clearly, they were not interested in accepting either British Pounds or US Dollars so it looked like my chances of staying in this hotel were nil. I collected my passport, credit card, picked up my bag and left the hotel; outside I stopped on the steps of the hotel and considered my next move.

I sat on the steps of the hotel to think through my options which were limited, it was now just after ten-thirty but at least the weather was kind as even for a mid-December night the temperature was not too bad at all and it was dry so it could've been a lot worse. Having now spent a bit of time in Spain in Bilbao and Sant Carles de la Rápita I knew that some Spanish bars stayed open all night so I thought my best bet would be to find an all-night bar and settle in until the morning. Across the road almost opposite the hotel there was a signpost showing Centro de la Ciudad; I wasn't absolutely sure what this meant but was hopeful that Centro meant, the centre of the town was that way. I slung my bag over my shoulder and set off walking hopefully into town with no real idea of how far away it was or indeed even what I was looking for really.

As I moved away from the hotel the time was now marching on and there didn't seem to be much going on at all. The place seemed totally deserted; I was surprised by the lack of people or indeed any sort of action at all because the times I had been to Spain before most things seemed to continue way into the night. I made my way into what I hoped would be the centre of this metropolis I was looking for something although I just didn't know what. I found myself wandering along a dirt road heading between ramshackle run-down houses, there were not many cars parked along the track, there were no streetlights, in short it was desolate. Before long I found I had picked up a pack of seven mangy looking dogs who had started following me circling around keeping their distance but always with their beady eyes fixed on me. Although I like dogs, I must say I found this a little unnerving to say the least, I continued walking and picked up a stick just in case, I thought it might come in handy if the dogs decided I was looking tasty.

I kept walking for another twenty minutes or so when I found myself on metalled road again, this led to a small square with a fountain in the middle, there was no water in the fountain but at least it looked a little more promising, there might be somewhere around here. I walked straight across the square continuing along a street where there were store fronts, I then saw lights a couple of hundred metres further along the street on the right, could this be the civilisation I was looking for?

As I approached the lights, I could see that it was indeed a bar and oh joy it was open; there was a small veranda with tables and chairs outside beside the street, the whole place was extremely dusty and looked none too clean but none of that mattered to me, after all it was open! There was a glazed entrance door to the right of the veranda, I pushed through the door to the sound of squeaky hinges and a jingling bell. I was relieved to see I was not going to be the only customer, the door swung closed behind me and I made my way to the bar, this was along the left wall of the bar.

My Spanish was of course very limited but I did know how to order a beer in Spanish, I was though served up a bottle of San Miguel in very short order, I took a pull of the beer settled onto one of the four bar stools and looked around at my surroundings. This turned out to be a nice little bar with the normal array of lighted signs for beers hanging on the walls; there were four booths along the right-hand wall each one had room for four people and as I say I was pleased to see there were five other customers in the bar, all were male, four were seated in pairs in the booths and the fifth was sitting on another of the bar stools to my right; when I came in, he had been chatting to the barman.

After a few minutes my fellow bar stool sitter caught my eye and to my surprise addressed me in English, the only accent discernible was Cockney, what a result! As the line from Casablanca says, 'of all the bars in all the world'; he was a scrawny looking individual who stood up to offer me a handshake, he was thin, suntanned with grey shoulder length hair and a big smile.

It seemed the Spanish I had used when ordering my beer was perhaps not as faultless as I had hoped and had given me away; we struck up a conversation as is often the case when two Brits meet in a bar in a foreign country. It seemed my new friend was living in the town and had been for quite some considerable time, he could speak what sounded to me like faultless Spanish, well it certainly seemed to work anyway. We shared a few beers and he of course asked what I was doing to end up in the bar at this time of night, I related my story to him explaining how I had hoped to pay for the hotel with a credit card. He found this hilarious and told me that he doubted I would find anywhere or anyone in Salou that would be willing or able to take payment for anything by credit card.

When he found out I was due offshore in the morning to go out to the Afortunada it seemed he knew the team well and had spent a lot of time with them over the previous few months; after we had been chatting and sharing stories for about an hour, he called the barman over and proceeded to pay the bill for both of us. I pulled out my wallet to pay a contribution but he would have none of it, it seemed he had enjoyed our chat and felt it was a nice change for him to find a fellow Brit to share some beers with. He asked what I was planning on doing now, I told him that I would probably stay in the bar until the morning then make my way to the airport. By now all the other customers had either left or were in the process of leaving, my new friend said the bar was going to close as soon as his locals had left.

I told him that I would probably take up residence at one of the tables on the veranda out front and see whether I could get a bit of sleep there; he would have none of that, he then pulled out his wallet again and peeled off enough Pesetas to cover a hotel room for the night at the hotel I had tried to book in to, he then asked whether I needed more for the taxi to the airport in the morning but I said that I already had enough to cover that.

I of course was stunned by this generosity and was not very keen on accepting his money as I had no way of repaying him; he waved this concern off with a flick of his right hand and said "when you get offshore tell the supervisor Graham Pitt that Shady Tree leant you the money, he'll pay me back the next time he's ashore". You could've knocked me over with a feather, he stuffed the money in my hand, put a hand on my shoulder shepherding me out the door so the barman could close up the bar, as soon as we were on the street, we shook hands, he turned around and wandered off down the street humming to himself walking a little unsteadily in the opposite direction to my hotel.

I turned around and made my way back to the hotel where the same desk clerk was clearly surprised to see me again so soon and with cash too? Clearly, I couldn't explain myself but she appeared to just put it all down to 'one of those things', I, of course had already done all the check-in procedures so was presented with a key without delay and found myself in a very reasonable hotel room with a bed and a bathroom without delay. I had a few hours' sleep and was able to find my way to breakfast and subsequently the heliport without further issues.

The Afortunada was another semi-submersible platform, this one was painted bright yellow and was operated by ENIEPSA the Spanish arm of Shell; as soon as I arrived on the platform, I found myself in the diver's cabin where I met the rest of the crew. There was the supervisor who was indeed Graham Pitt, and the divers were one Rhodesian (Zimbabwe now) Bruce; although Rhodesia ceased to exist in July 1980 Bruce still thought of himself as Rhodesian rather than adopting the new name for his country, there were also two Americans, Donnie and Morie as well as another Brit Gary. I was treated to the usual 'get to know you' session for the first half hour during which I related my story of being leant money by shady tree expecting to be ridiculed by the team only to find Graham saying 'oh yeah I know him, I'll give him his money back when I see him'. It seemed that he was a well-known character and this kind of behaviour was to be expected of him!

Gary was given the job of giving me the guided tour of the dive system, this took most of the afternoon, the system was very similar to the one I had been using in France. It was another Perry system consisting of single living chamber with an integrated 'wet pot' from which a trunking extended to which the bell would clamp for transfer under pressure; the bell was again a 'roll-over' affair with just the one door. This all was fine by me, the system looked to be well maintained and serviceable, Gary showed me where the hot water suits were stored and I was again able to select a suitable one for my use.

When we were back in dive control Graham came in with Donnie and Morie; he proceeded to tell us that there was a Coflexip operated ship working alongside the rig they were changing subsea hoses but that they had experienced a problem resulting in them dropping one of the hoses onto the seabed. We had been tasked with diving to attach strops to the dropped hose so that it could be recovered, this would involve us putting two divers in for what would hopefully be a short duration 'bounce' dive. As I was just covering for the diver who had gone home for Christmas I didn't expect to be chosen for the dive and I was right, Donnie and Morie had already been scheduled for the dive and were told to prepare the chamber for their dive.

I was to be teamed up with Bruce, we would be Life Support Technicians (LST) for the night shift, Graham and Gary would cover the day shift. We all started to prepare the system for diving, I was tasked with opening all the Heliox quads, this sounds like a simple task and it is but, there were six quads each consisting of sixteen bottles so, ninety-six bottles in total all of which had to be opened individually. This took me a good hour and I can tell you my wrists were knackered by the time all the valves were open! All was now ready for the dive to commence; I was given the role of handling the bell umbilical together with Gary; our American friends had already loaded their personal equipment into the chamber and Graham gave the order for the chamber to be closed prior to blowdown. As soon as the door was closed, I could hear gas being blown into the chamber, the drill was to take the chamber down to storage depth without anybody inside, the divers would then go down inside the bell at one atmosphere and would only pressurise when on the bottom in just the same way as we had done in France.

Donnie and Morie climbed into the bell and made ready, as soon as they were told to close the bottom door of the bell, I pushed the door up so that they could latch the dogs inside. We then attached the bell's drop weight before the bell was then lifted to that we could open the bell's moonpool. Bruce was handling the winch and started lowering the bell through the moonpool; as soon as the bell was beneath the rig's deck, we closed the moonpool cover again, Gary and I moved across to the bell's lift wire and started to attach the umbilical to the lift wire, this was done by wrapping chains around the lift wire and the umbilical binding the two together, it was a very simple and effective method of attaching the two together. Doing this meant that the umbilical would be supported by the bell's main lift wire reducing strain on the umbilical; again, this was exactly the same system we had used in France.

When the bell was at a depth just a few metres above the seabed the divers inside the bell were given the order to make ready to leave the bell and when ready to blow down the bell; this process should have taken just a few minutes but it seemed there was some kind of issue. The bell had been blown down to working depth in preparation for the diver locking out but, it took the first diver over forty minutes after the bell had been pressurised to leave the bell. This meant that the hopes of the dive being a short duration bounce dive were history. The client was jumping, as he had been expecting the job to take much less time than this. It did of course mean that this would not be a short bounce dive and that the divers would be in sat meaning the dive was going to be several days in duration however long the job actually took as the decompression would be some three days.

Eventually though the diver left the bell and made his way across to the job, the lifting strops had already been lowered and were waiting for him, the diver took about an hour to dig his way under the hose and to attach the lifting strops. The ship then took up the slack and as soon as the strop had been pulled up tight the diver was told to return to the bell and to prepare to leave bottom; this went without a hitch and very soon the bell was being lifted; Gary and I were once more handling the bell umbilical removing the chains as they appeared through the moonpool.

When the bell was on deck, we closed the moonpool, the bell was lowered so that we could detach the drop weight, once this was done the bell could be rotated through ninety degrees to allow mating to the chamber trunking. After about half an hour the bell was safely attached to the chamber, the trunking had been pressurised allowing the divers to open the doors in the bell and the chamber so that they could safely transfer through into the chamber. As soon as the divers had transferred through to the chamber, Graham told Bruce and I to stand down and get some rest and to return to take over LST duties at midnight. Over the next few days, we were looking after the decompression from midnight to midday and all went fine with us making multiple trips to the galley for tea, coffee, snacks and breakfast for the divers.

Everything the divers wanted Bruce or I had to get for them as obviously they couldn't get out of the chamber until their decompression was complete, everything would be passed into the chamber via the medical lock. This was exactly the same as the one I had used in France, we used it to transfer food and drinks into and out of the pressurised chamber. I was very careful to adhere strictly to the procedure for using the lock so as not to put anybody at risk.

On the second day of decompression, it was my turn to get the guy's breakfasts; once they were awake, I asked them what they would like for breakfast there was good deal of discussion inside the chamber but eventually I took their order and left Bruce in sat control while I went to the galley. I returned with a loaded tray with all they had requested, there were pancakes, bacon, maple syrup, coffee and a heap of sauces etc., it was now time for me to lock the breakfasts into the chamber.

Step one was for me to establish communications with Bruce, I did this by calling into a bullhorn alongside the lock, Bruce answered me confirming we had good communications. I then asked him whether I could take the lock, this meant that he would confirm with the divers that the lock's inner door was closed. Bruce confirmed to me that it was safe for me to take the lock, I told Bruce, 'I'm taking the lock'; I could hear him repeat this to the divers inside the chamber. I then opened the lock's drain valve, while watching the small gauge outside the lock that indicated pressure inside the lock and I could see that it dropped until it read zero, this should mean there was no pressure inside the lock but just to be sure I left the lock drain valve open.

Once I was sure the lock was empty, I started to undo the locking device; in this case the lock door was secured by a tubeturn device, this consisted of two semi-circular metal halves, they were attached to one another via a hinge on one side and a large bolt on the other. When the tubeturn was clamped around the outer door it would squeeze the door onto the outside flange of the lock thus making a seal and keeping the pressure contained safely inside the lock.

I was confident that there was no pressure inside the lock and that it was safe for me to open the lock, I removed the nut and bolt from the tubeturn and swung it away allowing the door to open. I removed a couple of cups from the lock that the divers had used the previous time they had coffees; wiped out the lock as it is very important that any spilt liquid or food is not left in the lock, this reduces the likelihood of infection. When the lock was empty and clean, I loaded the breakfasts making sure I removed the covers from the cups and made sure there were no sealed containers (if there were sealed containers they would be squeezed by the pressure and would either implode or be impossible to open once at depth).

I then closed the door replacing the tubeturn tightening the bolt back up; lastly, I closed the lock's vent valve before telling Bruce, 'Lock ready to be pressurised'; again, I could hear him repeating this to the divers inside so that they were kept updated on progress.

Once Bruce came back to me and told me I was authorised to pressurise the lock I slowly opened the valve allowing chamber atmosphere into the lock and watched the gauge rise until it read the same as that in the chamber. I told Bruce 'Lock pressurised' closed the valve and checked the gauge to ensure the pressure inside was not dropping this made sure there were no leaks. Once I was sure all was well, I told Bruce 'No leaks, safe to open'; he passed this on to the divers and they then opened the inner door, as soon as they had emptied the lock, they closed the inner door again. Bruce told me 'Inner door closed, take the lock'; I then again opened the drain valve and watched the gauge drop to zero. I told Bruce 'Lock on surface', I left the lock door closed and all valves closed as this was the safest condition for the divers.

During the next couple of days there was very little going on during the night shift, Bruce and I chatted about our lives outside of the diving world. It was very clear that Bruce was not at all happy with the new regime in Zimbabwe he told me a great deal about how the country was changing under the new regime particularly how the white farmers were being marginalised. Bruce's parents ran a farm just outside the capital Harare (formerly Salisbury).

During the last few hours of the decompression Bruce received some bad news from home it seemed that his father had been in dispute with the workers some of whom had been working on the farm for years but, with the new regime the workers felt they were entitled to more than they had been getting, this had resulted in their killing all of the family's dogs. Bruce told Graham that he had to leave and go home to help his family, Graham told him that he would get a replacement but that Bruce couldn't be spared until the replacement arrived which would be a couple of days. Although Bruce was clearly very upset, we continued with the rest of the decompression, this continued without incident and finished on the thirty first of December. Bruce's replacement a Scot called Josh McCrea arrived on the fourth of January enabling Bruce to finally make his way home.

After a few days on surface and before the crew had time to decamp to the beach there was another problem with the Cofexip hoses with another of them ending up on the seabed and needing to be recovered, this time the hose would need to be cut before it could be recovered. Graham briefed the team; Gary and I would be the divers with Danny and Morie carrying out the sat tech duties along with Josh and Graham. We were to set up an hydraulic cutting disk which would be lowered to the seabed to enable the cut. I was excited as I had not used a hydraulic cutting disk underwater before. Initially I helped set up the hydraulic hoses with the disk cutter; very soon Graham told me to get all my gear together in the chamber as we would be blowing down (starting the dive) in a couple of hours. I headed to my cabin to retrieve my washing kit, towels and books then as I was loading all my kit into the chamber Graham arrived and told Gary and I to come back out of the chamber; this was odd, what was going on?

As soon as we were back on deck standing beside the chamber Graham told us that we were not going to be diving, the divers would again be Danny and Morie! Gary and I exchanged puzzled looks, this was not right and seemed totally unfair, with any team I had worked with in the past the dives were cycled through the team so this should be our dive. It seemed that the issue came down to pay; the full-time crew consisting of six personnel who were operating as I had done in France carrying out one month on the beach standing by and two weeks on the rig were on salary. Gary and I who were covering for two members of the normal team who had gone home for Christmas were not on salary, we were being paid a day rate. Our day rate was more than the salary rate by some margin and it seemed that Danny and Morie were not prepared to act as our sat techs when they were not being paid as much as us! Apparently, they were threatening to walk off the job if they didn't get the dive. This now caused a big problem; Oceaneering clearly needed the dive to go ahead pronto and could not get replacement divers here for another couple of days at least.

Gary and I had no real choice other than to accede to their demands and so we removed our kit leaving the chamber for Danny and Morie, a bad day all round. I took Graham into his cabin and explained my views about how he as the supervisor should have put his foot down and although he said he could see my point of view he made it clear that he couldn't make them work if they didn't want too. I told him that I would carry out sat tech duties for the dive but as soon as the chamber was back on surface, I wanted a chopper waiting for me as I would be going home. A stand-up row ensued as he felt I was wrong to take this stance but I refused to go back on my statement, after a good fifteen minutes of very heated debate I left him to stew in his cabin and went to finish preparations for the dive.

I was working the deck with Gary when the dive started and as soon as the bell was at working depth, we started to rig the disk cutter and hydraulic hoses ready to send down to the divers. We had rigged everything to be lowered by an air powered winch termed a 'tugger', the tugger wire had been run through a pulley sheave above the moonpool; using short lengths of thin rope I attached the disk cutter to the tugger wire leaving about four metres of free hose to make it easier for the divers to manage getting the cutter to the job, I attached the whole assembly to one of the bell's guide wires using a shackle so that it would slide down the guide wire to the bell making it easy for the divers to find and started to lower the equipment through the moonpool.

Gary was paying out the tugger wire and as it descended, I attached the hydraulic hoses to the tugger wire every three metres or so, this would mean that the hydraulic hoses were supported by the tugger's wire rope in the same way that the bell's umbilical was supported by the lift wire and would be manageable both for me to handle on the surface and also by the divers on the seabed.

When all was on the seabed the diver easily managed to take the cutter to the Coflexip hose and started to cut however, it soon became clear that cutting the hose with the disk cutter was not going to work, it seemed the disk cutter didn't have sufficient power. Hydraulic tools either need high pressure or high flow to make them work properly, impact wrenches such as I had used on my diving course really need high pressure but relatively low flow to make them work properly. Disk cutters while needing a certain amount of pressure this was not the major factor what they really needed was high flow at a decent pressure to allow them to work properly. It seemed that because the hoses were so long there was too much back pressure in the hoses and this restricted the flow to a point that the disk cutter had virtually no power; in fact, the diver showed us that he could grip the turning disk and stop it from rotating!

The client decided a rethink was required so Graham told the diver to go back to the bell while the situation was discussed. There were limited options available for cutting these hoses, the disk cutter was the preferred option but as had been shown would not work. The next choice was to use Oxy-Arc cutting with Ultrathermic cutting rods, the miniature thermic lances. The client was not happy to use this hot cut as it's termed as the hoses had been carrying crude oil and he felt there would be residue in the hose that could cause fire or explosion. After a good deal of discussion, a plan emerged, the hoses had already been opened to the sea allowing seawater to flow through them; they were full of water so it was felt the risk of fire would be minimised to a point where it was acceptable.

The diver was told to lock out of the bell and make sure the disk cutter and hoses were ready to be recovered to the surface, Gary and I went back on deck to pull everything back up. By the time this was complete it was decided the divers needed to be recovered to the chamber on deck while the Oxy-Arc cutting gear was prepared. The bell was recovered and the divers transferred through into the living chamber where they would spend the night.

By the next morning, we together with the rig crew had prepared the Oxy-Arc cutting gear; this was then sent down to the divers using the same tugger wire system; as soon as all was ready the command 'make it hot' came over the coms Graham closed the heavy-duty knife switch thus supplying electrical power to the cutting torch. The diver struck an arc and pulled the trigger on the cutting torch allowing the flow of oxygen to run through the cutting rod and started to cut the hose, it soon became clear that this was working very well and quite quickly the hose was cut as required.

The job was eventually completed and with the divers safely ensconced in the living chamber decompression commenced, again I was on the night shift where I sat and seethed at how we had been treated. As the chamber neared surface some three days later, Graham informed me that my relief would be arriving the next day and I would be travelling home that day, I had been on the job for a month and three days.

The next day as I was just about to board the chopper, Graham took me to one side and told me he would do everything he could to ensure I never worked for Oceaneering again! As you can imagine this didn't fill me with anything but concern that maybe my offshore career was if not over then would be suffering a significant setback. As it turned out, he clearly didn't have anything like the amount of clout he thought he had, I arrived home on the seventeenth of January and was on my way to Abidjan in the Ivory Coast on twenty third of January!

CHAPTER FOURTEEN

For me 1982 started as the previous year had finished, after I returned home from Spain, I spent a bit of time with mum who had by now moved back to their hardware shop in Buckfastleigh. They had run this shop together for just a few years but clearly, she now would have to manage without him. We spent some time going through dad's things and when she came across his signet ring, she told me that dad had wanted me to wear it as I was now the senior male in the family (well in truth I was the only male now). I was touched by this and told mum I would love to wear his ring. Unfortunately, the ring was a little too big for my fingers, I knew that I would not have a chance to have it resized before I had to leave for my next job but I decided I would just need to be very careful with it. In truth, I really should have just left it at home until I had been able to get a jeweller to resize it properly but this is with the benefit of hindsight!

I was at home for just a few days during which time I teased and chided Chrissie my girlfriend for not even sending me a Christmas card while I was in Spain! She told me she had written every day and had definitely sent a Christmas card. I had decided that during this leave period I needed to look for a car, although I loved my motorbike. I didn't really want to have to ride it in the rain and in any case, there were times when a car would be much more sensible; I know, sensible, I never thought I would do anything sensible. I managed to find a Ford Fiesta 1.3 Sport in the local Ford dealership, the car had been won in a competition, evidently the winner didn't feel they wanted to run it so had sold it to the main Ford dealer in Torquay. I bought it with just two hundred miles on the clock, it was a nice little car that was perfect for me; it was finished in diamond white with fetching red flashes along the sides and four spoke alloy wheels; the interior was a bit garish for my liking with red and white checked upholstery but there's always something to compromise isn't there?

Anyway, I soon had to leave home again to cover another absence of a salaried team member, this time I would be on my way to Abidjan in the Ivory Coast or as it is now termed Côte d'Ivoire, the contract I was to be working was another rig support set up but this time the team were covering not one but five separate installations. We would be working from a supply boat and would be travelling around the various locations as needs arose; the water depth off Abidjan was quite deep with the maximum we may be faced with being two thousand two hundred and fifty feet (686 metres). This was beyond the depth capability of the Wasp as I understood it to be, I thought its maximum depth was two thousand feet (609 metres) but I had been assured that the suits had been reclassified just for this job and all was OK for the increased depth.

The whole contract was due to finish a month or so after I arrived so I would be helping with demobilisation. I travelled from London's Gatwick airport to Abidjan on a direct British Caledonian flight; B-Cal as they were termed was an independent Airline that unfortunately has disappeared along with many others since then. The Ivory Coast had been a French colony since 1893 there was a coup d'état in 1999, resulting in the country becoming a republic with the adoption of a new constitution in 2000. However, in 1982 when I was there the regime was fairly stable benefiting from a close liaison with France and other western democracies.

My flight arrived at what is now Félix Houphouët-Boigny International Airport early afternoon, as soon as I stepped out of the aircraft I was again greeted by that wonderful aroma of African rainforest, it was hot and very humid. I made my way down the steps of the aircraft safe in the knowledge that I had all the necessary information for any visa requirements; I joined the queue at passport control where I presented my documents for their scrutiny. In addition to my passport, I had proof of my yellow fever vaccination as this was an entry requirement; all was accepted, I received the stamp in my passport and was ushered through to baggage reclaim.

As with my trips to Angola again, I only had carry-on baggage so made my way directly to customs. When my turn came, I was invited to place my bag onto the table in front of the customs officer, now, being a seasoned traveller, (having been to a grand total of two African countries before) I had placed a number of packs of Marlborough cigarettes strategically in the bag. The customs officer unzipped my bag whereupon all my token gifts were presented for him; he totally ignored them, sweeping them out of the way so that he could delve into the bag properly. He removed my camera and wash bag, now I could understand why he would be interested in my camera but what did he want with my washbag? It turned out he didn't want anything with either of these, he had just removed them as they were making his search more difficult. After just a couple of minutes he shoved everything back in the bag including all the cigarettes, zipped it back up and gave me a wonderful big toothy smile before gesturing for me to carry on through to the arrivals area. In many ways the process had been very similar to that of entering any European country in the early eighties.

Diane had told me that I would be met at the airport by one of the team, so, as I entered the arrivals area I started to look around for my contact, of course Diane had not given me a name! I had thought ahead and was wearing a 'Rat-Hat Diver' 'T' shirt, this clearly worked as very soon another bear of a man clapped me on the shoulder and said "are you with Oceaneering", there was clearly no flies on him! He introduced himself as Roger and told me that he had a car, we made our way out of the terminal and walked about a hundred yards to the car park. He stopped next to a Toyota Hi-ace crew-bus unlocked the doors and told me to dump my stuff in the back. As we drove out of the airport Roger told me that Oceaneering had been working this contract for almost a year and were well set up, there was a staff house manned by a local cook/houseboy so we were apparently well looked after. It also seemed that the whole crew were ashore at the moment as the ship was off doing work that didn't require divers.

The airport was some fifteen kilometres outside the city of Abidjan and as we drove, I settled back to enjoy the ride; the roads were well maintained and not terribly overcrowded, on both sides of the road there was lush forest, it was quite beautiful. After about half an hour we were entering the suburbs; there was the usual array of run-down commercial plots and buildings with a few flashy car dealerships.

Finally, we made our way into a nice residential area, most of the houses seemed from the road to be single storey bungalow type buildings, all looked to be well maintained and on fairly large plots covered in lush vegetation. The staff house was on the left-hand side midway along a quiet street, there was a car port in front with another vehicle already in situ, we parked alongside the car, Roger turned off the ignition, we had arrived. We entered into a large open plan living area, there were three large sofas and a couple of arm chairs surrounding a low heavy wooden coffee table, the rest of the crew were chilling with beers, I sat down and was immediately given a beer as we started the normal 'get to know you' chat. As with the other Wasp jobs I had been on there were five personnel, these were two ADS pilots, two air divers and a supervisor. The supervisor this time was John Bryan who was quick to introduce himself (I had heard of John from when I was previously working with Wasps) the other pilot was Matt Chappel, the air divers were Roger and another Peter, Peter Shaw. We spent a nice couple of hours getting to know one another.

The chef/houseboy was working away in the kitchen but when he heard me arrive, he came in to see whether I needed anything; he was introduced by John as Jimmy although I know that wasn't his real name, he only spoke French with just a smattering of English. Jimmy was a native from Upper Volta (now Burkina Faso), he was a wiry individual about six foot tall; his face was marked with tribal marks, these were scars denoting his tribal heritage.

The house had three bedrooms, I would be sharing one of them with the Matt, the two air divers were in the second bedroom and of course John had the last one to himself. Dinner was served at about seven thirty and consisted of a very nice lamb stew served with rice, it was delicious, clearly, I would not starve on this trip! After dinner we all graduated to the decking at the rear of the property where we sat drinking beers and chatting all evening, the deck was a wooden affair, large enough for all of us to sit comfortably on very well upholstered rattan chairs, it was a lovely evening, the temperature had dropped to a comfortable level and there were very few mosquitos.

When initially driving along the road I had thought all the properties were single storey but I could now see that the houses on this side of the road had been built on a hill which fell away below the deck. John told me that the rooms on the lower level were the laundry, store rooms and Jimmy's accommodation; it was a very pleasant house indeed. We would spend quite a lot of our time on this balcony chilling out and watching the fireflies that we nicknamed B-Cal as they flashed a little like the wingtip lights of an airliner, we eventually wandered off to our various beds where I had a very good night's sleep.

The next day John made a call to the client who told him that we were not required for the next two days, it seemed there was nothing for us to do so here I was again in a wonderful location being paid to do nothing it really was a tough life. So, what would we do with the next couple of days? John suggested we take the crew-bus and visit Grand-Bassam this was the beach the team tended to use so we loaded the bus up with a crate of beers and off we went. Grand-Bassam was a town just a few kilometres east of Abidjan. It was originally the French colonial capital city until there was a significant bout of yellow fever forcing the French to relocate its capital further inland. When I was there in the early eighties the place was a ghost town, large sections had been abandoned for decades, Grand-Bassam was it seemed only inhabited by squatters.

Beginning in the late 1970s, the town began to revive as a tourist destination and craft centre although I was told that a lot of the locals would still not set foot in the place as there were lots of superstitions attached to it. We all piled into the crew-bus and made our way to the beach, yay! When we arrived, I was stunned by the place, it was wonderful, we parked alongside a palm tree lined beach facing the Gulf of Guinea. On the landward side of the road were a large number of grand old colonial buildings, the French had built their city on a grid pattern, the beach was long and straight with a wide road running alongside. As I walked along the road with the sea on my left, I could see a number of wide boulevards running north away from the beach road, this was completely empty of people, all of these wonderful villas had been abandoned, it seemed that the locals would go nowhere near them as the spectre of yellow fever still hung over them! It was an earie place to say the least.

We set ourselves up on the beach with towels, football and beers and set about enjoying the day we had everything except knotted hankies on our heads; Brits abroad eh. The beach was huge, maybe twenty metres wide but looking in either direction along the beach I couldn't see either end, I know now that the beach extends almost ten miles! However, on that day we had the beach pretty much to ourselves, there were only a few others to our left and nobody else. After a very short time of course the locals turned up trying to hawk their wares, although this was a little annoying it was really a small price to pay. One thing that I did take advantage of though was the guy selling fresh pineapples for the equivalent of fifteen pence each; he would cut them to order, he did this using a huge machete, he was very adept with his knife, he made it quite a spectacle. Once the pineapple was cut, he presented it to me in a banana leaf, it was great, very tasty if a little sticky to eat, still once I had finished eating, I just went for a swim all was good.

Late afternoon we decided to make our way back to the staff house but, on the way back to the crew-bus we stopped in a tiny bar next to the beach for much needed refreshment. We sat outside at one of the little tables overlooking the beach. While we were sitting there, I saw a local sitting by the side of the road with a tiny cooking set up, it looked like a primus stove, he was frying yams in a very small frying pan. I wandered over to see what he was doing and the smell of frying oil was lovely I decided I was a bit peckish so I bought a banana leaf filled with fried yam, it tasted great and finished off the day brilliantly or so I thought. As the sun was setting, we made our way back to the staff house where Jimmy produced another feast for us; all was well until we were again on the deck after our meal just finishing the day with another beer.

My stomach was churning and becoming a little uncomfortable, this continued until at about midnight I decided to retire to my bed; things did not improve and soon I was in the toilet where I spent the rest of the night! It had been a long time since I had felt so bad, I just couldn't leave the toilet, to say I had diarrhoea and vomiting would be an understatement, it was awful! It was just as well that there was another toilet in the house otherwise things could have become very messy; the next day I got worse and spent the whole of the next two days either in the toilet or in my bed, I really couldn't do anything, Jimmy kept me supplied with mineral water but I found even this difficult to keep down.

The following day it was decided I needed to see a doctor, I agreed but was very nervous about leaving the house, could the doctor be persuaded to come to the house? Not a chance; anyway, by now I really had nothing much left to throw up or pass the other way and so it was decided that I would be taken to Oceaneering's doctor who had a practice in downtown Abidjan. Matt was tasked with chauffeur duties, although I have to say he didn't look best pleased to have won this particular lottery; we were both very nervous for slightly different reasons as Matt and I made our way in to see the doctor. Matt pulled in to the kerb right next to the doctor's surgery, we had already agreed that I would go in on my own and he would park the crew-bus somewhere close by before joining me in the waiting room.

This was my first real experience of an African city although I now know that Abidjan was not really typical of African cities in the eighties, it was clear there was still a big French influence, it felt very French although there were significantly greater numbers of beggars here than any city I had been too in France.

The doctor's surgery was on the first floor above a row of shops, as I entered, I was greeted by a pretty young receptionist who addressed me in French, luckily, although my French could not be termed fluent by any stretch of the imagination I had just about enough to understand most of what she was saying. She wanted to know my name, so far so good, once she had this information, she located my name on a list and told me to sit down in the waiting room, luckily there was a toilet close by which I had to make use of. After a wait of just a few minutes I was ushered in to see the doctor, he was a very tall white chap who thankfully spoke good English. He spent a good ten minutes listening to my tales of woe and then had me lay down on a consulting couch where he prodded and poked me for another few minutes, as part of this examination I had explained what I was doing for a living even to the point that I may be required to be locked into a submersible with no access to toilet facilities for up to six hours at a time.

After this he gave me a sample tube and asked me whether I thought I could provide a stool sample; I told him I would give it a go and adjourned to the toilet again. Well to cut the story short, I managed to produce the requested sample which I gave to the nurse who was hovering outside the toilet door, this was something she was clearly used to and didn't bat an eyelid. The doctor wanted to see me again before I left so, in I went, he told me that results of the tests would take a few days and he would then want to see me again. I explained that I was due to go offshore the next day and that I really needed something to help me while I waited for the results; he clearly was used to this kind of request and produced a prescription for me.

He told me that these pills would certainly stop the diarrhoea and vomiting and should make me feel well enough to be able to work, I thanked him for his help and wandered back out to the waiting room. Matt was by then waiting for me, he stood up as soon as he saw me, I showed him the prescription and he said he knew where there was a pharmacy just a few minutes-walk away.

Again, the pharmacist spoke English and took very little time to provide me with the specified drugs, I got the impression it was not the first time he had a white guy in his shop suffering with my symptoms. I took the first pill as soon as we got back to the crew-bus and fingers crossed, I would start to feel better very soon. That evening and night passed with a lessening of my symptoms and by morning I felt almost human again even to the point of taking a little dry bread for breakfast, again, fingers firmly crossed about this. The whole team would be going offshore as Oceaneering wanted us to take some subsea video of the trials of a brand new remotely operated vehicle (ROV) called Scorpio, this was a work class vehicle and was apparently the first of many that Oceaneering planned to purchase.

We would be going offshore by boat so we all piled into the Toyota crew-bus together with our bags and John drove us down to the docks; this was not very far; as with most commercial docks we travelled through an industrial area to get there. Before long we arrived on a concrete dockside where we all decamped alongside our ship, John took off with the crew-bus to park it in a safe location while we were offshore. The ship we were to use was called the Arcadia Navigator, she was tied up alongside the dock, her portside against the wall, she was what looked to be a fairly newish supply boat with the familiar tall accommodation towards the bow leaving the rear deck open for payload and cargo.

Her hull was painted dark green with her accommodation being white. I wandered over to the side of the dock to look down at her rear deck where I could see our two Wasps and the associated A-frames, winches, hydraulic power pack and two ten-foot shipping containers; one of these I knew would hold our dive control and the other would be our workshop with spares and other equipment. Our equipment had been set up at the stern of the vessel and it was clear that when we launched the suits they would be dropped over the stern; it all looked fine to me.

Along the starboard side there were two twenty-foot containers positioned athwart ships (running port to starboard) with their doors opening onto the centre of the deck. They were painted in yellow and white, the Oceaneering colours, the Scorpio and its associated launch A-frame was sited between the containers arranged so that the ROV would be launched over the starboard side of the ship. This was the first work class ROV I had seen on a job although I had seen a few other work class ROVs at the Oceaneering site in Aberdeen. As I say the vehicle here was a Scorpio work class ROV manufactured by Perry Tritech in the USA, it was quite a large vehicle at 2.75 metres long, 1.8 metres high and 1.8 metres wide, it weighed some 1,650 Kg it had a maximum diving depth of 940 metres of seawater, its maximum forward speed would apparently be some four knots. This one was fitted with two manipulators, one of which was the very capable arm manufactured by General Electric (GE), this was the main arm that would be used for complex tasks. The second arm was a 'grabber' arm that would be used to hang on to a structure while the other arm was carrying out its tasks.

ROVs at that time consisted of an aluminium or plastic frame into which thrusters were fitted, these thrusters were arranged such that the vehicle could move in all directions as required. The Scorpio was a powerful beast. There were two video cameras fitted so that the pilots could see to manoeuvre and work with the arms as necessary, it also was fitted with a sophisticated sonar navigation system; our job would be to follow the Scorpio underwater videoing it at work.

We all made our way down the gangplank onto the rear deck of the ship, in common with all supply boats I had been on the deck was covered in heavy wood with lengths of steel running fore and aft at intervals across the deck. There were a number of steel rings set into the deck so that cargo and equipment could easily be secured, we wandered over to the Scorpio team to introduce ourselves, I didn't know any of the crew but it seemed John did know a couple of them. After we had said our hellos, we went into the accommodation where we were told there was not enough accommodation for all of us, it seemed that the Scorpio crew had taken all the available bunks and we would need to either 'hot-bunk' with them or kip on deck somewhere.

Clearly this was not an ideal situation but it was not something we could do anything about, it seemed that the plan was for us to sail today travelling a relatively short distance to find clear, deep water where we could carry out and film the trial and then to return to port the next day so it was only going to be just one night. I decided that I would be fine, I would sling a hammock on the rear deck and sleep under the stars; as we would be at sea there would be no mosquitos to contend with so I would be fine; in fact, I was looking forward to a night under the stars.

I have to say that the night was not the most comfortable or restful I have had but it was not too bad, my stomach was feeling quite a bit better, it seemed to have settled with the pills, this was just as well as I was due to dive the suit today and I certainly needed to be on form during this period of time. We had breakfast at just after five o'clock in the morning as was normal offshore and then adjourned to the rear bridge wing to watch the initial trials of the Scorpio.

The ROV crew could be seen buzzing around the vehicle preparing it for launch, when everything was ready, we saw the vehicle being lifted and the A-frame started to move the vehicle over the side of the ship. As soon as the A-frame had swung the vehicle over the side the main winch started to lower the vehicle into the water, all went well until the vehicle entered the water when it became clear all was not well! The vehicle was not responding to instructions and was being knocked against the ship's hull, the ROV crew lifted it back on board as quickly as possible; as soon as the vehicle was back on its launch skid the crew began looking for the problem. At this time ROVs had a bit of a reputation for being unreliable which I suppose could be expected after all putting an electrically powered vehicle into seawater did have the potential to end in tears didn't it?

We decided to wander down to offer our help, when we arrived though we were met by the Perry technician who told us that the problem was fixed as it had been caused by a connector not being properly seated. The vehicle was now ready for another launch; we stood by and watched the vehicle go through its launch procedure again and this time it did indeed go faultlessly.

I stood by the side of the ship and watched the vehicle enter the water, as soon as the weight came off the vehicle's umbilical, I saw the vertical thruster power up pushing seawater upwards and thrusting the vehicle down, it left surface at last. The first couple of hours were programmed to be the vehicle carrying out various trials of manoeuvrability and we had been told that we would just be getting in the way during this phase. This was programmed for the rest of the morning; we were told to prepare to dive early afternoon when the ROV would be diving to depth and where we would be required to video the vehicle going through its paces.

John told us we should prepare our system for the dive so that we were properly ready whenever they needed us; we wandered over to the Wasps and got to work. As I would be diving the suit I climbed in and checked that the floor was adjusted correctly for my height; the floor could be raised and lowered a few inches hydraulically, but it didn't need adjusting as it was just fine for me where it was. We spent the rest of the morning preparing for our dive, it was unusual for us to have lots of time prior to a dive as normally we were under pressure to dive as soon as possible after being told we were needed.

All was ready by twelve o'clock midday and we decided to go for lunch, as we walked past the Scorpio dive control, I poked my head in to have a look, it was a different world in there. The first sensation was that it was dark inside, it was also very quiet, in a normal dive control you could always hear the diver's breathing and there would be conversation. There were two guys sat in front of two large TV monitors which were displaying images from the vehicle's cameras. The right-hand seat was occupied by the guy who would be operating the vehicle's GE arm while in the left-hand seat the other pilot was responsible for flying the vehicle. There were other monitors one showing the display from the vehicle's sonar and another showing depth and heading information, as I say it was another world.

I decided to leave them to it and went off to find the galley and the rest of my team; as is the norm there was a wide variety of foods on offer for lunch and I decided to go for gumbo and rice. This was delicious and I ate quite a lot as I was actually hungry for the first time in days. After we had all finished our meals, we went back out to the dive system and stood by waiting to be called, John and I discussed what I was to do, he told me that the Scorpio would be on the seabed at around six hundred feet and I was to follow its umbilical down until I found it. This sounded simple enough, I had looked over the stern of the vessel where I saw the viz was very good, so finding and following Scorpio's bright yellow umbilical should be no problem; we checked the Wasp's video camera was working properly all was good.

At that time Wasps had a single camera mounted on the front of the chest just below the acrylic dome, it should be easy for me to keep the Scorpio in shot provided I made sure it was just in front of me, anyway John told me he would direct me. At two o'clock we were told to launch, I climbed into the suit and carried out all my pre-dive checks, when all was ready Matt closed the Wasp's dome and I was ready to go.

John kept me informed and I felt the suit tilt as the winch took the weight, I was lifted up into the A-frame which then started to winch me out over the stern of the ship; as soon as I was clear of the stern the winch operator started to lower the suit into the water. I was watching the water rise up to meet me but just as the dome was half submerged all stopped? I asked John what was going on and after a couple of minutes he told me that one of the A-frame's hydraulic hoses had burst. Oh dear, this meant that I couldn't go anywhere as the hydraulic system was common to both the A-frame and the main winch. I was stuck with the suit only partially submerged; the tropical sun was beating down on me through the acrylic dome and the suit was stuck in the splash zone being affected by the swell and wave action. The day was pretty much flat calm but, even so there was still a fair amount of movement making life quite uncomfortable for me plus it was becoming very hot in there, I had a small bottle of water but nothing else.

John told me that they would have things sorted shortly as they already had a replacement hose and would be fitting pronto! It was now that my stomach started to cramp, maybe it had not been such a good idea to eat such a large lunch! All I could do was wait, there was nothing for me to see or do but, it was becoming very uncomfortable, still John kept assuring me it wouldn't be long before they had me back on deck. As it turned out it took just over an hour before I was winched back on deck and the dome was opened, I can tell you it was a great relief to be out of the suit and sprinting up the deck to find the toilet which I reached just in time.

I was soon able to re-join the team on deck, while I was away it had been agreed that we would have to spend a second night offshore and try again tomorrow. Before we could knock off for the day, we needed to shut the system down properly and as we were going to be diving again tomorrow, we decided to make sure everything was ready. This included close inspection of all hydraulic hoses so that we wouldn't have a repeat of the problem in the morning. One of my jobs was to wash the suit down to remove as much of the salt from the suit as possible, corrosion was not such a big problem for the Wasps as it was for JIM suits as the torso of the hull was constructed from aluminium with the main body being constructed from glass fibre, but it was still sensible to wash the suits with fresh water and soap.

I wandered up to the accommodation armed with my bucket and found the laundry area where I filled the bucket with warm water and detergent. I then proceeded to wash the suit with the soapy water using a sponge, this didn't take long and when I had finished, I stood back to admire my work in the afternoon sunshine. We weren't very far offshore so I spent a few minutes leaning on the rail chatting to Matt about the coastline we could see across the glassy surface of the sea, it was very peaceful and pleasant. After about an hour everything was ready so we all stood down; I spent a bit of time refining my hammock to make the coming night more comfortable, then went to find the rest of the crew. Most of them were reading books in the common room just waiting for meal time; I decided to go back on deck to read my book as the common room was quite stuffy and full of smoke as in those days smoking was still common place and was certainly allowed in the common room.

When it was time for supper, I made my way to the galley and joined the rest of the crew, the Scorpio crew were also there and there was a good deal of light hearted banter about systems letting the side down as I'm sure you can imagine. After I had finished eating and was nursing a cup of coffee, I noticed that my signet ring was missing! Oh no, I had meant to remove it before I started work on deck but had forgotten and now it seemed it had slipped off my finger; I was cursing myself as I should not have been wearing it at all until, I had had it sized properly for my finger. I know it was just a tiny piece of gold but to me it was very significant as it was all I had left of my dad and I had promised mum I would wear it but now it was gone!

I left the galley and went out on deck and spent a couple of hours scouring the whole area around the suits and everywhere else I could remember going during the afternoon, I could remember twisting the ring on my finger at lunch so it must have, fallen off since then. I had to use a flashlight as by now it was dark, I looked very carefully inside the suit including taking off the right-hand manipulator sphere to check inside just in case, but I didn't find anything.

I was quite depressed about my stupidity but of course there was nothing I could do about it now. I had another night in the hammock trying to get some sleep, I did manage some fitful sleep but was kept awake by the distress I was feeling at losing dad's ring and how this would affect mum when she found out.

Anyway, the next morning after breakfast we had to set up for diving again, my job was to prepare the suit and to carry out the pre-dive checks. Of course, we had done the majority of the work required the day before but we hadn't been able to fill the CO_2 absorber cannister as the soda-lime needed to be in a sealed container until just before the dive otherwise it would have been partially contaminated by the CO_2 in the atmosphere. I made sure the oxygen bottles were still full and also the air bottle that was needed for the adjustable buoyancy system was also topped up, all was good.

The last thing on the checklist was to carry out a visual check all around the outside of the suit to make sure all cables were still connected correctly, the thruster propellors were freely rotating etc., as I worked my way around the suit, I didn't find any issues, I had started my visual inspection from the dome and was working my way clockwise around the suit, the starboard side was first, the Wasp had three thrusters on each side; two were arranged horizontally for forward and reverse with a third for vertical movement; these were all fine with everything as it should be.

I worked my way around to the port side which was the side where the sun was shining, as I started my inspection of the two horizontal thrusters, I started with the top one and noticed something was stuck between the thruster body and the main hull, the offending object was not very big and was glinting in the sunlight. I had a screwdriver with me which I used to pry the object free, when it popped into my hand I was stunned and overjoyed to find it was dad's signet ring! It must have slipped off my finger while I was washing the suit yesterday, well, to say I was pleased would be a massive understatement.

I immediately took the ring and put it safely in my wash bag where I knew it would be safe, I couldn't believe my luck, if I hadn't found it when I did it would surely have been gone forever as the suit was about to be dived and this would certainly have dislodged the ring! I never again wore any jewellery when on a job site; as soon as I arrived on a job, I would remove everything apart from my watch and wouldn't put them back on until I was on my way home, this was the way it should have been anyway as it is quite dangerous to wear rings when doing deck work as there have been a lot of instances of rings being caught and completely stripping flesh from the finger; this is a process termed degloving!

We completed the videoing without any further issues and were duly deposited back ashore that evening, the Scorpio was to be offloaded and would be making its way back to the UK the next day. The Scorpio crew were due to leave the next day as well so would not be joining us at the staff house, they were being put up in a hotel for the night and would supervise the loading of their system before flying out that evening. I for one was very glad to be back ashore as my stomach while much better was still not right. When we arrived back at the staff house there was an enormous package for me lying on the dining table, as I opened the package I could see that Chrissie's insistence that she had written every day while I was in Spain was true, there were some thirty-four letters and an enormous Christmas card; it seemed that these letters had been following me, they had been to Spain then back to Aberdeen and finally out to Abidjan, well, it was very nice to get to read them now, I would have to apologise to her when I saw her again!

The rig support contract we were on required us to be on a six-hour call-out so we had to be close at all times in case we were needed, the next day we decided to go to the beach again. This time it was decided to stay more local and chose the beach just to the east of the harbour; John decided he didn't want to come along with us so he stayed in the house but the rest of us loaded up the crew-bus with everything we thought we would need and off we went.

The beach was again lovely, soft sand lined with coconut palms, there was a fair swell sending waves onto the beach and we spent the morning playing football, swimming and body surfing it was great. Lunchtime came and we decamped to one of the bars that lined the beach, we bagged a table right next to the beach and settled with beers and some fried shrimp (nothing from street vendors for me!); we spent the next couple of hours just whiling away the time chatting and watching the world go by while fending off the local hawkers who were trying to flog us all sorts of 'genuine' rubbish! I was watching the sea when I noticed a supply boat leaving port, not just any supply boat but the Arcadia Navigator. We watched as she sailed away with the Wasps sitting serenely on the stern; we looked at each other as at least two of us should be on board whenever the ship went to sea with the Wasps onboard but the only person not with us was John?

We hurried back to the house to find John asleep on the deck with a few empty bottles on the table in front of him, clearly nobody from Oceaneering was accompanying the suits. John was not at all happy as he should have been told the ship was sailing and would have made sure a pair of us accompanied the suits. He called the client who clearly didn't see a problem and told him that the ship would be back in three days, oh well, I suppose that's up to the grownups, we would just go with the flow.

As we were off duty properly now it was decided we would make the most of the opportunity; our staff house was in an area where the majority of the ex-pats lived and was fairly civilised but, relatively close by there was an area of Abidjan known colloquially as 'Trashville' where the locals lived. The guys who had been in Abidjan for a few months were keen for us to go to the 'French' bar, this was a famed bar in the middle of this township. It was apparently run by a French woman and was the place for us to go to make a bit of a night of it. Off we went Roger was again the designated driver, I was in the back of the crew-bus on the right-hand side and spent the time watching the world slide by my window. The township was a few miles from the staff house we headed towards the docks along the route we had taken before but soon left the ordered streets behind and entered a different world; I could see how this place had got its nickname, there were hundreds of dwellings, I hesitate to call them houses but I suppose that is what they were.

These houses were crammed together with tiny tracks running between them allowing access to buildings behind the ones I could see alongside the road; these shacks were made of a random collection of corrugated iron, plastic sheeting all tied onto wooden frames; I had never seen anything like it before but of course I had not spent much time in Africa to that point.

There didn't seem to be much space between the homes, each one had a makeshift chimney emitting a steady stream of smoke, the combined emissions came together to create a smoky smog smelling of woodsmoke with a hint of cooking! We were making our way along an unmetalled road which at this time was little more than a dusty track but in the rainy season would probably turn into a quagmire. At the side of track was a gutter/ditch filled with an eclectic array of rubbish including dead animals and the perennial detritus of modern day living such as coke and beer bottles plastic bags and anything else that people didn't feel they had any use further for; it was filthy and more than a little smelly. However, there were kids playing in the putrid puddles in the ditches and even some women who appeared to be washing clothes? Strangely enough amongst this almost medieval backdrop there were a lot of really nice shiny cars and trucks, these were 'parked' (more like abandoned) very haphazardly, they seemed completely out of place but I was told that this was the norm in these places; very odd.

Eventually, we arrived at an open square lined by small ramshackle shops and cafes, Roger parked up in a small area that was evidently being utilised as a car park and we all piled out; I followed Matt who together with the others was making his way into one of the more substantial bars alongside the square. When I got inside the place was larger than I thought it would be, it was about five metres wide but extended a long way back, I really couldn't see the back wall although this was largely down to the fact that there was not much light. There were rough-hewn heavy tables with benches randomly placed with no clear logic to their position, the door through which we had entered was on the left-hand side of the front wall, alongside that were three glazed windows with heavy wooden shutters inside. Over to the right was the bar, it extended about six metres along the right-hand wall with bar stools placed along the front. The bar seemed to be very well stocked with wines, spirits and just about every kind of drink you could mention.

The vast majority of the clientele were obviously locals, dressed in a motley assortment of clothing most of which could probably trace its lineage back to clothing that had been in vogue a good few years ago. Some of the women were clearly dressed for the hunt with a good deal of flesh on display. There was a pervading aroma of body odour, cigarette smoke and stale beer, I am not making it sound like a pleasant place to spend an evening but in those days to me it was just another experience, I loved it.

We made our way to the bar which was manned by three young local ladies and an older woman who greeted us like long lost friends! This was the fabled French patron she introduced herself as Marie, she cleared a number of the bar stools for us, this involved her shooing the locals off the stools; I thought they might think this a bit rude but they just seemed to accept it as to be expected. So, we now, each set ourselves up on one of the stools, I really was taken aback by the whole place and spent a few minutes taking it all in, Roger nudged me and as I turned around to the bar, he shoved a beer bottle into my hand. We were the only whites in the bar apart from the patron and very soon we became quite popular especially when it became clear that we were buying!

We immediately had a bar full of new friends, some of whom seemed to want to sit on our laps; well, while I was enjoying the ambiance and loving the whole experience, I was not a fool and therefore, understood that the ladies who were trying to be our best friends were really interested in how much money we would spend on them.

We spent a very loud and raucous few hours with no real thought of time or much else, really; there was an impromptu band serenading the bar with truly awful music, although they were extremely enthusiastic and were clearly trying to play things that they thought we would like. At about midnight suddenly things changed, at first there was a subtle exodus of locals from the bar but then it became clear that our friendly patron was becoming concerned, she called a number of the larger remaining locals over and they huddled together for a few moments. We were still being served by the bar staff so didn't think much about what was going on until we noticed the shutters being closed over the windows, they were locked closed by slotting heavy lengths of timber across them forming strongbacks. At the same time the main door and the rear doors were closed and barred as well; we were locked in, the locals that had been in the huddle with Marie now took up positions by the doors and had armed themselves with heavy clubs and some had machetes.

Marie now came over to us and told us that there was nothing to worry about (easy for her to say!) but there was a bit of a disturbance outside, she had closed the bar so that she could ensure we were safe and remained unharmed. She was keen that we continue drinking but I have to say we were not so keen, she said we would be very unwise to leave so might as well carry on enjoying her hospitality. After another three quarters of an hour, we could hear commotion outside and it was clear things were escalating in the square, Marie seemed to also feel this was not going to end well and came back to talk to us again. She had apparently called the military who would apparently calm the crowd allowing us to leave. By now we could hear that the crowd outside was becoming a rowdy mob and I for one was becoming quite concerned.

Sometime later the front door was opened and a uniformed officer came into the bar, he was armed with a side arm and a swagger stick; he was very definitely the boss and acted the part! He was accompanied by two more soldiers who were carrying large rifles, Marie had a conversation in French with the officer, they then came across to us and Marie told us that we were to follow the officer who would escort us to our vehicle and would then escort us back to safety. I couldn't help thinking back to my arrest in Gabon and although that time everything worked out well, I had heard a lot of stories from others that had not ended so well, I was uncomfortable with this situation to say the least. We thanked her for all her help and hospitality and paid the bill although she didn't seem to want the money, we made her take it.

As we left the bar, we found ourselves surrounded by soldiers who were fending off some angry looking individuals who were clearly unhappy with our presence; we were taken to our crew-bus, when we were all inside and had locked the doors the officer indicated that we should drive up to the rear of an army truck which we were then to follow; behind us another army truck formed up to follow us very closely; the soldiers climbed into their respective trucks and our convoy moved off very slowly. The army stayed with us until we had reached the boundary of Trashville, where our convoy stopped, the officer came to the driver's window, in stilted English he told us that it would be best if we didn't return to the French bar for a few days, then he stood back and waved us off. We drove back to the house in silence, I for one was very grateful to have made it back unscathed, I never returned to the French bar.

The next couple of days were spent kicking our heels until the ship returned when we were told our equipment was due to be offloaded as the contract was due to finish. John had to go to another job and so was due to leave before the demobilisation was completed, his place was taken by Steve Walker another ADS supervisor who was returning from a job in South Africa and had agreed to relieve John for the demob. We spent the next couple of days readying the equipment for its trip back to the UK, the hydraulic hoses and cables together with the other odds and sods were packed into the dive control and workshop shipping containers. The suits themselves were due to be packaged into some additional larger shipping containers that would also be used to transport the hydraulic power pack, winches and winch control pods.

These were a couple of long, hot and hard day's work, it was now that I ran out of the medication, I had been given for my stomach problems; over the past week or so my stomach had been feeling a little more settled but by no means could it be said to be normal. The next day I woke up with stomach cramps again, clearly things were still not fixed; it was agreed that I should go back to the UK the following day, the rest of the crew would stay on for another day to get the equipment ready for shipment properly.

So, it was that on the twelfth of February I found myself in the queue at the airport checking in for the British Caledonian flight back to London Gatwick again. I was somewhat anxious as I was running to the loo again fairly frequently; I asked the pleasant young lady whether I could have an aisle seat; she checked and told me that unfortunately there were only seats in the middle of a row available. This would of course be less than ideal but the person who was outside of me would just have to put up with it. My flight was due to arrive in London at seventeen twenty-five in the evening and I was then booked on another flight from Heathrow back to Plymouth at nineteen fifty-five so should have plenty of time to make the transfer.

When I found my seat on the flight, in the aisle seat next to me was a young man who spoke good English. I explained my predicament, he was extremely understanding telling me he had experienced a similar problem just a few months before; he was more than happy to swap seats with me so that I could have the aisle seat; our row was just three rows from the toilets, ideal for me. I had to make many trips to the toilet during the flight so I think my companion was very glad to have swapped seats with me. As it turned out the flight arrived some fifteen minutes early, I was one of the first of the cattle class passengers to get off the aircraft, where I made my way to passport control via the toilets on the way.

Once I was safely through into the arrival's hall, I found the transfer desk to transfer across to Heathrow; in those days when we had a fairly tight connection, Oceaneering used to book us on the helicopter transfer so, with virtually no delays I was seated on another Sikorsky helicopter operated by British Airways for the short hop to Heathrow. This transfer went smoothly and saw me arriving at Heathrow at eighteen fifty-five, without any issues I found myself seated on a small propellor driven aircraft ready for the hour's flight to Plymouth. While at Heathrow I had called my mum to tell her I was back in the country, she knew I would have to find a way back to Torquay and she had offered to pick me up at the airport in Plymouth and ferry me home. I told her I could just get a taxi to the rail station but, I think she was secretly happy to be able to drive me that evening.

The flight took off on time and went without any kind of drama until we were coming in to land in Plymouth, in those days the airport in Plymouth was a small affair with very few facilities. The pilot told us that there was a significant cross wind at the airport which might cause us problems, he said that he would in his words "give it a go" but if it proved to be too dangerous, we would be on our way to Newquay where the ex-MOD airport was much better equipped. As we came in too land, I was looking out of the starboard window and everything seemed to be going just fine until we were just a few feet above the ground when suddenly I found myself staring along the runway, the plane had slewed, by ninety degrees and seemed to be travelling sideways. The pilot applied power and pulled out of the landing; he came back on the comms to tell us that he was sorry for the bumpy ride and that he would try once more, before heading off to Newquay.

As we came in on the second approach the plane was buffeted cruelly but, at the very last minute the pilot was able to straighten the plane up and bring it in to land; as soon as we touched down, he applied reverse power to kill our speed and although the landing was quite bumpy very soon, we were taxiing safely back towards the terminal, phew, what a trip.

When I entered the arrival's hall, mum was right there waiting and seemed very pleased to see me, as it was just two months since dad's death, I think she was pleased to be able to get out of her house to meet me. It was very nice to be back home after what had been for me an eventful trip but, all ended up OK in the end. The next day I made an appointment at my doctor to discuss my lingering stomach problems, when I was finally admitted to his office, I gave him the letter I had received from the doctor in Abidjan detailing the results from my tests. The doctor spent a few minutes studying these and checking a few things in one of his books before asking me to lie on the consulting bed, once he had poked and prodded me, he announced that I had suffered a mild bout of dysentery!

It seemed the medication I had been given had treated the symptoms but not the cause, I was put on a course of strong drugs and told to stay in the UK at least until I had completed the course. After a few days my symptoms cleared up never to return, thank goodness. I told Oceaneering that I would not be available for work for a couple of weeks and set about enjoying being back in Torquay with my girlfriend; I did apologise for berating her for not writing to me when in Spain; I think she has forgiven me now though. Our relationship was becoming serious to the point that she agreed to become my wife albeit this didn't happen for another couple of years. I would love to be able to say that I had planned a memorable scenario for popping the question but, unfortunately, I can't, I just asked her and she said yes! Maybe I should have made more of an effort but now, after thirty-eight plus years of being together it might be a bit late.

We spent the first week of my leave eating nice meals in the various pubs and restaurants around Torbay and the surrounding area, I remember one Sunday evening we spent hours traipsing around all the pubs we could think of only to be told, "we don't do food on Sundays!" How things have changed is truly amazing, back then food while being served in a lot of pubs was not the main attraction, the majority were still places, to go to find alcohol and company. I think it's true to say that a pub that doesn't serve food on Sunday evenings now would probably not be in business for long.

Chrissie had been suffering with significant issues medically for some considerable time, this had come to a bit of a head while I was in the Ivory Coast resulting in her having to go into hospital for some exploratory work. Unusually and luckily for me I happened to be still at home when she eventually was called to go into Torbay hospital for the tests. When I left her in the hospital ward, she looked lost and I felt extremely sorry for her; I decided to see about taking her on holiday when she came back out of hospital, I spent the rest of the day at various travel agents picking up brochures so that she could choose.

The next day I visited for the one hour allowed (in those days hospital visiting times were very short and strictly policed) and although I had the brochures with me Chrissie was still quite out of it from the anaesthetic so I didn't mention anything thinking I would leave it until the following day. So, when I arrived the next day, I stuck my head into the nurse's office which was on the right at the entrance to the ward, I told them about my plan to whisk her away for a few days; it seemed to go down very well and although I was cautioned to make sure she wasn't taxed too greatly I was given the green light to take her away.

I was pleased to see that Chrissie was sitting up in bed nursing a cup of tea on one of those silly tables on wheels specifically designed for the inhabitant to be able to eat from but not substantial enough to do so without liquids being spilt! She had a beaming smile of welcome, it was clear the procedure had gone well and she had been told that she would be fine after a period of rest; perfect, after being told this, I produced the holiday brochures with a flourish. Chrissie seemed more affected by this gesture than I was expecting, she flung her arms around me and hugged me tightly for significantly longer than felt comfortable as I was leaning across the bed at an unnatural angle. Eventually, she let me go and we started to look through the brochures; as I say the nurses had cautioned me to make sure it was a relaxing trip so I steered her away from the party destinations although in the early eighties there were not as many as there are these days.

Before I was chucked out at the end of the visiting hour, we had zeroed in on a couple of weeks in the Casino hotel (now the Pestana Casino), a lovely five-star hotel in Funchal, Madeira, overlooking the harbour. When I left the hospital, I went straight to the travel agent and booked the holiday commencing at the end of following week. I then called Diane at Oceaneering telling her that I would not be available for another three weeks, she was not impressed until I told her the reasons; as she and Chrissie were now on first name terms; although she gave me a hard time, she reluctantly agreed that I should go and look after her!

Anyway, we had a lovely, relaxing holiday; while we were away, we had made a conscious effort to avoid newspapers and the like so it was with some degree of surprise that when Chrissie called her mother from the airport on arrival back in London the first thing she said was "We're at war!" It seemed that on the second of April the Argentinian military junta headed by President Galtieri had invaded the Falkland Islands prompting our then prime minister Margaret Thatcher to declare war on Argentina. We were stunned by this news and I for one wondered how this might play out over the coming months. Anyway, as Chrissie had rested well in Madeira, she was nicely recovered and was able to go back to work just a few days after we returned home.

Speaking of which, I needed to go back to work as well, Chrissie was not at all keen on this as she had become quite clingy over the past few weeks and had definitely got used to my being at home. This was quite understandable given that she had been unwell but also, I knew that she had had a previous long-term relationship where her partner also working in the oil industry as a mechanic. He had been working in Nigeria towards the end of their relationship and had apparently 'gone bush' preferring to stay in Nigeria for his leave periods rather than come home to her? But of course, I couldn't just stop working; we had some uncomfortable evenings discussing how our relationship would progress from this point. I told her that I loved my job but was not going to treat her like her previous fella had, I told her that I didn't know what I could do for a job if I came home anyway?

After several fraught evenings of soul searching, it was decided that we should look for a business that we could run together; meanwhile I would continue working offshore to try to build up a better deposit for the purchase. I was less than pleased with this situation as I felt I had finally found in diving something that I was both good at and loved, I still couldn't really believe anyone would pay me to play with all this expensive kit all day while I was supposedly working. Oceaneering had clearly seen something in me as well as they always gave me work whenever I wanted it and had carried on my training, However, it was clear that if I wanted a long-term future with Chrissie continuing working offshore was not going to be an option.

I was not really qualified for anything other than diving so of course this limited our options. Chrissie though was a classically trained chef with several years' experience and was keen for us to look at buying a restaurant. I of course would be of no help at all with the catering side but felt I might be able to look after front of house? So it was that we visited estate agents in the Torbay area looking for restaurants or licenced premises. Once we were set up on the mailing lists with these agents, I called Diane at Oceaneering looking for work.

The very next day my friend working for the post office caught up with me, Diane had sent another telegram asking me to get in touch; I wandered over the road to the phone box and made the call. It seemed that Oceaneering had secured a year-long inspection job in Angola; the Cabinda field was up for sale and Gulf oil needed a report on the state of the structures. This was perfect for me as my Lloyds diver inspector qualification would be good enough to get me on the job although by now Lloyds, diver inspector had been largely superseded by a much higher-level qualification.

The new system was the Certification Scheme for Weldment Inspection Personnel (CSWIP), this was run by The Welding Institute (TWI) in Cambridge and had two levels. Level one was the 3.1U Diver Inspector; this individual would be proficient in visual, CCTV, photographic inspection as well as use of the Cathodic Potential (CP) meters and Digital Thickness Meters (DTM). Individuals who had this qualification would have undergone a two-week course at one of the dive schools, followed by an examination overseen by TWI. Level two was 3.2U, this was only available to individuals who had held a 3.1U for at least twelve months, they would then need to sit a second eight-day course followed by another examination. 3.2U divers would have been taught Magnetic Particle Inspection (MPI) to a higher degree than I had been taught, additionally they would be qualified to use an Ultrasonic A-Scan for more detailed assessment of the thickness of metal structures.

Being a job for one year I was able to sell this to Chrissie as she could see an end to it and of course it was hoped that by the end of the contract we would have found a business. The job had a six on four off leave rotation, so I would be away for a maximum of six weeks at a time, Chrissie seemed to be OK with this, well maybe on the surface but underneath it soon became clear that she was not at all happy! I was due to travel back to Cabinda on the eleventh of May, Chrissie booked the day off so that she could take me to Heathrow, sounds fine but in reality, it proved to be a very bad idea.

On the day I loaded up my carry-on bag as usual, ready for the trip, we were taking Chrissie's car as she was more comfortable driving it than she would be with my car. I drove and the whole trip was punctuated by sobs from the passenger seat but, eventually we arrived at Heathrow with about three quarters of an hour to spare; we found a spot in the short stay car park; I tried to get her to say goodbye in the car but she was having none of it. I had been told to go to the information desk where tickets and the rest of the team would be waiting; when we arrived, there was a group of four guys, I didn't know any of them but I knew the name of the supervisor, Reg Drake, I soon found him and introduced myself.

There were three others there with him Reg, Trevik Simms, Andrew Ward and Neil Haggar; we were to be the advanced guard tasked with setting up the job, another eight personnel would be joining us a week later.

Everyone started to chat about the job and I felt Chrissie was going to feel left out so I told the team I would be back in a few minutes and took Chrissie off to get a cup of coffee so we could say a proper goodbye.

I went back to the team, as I approached, I could see there was consternation, apparently the photo-tech had called to say he was no longer available for the job. This was a big issue as the job required a high level of photographic recording. Reg was discussing this with the team and he asked whether any of us had any photographic expertise? As you know I had an interest in photography and had acted as the photo-tech on the job in France although this had been only developing slides which were very easy to process. I told Reg this, he seemed delighted, I was at pains to emphasise that I had no experience with processing or developing of prints which I understood would be a requirement on this job. He told me he needed to talk to the office and disappeared off to find a phone, we were now getting close to the flight departure time and I was concerned we might all miss the flight. I needn't have worried; a few moments later Reg came back; he had spoken to the office who had agreed I could take the photo-tech position and they would send someone out to teach me how to process and print photographs.

Well, wonderful, I was chuffed with my new role, but even more so when Reg told me I would be given a pay increase for the more specialised role and even better the leave rotation was five on and five off, wow! I wished I could have told Chrissie as I was sure she would have been much happier with this situation but of course she was gone.

We made the flight to Paris with just minutes to spare, in Paris we transferred to an Angolan

Airways flight for the leg to Luanda, I was pleased that we were not staging in Gabon as I was not sure what reception I might find there after my last trip. The flight went without a hitch although the in-flight catering and entertainment left a lot to be desired but, they did at least seem to have unlimited supplies of beer so it could have been a lot worse. When moving along to the customs desks in Luanda I was able to supply packs of American cigarettes to everyone on the team so that they were all able to present these inside their bags for inspection by the customs officers thus ensuring nothing was going to disappear during the inspection of their bags.

From Luanda we were ushered onto another Angolan Airlines flight for the short hop up to Malongo, as I was the only one of our team who had been to Angola previously, I had briefed everyone about the mad dash from the terminal to ensure a seat on the plane. So it was that we had jostled through the crowd in the terminal and were in pole position when the doors opened; as soon as the doors were opened by an Angolan Airlines staff member, who I could see was putting himself off to one side where he would be able to safely enjoy the coming spectacle without being trampled in the stampede. I have to say that I have never been particularly gifted as far as running is concerned but I could certainly outpace women carrying babies and bags and old men also carrying huge bags; plus being at the front of the scrum we had a head start. So it was that the five of us made it to the steps of the plane relatively near the front of the queue, well I say queue, it was nothing of the sort really as the Africans didn't abide by the rules regarding queueing at all.

Again, I had briefed the crew and so we acted as a team of fit young men who managed to secure our position on the steps up to the plane without too much effort. When on the plane we all found seats together, then it was with some amusement that we sat and watched everyone else fighting their way to a steadily diminishing number of free seats.

Eventually, the few who hadn't been able to find a seat were ushered back off the plane, the doors were closed and we were off. The flight again was uneventful, very soon we were back on the ground in Malongo, where we transferred to the waiting American school bus for the trip to Cabinda camp. On arrival at the camp, we were all allocated rooms in the same accommodation block as the other Oceaneering divers who were still manning the routine oilfield maintenance team that I had been part of during my first trip to Angola. We were told that this situation was temporary, we, together with the rest of the inspection team would normally be living aboard the vessel from which we would be working.

The next morning, we assembled at five-thirty in the morning in the mess hall for breakfast, for me it was as though I had never been away. Once we had finished our breakfasts we assembled outside where I was able to point out the various points of interest; while I was doing this Reg wandered off to find the client to discuss where our equipment was. He soon returned driving another Chevrolet pick-up which apparently was going to be ours to use during the contract; we all piled in the back and off we went to find our equipment. Driving along the familiar crude oil surfaced roads we soon pulled off to the left into the main fabrication yard where there were several forty-foot shipping containers painted in the familiar yellow and white colours with large Oceaneering stickers along the sides.

As soon as the pickup stopped, we hopped off and moved across to the closest container, Reg had keys and was soon unlocking padlocks. Opening the doors revealed an Aladdin's cave filled with everything we were going to need equipment wise. We congregated around the opened container where Reg briefed us of the mobilisation plan; we now had three clear days where we would be preparing everything for transfer to the vessel, this vessel was to be arriving for us to onload our plant and equipment on day four. Sounded good but I could see that this meant we would have our work cut out over the next three days if we were going to be ready.

Helpfully, just inside the door of each container there was an inventory of contents, we spent the next hour with the four of us finding out which container held which equipment. Once we had a reasonable understanding of where everything was Reg delegated tasks to us all, as I was the photo-tech I was tasked with identifying all photographic equipment and starting to set up the dark room; Reg gave me a key and told me that I should find a smaller container set up as the dark room. I wandered around the various containers and soon found that behind the forty-foot containers there were two smaller ten-foot containers. On inspection I could see that one of these was fitted out as dive control and the other was the dark room, I quickly opened up the darkroom as I was eager to see what equipment was inside.

Of course, there was no electrical supply hooked up as yet so my first action was to go in search of a flashlight. Luckily, one of containers had a box near the door containing several flashlights; I returned to the dark room with my light to find it packed floor to ceiling with boxes. As with the other containers I found an inventory just inside the door from which I could see there were a lot of supplies other than just photographic inside; in addition, there were rolls of blue roll, various cleaning products as well as shirts and coveralls, for the whole team.

I made a pile of these boxes outside the dark room confident that they would not get wet as there was no hint of rain in fact it seemed rain was not expected for weeks. I was then faced with the photographic equipment and consumables; these included all the chemicals needed for developing. There were a large number of boxes containing film, again both slides (positive) and negatives for prints. The dark room had already been fitted out with benches, sink unit, drying cupboard and racks together with a colour enlarger needed for producing prints; I had never used most of this equipment but was reassured that my teacher would be arriving within the next couple of days.

I packed all the chemicals, boxes of film and other developing equipment in logical places so that I would be able to find it all again easily. I had found plastic 'Pelican' (waterproof boxes) boxes containing the cameras that I would be using, I had four Mk IV Nikon, Calypso cameras together with flash guns with their associated arms so that they could be set up to light the subject. These were exactly the same as the kit I had been using in France so should present no problem for me; there were also boxes of rechargeable AA size batteries for the flash guns together with their chargers. The cameras were fitted with standard thirty-five-millimetre focal length lenses and each had additional twenty-four-millimetre-wide-angle lenses and close up attachments; these would allow close up photographs of welds and any damage we found. In short, I had everything I needed for the job, of course chemicals and film may need to be replenished but this could be organised as required.

Having completed my work with the dark room I decided to see what everyone else was up to; as I exited the dark room it took my eyes a few seconds to adjust to the bright sunlight but when I wandered around the end of the nearest container I was faced with a hive of activity. The guys had located a Zodiac inflatable boat together with its outboard motor and associated equipment, the boat had by now been partially inflated with its aluminium deck boards being inserted. I couldn't see Reg but as I started to talk to Trevik and Andrew, he turned up dragging a length of very thick mooring rope, he proceeded to tell us that he wanted this rope to be attached along the sides of the Zodiac running from the stern along one side, around the bow and back down the other side. This would then act as a fender protecting the rubber boat from puncture by marine growth etc.

We soon had the boat fully inflated and started to fix the 'fender' around the waist of the boat using short lengths of twine tied to the eyes on the boat's side, these were threaded through the lay of the mooring rope and taken back to the eyes firmly securing the rope along the sides and around the bow.

Once this was finished Reg asked the fabricator foreman to come and have a look, he wanted them to build a launch cage for the boat so that it could be lifted into and out of the water easily, the fabrication team took the necessary measurements and assured us that it would be ready in two days. Our next two days were spent emptying the shipping containers and putting all equipment together as necessary.

As promised the launch/recovery cage for our Zodiac turned up at the end of day two, it was perfect, the boat fitted snugly into it and it had a very good lifting bridle attached so we could start setting up the boat properly now. The idea was that we would be using the boat to supply divers following flow lines etc. When following flow lines, the diver would descend on a riser then proceed hand over hand along the pipe on the seabed, this would be extremely difficult to achieve from a large vessel and traditionally would have been done using SCUBA.

SCUBA had been proven to be the cause of a great number of accidents and indeed deaths in the offshore world; so much so that it had been all but been outlawed in the offshore world, Oceaneering certainly did not want it to be used. This being the case we were going to be using Oceaneering's solution, we would be converting the inflatable boat into a SCUBA replacement system; this involved us fitting the boat with three large (fifty-litre) high pressure bottles these would be filled with air at two-hundred bar. Two of these bottles would be used for the diver's main breathing gas this gas would be supplied to him via his umbilical; the third bottle would be used as a standby bottle, while this is not an unlimited supply of gas it is certainly much improved over traditional SCUBA. The diver would also carry his normal 'bail-out' bottle on his back as well. We built a wooden frame into the boat and fitted the bottles into the frame, there was then a two-diver supply panel attached and two umbilicals supplying the main diver and the standby support diver. Over the course of the contract, we used this system a great number of times, it was extremely effective and easy to use.

On the morning of day four we were ready to start transferring our equipment to the vessel, flat-bed trucks turned up together with a crane, we marshalled the crew telling them which items needed to be loaded first and so it started. We left one of us to supervise loading of the trucks and the rest of our small team went down to the dock where our vessel was moored up. We were going to be using a small, self-propelled, tripod jack up platform called the Leon Grigsby; although it was not owned by Oceaneering it was fittingly painted yellow and white.

The rig's hull was an oblong with accommodation towards the rear of the deck; in front of that there was a clear deck area where our equipment would sit; towards the front edge of the work deck there was a crane on the starboard side. It all looked fine to me and although not large it would I thought be big enough for our purposes; we went onboard where we met the skipper and chief engineer both of them British although the deck crew were all Nigerian.

We discussed what equipment would be brought on board and where it needed to be positioned, as we were finishing our discussion the first of the trucks arrived along with a motley crew of white men. These were the rest of our team who had just arrived from the UK, they came aboard and were shown the accommodation where they left their bags and changed into work clothes. I went along with them being very pleased to see that two of them were old friends from my BAD course at Bovisand; these were Adrian Fricker and Paul Sims, happy days.

I had not seen the accommodation until now either and, well to say it was not palatial would be an understatement! The living accommodation was situated on the first floor with the deck level accommodating the galley, mess room and engineering spaces. It seemed that on the first floor there were basically two bunk rooms, one of these was being used by the Nigerian deck crew and the other had been set aside for us; the room was large enough for five sets of bunks. Each set of bunks consisted of two beds one above the other so in all there was space for ten of us, apparently Reg would be going ashore every night but the rest of us would be housed in this room. Well, it could be worse, at least we each had our own bunk, the room was air conditioned so at least we would be comfortable, or so I thought.

We later found that the temperature of the air conditioning was fixed far too low to be comfortable and couldn't be altered so in order to maintain a comfortable temperature we had to leave the windows open! Very environmentally unfriendly.

When we arrived back on deck loading had already started with the shipping containers that we were going to be using as stores and workshop being positioned immediately in front of the accommodation, the Zodiac installed in its launch/recovery frame sat on top of the workshop container with my photo lab being placed on the starboard side of the deck just behind dive control. Compressors, water jetting equipment and all our other ancillaries were placed in a logical order making them easily accessible.

We spent the rest of the day welding the equipment to the deck and starting to set up the dive spread and inspection equipment; we worked until six o'clock in the evening when the light was fading as is always the case in the tropics. Cabinda being situated just a few degrees south of the equator it was firmly in the tropics; where there is pretty much twelve hours of daylight from six a.m. to six p.m. or thereabouts regardless of the time of year.

For us though it was the end of a very long day and I was ready for some food and a catch up with my old friends. We were fed a really nice curry by our Nigerian cook, I then sat on deck with Adrian, Paul and a few of the others catching up on old times and learning a bit more about each other before we headed up to our bunk room where as I say we sorted out how to keep the temperature at an acceptable level.

The next morning, we were all up for breakfast at five-thirty in the morning and on deck by six, most of the guys continued with setting up the dive system and inspection gear but, I had learning to do. My tutor had arrived with the other guys yesterday, he turned out to be a tall, thin, very affable Scot with dark curly hair, his name was Mungo Ross, he was one of Oceaneering's senior photo-techs although I had not met him before we quickly hit it off. After introductions had been made, we headed for the photo lab where he showed me what all the equipment was for and how to operate it. We spent the second half of the morning making up the various solutions to enable development of positive and negative films as well as for developing prints. I made lots of notes but I must confess I was nervous as I only had his help for the next four days, not long to learn a totally new trade in my opinion! The positive development process was termed 'E6', the process for developing colour negatives being 'C41', luckily Mungo had brought very specific procedures for all the development processes that should be fairly straightforward for me to follow even when I was alone.

We came to agreement that there was nothing like doing the job to be able to learn it properly so we went on deck and shot a reel of colour negative film of the crew setting up the systems. Once this was done and the film had been safely wound back into its cassette inside the camera, we locked ourselves inside the photo lab to start the developing process. The first issue I had to master was to remove the film from its cassette in the camera, this shouldn't be too bad as I had already mastered the technique while I was in France.

Of course, the film had to be transferred under total darkness as obviously any light hitting the film would ruin the photographs; I had a black transfer bag to facilitate the transfer of the film from its cassette into a lightproof developing tank where the chemicals could be administered. But I was not going to use the bag unless I really had to, first with the lights on I organised all my equipment on the work surface, I made sure I had the developing tank, plastic spiral (film developing reel) onto which the film would be wound prior to being fitted into the developing tank and lastly a pair of scissors. I made sure everything was clean and dry then made a mental note of where everything was on the bench, before removing the cassette from the camera and working on the bench with all the lights switched off, we were now in total darkness.

As I say, I had done this a lot of times before in France; so, by feel I easily found the entrance of the spiral and fed the end of the film onto it. Inside the spiral there were a couple of ball bearings, these would grip the film, allowing the film to be wound into the spiral. The two halves of the spiral could be moved independently so that each side of the film would be gripped in the groove. I gripped both sides of the spiral and as I alternated my right and left hands wound the film onto the spiral, all went as expected, eventually I felt the adhesive tape that had been used to fix the film to the cassette I cut the film again continuing to wind the film onto the spiral until I was sure the whole film was loaded. I then put the loaded spiral into the developing tank, found the tank's top which I wound onto the tank, this now meant that the film was in the tank correctly and was protected from light so the lights could be turned back on.

Mungo then helped me to follow the instructions to complete the development process, it actually proved to be quite easy and was very similar to the process for developing positives such as I had used before; the main differences were temperature and timings. Once we had completed the process, I opened up the developing tank, separated the two halves of the film spiral, I could see that there were images on the film, so, success? We would see how good they were when we printed from them. That was the next procedure but this could not be completed until the film was fully dried off, I used the double-sided squeegee provided to remove most of the water from both sides of the film, I then hung the film inside the drying cabinet and we went for a cup of tea.

When we returned the film was nicely dry and Mungo led me through the process of using the enlarger to shine light through the negative onto photographic paper; he showed me how to set up the enlarger and how to carry out test exposures to learn how long to expose the paper in order to get a good image. Once the film had been exposed the paper needed to be loaded into another larger developing tank as, again the paper needed to go through a chemical development process; all of this had to be done in total darkness! Quite quickly I got to know my way around the photo lab, I knew where everything I needed was without needing to be able to see, another example of 'a place for everything and everything in its place'. We spent the rest of the day practicing and refining my technique until in the evening I had managed to produce good quality prints from the negatives.

The next day was a re-run with me taking and developing films both colour and monochrome (black and white), negative and positive films and printing from both. At the end of this second day, I was beginning to feel much more confident, Mungo was a very good teacher. The next day, we were due to leave harbour, move out to start inspecting the first structure.

First thing in the morning we all assembled on deck just after breakfast, we had been told that when the rig was going to be jacking up its legs to allow it to move location, we all had to be on deck? We weren't told why but as we were about to start work, we were all on deck anyway; I was standing with Paul by the starboard rail alongside the galley door almost at the stern of the vessel when the legs started to be jacked up. I glanced into the galley and saw the chef putting all the pans with any liquids inside onto the floor?

The rig moved down towards the surface of the sea, as the hull reached the water and started to gain buoyancy all was fine until suddenly the whole rig lurched alarmingly to starboard; I found myself looking at water coming over the rail, it was quickly heading towards us, Paul and I started to climb onto the rail and up into the rigging aiming to stay above the water; we could hear pots and pans falling in the galley. The deck was now canted alarmingly with the bow and the port side raised up with the stern, and starboard side gradually sinking below the surface; there was a bit of a swell in the harbour which was adding to the problem, as the rig fell into the trough of the waves the rig would start to right itself but then as the next crest came through the deck would rise again. Anything that had not been properly secured became a missile so we were dodging oil drums etc., then all of a sudden, the rig righted itself and normality returned to the deck.

What had caused this? Well, as I said the Leon Grigsby was a jack up structure which had three legs, when jacked up its three feet were sitting on the seabed and as the seabed in the harbour was soft mud, they had sunk into the mud, it seemed that when the legs were being jacked back up, the rear, starboard leg had stuck in the mud while the other two had come loose this caused the issue, as soon as the stuck foot broke free everything returned to normal! This had been alarming to those of us who had not experienced it before, I thought it was just as well that we had welded all our equipment onto the deck otherwise we would have had compressors, containers and goodness knows what else hurtling around the deck. We soon came to realise that this was routine, whenever we were jacking down to move location the same thing would happen to a greater or lesser extent depending on the seabed. So, we just made sure everything was properly secured and made ready to climb if necessary whenever we were jacking down to move location.

We left the harbour and the skipper set a heading for the structure we would be working on today, as was the norm for that part of the world, just a few miles south of the equator an area known as the doldrums; the sky was overcast and there was very little wind. In the days of sail power, it would not have been uncommon for ships to be becalmed for days in these latitudes sometimes they would even lower small boats with men who would row towing the ship! Although there was almost no breeze, there was a fair groundswell running from the west to the east, this was again the normal Atlantic oceanic swell.

Today was going to be our first day of inspection and was going to be used as an opportunity to use all the kit and to make sure everything was working and set up correctly. I was going to be photographing the structure and risers, including the tube turns where the vertical riser turns to run along the seabed; I would also be photographing riser clamps and anodes. All of these were to be photographed before cleaning as assessment of marine growth accumulation at different depths was an important part of the job. As we started motoring out of the harbour, Mungo and I set to work in the photo lab getting ready for my dive; Mungo told me to carry on with preparation, he would observe and let me know if he felt I had missed anything.

I set up the necessary identification (ident) boards in order to ensure all photographs were easily identified as to location and subject. These boards consisted of a flat face screwed onto a small magnet giving them the ability to adhere to the structure.

The specific structure I was to be photographing was one of the numerous tripod structures carrying a single well; this one's identification number was CABGOC (short for Cabinda Gulf Oil Company) 73/18 so that went onto the board. I made up boards for each of the significant features I had been asked to photograph, once I had finished the boards I had quite a collection. I would need to carry all of these boards, other identification markers such as tape measures, arrows for defects and clock position markers; this was looking like being a mammoth amount of 'stuff' I would have to juggle in the water. I decided that the smaller items such as magnetic arrows and clock position markers could be transported by being stuck to a small flat metal plate. This actually worked very well, I had a painted steel plate about 150 millimetres square which I attached another lanyard to; I was able to put a plethora of ID markers onto this plate that I could just pick off when necessary.

I then moved on to setting up the camera and strobes; I was going to be taking stand-off general shots so would not be needing the close-up attachments. I knew that the structure was quite close to the shore and so was in just forty-four feet (13.4 metres) of water; I also knew from my previous trip to Angola that the top three metres or so would not have good visibility due to fresh water from the Congo River just to the south of us. In addition to this problem, I also knew that about four to six feet (1 – 2 metres) from the bottom visibility would again be very poor.

With this in mind I decided to fit the twenty-four mm wide angle lens, this would allow me to get in close to the subject but still photograph a reasonable area of the subject, the closer I could get the less silt would be between the camera and subject well that was the theory anyway. I was using a single strobe flash this was attached to the camera using an articulated arm so that I would be able to angle the strobe as appropriate for each shot.

Once everything was ready and Mungo agreed with all my choices I felt properly prepared for the dive; we went out on deck and very quickly it became evident that all was not well. We were under way and were by now some distance from the harbour; as we exited the photo lab, we stepped onto the deck which seemed to be awash to a depth of a few centimetres! What was going on? We turned right to make our way toward the bow, dive control and the main working deck area, as we came around the end of the workshop container, we could see that the whole of the main working deck area was under water and as the bow pushed through the swells more water was finding its way onto the deck. I saw that the rest of our team had decamped to the companionway on the first floor in front of the accommodation where they were drinking coffee and smoking, we decided to join them.

As we arrived to join the crowd Reg was just returning from the bridge where he had been discussing the situation with the captain; it seemed that our equipment was heavier than had been expected and was very close to Leon Grigsby's maximum payload the result was that there was almost no freeboard to speak of.

As soon as we started making way the bow wave had overcome the freeboard resulting in the deck becoming awash; the main worry for us at this time was that the video recording equipment was in dive control on a shelf very low down. Before long we arrived on location, the rigs legs were jacked down the hull rose out of the water; when the hull was some four or five metres clear of the water and had been stable for half-hour, we were given the all clear from the skipper so diving could commence. By now of course all the water had drained from the deck and it was almost dry, Reg asked me to go with him to have a look at the video equipment; when we arrived in dive control it was clear that some water had found its way inside but luckily had not reached the VCR thank goodness!

It was mid-afternoon before it was my turn to dive, I spent the morning with the other guy's prepping air tools and the LP tools compressor as well as the HP water jetting equipment. My turn to dive came at just after fifteen hundred hours, we had constructed and fitted a metal staircase to the bow of the rig so that we could walk to and from the water. This set of stairs was hinged so that when the rig was due to be moving the stairs were stowed at deck level and when rigged for diving, they were lowered, it was a very effective and simple system.

So it was that I was kitted up using a Kirby Morgan Bandmask (KMB 18), I walked down the staircase when I was up to my knees in the water, I turned to take the camera system from Adrian; I already had the ident boards clipped to my harness. I confirmed with Reg that I was clear for the water, he told me I could go when ready and off I stepped. There was a downline leading to the riser I was to photograph, having told Reg "Diver two leaving surface" I dipped my head and started to follow the downline.

Again, I was engulfed in very poor visibility until I dropped through the fresh water layer; as I fell out of the fresh water layer as expected the visibility improved immensely, I could again see all three legs of the structure together with three horizontal braces connecting the legs; additionally, there were three vertical/diagonal braces running between the horizontal level towards the surface and another three descending towards the seabed. I could see the downline had been attached at or very near the seabed as I could see it disappearing into the murk just above the seabed; the visibility again decreased almost to zero as I neared the seabed. I reached the bottom of the line and transferred from there to the riser continuing my descent another couple of feet to the seabed. Once on the bottom I informed Reg who started the process of checking my depth; there was almost no visibility now as the silt near the seabed always was a problem in Angola, by the time depth had been checked and confirmed and I was ready for work I felt could see enough though.

I rummaged through my ident boards until I found the correct one which I positioned against the riser tube turn where it sat against the seabed; I set up the flash to illuminate the subject from the side to try and reduce light scattering from suspended particles and took the required photos. I relayed what I had done over the comms and Simon who was now monitoring my comms and was writing a log of the photos taken for me. I then climbed up the riser; as I passed clamps holding the riser to the structure, I would photograph marine growth as well as bolts both fixing the riser into the clamps and also where the clamp was attached to the horizontal bracing of the structure.

As I swum up the riser, I took a number of photos at ten-foot intervals this would show how levels of marine growth varied with depth; at thirty feet the dominant growth seemed to be large oysters that had grown to form around the riser, they had clearly been there for years, at twenty-feet the predominant growth were seaweeds over a few oysters and some mussels. I then moved on to photograph anodes and their attachment points, I could only find one anode close to the riser just off to the left on the horizontal brace at thirty-two feet water depth. The anode was severely corroded which of course was a good thing as it showed it was working. Once I had general photos of the anode's condition and had a few of the attachments I was done for this dive. I told topside I was leaving bottom and made my way back to the steps where I handed the camera to Adrian again, I walked up the steps. When on deck Adrian helped me to take the diving gear off, as soon as I removed the Kirby, I confirmed to him that I was well; it was always important to confirm this to your tender as soon as you arrived on deck.

As soon as I was out of my gear and was dressed, I went to find Mungo so that we could start developing the film; I found him in dive control where he was watching another diver who was carrying out a general video survey of the horizontal braces. Mungo and I went off to the photo lab where, this morning I had placed the required chemicals in a temperature-controlled water bath to bring them up to the correct temperature. we checked the temperature was correct and that I had arranged all required equipment making it easy to find when the lights were out; I was ready. Again, Mungo had told me he would not get involved unless he felt I was doing something incorrectly so, with him watching I started the process.

When the pictures were finished Mungo announced that it was a good job and told me that he was happy for me to carry on without him; this was very good news for me as it confirmed that I was now a qualified offshore photo tech. Mungo was due to leave in two days so I had one more day with him to help should I need it, luckily, I didn't need him and he did leave on schedule.

I spent the rest of my five-week trip not always photographing but also carrying out lots of other tasks associated with inspection such as cleaning marine growth from the structures using HP water jet, air tools and the trusty old hand scraper. Of course, I would carry out photography of any defects found by any of the team. From time to time, I carried out MPI of welds checking for cracks which I would then photograph; it was a lot of fun with the team gelling very well such that we were able to completely inspect one of the little tripod structures in just a couple of days.

As we progressed, we became accustomed to sea life around us but, I never tired of seeing all these wonderful marine tropical fish who would shoal around us especially when we were cleaning the structures providing a terrific free lunch for them. Midwater where the visibility was always good, I was able to take some lovely photos of Angel fish, Parrot fish, Barracuda (they always looked so menacing hunting around the structures in shoals), Wrasse and the odd Moray eel. I think my favourites were Clownfish, I loved watching them swimming in and around toxic anemone fronds apparently using the anemones sting cells as protection from their own predators. They would allow the anemone tentacles to stroke their bodies oblivious to the sting cells that would kill other fish, they were wonderful and so photogenic.

All of us spent some time during our respective dives collecting some of the abundant crayfish so that whenever one of us was due to fly home we had enough frozen fish to take home with us. After I had been on the job for three and a half weeks, I received a telex from Diane in Aberdeen informing me that I would not be able to come home as planned at the end of week five as Chrissie had apparently called to tell her that she wouldn't be able to meet me at the airport! I would have to stay for an extra week making it a six-week trip, well, I thought there's no way that's happening!

It may seem childish but I used to count the days to my next leave as although I loved what I was doing, being on leave still had the edge; the day I received the telex was a bad day, I was in a foul mood all day, luckily for the rest of the crew I had a lot of developing to do so spent much of the day holed up in the photo lab. I smelt a rat as I knew Chrissie wouldn't have called Diane to ask me to stay away, I knew Chrissie and Diane had become friends but still didn't believe it and, in any case, I thought I could find my own way from Heathrow to Torquay without too much problem as I had managed OK in the past. I discussed this with Reg who agreed that this was not going to happen; he told me not to worry and that he would arrange for me to fly home with him as we were both on the five-on-five-off rota; sorted!

On the day I was due to fly home my bag had been stolen, luckily, I had my passport and travel tickets in my briefcase but it meant that I would have to travel home wearing shorts, T-shirt and flip flops, this was not really a problem other than these clothes had been worn while I was working and so were not very clean, to say the least! Also, on the day of arrival in the UK I was greeted by weather that really did not suit my attire! I remember standing on Reading railway station with horizontal driving rain barrelling along the platform at a temperature not far above freezing with most of the rest of the passengers avoiding eye contact with the nutter; I was freezing! Even in the pub for my routine first pint the barmaid seemed reluctant to serve me, I must have looked a real sight for sure.

Other than this my trip home had no negative issues, I arrived home to a very nice welcome from Chrissie; she tried to tell me she was happy to see me but I was not so sure; maybe it was my goody bag full of defrosting crayfish that was the real star. She was somewhat confused by my tale of woe regards being told to stay an extra week and confirmed that she had not spoken to Diane at all, it was probably just a ploy to keep me there for an extra week, anyway, it didn't work!

My leave period of course went like a flash, Chrissie was working as a chef at the Highweek Inn in Newton Abbot so I had a fair amount of free time to fill. I managed this by playing with my motorbike and a fair amount of shopping for electrical kit like stereo systems, cameras and the like; at this time, I didn't have a TV in my house as I just didn't want to watch anything, evenings were much too valuable to waste with TV. I was somewhat amused that while I was away my housemates had received a letter addressed to 'the occupier', it was from the TV licencing authority who were apparently going to be visiting as the property didn't have a TV licence registered. Well, I was looking forward to this, as far as I was concerned if they wanted to waste their time on me then fine; as it turned out they never arrived and we never received any other correspondence, shame.

All too soon my leave was coming to an end, I told Chrissie that we would be saying goodbye at home and that I would travel to the airport by rail; she was not happy about this but I thought it would be better for us both this way.

The five-on-five-off routine was great, it was the first time since I left ICI that I could plan things, what a treat; this made my leave periods even more satisfying. Anyway, at the beginning of April the Falklands war was coming to a head, our prime minister Margaret Thatcher had mobilised a task force to sail from Portsmouth to retake the islands from the Argentinians. On the fifth of April we watched the TV show pictures of ships leaving Portsmouth harbour led by the aircraft carrier or through deck cruiser, (apparently that was what it was called) HMS Invincible, it looked like an aircraft carrier to me? There were lines of ratings arranged on the flight deck with a Harrier jump jet standing proudly on the ski-jump at the bow; it was a stirring site.

The task force would take some six weeks to reach the Falklands and be ready to undertake the mission; in fact, the force landed on East Falkland on the twenty-first of May; the whole country watched with interest and some anxiety for the guys who would actually be fighting. I was due to fly back to work before the task force would reach the Falklands so effectively was out of contact during the first part of the conflict.

As I've said at this time Angola was engaged in civil war and was being supported by the Soviet Union and their allies such as Cuba, they were also firmly on the side of Argentina in their fight against us, the Brits. Being slightly naïve I didn't really give it much thought as to how this might affect me or the rest of the Brits on the job with me. Travel this time was again via Luanda which thankfully had become the preferred route now, in fact, I never had to run the gauntlet of Gabon again so that little problem never raised its ugly head for me.

As we came in to land at Luanda, I could see a large group of silver aircraft on the ground, these looked menacing, they appeared to be large bomber type aircraft; they had a slim fuselage and four engines sporting propellors. I later found out that they were Tupolev Tu-142 this was a Soviet/Russian maritime reconnaissance and anti-submarine warfare aircraft that was derived from their turboprop strategic bomber. It seemed that these aircraft were tasked with long-range communications duties for the Soviet Union; they were currently based at Luanda assisting the Argentinian's, by providing them with high altitude surveillance of the UK's forces around the Falklands during the conflict.

As we taxied past them, I was aware that one of the passengers on our plane had left his seat in the central part of the aircraft and was leaning across the row of seats in front of me in order to get a good look at the Tupolevs; he was also taking photographs with a very nice-looking camera. I didn't really think much more about it but, when we came to a halt and started to disembark, he was just a couple of feet in front of me continuing to take photos of the silver aircraft as he was walking down the steps from our plane. I again didn't give this much thought and concentrated on getting through customs and immigration, for me this went without a hitch again thanks to Marlboro, I was soon chatting to Reg in the queue for the internal flight up to Cabinda, when, there was a commotion behind us.

Looking around, we saw the guy who had been taking the photographs was being led away by uniformed personnel; I didn't know it at the time but later found out that he was a professional photographer working for Oceaneering, he had been contracted to cover the opening of a new platform in the Cabinda field.

His interest in the Soviet planes had been noticed and he had been arrested for spying, the powers that be had taken a very dim view of his taking photos of the Russian planes; he obviously missed the flight to Cabinda and, indeed nobody saw him for almost a week.

On arrival at Cabinda, we were introduced to a new member of the team, Charlie, he was an African Grey parrot, it seemed he had adopted the inspection team and was living ashore with our superintendent. Charlie would travel around the camp standing on the steering wheel of our pickup truck, it was amusing to see him dance to stay vertical whenever the wheel was turned to negotiate corners. He didn't seem to care so long as there were sufficient peanuts available, he would be given nuts in their shells and of course was very adept at cracking the shell to get at the nut inside he had extraordinary dexterity with his beak and feet, sometimes standing on one leg gripping nuts. All of this while hoping around the steering wheel!

Charlie became a valued member of our team over the coming weeks, he kept our spirits up and although he didn't seem to want to talk maybe this was not a bad thing as I'm sure phrases he was being encouraged to say would not have been welcomed in polite society not that there was much of that in evidence in Angola either.

When the photographer did eventually turn up Reg told us that all his photographic equipment had been confiscated; he had been interrogated for some three days before they let him continue his journey. Well, when he did arrive, he was obviously quite shaken up and, in any case had no cameras or equipment and so was not in a position to carry out the job he had been tasked with. He just turned around and went home as soon as his travel could be organised; this left Oceaneering with a bit of a problem, they had evidently agreed to provide photographic cover of the official opening for this new offshore facility and now couldn't get a photographer out to Angola in time for the event which was scheduled to take place in a couple of days.

There were a lot of local dignitaries scheduled to attend including a government minister, all the arrangements had been made meaning that Oceaneering needed to find a way to cover the event. Well, you've probably guessed what happened next; I was taken to one side by Reg who informed me that as the on-site photo tech, I would have to cover the event! Now, I wasn't against doing this other than the photographic equipment I had available was not really designed for this kind of job. I had a few Nikonos-4 sub-sea-thirty-five-millimetre cameras and strobes and my own Canon camera. I hadn't brought a flash with me for the topside camera either; still, I would do my best.

The day of the shoot arrived, it was the second of June and the weather was playing ball, there was not a breath of wind and unusually the cloud cover had become quite broken so there were large areas of blue sky. I had been presented with brand new short sleeved coveralls with prominent Oceaneering patches on the left breast and back; although I say it myself, I felt I was a smart advertisement for Oceaneering. The day was to mark the official opening of the Juliet platform in the Cabinda field, I turned up at the heliport armed with two Nikonos cameras and my Canon, I had decided to take some colour and monochrome negatives. I was armed with enough spare films to ensure I would not run out; I was ushered onto one of the little jet-ranger choppers together with the junior Gulf Oil client rep, and we were off.

The new structure was to the western edge of the Cabinda field and so was some distance from the beach, even so, it only took about twenty minutes flying time to get there. We were deposited on the Juliet platform's helideck at a little after eight in the morning; from there the rep showed me around indicating where the significant events would be taking place.

There were to be some shots of the dignitaries arriving on the helideck, then some general shots of them being shown around the facility. Finishing off with shots of them throwing the switch to activate the systems bringing the facility on line; of course, this was all for show as the facility had been producing for some time already without being officially opened. While I was being shown around our chopper had left leaving the helipad empty for the dignitaries arrival; we had an hour or so before their arrival so I spent the time checking light levels in the various locations, making a note so that when we got there, I would have an idea of the correct settings to use.

When I was finished with my preparations, we made our way back up to the helideck to wait; looking around I saw there was one of the larger supply boats sitting alongside the platform, the rep told me that the dignitaries would be transferred to the boat for lunch. At about ten-fifteen I saw the Huey helicopter approaching and got ready to start taking pictures with my Canon; when the chopper settled onto the helideck the pilot cut power and the rotors slowed to a standstill.

Once all was quiet the welcoming party was ushered onto the helideck and I went with them positioning myself with the sun at my back. The doors to the passenger compartment were opened and out climbed the senior client rep along with the local dignitaries, I was not introduced to them but was told later that they were government officials and their entourage. The minister was not very tall and despite the temperature of the day being in the low thirties Celsius was wearing a thick black leather coat, a Homburg hat, fine trousers and highly polished brown shoes.

He looked uncomfortably hot and was sweating profusely, but I suppose he felt his clothing would indicate his sophistication and bearing or something of that nature? He was accompanied by a stunningly beautiful African lady probably half his age who was wearing a wonderfully bright and colourful dress together with an extremely large and equally brightly coloured headdress adorned with some beautiful feathers; I thought the feathers probably would have looked better if they were still on the bird that grew them, but that's the way it goes I suppose. There were another few men together with their wives or girlfriends in the party all wearing their finery, most of the women were wearing footwear with very high heels which I felt would be challenging as a number of the decks were constructed using 'Texas Walkway Grating' the galvanised steel grating commonly used offshore for deck plates. As I say though I thought this would prove difficult for someone wearing high heels! Anyway, as each person left the helicopter, I took lots of photos; there was a lot of hand shaking and I was instructed to take some group shots with the helicopter in the background.

The group then started to leave the helideck, I was way ahead of them as I knew where they would be going; I took photos of them coming down the steps, along the walkways and with them being shown various pieces of equipment. I was amazed by how well the women seemed able to cope with the walkways by walking on the balls of their feet; awesome! Some of the ladies were really playing up to the camera and I was happy to oblige them.

I had now used all the film in the cameras and had to reload, everyone seemed very happy to just stand around and talk amongst themselves while I did this, then we were off again. The next point of interest was the main event, the main man was going to throw the switch in the control room; I was positioned in the doorway and was happy that the government official was well illuminated, no flash needed. I took several shots of him with his arm raised, hand on the switch and then more with him throwing the switch; once he had completed this I was happy that I had what I needed. The company man had other ideas, he wanted to make absolutely sure and had the minister go through the actions again with me using a second camera.

Once everyone was happy the party moved back to the helideck where they again boarded the helicopter and were transferred the very short distance to the helideck on the supply boat sitting alongside the platform. The junior client rep had stayed with me and was arranging another helicopter to ferry us back to the beach; while I was waiting, I watched the party getting started on the rear deck of the supply boat. A couple of marquees without sides had been erected to provide shade for the celebrations, I could see a lot of glad-handing going on with champagne being handed around, it looked like they were set for a pretty good time. I on the other hand would be going back to the beach to develop the photos, oh well, that's the way of things, isn't it?

My chopper turned up after just a short time and I was taken back to the beach where I cadged a lift in a pickup truck back to the Leon Grigsby that was still in harbour. I then closeted myself in the photo lab; in my haste to start the developing process I didn't check the temperature of the chemicals properly which I'm afraid was an enormous oversight! I developed all the films and started printing from the negatives, the monochrome prints came out really well and I was very happy with the results.

The colour prints were not so much of a success though! They all came out very well from the point of subject framing, focus and lighting but they all had a greyish taint making the colours all wrong? I couldn't understand it, what had I done wrong? It was then that I realised that the water bath where the chemicals had been brought up to temperature was set at the correct temperature for the E6 Ektachrome process for slides. This temperature was however incorrect for the C41 negative process and this had led to the problem, it was all my fault and of course there was no way I could ask to do it again! This was a disaster I had been told that the minister would like to take some photos away with him when he left so I had to produce something. In the end I printed some of the better monochrome pictures and they were presented to him which apparently, he was very happy with, I suppose he might've thought that's all I took?

The films I had messed up were sent back to Mungo in Aberdeen who was able with his much greater knowledge and experience correct the colour problems and did manage to produce photos of an acceptable quality thank goodness. I though was glad to go back to my day job, I had learned an important lesson though and from then on always double-checked temperatures before starting developing!

We spent the next few weeks working around the field inspecting all the structures as we came to them in a logical sequence. Eventually, we arrived at Charlie platform, this was another larger platform used as a gathering station, much the same as the Juliet platform the location of my fopah! The gathering stations collected oil from a number of the small tripod structures consolidating their input into a larger pipeline that then carried the oil ashore to the storage area. I had been on Charlie before when I was working with the maintenance crew during my first trip to Cabinda.

I knew that the platform was one of the first to have been installed and so was some twenty-plus years old, I was expecting to find a fair amount of deterioration. My first dive on Charlie was to clean a horizontal brace at the fifteen-foot level, this was going to take a lot of cleaning as the growth at this shallow level was always major. I was to take the down line with me and attach it to the brace thus making things easier for the guys following to get to the work site. I was using a Rat-Hat and entered the water by jumping, I swum on the surface to the nearest of Charlie's legs and left surface to work down the leg.

I moved around the leg so that I was dropping down the side of the leg where the brace would be attached; as usual for the first few feet the viz was awful but I soon dropped out of the murk and from my vantage point at one corner of the rig I could see all of the structure's legs. As I looked down towards the brace I was to be working on that should have been some five or six feet below me, I couldn't see it? I moved around the leg and could see a brace extending north at the expected depth level towards the other leg; but moving back around to locate the brace, I was due to be cleaning which should have been running west towards the leg in the distance, there was nothing there? I descended to the position where the brace should be and started to clean the marine growth from the leg; I soon discovered the weld that should have been securing the brace in position but it was clear the brace was no longer there.

I informed topside of my findings and they told me to sit tight while they checked the as-built drawings to confirm the brace had actually been fitted originally. After a few minutes they came back to me confirming that the brace had been fitted so it must have fallen off! As I was there, I was told to clean the area around the weld and they would send me a camera so that I could photograph the stub. I managed to complete this without too much problem and found myself photographing a badly corroded stub of the brace; it looked like it had simply corroded and fallen out. One of the other divers later found the brace on the seabed sporting sizeable impact damage in the form of a large dent, so, it was likely there had been a lot of corrosion and then an object had been dropped onto it knocking the brace out. All in all, we spent a lot of time on Charlie, both because it was one of the larger structures and also because we found a good deal of damage and deterioration.

While on the surface one of the guys called for us to come over to the rail, a few of us wandered over to be faced with quite a spectacle, there was a floating 'island' of logs, shrubs and a great deal of nasty looking debris and rubbish passing us pushed along by the Congo-river water which in that region always created a northerly flow. This particular island was not especially large at perhaps twenty metres diameter but what made it memorable was that there in the middle of the island was a beautiful antelope; the poor little soul was destined to stay on the island until it either broke up or ran aground somewhere to the north. This was not especially unusual as these islands were often emitted from the mouth of the Congo but, it was unusual to see wildlife marooned on them like that.

Accompanying the island was a large pod of dolphins, there must have been over a hundred of them including some very young ones, it was lovely to see them trying desperately to keep up and being encouraged by the larger animals, I especially liked to see dolphins as when they were about you were less likely to see sharks.

That evening we were moored up at the end of a jetty enabling us to get ashore; we made our way up to the mess hall to have our meal where we were given news of the Falklands conflict by one of the shore-based Gulf oil workers. It seemed that the local news was broadcasting updates on the war on a daily basis but these were definitely from an Argentine viewpoint. The news we were given was that the UK task force had lost six ships to French supplied Exocet missiles fired from Argentine Mirage fighters on that day alone! Clearly this was awful news and gave us the impression that the conflict was going very badly for the UK task force.

We later found out via the BBC World Service that indeed the task force had lost six ships but this was in total over the whole conflict and not all on the one day; still awful but not as bad as we had been led to believe.

We tried to get ashore whenever we could as when we were ashore, we would be able to purchase our four cans of beer each, this was a nice benefit but as we were normally too far offshore for the majority of the time, we only managed it periodically. We tried to be close to shore on Sundays though as Sunday was a half day for the camp and we liked to use the morning to maintain our equipment or in my case catch up on developing; then in the afternoon wander ashore. We would normally watch or even take part in an organised softball match and of course looked forward to the bar-b-que in the evening for one of the wonderful steaks; Malongo camp really was a small piece of America plonked down in Africa.

For the next few days, we were tasked with buoying flowlines prior to a jack up rig coming in to work over one of the structures; the jack up would be floating in to the side of the structure where it would lower its legs to the seabed before jacking the hull clear of the water. As usual it was important that all flowlines on the seabed were buoyed so that the feet could avoid standing on anything important; for this we would be 'live boating' with the SCUBA replacement system. We prepared by loading up the zodiac, while the rest of the team would stay on the Leon Grigsby cleaning the jacket prior to inspection.

I was to be the first diver; Neil would be the standby diver and Trevik would be along as coxswain; Reg would be the supervisor. Although the boat was quite large as inflatables go it was still very cramped and crowded what with the three large bottles in a frame, two diver's umbilicals, all personal gear for both divers, harnesses, bail-out bottles and a number of ropes including a couple of buoy lines. The four of us were perched on top of the equipment rather than sitting in the boat, still, we were winched over the side of the Leon Grigsby and into the water.

As soon as the boat floated in the frame Trevik started the outboard motor and selected reverse, we glided out of the launch frame, it worked like a dream. Trevik motored over to the first riser and I made ready for the water, carrying out all my pre-dive checks; I then rolled backwards into the water. Neil pulled me back to the surface and I swum over to the riser; it was a six-inch diameter pipe and of course was covered in heaps of marine growth. I had the buoy line in my left hand and made sure the buoy was being trailed away from me in the current. I then told Reg I was leaving surface, down I went, as always, I couldn't see much for the first few feet before clearing when I fell through into the clear seawater, I saw one of the other divers working with a waterjet on the other side of the jacket. He was engulfed in shoals of fish taking advantage of the free feast, as I made my way down the riser, I could see a large number of beautiful blue crayfish scurrying away from me; they were safe from me today but of course they didn't know that.

When I reached the seabed, I told Reg I was at my deepest point and he took my depth with the pneumo; he came back and told me I was at sixty-four feet (19.5 metres). I then sorted myself out to make sure the buoy line was not snagged around anything and started out along the flowline, as expected the visibility was zero which of course meant I was following the pipe by feel. All was well for the first fifteen-feet or so as the line was suspended above the seabed. After it touched down onto the seabed initially, I found that I was able to follow it quite easily as it was not completely buried, but of course before long it disappeared into the mud and I had to dig into the soft silt to keep in contact with the pipe.

The brief was that I was to carry on like this until the pipe became buried deeper than about eighteen inches (about half a metre); in fact, it never got to that point and some distance further on it was again back on the surface of the mud. I was running my hands along the pipe wearing a pair of thin cotton, polka dot work gloves so would be to some extent protected from sea urchins and the like but as with any work in black water my mind was playing tricks on me. I was imagining all sorts of nasties like Moray eels and the like, again, none of these materialised; I was fine, eventually Reg came across the comms telling me I had gone far enough and I was to tie the buoy line off and prepare to come back to surface.

Now, I had been told that I had gone far enough but, when the rig came in it may be that the pilot would ask for the flowline to be buoyed further along so, with this in mind I wanted to tie the line so that another diver descending on the buoy line would know which direction they had to go to swim the line away from the jacket. The flow-line was partially buried at this point so I dug away at the seabed to enable me to pass the buoy line underneath the pipe. When I had space to pass the line under the pipe I took the buoy line down the right-hand side of the pipe, underneath and back up the other side, I pulled the line through until it was almost vertical then took another turn before securely tying it back off to itself using two half-hitches. I coiled the loose buoy line and tied it so that it was in a nice neat coil, this would mean that when we came to undo it for recovery or to go further along the line it would be a straightforward job.

I left bottom and made my way back to the surface using the buoy line, Neil was coiling down my umbilical in a nice figure of eight in the bow of the boat. Trevik had done a great job of following me with the boat, I had not felt any tugging of my umbilical to speak of; when I was back in the boat, I looked back at the jacket to see I had swum about a hundred and fifty metres. We spent the next two days buoying all the flowlines on that side of the jacket, when finished there were several buoys showing clearly where the flowlines were, good job.

Soon it was time for me to go on leave again, for the last few days we were billeted on the beach so had left the Leon Grigsby a couple of days before I was due to leave. I used the time to carry out some much needed maintenance on the equipment. This time I was again to be transferred from Cabinda to Malongo airport in the Huey helicopter this time though it was because there had been a little unrest and they were worried we might become a target. I had wondered what was going on, for the past few days we had seen bush fires raging outside the camp off to the east, apparently these had been started by rebels.

We also heard some small arms fire one evening and were briefed that, if necessary, to head for the harbour where we would board supply boats which would take us to safety; again, I was so naïve to have thought I could spend nearly a year in the middle of a civil war without seeing any evidence of it. The Cuban soldiers caught three rebels who were labelled as responsible and their bodies were left strung up by the camp's entrance as a gruesome warning.

On the day of departure, I boarded the Huey and was whisked to the airport without any issues, I disembarked and headed for the terminal. Once formalities had been completed, I was again standing in the departure lounge; well, as always it was not so much a lounge, it was a departure room really, there was nothing about comfort here! While I was waiting a big Russian bi-plane was taxiing along the runway, we had seen this plane from time to time patrolling the skies over the oilfield, heaven knows what it was looking for? Anyway, I was astonished when it lined itself up on the runway and started its take-off run, it seemed to be going at little more than a fast trot when it lifted off, it almost seemed to float away, amazing.

After what had been an eventful five week's I arrived home on the seventeenth of June to see the newspapers full of the Argentinian surrender, this had happened at twenty-one hundred hours on the fourteenth of June; the mood in London was very buoyant, it made for a nice homecoming.

I spent a lovely few weeks at home again playing with my motorbike and partying with my friends; Chrissie had lined up all sorts of businesses for us to view, mostly small restaurants but there was also a large run-down pub in Mortonhampstead called the White Hart. I must confess that I was not seeing anything I would want to run at all although if I had to choose then I could see the White Hart had great potential. With the benefit of hindsight, we should have gone for the pub but, well, we didn't. Anyway, without any decisions being made and all too soon it was time to head back to Angola, after an uneventful trip I arrived again on the Leon Grigsby which was at the time jacked up in Cabinda's harbour.

The evening was spent catching up on where the job had progressed while I was away and it seemed that as we had now been on the job for some five month's we had worked our way through almost half of the structures. This was very good in one way but unfortunately, we had identified so many problems and issues that a rethink was being undertaken by the grown-ups at Gulf.

Cabinda's oilfield had been looked after by the Russians, for some twenty years prior to Gulf Oil getting involved and it was clear that although they had kept on top of some issues others had been left, the result was that the field was in a dreadful state! We didn't know it at the time but the result was that the field was eventually sold to Chevron quite soon after we left.

One morning when we were again onboard having been jacked up inside the harbour for the night, we had just finished breakfast. I was leaning on the starboard rail close to the galley's doorway chatting to Paul and Adrian when we noticed thick black smoke coming from the engineering space's ventilation louvers; we dashed around to the engineering space's door to find the whole electrical panel in flames! The place had obviously been burning for some time and was well alight, there was a great deal of flame and black smoke billowing out the door. Clearly, this was a very bad situation, I collared a couple of the deck crew and told one of them to organise a fire hose and the other to go to find the rig's engineer.

Paul and Adrian worked with the deck crew bringing fire hoses into action and I started to try to fight the fire with a single CO_2 fire extinguisher, this had almost no effect but maybe did slow the spread of the fire. By the time the extinguisher was exhausted the engineer had arrived and took control; he was very quickly able to isolate the electrical power allowing the sea water fire hoses to be brought to bear.

Paul, Adrian and I backed off and left them to it as they clearly had practiced for this situation, within half an hour the fire was extinguished but, the whole electrical distribution board was finished and would need to be replaced. Clearly this meant the rig would be out of action for a few days, so, what could we do in the meantime? After some hurried negotiations it was decided we would transfer some of our gear onto a supply boat the Birch Tide II; this was accomplished in a little over a day and off we went again to continue our work.

Working from a supply boat again was nice as there was a lot more space for our equipment and getting in and out of the water was easier than it had been from the deck of the Leon Grigsby. I had about another three weeks of my stint left and this was all to be carried out from the supply boat. Towards the end of my stint, we found ourselves tied up to the Single Buoy Mooring (SBM) situated some distance offshore towards the western edge of the field. I had been on SBM's before and so knew what to expect. These buoys were designed for tankers to tie up to periodically, once the ships were at the buoy, they would pick up floating hoses attached to the buoy enabling them to take oil onboard from the buoy; for Cabinda, this was their only export method available so was extremely important.

The first day we were on the buoy we checked the anodes and took CP readings of the main buoy. We also checked the angles of the buoy chains; if the buoy had been dragged off station, then at least some of the chain angles would be changed. I measured all the other chains noting the angles were all very similar meaning the buoy had not been dragged off station, once I had measured all chain angles topside called me back to the surface.

My last dive before going on leave and indeed although I didn't know it at the time my last dive on this job would be to carry out CP readings and visual inspection of the SBM's Pipe-Line End Manifold (PLEM). We were tied up stern on to the SBM, being tied up by the stern meant that when we entered the water we didn't have very far to swim to the job. I jumped in and made my way across to the buoy, as soon as I got there, I told Reg I was "ready to leave surface"; he told me "Leave surface", I ducked under the buoy saying "Left surface", I found one of the large flexible subsea hoses running down from the centre of the buoy; down I went following the hose. As with SBM's in general the subsea hose had to be able to deal with rise and fall of the main buoy on the surface, this could be due to with wave action or tidal variations. It was not a good thing for hoses to be allowed to lay onto the seabed at low water as this may mean that when the tide turned and started to rise again the hose could become trapped on the PLEM or some other obstruction causing damage to either the hose or the PLEM.

Normally hoses were arranged in a 'lazy-S' configuration, there would be buoyancy fitted to the hose sufficient that the hose would be kept under tension from the PLEM to the buoyancy. The hose then would gradually bend over the buoyancy and a loop would be created before the hose finally made its way up to the buoy, any rise and fall would then be accommodated by the mid-water section of hose without risk. So, there I was following the hose which would lead me directly to the PLEM, as I descended, I soon reached the point at the bottom of the loop, continuing along the hose I could feel that it was rising. Quite soon I came across the first syntactic buoyancy collars, I hadn't seen any of these since my abortive attempt to cut one up with a chainsaw in Aberdeen, I climbed the hose up to the apex of the loop noting and reporting on the condition of the buoyancy collars as I went. Descending past the end of the buoyancy collars, I could see the hose disappearing into the murk near the bottom; quite soon the visibility reduced considerably, and when I eventually found the flange marking the end of the subsea hose where it joined the PLEM the viz had reduced to about a foot (30 centimetres).

Before the dive I had seen drawings of the PLEM so knew where I had arrived and where to go from there; I made my first CP reading on the steel pipe immediately the other side of the subsea hose flange, this was a good reading of -0.91 V protected. I was relaying all my readings and visual findings up to Reg on the surface where he recorded them; I worked my way around the PLEM visually inspecting and taking CP readings at pre-determined points. There were a number of large valves and flanges on the PLEM together with some sacrificial anodes all of which needed to be inspected; finally, I had to make my way a short way along the main thirty-six-inch flowline, this was the main supply pipe to the PLEM. I had to make sure the seabed was not undermined and that the PLEM was properly supported on the seabed; I knew that this would be a very attractive location for moray eels and the like, but I also knew that they would leave me alone unless I gave them no option. I made a lot of noise moving around and although I saw a few eel heads none of them gave me any cause for concern.

After fifty-nine minutes at a maximum depth of seventy-six feet I was ready to leave bottom, as I started my ascent, I was careful to ascend at the rate as appropriate for surface decompression using oxygen, this was twenty-five feet per minute. I completed all my in-water decompression made my way up onto the deck again, the team helped me to remove my diving equipment then I was again in the deck decompression chamber being blown down to forty-feet to complete the rest of my decompression breathing oxygen.

Following this dive and my subsequent twenty-four-hour period of 'bend-watch' I was able to make my way home together with my bag of frozen crayfish. Again, this trip was largely without incident other than when I arrived in Paris, I had been expecting a two-hour wait for my ongoing flight to London but, owing to fog in London the previous flight had been delayed by several hours and was due to leave just as I arrived at the terminal, luckily there was space on the flight and so I was able to virtually walk onto it without any wait! This resulted in my arriving home a good couple of hours early, what a result.

While I had been away Chrissie and my mother had been busy; it seemed that mum had decided that the hardware, pet and garden shop that mum and dad had run together was now proving too much for her on her own although she had been running it with my sister since dad died. Chrissie was very keen that we buy the shop from mum so that she could retire; I have to say, I was less keen as I didn't really see myself as a shopkeeper! We had a frank discussion that evening where I put forward that I still had six-months of this Angolan contract to go and that as it was an equal time contract that meant I would only be away for three of those months. This didn't cut much ice and I was faced with an ultimatum; do I want Chrissie or not? If I continued with the contract, it was likely she wouldn't wait for me, so, it looked as though I would have to stop diving and become a shopkeeper after all!

I spent a few days where I distanced myself, I was analysing the situation and looking back over the past few years and I have to say. I had been extremely lucky; I had been diving with ICI for some five years where I had been taken to some lovely locations all around the British Isles to dive in places where admittedly the diving sometimes turned out to be less than optimal, but some were wonderful like the west coast of Scotland and Whitby. Then I had gone on my BAD course at Fort Bovisand where I found that I seemed to have a talent for the kind of work I would be expected to carry out offshore. I walked into a job with the top offshore diving contractor straight from my course and then after only six months was saturation diving in France!

At the time this progression was unheard of and from there I had been sent to wonderful locations around the world where I seemed to always be able to secure coveted positions. In short, I had found a job that I loved and I seemed to be recognised as being quite capable. In the early eighties the job paid handsomely and as I say I was encouraged to play with a very wide range of expensive and sophisticated kit in far off locations carrying out a job that in truth I probably would have done for nothing. I had loved it, what a way to earn a living! Still all good things have to come to an end don't they.

I certainly felt that it was a life for young single individuals and certainly at that time the offshore world was littered with bitter men who were paying the price of divorce (sometimes more than one); it was clear to me that the majority of these divorces were brought about by the job. I had from day one resolved that when and if I found the right lady, I would have to find work closer to home as I couldn't really see the point of being married only to spend the majority of time away from home especially if kids came along as I certainly would want to be there to see them grow up.

A few days into my leave I received a telegram from Oceaneering, it seemed that we had been somewhat too effective with our inspections of the Cabinda field. We had found so much damage and deterioration that maybe the client didn't want to know about any more; the contract had been terminated six months early, I called Diane to chat about what happens next for me. She told me not to worry, in the short term I had been scheduled to go back to the maintenance team at Cabinda and she would be looking to get me onto a routine sat job as soon as she could. Oh well, at least I had a job to go back to for now.

So, it was that I picked Chrissie up and we drove out to Buckfastleigh to discuss everything with mum. Chrissie and I had originally agreed that I would work offshore until I had been able to build up sufficient capital enabling us to buy a business without needing a big loan. However, at this time I had not had enough time to build up the pot; this meant we would need a sizeable loan for any purchase. Being a Wednesday, the shop would be closed in the afternoon, in those days Wednesday's in Buckfastleigh was early closing for all shops, it was a different world in those days. We sat down in the flat above the shop with a nice cup of tea and started our discussions; I tried to be as positive as I could and after just a couple of hours, we had thrashed out a deal. We would need to borrow some thirty-thousand pounds, this might seem a paltry sum now but, in those days, it was a lot of money as you could have bought a really nice five bedroomed house in Torquay for that sort of money.

As we walked back to the car Chrissie was jubilant, she was extremely excited about the prospect of us working together and being shopkeepers! I tried to put the right face on it so as not to burst her bubble. Before leaving Buckfastleigh I went into the Nat-West bank in the main street where the shop banked and arranged to see David the bank manager to discuss a business loan. This was arranged for the following Friday at midday; I was not really sure what would be needed for this meeting so I also arranged to meet with my accountant James Forbes-Smythe who had an office in Ashburton to discuss all of this.

Friday came and there I was in the bank manager's office; you have to understand that in those days bank managers were seen as major individuals with a lot of power and I had to come across as a credible individual who could be relied on. As I say, the shop had been banking at this branch for years so, they knew the state of the business (certainly better than I did). Up until this time I had been steering clear of corporate and authority figures and when I sat down in the manager's office, I felt much the same as I always had when I had been summoned to the headmaster's office at school. It was clear right from the start that he had been briefed by mum, he knew all about our plans and had I think prepared his spiel, it consisted of my being told, that I needed to become a 'pillar of the community' as people would rely on me.

I played my part trying to come across as a business man it was clear that he didn't want to lose the account; I explained that I had always banked at the Midland bank who also wanted the business. Before long we came to an agreement for us to borrow the required funds as an overdraft on the business at quite a favourable interest rate; so, the deal was done. I was a Nat-West customer, I explained that we wouldn't be in a position to take over the business for some three months or so and he accepted this without question, he told me the funds would be ready for us whenever we needed them.

Chrissie was of course overjoyed as was mum, my sister; less so as she was effectively out of a job! She seemed to take this well though, all seemed well. We agreed that I would do one last trip to Angola and would tell Oceaneering that I was no longer available after that!

I left for my last offshore trip back down to Cabinda on the seventeenth of September, I was to be there for six weeks so would be due to fly home in late October or early November. When I arrived, I found that the maintenance team were not working from their normal supply boat, apparently a jack-up rig had caused significant damage to flowlines alongside one of the tripod structures meaning that the team were working to resolve the damage. The team were working from a McDermott barge, at the time (and even now) McDermott was a large offshore company principally engaged in construction and repair of offshore structures. We would be working from the McDermott Dredge Barge DB14, this had been positioned above the area where the damaged pipelines were situated.

The barge had been positioned using a four-point mooring; with four anchors put out, one from each corner of the barge. These anchor lines had been tensioned such that the barge would more or less stay in position regardless of tide, current flow or wind. I was flown out to the nearest tripod structure and from there was ferried to the DB14 by Bart using the inflatable that the maintenance team had inherited from the inspection contract.

I knew Bart from my previous trips with the maintenance team; it was nice to see him again, he was a real gent, always saw the best in people and never seemed to get flustered or angry about anything. When we came alongside the DB14 it was clear this was a real workhorse, the hull was painted black with the accommodation being white, well I say the paint was black and white, this was how it would have been originally although I'm not sure how much paint remained, there was a lot of rust visible; the barge's sides were lined with old tractor tyres running along at water level acting as fenders. The decks were full of equipment, all our diving kit including the decompression chamber was on the port side but the rest of the barge had been set up with fabrication units for welders and fabrication of metal work.

As soon as I made it on board Bart took me along to the accommodation where the others on the team were waiting as there was no diving being required at the moment. The normal supervisor Richard (Rick) Newman was on leave at this time so Bart was the acting supervisor and in charge, Byron Gibson who had been on the inspection contract with me was there as well as Alex Gray a young Canadian lad who I had worked with in France, he had been an apprentice diver back then but now was a fully-fledged air diver.

As was the norm, we chatted for half an hour or so about the job and mutual acquaintances, it felt nice to be back with them. My bunk was in a cabin of four, I was assigned the lower bunk on the left-hand side, the cabin was windowless and lined with plywood walls, this gave it a fairly dark ambience but hey, all I would do was sleep there.

I spent the rest of the day being shown around the dive system and being made aware of how we worked together with the barge crew, as we were wandering around, I was very glad to see that our African Grey parrot Charlie had been adopted by the maintenance crew and was on board with us. Bart told me that Charlie was not in a very good mood these days as the deck crew that consisted mostly of Nigerians had taken to pulling out his tail feathers for some reason; I later found that African Grey parrot tail feathers were much treasured by Nigerians.

Charlie had decided that anyone who wasn't white was an enemy and from time to time he could be found sitting above a doorway ready to leap onto a Nigerian shoulder where he would nip at their ears! I can tell you having seen him opening nuts there is no way I would want him biting my ear.

Bart told me that Charlie was really not able to fly very far without this tail feathers and so was in a bit of a precarious position being on a barge some miles from land. This was demonstrated to me within a couple of days when I saw him flapping away from the barge only to lose height until he ditched in the sea immediately alongside the barge; African Grey parrots are really not equipped for life at sea and cannot swim but the poor little guy did eventually manage to make his way to one of the tractor tyres where using his beak and talons he was able to climb back on board. He looked a sight, feathers all soaked and sticking out all over the place, we managed to sit him in the sun on the top of the decompression chamber where he could dry off, he spent a good couple of hours preening himself until be started to look himself again.

This was not an isolated event one time he was seen to be flapping like crazy only to ditch in the sea some twenty-feet or so off to the side of the barge. This time he was really in trouble and although he was keeping his head above water, he was clearly fighting a losing battle, we were diving at the time and were able to jump our standby diver to go and rescue him, it looked very funny seeing him sitting on the diver's head while being brought back to the barge.

The first day of my trip started at five-thirty in the morning with breakfast, this was in the mess room together with the rest of the dive team and a good few of the deck crew. I decided to go for cereal and was digging into the bin with corn flakes when I saw tiny black bugs running around in the bin, these turned out to be a kind of weevil which, while not dangerous to us did make me feel less inclined to partake, I decided to go for eggs instead.

We were buoying flowlines and my first few dives were to locate and follow a twelve-inch (30 centimetre) line at a depth of ninety-five to one hundred feet (29-31 metres), this went fine but of course they were not particularly pleasant dives as being on the seabed there was absolutely no viz. This continued for a few days until we found the twelve-inch line was crossed by a six-inch line laying beneath, the two lines were in contact with each other. This was very bad news and needed to be rectified, it was decided that because the seabed consisted of very soft mud, we would use a low-pressure water-jet to dig a gulley below the six-inch line so that it fell away from the larger line above it.

Over the next few days, we set about jetting under the six-inch line trenching to a distance of some thirty-feet or so either side of the crossover, now, as I'm sure you can appreciate, this is not a lovely job but once you get in position and start up the water-jet it is quite mindless, it became somewhat boring but eventually the trench was dug and the smaller pipe settled nicely into the trench leaving a gap between the two pipes. All we had to do then was to ensure the lines had not been damaged, I was given the task of assessing the damage which had to be done completely by touch and feel; I could feel that where the lines had been in contact, they had been kept clean of marine growth and were very smooth. I cleaned some distance either side of this clean patch and with the aid of a calliper was able to measure the diameters from either side of the contact patch and actually on the contact point.

These measurements showed that although there had been some wear, it was not significant so, all we had to do now was to place sandbags between the two pipes so that as the twelve-inch pipe settled it would not come back into contact with the six-inch line beneath.

We spent the next few days following and buoying flowlines and where we found crossovers jetting and bagging the crossovers as before, while the diving conditions were not particularly pleasant, the work was quite satisfying, I was enjoying myself. Eventually we came across a six-inch line that had been broken by the jack-up rig jacking standing on the pipe. Byron had followed the flowline out from the jacket and had left a buoy at the point where the flowline had been bent upwards. I was to dive next; I was tasked to follow the flowline along to the point where the break was and to place another buoy at that point. I descended the buoy line left by Byron and when I reached the bottom Bart gauged my depth with the pneumo; I was at ninety-five feet.

I knew which way I had to travel because Byron had wrapped the buoy line properly, so, leaving that line in place I set off making sure my umbilical and the second buoy line I was carrying were not fouled around Byron's buoy line. As I moved along the flowline, I could tell that the pipe was no longer in contact with the seabed, indeed it had been badly bent and was rising at an angle of about thirty degrees; as I continued along the pipe the angle increased until it was climbing steeply; as I followed the pipe, I climbed out of the zero viz and into clearer water. Eventually, I came to the pipe's jagged severed end which was mid-water; I told Bart what I had found and he instructed me to tie off the buoy line and prepare to leave bottom.

Once I was back on deck the next diver, Alex, was tasked with finding the other end of the pipe, this didn't take very long and quite soon we had buoys indicating both ends of the broken pipe. As a small team of just four divers, we were now dived out for the day and retired to consider our next move tomorrow. As luck would have it, bad weather came in overnight so there was no diving for the next two days. This of course gave us lots of time to decide on our next move, when we did get back to the job it had been decided that we would cut both ends of pipe where they were flat on the seabed. Once the bent parts of pipe had been removed, these would be recovered to the surface and the distance between the pipe ends would be measured so that a replacement pipe (spool-piece) could be fabricated; we would then be able to repair the broken pipe.

I was to start cutting the pipe end closest to the jacket first, the cutting method was to be Ultrathermic oxy-arc (Broco rods); I was quite looking forward to the job as it was fiery and fast. When I arrived on the bottom, I set up with earthing clamp making good electrical contact with the pipe, I then fitted my first Broco rod into the oxy-arc torch and squeezed the trigger to see that enough oxygen was coming through the rod. All was working well, I called "Make it hot", the response was "It's hot"; I moved in to start cutting. Squeezing the trigger again I saw oxygen rushing out of the end of the rod in a fierce bubbling flow; as soon as the flow was established, I pulled my welding mask down over my eyes so that I would not be blinded by the bright arc. Touching the tip of the rod against the flowline, Bam, my world was suddenly illuminated with a fierce blue-white light from the arc, as the visibility was still very poor, I could not really see much of what I was doing but, I could see enough to know where the cut was beginning.

I was conscious of the danger of trapped gas causing explosion, this had killed or seriously injured divers in the past, to ensure this couldn't happen I first needed to punch a hole in the top of the pipe ensuring that any gas inside would be able to bubble away harmlessly. Broco is extremely efficient and the metal of the pipe just seemed to be blown away, the rod punched straight through, I now had the required vent hole at the top of the pipe. I pulled the rod back and moved down to the bottom of the pipe where I started to work my way around the pipe, all went well until I had completed cutting just over three quarters of the circumference when the weight of the damage pipe free end started to bend the remaining metal. I stood back from the cut and watched as the pipe settled onto the seabed; I had a length of rope with me which I had already tied on to the pipe about six-feet back from where I was cutting.

I put the cutting set down on the seabed and tied the other end of the rope onto what would be the cut end of the pipe again about six-feet from the cut; this would mean that we would be easily able to locate both ends of the pipe. Once this was done, I returned and picked up the cutting rig again to continue the cut; I was very aware that the small section of pipe still attached would be under significant tension and so made sure that I positioned myself clear of where I felt the pipe may spring when I completed the cut. As I started the final cut, I could hear some wrenching noises and even before I had properly completed the cut the small section of remaining metal separated; the pipe sprung upwards by a couple of feet very quickly, I was glad I had not been sitting on top of the pipe. The other end fell harmlessly onto the seabed and I noted that my umbilical, the oxygen hose and electrical cable of the cutting rig were all free and running directly back to the surface; job done.

The pipe would eventually be repaired with the replacement spool piece but this would be done by another crew as it was not ready before I left.

For the next few days, we went back to tracing flow lines and identifying where lines crossed one another; it was amazing how many flowlines ran across the field, there didn't seem to have been any plan to setting out the field and subsequently nobody knew where flowlines crossed. Still, this kept me and Oceaneering employed so not all was bad; however, it was on one of these crossovers where the next significant event took place.

Alex had been jetting to create a trench below another six-inch flowline, his dive was without incident and he completed his surface decompression at five-past-six in the evening, when he came out of the chamber he had reported well, we then stripped down the dive gear and made ready for diving to commence again in the morning. When this was done, we all made our way to the galley for supper; all was fine until about one-thirty of the following morning when I was woken by Alex's moaning, he was clearly in pain. Alex was in the top bunk across from mine, I got out of my bunk and went across and asked him what was wrong, he told me that he had a bad pain in his knee. I immediately thought he was suffering a likely DCI from his last dive; I roused Byron and told him to help Alex to make his way out to the decompression chamber on deck, while I went to get Bart up; he was in the cabin next door to ours.

Bart was understandably very concerned for Alex and told me he would rouse the rest of the team and asked me to prepare the chamber to treat Alex. I went out on deck where I found Alex by the chamber, he was looking very pale and was clearly in a good deal of pain.

I had been the first diver on the previous days diving so it was decided that I should accompany Alex as the attendant during his therapeutic dive, Bart told us that we would be carrying out a US Navy (USN) therapeutic recompression using table six. This was the routine first step in treatment of pain only DCI; it meant that we would be in the chamber for at least the next four and a half hours. I loaded the chamber up with bottles of water, blankets and pillows; the chamber was a relatively small air diving chamber and so was not equipped for long stays at depth; I therefore put a bucket and some toilet rolls in as well just in case.

We left surface at four-forty-five in the morning and immediately went to the treatment depth of sixty-feet (18 metres) where Alex was put onto oxygen (O_2) via the built-in breathing supply (BiBS) mask; as soon as we got to depth Bart asked me to carry out an assessment of Alex to see whether his pain had reduced. Alex said that he did feel the pain had subsided a bit but had not gone altogether; Alex continued breathing oxygen according to the USN protocol with cycles of twenty-minutes on O_2 interspersed with five-minute air breaks during which he removed the BiBS mask and breathed the chamber atmosphere. The USN table allowed for extensions to be undertaken for symptoms that were not improving, Alex's table was fully extended.

During the final part of the decompression from the table six protocol the attendant (me) was also required to breathe O_2 along with the patient, I did this without any issue and we arrived on surface some six hours after leaving surface. Alex reported that he was feeling much better and we all dispersed to our various bunks to try to catch up on lost sleep; diving was of course cancelled for the day.

All was well until sometime later when again Alex told me that he was feeling the pain in his knee was back again; again, I roused Bart and the rest of the crew and we geared up for a retreatment. Bart decided that the oxygen should be analysed, Byron was dispatched with the oxygen analyser and within a few minutes returned with bad news, it seemed that the oxygen quad we had been using was in fact filled with air! This was extremely bad news as not only had Alex been wrongly decompressed from his original dive and the subsequent therapeutic treatment but also as I should have been breathing O_2 for the last part of my decompression I had also been incorrectly decompressed! I had no symptoms but would now need to be treated using a therapeutic table as a precautionary measure.

So, it was at two-thirty-eight Alex and I were again recompressed to carry out another therapeutic recompression, this time using oxygen from a bottle that had been properly analysed! This time all went well and we were both decompressed without any further issues. As is the protocol, I was not dived for the next seven days just to be on the safe side,

Alex was relieved and went home as soon as it was safe for him to fly.

Bart felt terrible about the issue as he was the supervisor but at the time there was no requirement to analyse gas while it was being breathed, this is no longer the case and so this sort of problem should not be able to occur nowadays. I did have a close look at the oxygen quad we had originally been using and although it had been painted in the correct colours for a quad containing oxygen; with the cylinders being painted properly for diving oxygen; black body with white shoulders I found that someone had scratched Air on some of the bottles; I'm sure this made sense to someone but there you go, this was diving in Africa in the eighties! Alex did not suffer any long-term consequences as far as I know and did return to diving with Oceaneering.

Following this incident, our world returned to normal with Rick Newman returning from leave meaning that Bart reverted to lead diver; he told me that he was very glad to have been relieved as supervisor as he had not enjoyed the responsibility. The team continued on the DB14 for the rest of my trip; we were swimming and buoying flowlines, fitting clamps to risers, connecting flowlines together and other general construction jobs, I loved it. I always enjoyed construction as no two days were ever the same, there was always a tremendous feeling of achievement when even small tasks were completed well.

One of the last dives of this trip was also one of my most memorable; the job was to fit a clamp onto a horizontal brace and then to pull the riser into the clamp securing it in place. The dive commenced at eight minutes past seven in the evening which in Angola meant that it was to be a night dive; as I've said before I have always loved diving at night as the sub-sea world seemed to really come to life during the hours of darkness. I left surface carrying a lamp following the downline to the job, dropping through the poor viz layer I was greeted by the usual vista afforded by the clearer water with my being able to see all three of the jacket's legs, there were crayfish scuttling around on the braces, angel and clown fish showing off their brilliance.

With the brace I was to be working on being at only twelve feet water depth there was no rush, I could stay there for hours if necessary. I can't tell you how lucky I felt again, I was truly privileged to be given the chance to be there and I knew it; being that this was to be one of my final offshore dives I spent a bit more time just enjoying the spectacle and the marine life seemed happy to oblige me, it was great. The area of the brace where the clamp was to be fitted had already been cleaned so I didn't really need to do any more cleaning but, I knew that if I did knock some marine growth off, I would be joined by even more colourful fish so, I set to work knocking off a few oysters.

I was not disappointed, huge numbers of tiny silver fish turned up starting to gorge themselves; eventually though I had to get back to work and asked for the clamp to be sent down. Within minutes I had settled the clamp onto the brace and was concentrating on attaching the securing face plate with six large bolts. This took about three quarters of an hour, I then called for the riser to be lowered and guided it into place. Once the new riser was in position, I bolted the clamping face on with four bolts completing the job; all that remained for me to do then was to clear up the worksite and send everything back to the surface. I attached the spanners to the workline and signalled for it to be recovered then untied the downline, told Rick that I was ready to leave bottom and made my way back to the surface.

My last journey home from Angola was tinged with sadness, not so much for leaving Angola as knowing that I would no longer be an offshore commercial diver, I had loved pretty much the whole time although as I've already said there were a few times that I could have done without. Anyway, as we lifted off in the Huey for the short hop to Malongo airport I was glad that the pilot circled the field for a short time as it gave me a last look at the field where I had spent almost a year of my working life. The trip home was uneventful, when boarding the train for the final stretch of the journey I looked for a seat on the left-hand side as was usual for me. I loved to be on that side of the train as it gave the best view of the Exe estuary, the beaches between the Exe and Teignmouth and finally all the way up the Teign estuary before depositing me at Newton Abbot station; this always reminded me of why I lived in this part of the world and made me feel very happy to be home.

As soon as I was home, I contacted Chrissie who it became clear had been very busy while I was away; solicitors had been working away with all required paperwork for us to take over the shop in Buckfastleigh. My first job the next day was to call Ian Little at Oceaneering to tell him that I would no longer be available for work, he was I think quite shocked as he had felt I was going to be a long-term stalwart of the offshore world. Anyway, he eventually wished me well and told me when (not if) I got bored with home life I would be welcomed back. So, there I was jobless again, I now had to make this work; I put my house on the market (Chrissie's had already been up for sale for a few weeks).

PHOTOS FROM ANGOLA

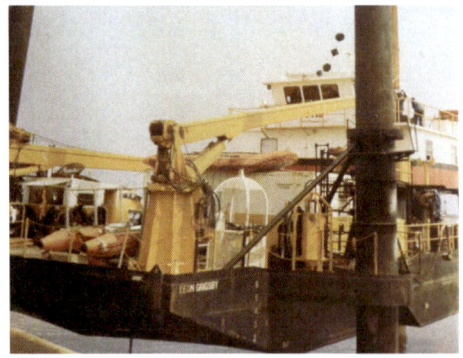

The Leon Grigsby Tripod 'jack-up' rig that became our home for the Cabinda Gulf Oil Company inspection contract in 1982-83.

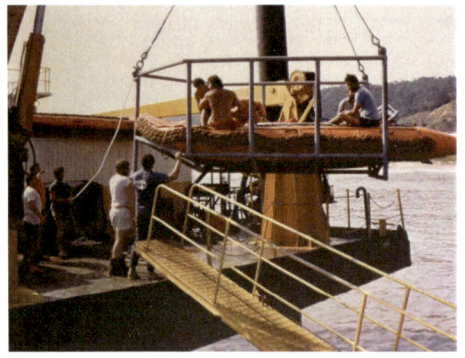

Our inflatable workboat fitted into the lifting frame that had just been fabricated for us.

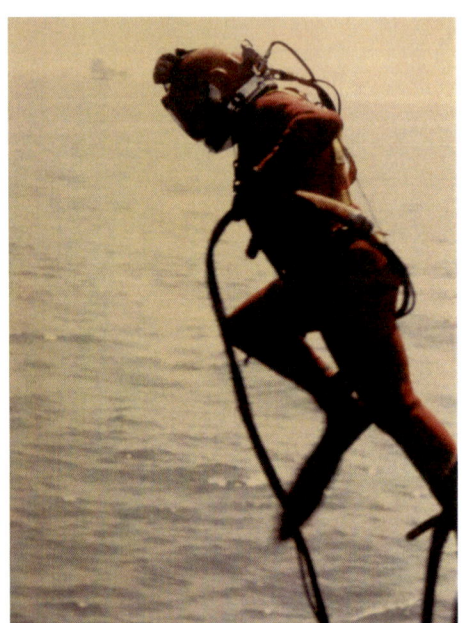

Entering the water going to work.

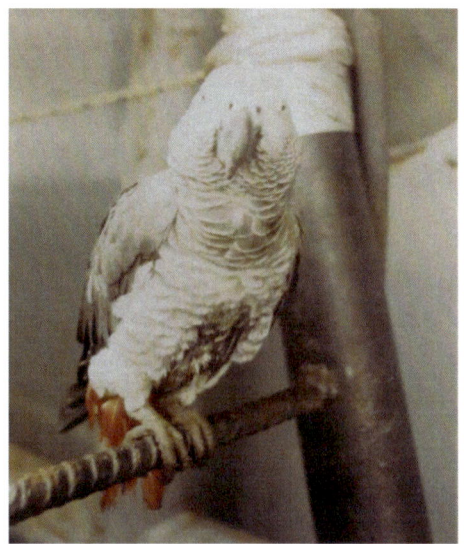

Charlie with very few tail feathers.

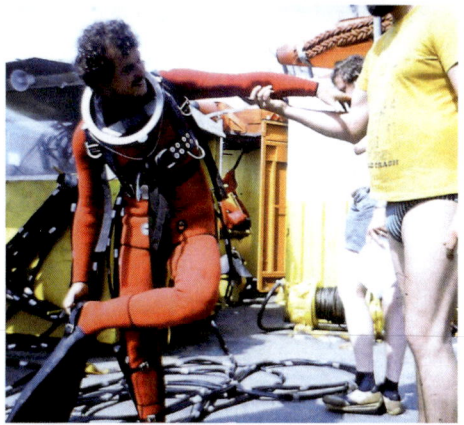

Preparing for another dive as photo-tech on the Leon Grigsby.

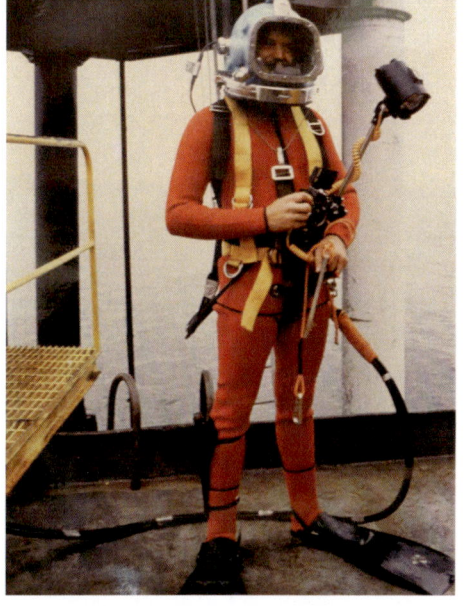

Ready to go now wearing a Rat-Hat and carrying the Nikonos 4 camera system.

Part Five

CHAPTER FIFTEEN

Shopkeeper and Beyond - 1983 to 88

Almost as soon as I arrived home from my last trip, I started to work in the shop learning the trade as it were, while I was definitely not very keen on being a shopkeeper, I had made my choice and knew I really had to make a go of it; I therefore, did my best to put a positive face on it for the customers and of course for Chrissie. I did however really like Buckfastleigh; we soon made some very good friends and the local pub, the King's Arms that was just a few doors along Fore Street, from our shop was at the time run by a lovely couple who made the pub the centre of the village.

Before long all was settled with both houses being sold and moneys transferred to mum completing our purchase of the shop, Johnsons Hardware, Pet and Garden. At the time shops were generally open in Buckfastleigh Monday to Saturday with a half day on Wednesday; we settled into the flat above the shop and started to make our mark on the shop. While mum and Sue had been running the shop there had been a focus on small gifts and tourist stuff, I was not at all interested in this and in the first few weeks of our being there I could see that the number of sales didn't warrant the cost of stock so wanted to move away from this. I started to stock more in the way of DIY equipment such as wood, plumbing fittings, pipe, sand and cement etc. Of course, this would take some time to take off but I felt Buckfastleigh needed this much more than the tourism tat!

One of the first steep learning curves for me was mixing paint, the shop already had a Dulux Mix Lab, this was a machine enabling us to stock a huge variety of paint colours and finishes, gloss, emulsion, silk and matt without needing a massive stock of individual colours. The process was for the customer to choose the finish for example gloss and then choose from the wide range of colours picked from the normal colour chart. Once chosen, I had a recipe book detailing which base colour to use, I would select the appropriately sized can of base and then would add the required millilitres of the appropriate concentrate colour(s) as dictated by the recipe book.

Once these colours had been added the top of the can was replaced, the can was fitted into the machine which rotated and basically shook the can for some time in order to mix everything together. It was a very good system and although we never sold a huge amount it did allow us to stock paints in sufficient variety to be of use; we were however never cheap and couldn't compete with the big boys so tended to only be used for small jobs by the locals.

During our first year in the shop, we decided to make a special effort with sale of bedding, fruit and veg plants; I knew nothing at all about plants so again I had to learn a lot very quickly, I built some trolleys on casters on which to display the plants allowing us to roll them out onto the pavement in the morning and back into the shop at night. This proved to be a big success with us finding it difficult to keep up with demand, but of course this is a nice problem to have and it had the added bonus that the profit margin was very good.

Chrissie had by now agreed to become my wife and we set about organising this although it took us until September to make this happen. Chrissie had been told by numerous doctors that she was extremely unlikely to be able to conceive or carry children, this was a really big issue for her, I would have been sorry not to have kids but I didn't want it to ruin our lives. We decided that in the absence of kids we would get a dog! As soon as I made it common knowledge in the village that we wanted a puppy we were made aware of a farmer who had a Welsh Springer Spaniel that was pregnant. When the puppies were born, we went to have a look and one in particular decided my shoe was special, she proceeded to lay into chewing my toe. The decision was made, she was the one, I don't think we had much to do with this, she had chosen us.

When she was able to leave her mum, we took her home where she set about making herself at home, first on her list was to make the acquaintance of Chrissie's cat Scamp; Scamp was a Siamese cross who was fiery at the best of times and was less than impressed with the new arrival! The first time they met Scamp was asleep in front of the fire, the puppy decided to give Scamp's tail a playful nip! Scamp came awake in an instant, leapt up turning in flight and gave the puppy a swipe with fully bared claws, blood was drawn, the puppy treated Scamp with respect from then on. Naming the new addition to our family took us a couple of days but we eventually settled on Tess and she was a darling, I loved that dog and I think the feeling was mutual.

Over the coming months we settled into a comfortable routine, I would open up the shop and see to customers with Chrissie joining me once she had done housework etc. On our Wednesday afternoons off we would go up onto Dartmoor where we would walk with Tess it was a lovely time; on one of these afternoons, we made our way up to the Avon Dam where I decided it was time for Tess to learn to swim. I stripped off my jeans and waded out into the reservoir where I called Tess to me, she dipped her feet in the water but that was clearly going to be as far as she was prepared to go! I waded ashore picked her up, carrying her back out to where I had been and put her down in the water; her legs were windmilling before they even touched the water but she quickly realised she was floating and was able to make her way back to the beach.

From then on there was no stopping her, whenever we were near a river, lake or the sea she would be gone into the water, she loved chasing sticks and bringing them back to the beach for us. She really loved the water, however, if I had the audacity to try to take her out for a walk in the rain, she would follow behind me with her head down looking miserable until she was soaked through, then she would stop and sit down, it would be very clear that she was not interested in continuing. I often would be forced to carry her back to the car as once she put on the brakes, she could not be coaxed or cajoled into movement again.

The first few months of our running the shop were a little worrisome, it seemed the takings just about covered the outgoings but there was never enough to start paying off the overdraft. The bank manager started to make noises about this being a problem, however, my accountant was much less concerned, his words were "what's he banging on about, it's his job to lend businesses money!" Well, I have to say I was quite worried but all I could do was to keep opening the door and hope business would pick up. By April, the bedding plants and other garden accessories had really started to make a difference and we were beginning to see people coming to us for their DIY projects; by the time summer came it was clear that we were going to be able to make some payments to reduce our overdraft, this of course made the bank manager very happy.

While our new lines were going well, I was conscious that I needed to keep the old customers happy as well if at all possible; in a small village with everyone knowing everyone else this was especially important, we couldn't upset anyone, if we did then all their friends and family tended to vote with their feet! To this end I started to do a lot of deliveries particularly to elderly customers, this went down very well and for me had an added bonus as it meant that I was not stuck in the shop all day. It did however mean that Chrissie had to spend more time in the shop which was not popular, we decided to take on a part time shop assistant.

It was not difficult to find people for the role but it proved to be a lot more difficult to find someone who fitted in and was right for the role, after a few false starts we came across Barbera Bray, she was a ray of sunshine and became a real crutch for us to lean on; she was perfect. With Barbera on board things really started to settle down, she was Buckfastleigh born and bred and knew everyone, most often this resulted in higher levels of sales for us, great. I found I was beginning to enjoy the role a bit more, I especially liked the banter with the customers and being able to help people out.

Sunday was our day of rest, we had taken to getting up late, I would take Tess for a short walk then we would head to the King's Arms for lunch; with Tess being just a few months old and still a very boisterous puppy we didn't take her with us leaving her with the run of the flat. On one particular Sunday we returned from the pub at just after two o'clock in the afternoon when pubs had to close in those days, as we arrived back at the flat the living room looked as though a hurricane had passed through! There were books and magazines torn up and strewn on the floor, wires had been pulled out from behind the TV and chewed through; ornaments were lying on the floor smashed to bits, all cushions had been pulled off the lounge suite, one of these had also been chewed with stuffing being distributed all around the place!

In the middle of all this carnage was a very happy puppy who ran to us welcoming us home; she was so very pleased with herself; she couldn't really deny being responsible as there was cushion stuffing caught in her mouth and ears. It took us quite some time to clear up the mess and to repair cables etc., we then took her out for a long walk to tire her out. The net result of all this was that she was not left alone in the flat for a prolonged period; she came with us to the pub each Sunday from then on, when with us in the pub or anywhere else she was an angel, she would curl up under the table and not make a sound; well, she'd got her way hadn't she, we had learned our lesson!

Seventeenth of September nineteen-eighty-three was very memorable for us as that was the day we were married; Chrissie was still resident in Paignton as far as the government was concerned, this meant we could marry in the Paignton registry office that was at that time housed in Oldway Mansion. Oldway was the wonderful almost stately home of Mr Singer who made his fortune from sewing machines, at the time of our marriage it was still being looked after and used by Torbay Council so the gardens were wonderful. We had decided to have just a small affair with some thirty friends and family; Chrissie was looking radiant in a beautiful blue dress with a white hat. By the end of the day her hat looked very second hand as I seemed to be quite good at knocking it off whenever I put my arm around her.

At the allotted time we were all settled in the registrar's room ready when, the registrar asked me who my best man was? I hadn't even thought about needing a best man and so hadn't asked anyone; she clearly felt I did need one so I collared Phil Pope who thankfully agreed to fill that role although it wouldn't be as challenging as it normally would be. From then on all went well, we were very soon pronounced man and wife and I was invited to kiss the bride, promptly knocking her hat off!

We then adjourned to the gardens to have some photographs taken, we couldn't afford a professional photographer so all our friends took photos and did a great job. Luckily the sun had come out making the photos look great with all the colourful flowers and the ladies, finery being very vibrant. Then it was off to the reception which was held in the lounge bar of the King's Arms, there was a small buffet table with bubbly that the landlord told me in a stage whisper that he had removed the labels so that nobody knew it wasn't champagne. We had a lovely afternoon with our friends and families before we left for our honeymoon which was a single night in the post-house hotel on Plymouth Hoe where I watched the Sweeney film while Chrissie slept!

On the following Monday I was again in the shop serving customers when one of our regulars a little old lady came in, she wanted her regular dog meat order which I fetched for her; she then asked where I had been on the previous Saturday as she had been in and was surprised, I was not there. I explained that Chrissie and I had been married that day, and had therefore taken the day off; her expression became one of a bulldog chewing on a wasp, she was horrified. "What! I thought you must have already been married, as you have been living together, haven't you?" I confirmed that yes, we had been living together for a few months but that this was the first date we could arrange for the wedding. To say she was not impressed would be an understatement; I don't think I ever saw her in the shop again, small town, small minded?

We did have a longer honeymoon but as with my whole life, I never seemed to do things the conventional way. Anyway, it had to be a couple of weeks before we were married; mum agreed to look after the shop and we flew to Jersey for a week. When we arrived at our guest house in St Hellier the landlady was not amused to hear that we had not as yet tied the knot and was reluctant to let us sleep in the same room. Eventually she saw sense and all was well until later that day I went to get some money out of an ATM only to find that the machine decided to eat my card! From then on, we had to eat in places that accepted credit cards, in those days in Jersey this meant we could only eat in the more expensive restaurants, while this was very nice, we hadn't budgeted for this expense.

On the second day we hit the shops where we bought Chrissie's wedding ring, I didn't need one as I was going to use dad's signet ring as a wedding ring. We had a lovely week although it took us quite some time to pay for it when we got back.

One Tuesday morning in April of nineteen-eighty-four Chrissie told me she had to go to the doctor but was evasive about why, I didn't think much more about it as she didn't appear ill to me and I was busy with a delivery. After an hour or so she returned to find me with a shop full of customers; she had a huge grin on her face; then standing just inside the main door to the shop using an uncharacteristically loud voice she proceeded to announce to the whole shop "I'm pregnant!"

You could have heard a pin drop for a few seconds until one of the older ladies broke the silence with her congratulations, the whole shop took on a party atmosphere although I was a little stunned as I was under the impression that this couldn't happen! Anyway, once the shock wore off, I was overjoyed with the news, Chrissie didn't come down off her cloud for the rest of her pregnancy apart from the time when she was maybe eight months and therefore quite big, while visiting a friend on a farm she was chased by geese; I wish I'd been there to see that.

Most of our customers were very nice but some would from time to time try my patience, we used to sell Calor gas and certainly in the colder months did a roaring trade in all fuels such as gas, paraffin, coal and logs. Bank holidays were very special to us as the shop was closed for the day, you might be forgiven for thinking that this would be a bad thing from the point of view of bottom-line sales but, that was really not the case. The last working day before a holiday would be manic, it would be common for us to sell twice as much as we would normally move so averaged pretty much the same turnover; sometimes you would think we were going to be closed for weeks not just the one day.

Anyway, on one of the May bank holidays, I was having a lie-in before looking forward to a leisurely breakfast when at eight-thirty the doorbell rang, not only did it ring but it was clear someone was extremely agitated as the bell was being pressed repeatedly. I ran downstairs to answer the door and was confronted by an irate customer who had been in the shop on the previous Saturday but, they had clearly forgotten that there was a bank holiday coming. He was very unhappy that we were not open as he needed a bottle of gas, I explained about the bank holiday but he was having none of it. Eventually I went to get him a bottle of gas only to find he hadn't got the right money and wasn't happy to give me extra, he just said, "I'll pay you the next time I'm in" and left with his gas, I was dumbfounded with his cheek but there you go, in a small town this was expected.

Another example of customers not thinking about anything but their own needs was a little old lady who had been a frequent customer although she seldom bought anything more than the minimum. Indeed, it would be quite usual for her to come in with a basket loaded with cat food purchased from one of our competitors and although we sold the same food at a very similar price, she wouldn't buy it from us. On this day she brought in a broom head and handle that she had bought in our competitor's shop, she asked me to fit the handle for her which I was happy to do for her, it didn't take long, just a few minutes really; the handle had to be pushed into the broom head and a nail knocked in to keep it in place.

Job done very quickly, I gave her back the broom and asked her to make a small contribution for the time taken and nail used; she looked as though I had slapped her, turned on her heel and stormed out with her broom; we didn't see her again for months.

October the third was a Wednesday, in the afternoon I was out picking rose-hips to make wine. Mike, Chrissie's brother who was home from the army was sitting with Chrissie so I was not bothered that she was so close to her due date. We had had a false alarm the previous weekend when we had dashed to Torbay hospital only to be told nothing was actually happening and to go back home. By now Chrissie had really had enough of being pregnant and just wanted it all to be over. So, there I was gaily picking rose hips all on my own apart from Tess of course and completely out of contact with mobile phones not being an option in those days.

After a couple of hours, I felt I had enough rose-hips and headed back to the flat; as soon as I opened the door, I was met by a very red-faced Mike who informed me that Chrissie's waters had broken. Now, we had been assured during our anti-natal classes that there was no rush and so I told Chrissie I would just prepare the rose-hips and make some sandwiches (we had been told to take sandwiches but no mention was made of rose-hips). I received significant glares but as I said, I'm just doing what I was told to do; eventually, we arrived at the hospital and made our way to the maternity unit.

At this time, I was suffering from a chest infection and the midwife was not at all impressed, she had me wear a surgical mask whenever I was in the delivery room; Chrissie was having a bit of a difficult time and although things were progressing it was a very slow process. At about six o'clock I was getting hungry so decided to have one of my sandwiches; the midwife was not in the delivery room at this time but while I was eating, she returned. She gave me a strict telling off shooing me out of the room until I had finished my meal; apparently, this was not the done-thing as far as she was concerned.

Later on, that evening at about eleven o'clock the midwife returning to the delivery room took one look at me and told me I needed to go and lie down, clearly, I was not looking well. Chrissie gave everyone in the room thunderous glares but the midwife was adamant and I was dispatched to one of the doctor's on-call rooms to get my head down; I managed to get a few hours sleep until about six in the morning. I then went back to find how Chrissie was doing; well! Not very well it seemed she had been calling for me most of the night but the midwives kept telling her that I needed my sleep and that I was not to be disturbed; as you can imagine this hadn't gone down very well with my darling wife.

Eventually after some twenty-four hours of labour things were clearly coming to a head and the doctors were preparing forceps to deliver the baby, I was holding Chrissie's hand when she had a bit of a meltdown and told me in no uncertain terms what she thought of me! The doctor leant across her and told me it was probably best if I left and he would come to get me once baby had arrived. I went out of the room and sat on the stairs, I was quite distressed, then a lovely Cypriot healthcare assistant took pity on me bringing me a cup of tea, she sat with me telling me this was all normal, it happened all the time; she was lovely.

After a few more minutes the doctor came out to tell me my first child a son Steven was born, I rushed back in to see he was perfect in every way but didn't look very happy to be here. Chrissie looked very relieved and a little washed out but OK, almost as soon as the midwife had presented Steven to Chrissie my mother-in-law burst into the delivery room. You may be wondering how she got there so quickly but she was in fact already there, my father-in-law had had a heart attack a few days before and was in a ward just one floor above so Margaret didn't have far to go when the nurses had told her the birth had happened.

I went out to telephone my mum and also Barbera at the shop with the news, then went back to Chrissie; I couldn't stay long as I had to get back to the shop as Thursdays was delivery day for dog meat which had to be cut up into saleable lumps. So, I spent the rest of the afternoon up to my elbows in cooked dog meat cutting it into one-pound portions which I then put into the freezer to be ready for sale.

As was the norm in those days, Chrissie stayed in hospital for a few days until they were happy mum and baby were doing well, I picked them both up in our van with Steven being placed in a carry-cot in the back. This would not be considered safe now and indeed it wasn't but that was the way things were done in those days. The next few months went by with Chrissie looking after the baby and me trying to run the shop on my own with Sharon, who was an absolute star making it possible.

I was not really enjoying life as a shopkeeper although I did enjoy living in Buckfastleigh, living above the shop was definitely something that we didn't enjoy; we started looking for a house. It soon became clear that we couldn't afford property in Buckfastleigh and so started to look at houses in Paignton, at the time property was moving extremely fast, if you saw something you liked you pretty much had to make an offer on the spot! Eventually we found a small end of terrace house in Paignton which fit the bill perfectly. One issue with this was that if I was living in Paignton and still running the shop, I would need transport. At the time we had a cheap run around car but it was felt Chrissie would need this in Paignton so I needed a second vehicle. As luck would have it one of our customers came into the shop with a card he wanted to display in the window, he wanted to sell his motorbike. Well, we chatted for a few minutes and wandered outside where he introduced me to his Honda CX500, it was already quite long in the tooth and certainly looked a little tired but it was cheap. He let me have a ride and although it was nowhere near as exciting to ride as the bikes I had previously run it felt sound. When I got back to the shop, he was keen to point out the positives of the CX in that it was shaft drive so no troublesome chains; I hadn't felt chains were troublesome before but at least shaft drive was reliable. Well to cut to the chase, I very soon became the proud owner of a black(ish) Honda CX500 which would be great for commuting.

At around the same time we received an offer that made us think again about our future; Marvin who was the chap who normally delivered Calor gas to us asked me whether I would be interested in selling the business. At the time Marvin was working for another hardware store in the neighbouring town of Ashburton; he had been working for them for years and was now looking to go his own way; he felt that our shop would be perfect for him and his wife. I told him that I would discuss his proposition with Chrissie and would let him know; that evening we discussed Marvin's offer, Chrissie knew that I was not enjoying being a shopkeeper and agreed that it was too good to miss.

The next day I asked Marvin and his wife to meet with us to discuss in detail what he was proposing and how we could move this ahead. Over the next few days, we met with Marvin and his wife a few times and were able to hammer out a deal, it was agreed that Marvin would buy the shop as soon as he could; I was very happy.

Over the past couple of years, we had built the business up to a point where it was easily funding itself and giving us a modest return but it was clear to me that without significant extra investment we would always be at risk, we would never be able to compete with the major players in the market. In fact, I could buy named brand paint from a local big fish, Trago Mills cheaper than I could get it from our wholesalers; it was a bitter pill and to me showed how fragile the business was always going to be. We decided to accept Marvin's offer and walk away; over the two years we had been running the business the property world had started to go ballistic, this meant that financially selling at this time made very good sense and we were able to realise a significant profit.

Again, it was with some degree of anxiety that I handed Marvin the keys to the shop walking away from the business, I knew it was the right thing to do but was not sure what would be my next move. The overdraft from the business had been paid off by the sale but I now had a wife and a six-month-old son who were completely dependent on me, Chrissie was not working we both wanted her to stay at home with Steven at least until he went to school. We also had a mortgage on our house which while not huge by today's standards still would be a significant drain on finances; I needed a job! First though, we needed to find a way of limiting capital gains tax (CGT) from the sale of our business, CGT would be payable on profit made from the sale of the shop unless we could roll it across to another business. However, I had no clue as to what business would be appropriate, I really had no skills other than diving and there was no way I could start a diving business at that time as the investment required would be much more than I could afford.

My mother had been running a block of residential flats for a number of years and I could see that this might be an option for us; we started trawling estate agents looking for blocks of flats. There were a few options available that were in our price range and after just a couple of weeks we had focussed in on a semi-detached Victorian villa in Tor Hill Road, Torquay. This was already divided into ten units, there were two one-bedroom flats and eight bed sits; it had been run like this for some years and had all units let so was producing income already. Before long the deal was done and we had taken possession of the building thus negating any requirement for CGT and securing a small but important income. This was in May of 1985, I now needed to find a job, but where to look?

The obvious route was to look at local diving companies of which there were a few, I approached all the ones I could find within a sensible commutable distance including the council divers, without any success, it seemed nobody was hiring. Back to the drawing board, one of my long-term plans had always been that whenever I gave up working offshore maybe I could become an instructor at Fort Bovisand so I thought it would be worth a trip down to Bovisand on the off-chance. So, it was on a nice sunny morning in late May, I made my way down to Plymouth and parked my trusty CX500 in front of the Fort; as I walked over to the wall overlooking the harbour, I could see a number of people working away on the jetty. It looked as though another course of BAD lads were setting up for diving, this really brought back memories, I hoped I would be able to fit into some role here.

As I made my way into the fort, walking up the lane nodding to a few individuals I remembered from my time there, as I turned the corner and was passing the café on the left, I heard a female scream "Pete!" I looked up to find Susie running down the hill from the office.

She showed no sign of slowing as she neared me and indeed when she was a few feet from me she launched herself into my arms. She gave me a nice hug and a peck on the cheek before saying, "It's great to see you Pete, what are you doing here?" Well, we chatted for a few minutes about how things were going for both of us, she told me she was still working in the office and Hazel was also still in the bar. I explained that I was looking for work, she looked pensive while she thought about it; "Alan's down on the jetty, why not go down and see what he says about it".

I left Susie and made my way back down towards the jetty, emerging from the bottom of the Fort, I saw Alan Bax the director of the school standing on the slipway talking to another man who I didn't know. I wandered over and stood near to them and made a show of looking out over the harbour; the BAD course was now diving and I watched a couple of them jump off the jetty, they were using SCUBA so I thought they were probably in their second week maybe practicing rope signals? Quite soon, Alan finished his conversation with the other chap walking off to his car, I approached Alan, introduced myself and asked whether he remembered me.

It was clear he had no memory of me but seemed happy to chat, I explained that I was an old BAD lad and had been working offshore with Oceaneering since I had left my course (I didn't mention that for the last year or so I had been a shopkeeper) and was looking for work. He asked whether I had been supervising in the north-sea and when I told him that no although I had been supervising for a short period but it had been in Africa, he didn't seem impressed. He told me that he appreciated my coming to see him but, at this time there was no work available. I was not surprised but was a little disappointed nonetheless, Alan strode away back up through the Fort. I decided to wander back up to the office to say goodbye to Susie, it really was a lovely day and as I strode up through the Fort with the sun on my back it was really quite warm and pleasant.

I made my way up the hill to the office which was still housed in the small brick-built block on the left, I went straight in to find Susie sitting at the desk right in front of the door. She introduced me to another woman who I hadn't met before she was working at the desk to Susie's left, she was introduced as Lisa James who I later found out was now handling the admin for the BAD courses. We all chatted for a short while, I told her what Alan had told me then said goodbye to them before making my way back home.

As I drove away up the hill, I was a little miserable as I had secretly been sure there would be something for me at Bovisand, still never mind, I spent the rest of the trip back to Paignton thinking about my next move: maybe I needed to forget about diving and find something else. About three quarters of an hour later I parked up alongside our bright red,

Datsun Cherry on our car port and made my way down the steps, I let myself in through the front door to be greeted by Chrissie and Steven; Chrissie was cradling Steven who was chuntering on in the way six-month old babies do.

Chrissie said, "you've got to ring Susie at Bovisand straight away"; I said "I've just left her at Bovi, what does she want?" Chrissie didn't know so I made the call, luckily, we now had a phone in the house on the wall just inside the front door. When I was put through to Susie she said "you've got three day's work starting tomorrow if you want it?" I asked her "What would I be doing?" She told me that I would be standby diver on the Breakwater Fort; I told her that I would be very happy to take that job, we talked about when I needed to be there, where I was to report and who I would be working for, I then thanked her and put the phone down.

So, there I was a working commercial diver again, this was great; I was very relieved to at least have some work. The next day I reported for work in the Fort's dive store where I met Kevin Salter who was to be the supervisor, I was issued with a life jacket and was told to carry some equipment down to the jetty. Off I went carrying an ultrasonic A-Scan, when I arrived at the jetty Kevin beckoned to a Zodiac that was milling around in the harbour, this then came in to pick us up. There were five other guys boarding with me, I later discovered that these were four candidates who would be taking their CSWIP diver inspector examination which at the time were all conducted from the Fort Bovisand, Breakwater Fort facility. The other chap was the CSWIP examiner for the week, I later found out he was Ken Jackson, I got to know Ken quite well over the next few years.

Once we were all on board, the coxswain who was Fred motored out of the harbour, as we cleared the jetty wall we turned slightly to the left and headed straight for the Breakwater Fort, although I was pleased to be at sea again on my way to the breakwater fort, I still didn't really know what was going to be expected of me.

I had not been anywhere near this structure since my BAD course and was quite keen to see how it had changed. Before long, we arrived at a very badly corroded set of steps leading up the side of the broadly elliptical fort, these steps were on the north side of the fort the most weather protected side. I along with all the others stepped off the boat onto the landing stage; we made our way up the steps; as I say I hadn't been on the fort for years but was glad to see that it was still being used. What a structure it was, it had been built using large blocks each shaped by masons so that they fitted together beautifully, it was and still is really a work of art. As I reached the top of the steps, Kevin Salter was unlocking large double doors at the top, these opened up into the main body of the fort. There were three diver's umbilicals coiled down in figure of eights laying on the floor together with Kirby Morgan Superlite Seventeen helmets on two of them with the third sporting a Kirby Morgan Bandmask Ten (KMB10).

Kevin and the CSWIP examiner turned right into dive control which was a wooden shed that had been built into one of the gun rooms, I was later told that most of the rooms leaked rain-water like sieves and this was the only way to ensure a dry area for dive control.

Fred who I now found was called Fred Small and was the coxswain of the boat had secured the boat to a buoy where it would be safe and had followed us up to the dive station, he then took the four candidates through into another room where they could get changed. He then carried on into the engineering room where he fired up the electrical generator and LP compressor. The CSWIP examiner followed them, he would have two of them start their written papers while the other two would change ready to dive. Kevin told me to get kitted up in my dry suit and to get my standby diver kit ready; my kit was the third of the umbilicals set on the right-hand side of the corridor, I was to use the KMB10 which was sitting on the umbilical. I set to work checking all was well and carrying out the pre-dive checks, I was pleased to find that I had not forgotten much about how to carry this out and was very soon ready.

While I was waiting, I wandered through the corridor past an old electric winch, I continued through another set of doors where I found myself in the inner courtyard of the fort. This was an area some sixty-feet long by forty-feet wide, elliptical in shape. Around the circumference were casemates or rooms some of which had been refurbished as class, changing and drying rooms. It was all in a bit of a state and while it was serviceable it looked to be a bit tired to say the least, it was something of a mess with all the window frames looking to be rotten and in danger of falling to bits.

Straight across this area were another set of double doors, these led into the engineering space where I found two large diesel generators for electrical power, a very old and noisy Low-Pressure compressor and a smaller High-Pressure compressor. The noise in this area was incredible when everything was running, but of course we didn't need to be in there much.

I made my way back to the dive site to find the first two divers almost ready for the water. They were kitted up in hot-water suits, I was impressed, when I had last been here there had certainly never been any hot-water suits! The divers were readying their personal kit. I later found that the hot-water supply for the suits was not really adequate resulting in cold divers and therefore complaints as the guys were paying a lot of money for these exams. I was to act as tender for one of these chaps and so started to help him with his kit; the CSWIP examiner was lugging test-pieces through and out to the diver's basket that was suspended from a gantry above the entrance way. The basket was supported by a main lift wire and was attached to two guide wires, one either side of the entrance to the basket, these were secured to the basket by shackles that would run freely up and down the guide wires thus guiding the basket down to the right position on the seabed.

Soon all was ready, my diver had completed his pre-dive checks and I led him to the basket where he stood waiting for the other diver. As soon as they were both installed, I clipped the chain across the front of the basket and slid a scaffold pole across so that it formed a rail for the topside crew; I then received a thumbs up from both the divers I called to

Kevin via a bullhorn telling him that the divers were both in the basket and were ready for the water. My fellow tender Fred Small had left me with both umbilicals while he went to man the winch, he started lowering the basket while I paid out the umbilicals; very soon the divers were on the bottom, the winch stopped and my fellow tender arrived to take one of the umbilicals.

The divers then made their way across to the job, apparently since I had last been here CSWIP had installed a section of conductor guide frame from an offshore structure which the candidates would now set themselves up on, they would be working there for a good couple of hours.

The rest of the day progressed with the first two divers completing their practical assessments and swapping with the other two when they finished their theory exams. All went smoothly and by mid-afternoon we were squared away and, on our way, back to Bovisand before four o'clock in the afternoon; the candidates were dismissed as soon as we arrived back in harbour with the examiner also disappearing back to his hotel. We, the crew recovered the Zodiac to the quayside using an old hand-powered davit on the inner arm of the quayside, returning the inspection equipment and life-jackets to the store. The battery powered equipment would be put on charge for use the following day, I was then dismissed and was on my way up the road well before five o'clock, home in time for tea, wonderful. This was a great day and I was really feeling buoyed up and very positive for the first time in weeks.

The next couple of days went by in much the same way, more candidates would arrive, be ferried out to the fort where they would undertake their exams. On one of the days one of the divers experienced a problem with his communications so when he returned to the surface, I stripped down the comms system in the hat replacing the microphone and speakers. This apparently impressed Kevin Salter, I later heard that he was not accustomed to 'day-raters thinking for themselves'! As the end of the week arrived, I was thinking that I would need to start looking for a job again but before I left on the Friday I was called up to the office where I was told I would be required for the next two weeks. This was totally unexpected but of course was great news, I had a weekend off, two days to do whatever I wanted, this was a real luxury and had not been something I was used to since we had taken on the shop.

Over the next two weeks every day was pretty much the same as the first day apart from the Monday's when there were no exams, this was the maintenance day for us. We spent those days cleaning floors and toilets as well as fixing problems identified the previous week, I loved it. Speaking of toilets, there was only the one functional on the fort, this was situated up on the top deck above the crane gantry. It was not what you would term luxurious, indeed in the winter it must have been awful, there was no heating, there was a door although it didn't fit well and was nearly always left open. However, it had the best view of any toilet I had ever used, on a sunny clear day you would be treated to a wonderful vista of Plymouth Sound with the backdrop of Plymouth Hoe and Drake's

Island. In the foreground it was not unusual to find a large number of pleasure craft as well as Naval ships, car ferries and other commercial vessels milling around.

Very soon the two weeks were up, during that time I had been working tirelessly in my normal way, tidying up and carrying out running repairs as they became necessary. I learned that Kevin Salter was about to leave to start his own dive school training saturation techniques, I didn't know it initially but it became obvious that this was happening imminently. It seemed that Salter and Bax had had something of a falling out, this resulted in Kevin leaving; I was not unduly worried by this as I knew there would be others who could take over without too much of a problem. Well, on the Friday before Kevin was to leave, I was summoned to Alan's office; I was a little apprehensive but was hoping he was going to offer me to come back as standby diver the following week.

When I was admitted to his office, he immediately asked me to sit down; this was unusual; Alan as I said before was an ex-Lt-Commander from the Royal Navy and I knew that he very seldom asked anyone to sit in his office?

What came next really knocked the wind from my sails! Alan told me that Kevin had been very impressed with me and had recommended that I be offered the job of supervisor of the breakwater fort and diving instructor; as I say, this was totally unexpected but very welcome. We talked about pay and conditions for a good hour following which I accepted; as I walked back down the hill towards the entrance to the fort, I poked my head around the door of the office as I passed to let Susie know the news. She was extremely happy that I would be with them for some time to come, I got the impression she already knew anyway, I still couldn't believe it. Two and a half weeks ago I had been told there was no job, but on returning home, I had been given three days which turned into an extra two weeks and now I had a full-time job as supervisor of diving and Bovisand instructor, it's a funny old world!

Monday of the next week, I turned up as usual and was issued with the Bovisand instructor's overalls and given a locker in the instructor's 'grot' (this was the term used for the instructor's office) situated in a small blockhouse between the access road and the sea. I spent the day with Fred Small who hadn't been told of my escalation to supervisor, to say he was sceptical would be an understatement; it was clear I would have my work cut out to convince him I was worthy. Indeed, this took about three months but eventually we forged a good working relationship with him accepting me as his boss.

As supervisor I had to take charge of the dives, this of course involved being the main communicator with the divers. I also would be responsible for driving them through their examinations, by this I mean each of them had specific tasks to be completed; these each needed to be timed. For instance, they would be given ten-minutes each for carrying out Cathodic Potential and Digital Thickness Meter readings, fixed timing for CCTV inspection and Photography. I was not required to log any readings as the divers had to record these on scratchboards, I did though have to ensure that CCTV inspections were recorded on the correct video tapes. All this needed to be done for two divers at a time; now I was used to having two divers in the water at a time but this was a bit different. Because each diver was being driven through their individual examination including recording of audio on the video tape, they each had their own communications box.

I was faced with two comms boxes both of which I had to be keeping up with all the time; I had two sets of paperwork detailing timings for each of the divers, two microphones, one for each comms box and other people asking me questions.

For the first couple of weeks, I found it exhausting, but after that I found, I could easily listen to the two divers, carry out two conversations while making notes as required. It was with some relief though that I completed my first week as supervisor without any major errors or omissions.

I was very happy with the way things had turned out; I had a job that was in the field I enjoyed albeit I didn't get into the water as much as I would have liked; day to day, we handled CSWIP candidates of which there were hundreds, it really became something of a production line. From time to time there were exceptions though such as when Bovisand was contacted by a shipping company. On this day it seemed there was a small cargo ship that needed a CCTV inspection of its hull for a Lloyds interim survey, this would extend the period between dry docking of the ship which of course saved the company a lot of money. The job was given to the Breakwater Fort crew as there were no scheduled CSWIP examinations for the allotted day. We boarded Bovisand's old tug 'Deepwater', I had not been onboard her since my diving course but she had not changed at all. The ship we were to be inspecting was anchored in the sound just inside the breakwater; we tied up alongside and started to rig for diving.

The ship's engineer came on board and started chatting to the Lloyds inspector who was here to witness the inspection; I was due to be the supervisor and so would not be diving, however, the Lloyds inspector was not happy with this as he wanted the diver to have an inspection qualification and I was the only one who had one!

It was decided that I would hand over supervision to one of the others on the team and would carry out the dive; I was not unhappy about this as I was keen to be getting in the water again. The kit I was to use was a Kirby Morgan Superlite 17 helmet so that I could give a running commentary for the video we were going to be producing; when we were ready to dive the Lloyd's, inspector briefed me as to what he wanted me to look for, and video. It was all quite straightforward, I left surface carrying the CCTV camera and having established that the inspector wanted me to commence the inspection at the ships bow I made my way along the starboard side of the vessel. I spent the next couple of hours moving from point to point as requested taking video of all the significant points, it was a small ship but working mid-water along the side and underneath the ship was quite exhausting, especially as I hadn't been in the water for some time. Once the inspector was happy the CCTV camera was recovered and I made my way back on board.

Another day when we had no CSWIP exams I was told there was a beached whale in Hope Cove; Hope Cove is a small secluded beach just up the coast from Plymouth near Salcombe; a chap from South Hams Council contacted Bovisand to tell us that there was the body of a whale washed up on the beach and would we be interested in helping them remove it. It seemed that normally, removal would be done by council workers attacking the carcass with chainsaws, this was a horrible job and the council was looking for a better way of getting rid of the body. Some bright spark had come up with the idea of using explosives to blow it up!

We at Bovisand were one of the few companies authorised to carry out demolition using explosives so had got the job; now it must be said that my level of experience with explosives was very limited; in fact, the only time I had ever used them was on my BAD course and even then, only for half a day! But never mind, this clearly hadn't phased anyone so, I together with my intrepid band booked out a quantity of submarine blasting gelatine together with the necessary detonators, wire and electrical blasting machine. Off we went in the company's van to Hope Cove; it was a beautiful summer's day with just a light on-shore breeze. When we arrived, we were met by a council official who came with us to survey the site, at first, we found it hard to find the carcass but eventually it was found, wedged in a gulley between a couple of rocky outcrops on the left-hand side of the beach.

I turned to look out over a very crowded beach, as I say it was a beautiful, warm, sunny, summer's day, the beach was packed with tourists having a lovely day out at the beach. There were hundreds of them, kids running around, some building sand castles, others trying to fly kites although there wasn't really enough of a breeze. Lots of people were just sunbathing, it was a nightmare scenario, I told the council official that they would have to clear the beach; he was not keen but I explained that there was no way we could carry out a controlled explosion with all these people in the apparent firing line! Eventually he agreed to have the beach cleared and we set to work while his crew were clearing the beach; we had brought quite a lot of explosives so I was not concerned that we didn't have enough; I was looking at the carcass trying to decide how to pack it with explosive to achieve the best result.

Finally, having called on all of my 'extensive' knowledge we had packed all the explosives we had brought with us in, under and around the whale's carcass, I then inserted several electrical detonators, connected the wires that would lead back to our safe position, we were ready.

As I say we had identified a safe location from where we would fire the charge, I left the rest of my crew to run the cable out to the chosen safe position on the headland; I wandered around the beach making sure everyone had been moved off only to find one individual who was sitting in his little deck chair right in the middle of the beach reading his newspaper. I thought his position would be directly in the line of fire and nowhere near far enough away so, I walked up to him to be faced with a belligerent chap from

Birmingham; he proceeded to tell me he had driven two hundred miles so that he could sit on this beach and there was no way he was going to miss this wonderful sunny day for anyone!

I explained the situation but he was having none of it, the council boss joined us and told him that either he moved voluntarily or he would be arrested! Eventually, he agreed to move up to the headland where he set up his deckchair again and proceeded to tell anyone and everyone how unfairly he had been treated.

All was now ready, we retreated to our safe position where the boys had set up the blasting machine, before the wire had been connected to the detonators, I had twisted the two wires together so that there would be no possibility of a charge building up in the wires that could explode the charges prematurely. I separated the two wires, attaching them to the terminals of the blasting machine; once this was done, I had a last look around at the beach, all looked fine with the beach being completely deserted.

The headland was packed with spectators including our Brummy friend who was still spouting off to anyone who would listen. I put the whistle to my lips and gave three long blasts to signify we were about to set off the charge, I bent down and wound the charging handle on the blasting machine, to build up the required charge. Then had another quick look around, pulled up the 'T-bar' handle before plunging it back down, immediately there was a massive boom, a huge cloud of smoke erupted from the gulley where the whale's carcass had been and I watched as atomised whale was evenly distributed across the whole beach. As the slight on-shore breeze wafted the smoke towards us it was accompanied by the most horrendous smell of rotting whale! It was awful, as I looked across the previously pristine, beautiful beach, I could see that it was now liberally coated in small lumps of stinking, rotten whale.

The largest lump remaining was something resembling the animal's tongue which had been launched right into the middle of the beach and had landed almost exactly where our Brummy friend had been sitting, I looked around for him but he was nowhere to be seen! There would definitely not be any more carefree playing on this beach for holiday makers today, the council official didn't look best pleased but, I wasn't sure what he was expecting, where did he think the pieces of whale would go? Of course, when the tide came in it would wash the beach clean and before that a flock of seagulls were doing their best to help out as well, they'll eat anything won't they?

We cleared up everything and checked that there were no unexploded explosives left where the carcass had been before making our way back to Bovisand; I never heard anything more about this job but maybe that's for the best as I don't think Bovisand were ever asked to blow up any more beached sea mammals again.

When I had been looking after the CSWIP exams for a year or so CSWIP decided to add a supplementary qualification involving inspection of concrete structures. There were and still are a number of very large, ageing, deep-water concrete structures that clearly were in need of being inspected by properly qualified divers. CSWIP needed a concrete structure on which known defects could be used for the test; CSWIP decided to commission two concrete blocks from a large civil engineering company (Taylor Woodrow). Bovisand was contracted to site the concrete blocks, the position chosen was slightly to the east of the metal CSWIP test structure, firstly the site had to be inspected and cleared of any subsea obstructions. My team were given a week to prepare the seabed; we set to work clearing the area of all sorts of random junk that had probably been jettisoned from passing boats over the years.

After this we made sure the seabed was levelled off; when everything was ready, we headed off to Victoria Wharf situated in the Cattedown area on the Plym River where Bovisand's contracts department headed by Arti Shaw had been constructing a couple of concrete bases on which the CSWIP blocks would be placed.

When we arrived, we could see that the bases had been poured and were ready to be moved out to the chosen location; we were not involved with this move but watched as the blocks were craned into the harbour. At low tide a barge was floated over the top from which four Tirfor winch wires were suspended, these wires were attached to the blocks, the slack was taken up. As the tide came in the barge of course rose and the blocks were automatically lifted off the seabed, the barge was then towed out to the Breakwater Fort where we were waiting for them. The barge was anchored with a four-point mooring directly over the seabed we had prepared and the Tirfors were winched down to lower the blocks into position. I had one of my divers sitting on the seabed ready to make sure the base blocks both settled into the correct locations; this went like a dream and very soon both base blocks were in position ready.

The barge then returned to Victoria Wharf to pick up the CSWIP blocks one at a time in much the same way; of course, they had to wait for the next low water period so that the block again could be lifted by the rising tide. It was decided to wait until the next day so that we could continue to carry out the task in daylight. The CSWIP blocks were much bigger than the base blocks, they were about four metres tall, three metres wide and two metres deep. Although they were not solid, they had been constructed with a hollow central well, the walls were about thirty centimetres thick, this meant that each block weighed in at about twenty tonnes; they were significant lumps!

The blocks were to be moved individually, the first one was craned into the harbour and was suspended under the barge using four, five tonne Tirfor winches; in theory this should be fine and indeed all went well. The barge lifted the blocks as the tide came in and was towed out and positioned immediately above the first of the bases; the crew on top of the barge started to winch the Tirfors down lowering the block onto the base block; my diver reported that it had settled exactly in the centre of the base block and was sitting nicely vertical on the base. I asked him to remove the Tirfor wires so that they could be recovered; this was achieved very rapidly and the barge was taken back to collect the second CSWIP block on the next tide.

Again, it had been decided to pick up the next block the following day to make use of daylight; the weather had been flat calm and perfect for moving the first block and although it was still good the next day. When I saw the barge emerging from the Cattewater around the end of the Mount Batten breakwater, I could see that there was slightly more of a southerly breeze, this was whipping up a bit of a chop in the sound. We watched from the dive platform on the Breakwater Fort as the barge progressed slowly towards us; I could see that wave action was causing the barge to move about quite a bit more than it had with the first block. When the barge eventually arrived and was anchored above the second base block, Arti contacted us by radio, it seemed that things had not gone quite so well with the passage of the second block.

While it was true that each block weighed twenty tonnes and was supported by four, five tonne Tirfor winches which in theory should have been fine, this did not take account of movement of the barge due to wave action. This movement had resulted in three of the four Tirfor wires becoming overloaded and parting, they had snapped! The block had arrived at its desired location but was now being supported by just one Tirfor it was significantly overloaded to say the least. In fact, the Tirfor was so overloaded that it was impossible to move meaning that the block could not be winched down to the seabed; what were our options?

We could just cut the remaining Tirfor wire dropping the block onto the seabed; this may be a viable option as the seabed was very soft and the block would very likely survive but then we would still have the problem of how to lift it into position on the base block. This option was quickly discounted in favour of attaching a twenty-tonne lifting bag to the block; this would mean that the majority of the weight could be supported by the lift bag allowing us to manoeuvre the block into position. A couple of Arti's team were dispatched to get an appropriate lift bag and while we waited, I briefed my team. By this time of the day, I was the only one of the team who had not dived and so I told them that I would be attaching the lift bag when it arrived.

When the bag arrived the crew on the barge could be seen unfurling it and getting ready to deploy it down to the block, I prepared to dive and was sent down in the basket. When I reached bottom, I left the basket by squeezing between the left-hand guide wire and the fort's wall then located the line that I knew was attached to the base block onto which the second CSWIP block was to be settled.

The visibility was good, I could see a good seven or eight metres, I looked up and could see the CSWIP block hanging at an alarming angle some distance above me, I certainly did not want to stay below it any longer than was necessary and so swum up alongside until I reached the top of the block. I could see the lifting bag hanging below the barge and was able to quickly locate the four shackles that needed to be attached to the rings at each corner of the block these had been cast into the top of the block for this purpose. The first three were very easy and were attached very quickly, the fourth one though had to be attached to the ring where the remaining Tirfor wire was still attached, I was very nervous of being close to this very overloaded wire but it had to be done.

I made sure that I was above and off to one side and that my umbilical was clear should the wire part as, if this were to happen it would result in the block dropping uncontrolled, I then set about securing the last shackle, there was just room for the shackle pin to fit through the ring, before long the last shackle had been secured. All that was left to do now was to connect the low-pressure air-line to the lift bag's inlet valve and to inflate the bag; the LP hose had a 'Chicago' coupling, that I quickly connected. Once this was done, I returned to the basket and back to the surface to watch as the bag was inflated.

Arti called for us to turn on the air supply to fill the bag which we did, opening the valve so that air entered the bag reasonably slowly; eventually, we could see the bag was inflating with its twenty cubic metres of air, when completely full this would result in giving twenty point six tonnes of lift.

When the bag was almost full Arti called for us to stop the air flow as he had found the remaining Tirfor winch was now operable, his team could now be seen frantically lowering the block by slacking the Tirfor wire. I went back in the water when Arti indicated that the block should be just about at the correct depth; as I approached the block, I could see that it was almost perfect and called for them to "keep coming down". Very soon, the block was safely settled in the correct position on the base block, thank goodness; I then went back to the lift bag where I vented the air to deflate it before derigging the bag from the block and removing all the Tirfor lift wire shackles which were sent back to the surface.

The next day all we had to do was to video the blocks to show CSWIP that they were correctly and securely in position and ready to be used for examination; part of this was also to video both blocks showing all of the manufactured faults and defects so that they had an in-situ video record; I can tell you I was very relieved when this job was complete.

Supervising the CSWIP exams was never dull, I always had to tread a thin line of being off to one side with respect of CSWIP as far as the candidates were concerned; I had to make it clear that whilst it was my job to drive them through their examination it was the CSWIP examiner who passed or failed them. I soon became aware of rumours circulating offshore with respect to the exams; one of these related to the photography section, Bovisand did not use industry standard cameras, these would have been the Nikonos such as I had used in my time with Oceaneering. Rather they used small yellow plastic cameras manufactured by a company called Sea and Sea; now these cameras were really perfect for the job in that they were small, making access to the relatively small welds easy. They were also cheap, and almost fool-proof; however, the rumour circulating offshore was that the cameras were prone to flooding.

This really wasn't true but we had had a couple of times when a camera had flooded; anyway, the rumour was that a flooded camera would guarantee a free retest if the photographs recorded on the film were no good. Unfortunately, this led to an increase in the number of flooded cameras, we were at a bit of a loss as to why so many cameras seemed to be failing and even called the manufacturer down to discuss.

At this time, we were using one hand held CCTV camera for both divers, when not being used the camera was hooked onto a workline at the top of one of the structures legs, in this position it would be available to either diver when they needed it. Well, on this particular day the CCTV camera was sitting at the top of the leg looking down towards a diver who was taking his photographs, he seemed to complete his pictures and then I saw him start belting the structure with the camera; clearly, he was hoping to cause the camera to flood! I immediately contacted the diver in question informing him to look up where he would see the video camera above him. I told him the CSWIP examiner was also watching what he was doing, he apologised and just carried on with the next part of his exam. The number of flooded cameras reduced markedly following this episode,

From time to time, the CSWIP management board would come to visit us for audit purposes, this was always a difficult day but was of course a necessary evil. The first time this happened while I was in control there were three auditors, two of them were senior members of offshore diving company NDT departments and the third was the main man from The Welding Institute (TWI) who were responsible for management of the CSWIP exams. On the day, we had four candidates going through the exams and I went out with my team to get them started; about ten o'clock the auditors arrived, I was a little nervous but that was nothing compared to how the CSWIP examiner of the day felt, he was clearly extremely agitated and was like a bear with a sore head all day.

The auditors were shown around the fort by Alan Bax, then they were shown into dive control to see how the exams were being conducted, one of the auditors produced an hip flask and offered it around to all of us. He told us it contained brandy which he proceeded to put in his coffee; I was glad to see all my team refused his offer; I'm convinced this was a test to see whether we would take alcohol while carrying out diving operations; sneaky?

After diving was complete, I was asked to go back to the main fort with the auditors where I was grilled about how I thought the exams were perceived and what I felt could be done to improve them. I spent a good hour with them discussing what I knew to be things the divers were unhappy about including the fact of the hot water machine not being up to offshore standards. I asked whether one of the offshore companies could be persuaded to donate a machine to Bovisand? This however, clearly fell on deaf ears as nothing ever materialised; they were clearly amused by my anecdote about the camera flooding episode though. A few days after the audit Alan handed me a copy of a letter, he had received from the more senior auditor from Comex who complimented me on my attitude and abilities demonstrated on the day of the audit, very nice and totally unexpected.

I had been looking after the CSWIP exams for nearly two years when one morning at eight-thirty on arrival at work, Alan was waiting for me at the entrance to the fort; he proceeded to tell me that his NDT instructor had suddenly left and this was a big problem as there was a CSWIP 3.1U preparatory course due to start at nine o'clock that morning. He told me that I was the only person on the staff who he felt would be capable of instructing this course and would I do it? I was not at all sure I could do this to the required level as the only NDT training, I had received was the three days on my Lloyd's diver inspector course, this was of course at a much lesser level than that required by CSWIP as the 3.1U course was ten days and of course my Lloyds course was completed some years before!

The only saving grace was that the 3.1U covered visual inspection, CCTV inspection, photography, cathodic potential and ultrasonic digital thickness readings. All of these I had been carrying out offshore for several years and had clearly been overseeing on the Breakwater Fort for another two; anyway, I was really left with no option, I couldn't really say no.

The first day of the 3.1U course was fairly basic and I felt I could make a decent fist of it, but I would be lying if I said that when I went to pick up the ten candidates in reception at nine o'clock, I wasn't very nervous! These guys had paid a lot of money to be taught how to carry out inspection properly and of course to pass the CSWIP exam; they had every right to expect the instructor to be something of an expert! Luckily, I didn't know any of the guys on the course so there was nobody who knew my background and how much of a fraud I was. I led them down to the NDT classroom (Mag 16) where they all took seats and looked expectantly towards me.

I went through the course admin that was the same for all courses, I tried to build up some kind of rapport with them; this was all done by nine-thirty and I then had to launch into the course material. Each of the course members had been issued with a book written by the previous instructor and I also had a copy of this book from my Lloyds course, other than that there was virtually no prepared information, there were no slides for the overhead project to speak of. I spent the first hour basically winging it discussing stuff they probably all already knew as they were all experienced offshore divers, by ten-thirty I had run out of things to say and we broke for coffee.

When we returned, I had reread the chapter on visual inspection and decided to give that a go, that is how the whole day went, each time we broke for lunch or coffee I would read the next chapter and then try to regurgitate to them. I'm sure none of them were fooled, but by the end of the day I had managed to get some of them to provide tales of their own experiences of inspection and had been able to angle these towards what I felt they needed to know.

When I went home at the end of the day, I took all the books and handouts Susie, Lisa and I could find and proceeded to spend the evening and a good part of the night swatting up on what I needed to tell the course next day. This was how it went for the full five days of week one; at the end of the week the last thing they had to do was to sit Bovisand's theory examination. I don't know about them but I was certainly very nervous about how they would feel when faced with these questions; when they had all completed the exam, I marked them and luckily, they had all surpassed the required mark of sixty percent, in fact, they had all passed with good grades the lowest was seventy-five percent; I was extremely relieved to say the least.

The second week was practical where the guys put into practice what they had learned the previous week. I was much happier with this as I just made them do what they would be expected to do when on the CSWIP exam. In the intervening period since my courses Bovisand had expanded a lot, there had been a large new accommodation block built to the north side of the fort's entrance, beneath this there was an impressive facility housing the Diving Diseases Research Centre (DDRC). DDRC had several ex-offshore saturation chambers apparently donated by Comex Houlder; these were being used for research purposes and to treat divers suffering DCI. This facility was run by Maurice Cross, the same doctor who had carried out research on me during my BAD course.

The inspection course practical was carried out in a small tank situated in front of DDRC, this again had not been there when I was on my courses, on the face of it, this seemed like a good facility but after only a few minutes of divers being in the pool the visibility reduced to almost zero making visual inspection and CCTV very difficult. Anyway, it was what it was and we had to deal with it, at the end of the week all the guys seemed to go away happy and I heard that they did all pass their CSWIP exams so I must have been doing something right.

I went to see Alan at the end of the week and told him that whilst I felt I could do the 3.1U courses I was not as confident with the 3.2U course as that course included MPI at a much higher level than I had been taught as well as Ultrasonic inspection using A-Scan for which I had received no training in at all. Alan told me that as far as the ultrasonics were concerned, I needn't worry as this was taught by a college professor so I didn't need to know much about that; I accepted that this may be okay but I told Alan that I would only teach the 3.2U if he paid for me to be trained in MPI at a higher level.

He agreed to this straight off which was not like Alan but there you go I had set out my stall now; I was subsequently booked on to a topside MPI supervisor's course at TWI in Cambridge where all the CSWIP examiners I worked with were based. Following my course and subsequent passing of the examinations I felt much more prepared and more to the point I felt the students I taught could be assured that I could answer their queries with a reasonable level of authority.

In 1987 my second son James made his entrance into the world, despite Chrissie being told following her pregnancy with Steven that this had been a miracle and would never be repeated she did in fact manage a second conception. After a fairly routine pregnancy she eventually went into labour on my birthday, twenty-eighth of April and after another fairly torrid twenty-four hours James made his appearance, so now we had a brace of boys. Poor James was eventually delivered by application of a Ventouse system (a vacuum cup); the poor lad emerged looking very much like he was wearing a policeman's helmet! As far as Tess the dog was concerned, she definitely hadn't signed up for dealing with babies or more to the point toddlers, she was really not impressed with this development! Before long she made the decision to leave home and go to live with my mum and her dog.

I never returned to the Breakwater Fort exam supervision, over the next couple of years, I was employed nearly full-time teaching inspection courses; I came to realise that whilst I had no formal training in ultrasonics it was clear that the professor who was teaching the students really couldn't speak about the subject at their level. I would normally spend at least an hour after the prof had left defusing some of the confusion, the level required was really not all that high but when theories, algebraic equations and formulae were put up on the board a lot of the guys would just switch off. I don't think this was anyone's fault but it soon became clear to me that I needed to learn enough so that we could do without the prof, I also found that I needed to produce some clearer handouts for the students.

My first attempt at this consisted of a bunch of handwritten sheets that the girls in the office would photocopy for me; these seemed to be well received and made me feel that perhaps I should take it further.

Handwritten sheets are OK but I thought the next logical step would be to improve all the handouts and teaching materials, I needed to start to use a computer, now, we didn't have a computer at home and to be honest personal computers were only just starting to find their way into private homes. Computers were expensive, even the entry level first step one was going to cost us upwards of six-hundred pounds; this was money we just didn't have and certainly I couldn't justify for what I needed. How could I fund it?

Well, over the past year or so I had been looking in on the staff at DDRC, I had become a frequent visitor. Indeed, I had been working with them from time to time carrying out treatments for recreational divers who had been unlucky enough to be needing therapeutic treatments following sport dives.

Eddy Johnson the centre manager, Dr Maurice Cross and others knew my background to the point that one day they asked whether I would be prepared to help them out with a couple of planned saturation dives they were going to be running as part of one of their research projects. Over the next couple of weeks, we came to an understanding that I would be their senior Life Support Technician (LST) for the night shift, I would be accompanied by one of their engineers Jim Walker who would be my assistant.

The dives were to be to a depth of one hundred metres and would be manned by college students who would be inside taking their own blood and other tests while under pressure. The trial would be conducted over two-weeks, each week there would be a five-day sat dive interspersed by two days off at the weekend in between. This all seemed fine to me but the only slight fly in the ointment was that I couldn't get the time off work from my day job at Bovisand! What to do? I really needed the extra money that the DDRC job would give me so that we could buy the computer; well, I decided there was nothing else for it I would have to do both!

My shift at DDRC would be twelve hours, six pm through to six am, I would then have a couple of hours off until my normal day shift started at eight-thirty and another hour at the end of the day when I finished my day job at five pm before starting again with DDRC at six pm. Simple, I was sure I could do this, I explained my plan to Eddy who agreed we should give it a try but that if I really felt I couldn't cope I was to call him and he would come in to take over from me.

Very soon the first dive's day dawned, I said goodbye to Chrissie and the boys telling them I would see them again on Friday. The first day went really well and I didn't feel too bad at all, I managed to get a good hour's sleep between the end of my day job and starting the night shift and even days two and three were not too bad. By Thursday though I was definitely beginning to flag a bit, in fact I fell asleep on the wall by the harbour at lunchtime only to be woken up by one of the other instructors who saw Alan coming towards me. The dive completed on Friday freeing me up to drive home Friday evening, I took a couple of hours to rest before making the drive home but even with that I was completely knackered when I got home. I went straight to bed and slept until ten o'clock the following morning when I was woken by a very excited three-year-old.

The second week was much more of a challenge although I did manage to complete it without issue and never fell asleep on the job much to my own surprise. Once this was over, I vowed never to do something as stupid as this again as it was really too much and indeed, if there had been a problem, I wouldn't have been able to defend my actions, even if I wasn't really responsible, I probably would have been seen as at fault, truthfully, as I say it was a stupid thing to have attempted but there you go, it wasn't the first or last stupid thing I've done. We did though have enough money to buy our first computer and also a dot-matrix printer. Being totally ignorant of how computers worked once I had the computer set up, I found I was looking at the homepage of Microsoft Window 3.1; there were a number of icons that meant absolutely nothing to me, after a couple of hours clicking on the various icons it became clear that although I had the computer, I needed something else before it would become useful to me but what?

The next day, I made my way up to the office to discuss the problem with Susie and Lisa, both were very kind but it was clear that they found it quite amusing to hear that I didn't know what I needed! It seemed that I needed another 'Programme', what was that? Lisa who was the expert, told me that the basic Microsoft package included a very basic word processing package called 'Notepad' but apparently this would be of little use to me; I needed a proper word processing programme. It seemed these were not cheap but luckily Lisa could point me towards an appropriate programme, this was 'Wordperfect', she told me it would fit the bill perfectly. Well, Wordperfect came on a set of some nine three-point-five-inch floppy disks which had to be fed into the machine in order; once this had been done a page for a new document opened up and I was away!

The next thing I had to master was typing, I bought a Pitman's teach yourself touch-typing book and proceeded to try to teach myself, this was not the first time I had started to learn to type as when I left school, I had enrolled at college to be a marine radio and radar technician and part of this involved learning to type. I didn't stay at college for long due to writing off my sister's car so really this was the first time I seriously tried to learn to type. Although the book was great and took me step by step through how to learn it took quite a long time as I never seemed to be able to put enough uninterrupted time into it but eventually, I achieved something of a level of proficiency. However, I never became super proficient, eventually was able at my maximum to type at about forty words per minute without too many mistakes which was good enough for me.

By now we had moved to a slightly larger semi-detached house; when we moved in there was quite a lot of work to do but we had managed to negotiate a good price as it was seen as a do-it-upper; we didn't realise though how bad it was until the day we moved in. One of the first things to happen was that as we were loading things into the wall cupboards in the kitchen, the cupboard fell off the wall bringing a good part of the wall down with it! So, the first thing I had to do was to install a new kitchen complete with replacement wall.

Over the next couple of years, I changed the horrible 'avocado' bathroom suite to one that was not so hideous, installed central heating and redecorated the whole house. Once this was done, we settled back to enjoy the house for a while.

Meanwhile at our flats one of the tenants who had the best flat, the one in the attic of the house, which I thought was a nice place, there was a lounge, bathroom, kitchen and bedroom all nicely decorated and bright with good windows. One Friday she told me she was not happy with the amount of money she was being required to pay for rent and had asked for a rent review. This was the first time she had mentioned this to me and I was horrified; anyway, I had no say in the process other than to specify what the rent covered. The flat was furnished so I wrote a list of all the furniture, kitchen implements, white goods, curtains and floor coverings. Once I had sent this off to the authorities, I sat back to wait, after two weeks I received a letter detailing their findings and was stunned to find that following their review I was to put the rent up by ten-pounds per week! To say I was surprised would be an understatement, the next time I saw the tenant she said nothing other than she would comply agreeing to the rent increase, amazing.

We decided though that it was time for us to sell the flats. We put them on the market when they were fully let this took us about a month; luckily, we found a buyer very quickly in fact, within a month. We had owned the flats for a little over three years and during this period the price of property had again skyrocketed. We effectively doubled our money, I could say it was all worth it but I have to say that I don't feel it was; if I had to do it again, I would have just bought a couple of residential properties; this would have given us a similar return without any of the agro.

Anyway, back to my day job, I was now well up to speed running the CSWIP 3.1U and 3.2U courses, I had started to write comprehensive handouts for the students and although I wasn't ready yet I started to think about writing an inspection manual specifically for CSWIP candidates.

During 1988 the Association of Offshore Diving Contractors (AODC) had finally managed to formalise diving supervisor qualifications; as I had been supervising offshore while in Angola, I was eligible for their grandfathering scheme. I later learned that personnel working as diving instructors at eligible schools could also apply, so I was eligible on two fronts. All I had to do was apply with details of my experience and if accepted I would be authorised to sit the AODC theory examination. I applied in May of 1988 and was accepted by early June; I alongside my fellow Bovisand instructors were scheduled to sit the examination at the Plymouth College of Further Education in mid-June.

On the day, we all turned up in the college's reception where we were asked to sign in before being led into one of their large halls, as we entered, we were faced with several rows of single desks with chairs. It seemed we were to be in a room where a lot of different examinations were being administered simultaneously, as well as the AODC exams there were people taking a number of other qualifications.

We each found a seat where before long we were presented with our papers; the invigilator told us how long we would have for the exam; she also told us that were we to finish before the allotted time we were to leave our papers on the desk and leave quietly by the back door. We were not allowed to bring in anything other than a couple of pens and a calculator, we were though presented with a few sheets of blank paper that we could use for calculations etc., these also needed to be left on the desk when we left. We had been led through what to expect by one of our friends who had recently successfully sat the exam so knew what to expect to some extent.

He had told us that we would need to be able to convert from Imperial to metric units for temperatures, pressures, length and density; we had been told that although programmable calculators were not allowed it was acceptable to use a metric convertor calculator. This seemed odd to me as surely this was a programmable calculator? Anyway, we each had bought one of the accepted calculators so, we were all as prepared as we could be.

As I turned over the paper, I was faced with eighty multiple-choice questions and off I went, I had been advised to start with the calculations as they would take the longest time. Luckily, all the questions had been segregated into sections and it was easy to find the physics section where the calculations would be found. By this time in my career, I had been teaching diving for quite some time so I was quite used to working through diving related physics questions, because of this I found this section relatively straightforward or at least I felt it was OK anyway!

I worked methodically through all the questions with only a few posing problems, with the ones I really didn't know the answer for, I went for option 'C' as correct (statistically this was the most likely to be correct apparently). I finished the whole paper with some forty-five minutes of time remaining: I spent some of that time going back over the paper to ensure I had not missed any questions although, I was conscious of being careful not to change answers unless I was absolutely certain of the change. I then left my paper on the desk and made my way out of the hall to wait for my friends in the college's reception area; everyone finished before the allotted time and as we had a bit of a debrief, we seemed to feel we had all done OK; well, we would see wouldn't we.

There was an anxious wait of just a couple of days before we were all told the good news that we had passed our examinations, consequently on the first of July 1988 when the scheme went live, we were all AODC qualified air diving supervisors, my certificate number was 5208, so there were a lot of us!

My work at Fort Bovisand although OK, was not very fulfilling, I felt I was not being able to provide courses to a high enough standard as the equipment we had to use was very old, not current to that being used offshore and kept breaking down. It was not at all unusual for me to spend an afternoon taking subsea MPI units to pieces in order to make one fully functioning unit out of two units that had different faults; all the time being watched by the paying students, not good at all. This came to a head when I was supervising Lloyds, diver inspector examinations, I knew the examiner Glynn Palmer quite well by then but he spent a very boring three hours pacing the floor of dive control while I again attempted to fix the MPI unit. I did eventually get it working but by the time I did we were nearing the end of the working day and had to work into the evening to get everyone through the exam; we did this and they all passed but, I was nearing the end of my tether.

I don't think I was ever very good at hiding my feelings, it was quite clear I was grumpy to say the least! So it was that towards the end of 1988 I decided to part company with Fort Bovisand for the time being anyway; Bovisand did though from time to time become my stop gap part time employer over the coming years but never again on a full-time basis.

CHAPTER SIXTEEN

The Next Steps – 1989 to 1994

Chrissie was now ready to start thinking about going back to work but didn't feel she wanted to carry on with being a chef, principally this was so that she wouldn't have to work unsociable hours. Indeed, it would have been extremely difficult particularly as I was not always at home every night, she enrolled in an RSA Business Management course which she of course aced; armed with her new certificate RSAdip (I told her she had always seemed dippy to me!); she looked for a job and seemingly without much effort landed a plum job at the local school as PA to the head master. This was great for all of us as she didn't have to work during school holidays making childcare much easier.

Anyway, as far as I was concerned at the end of 1988, I was effectively out of work again although I saw it in a different way though, I had decided to become self-employed. I was looking to build on my contacts to provide supervision and consultancy for civil engineering diving projects in south-west Devon and Cornwall. Before handing in my notice to Bovisand I had met with and had positive discussions with Kevin Salter; Kevin's leaving Bovisand had been the catalyst for my getting the job on the breakwater fort in the first place. Since then, Kevin had been running a company called Interdive. Interdive had principally been running HSE Part two courses, these were courses for experience air divers who wanted to move into saturation and mixed gas diving. When I had made this transition there had been no requirement for extra qualifications but in the meantime this had become mandatory. It sounded like Kevin's company was doing very well and he had decided to take the next step in his quest to eventually offer all levels of diver training.

His second step had already been taken by his offering Diver Medic Technician (DMT) courses; he now wanted to venture into the field of diver inspection training. He wanted to be able to offer CSWIP 3.1U and 3.2U courses as soon as possible with a view to provision of 3.3U and 3.4U courses in the next couple of years. 3.3U was a qualification for Remotely Operated Vehicle (ROV) pilots this was effectively a 3.1U carried out remotely; 3.4U was offshore inspection controller, these were the people who ran the jobs and were top dog on larger inspection contracts.

1989 was a whirl of setting up CSWIP inspection courses for Interdive, these would be run at City University. Jim Sheppard was the manager at the university, we didn't know each other at all at the time though.

Kevin had already been in talks with City University to use their tank for the practical aspects of the course, we both saw this as a big step forward as far as quality was concerned. As I say Jim Sheppard, was now the diving supervisor at City University, I had heard a lot of good things about him as he used to work at Bovisand, my relationship with Jim was a bit rocky to begin with but eventually we came to work well together, more of that later. Initially, Kevin suggested that I sit at home and produce the necessary paperwork to start the 3.1U and 3.2U courses, he didn't however pay me for this which meant that everything I produced would continue to be my own intellectual property.

I sat at home producing homework, examinations, programmes, dive logs and the associated overhead projection acetates. I had the CSWIP div 7 booklet to work from; this contained the syllabus needing to be taught, it detailed subjects, expected levels of achievement as well as all the necessary additional information. It took me a good two weeks of solid work at home before I felt I was ready; all of this then had to be submitted to CSWIP who would visit our first courses before they would accept and accredit our courses as satisfactory.

Before long I was heading up to City University to run our first 3.1U course, we had just one candidate but CSWIP had told us this would be acceptable for the audit. On arrival the day before the course I met with Jim who was enthusiastic, he showed me the classroom we would be using which was a bright and airy room, very far removed from the magazines at Bovisand. He showed me where I needed to go to pick up the required TV and video player as well as a topside hand-held video camera, we would be using this to practice video inspection on the surface before the students progressed to underwater. The topside video camera was by today's standards huge, it made video inspection much more difficult than it would be underwater but it was all that was available in those days; today of course everyone has a video camera on their phone but not then.

The next day my single student turned up and we got down to business, I had been told the CSWIP auditors would not be with us until the second week when diving was taking place. The first week was quite laid back with me running though the course using my new acetate overhead projection slides but we were still using the same course book as I had been using at Bovisand. All went well with my noting some alterations that needed to be made but there was nothing major, I had arranged that as I was going to need to be in London for the whole course, we would not be taking the weekend off; I generally found that students also liked this as they didn't want to waste time kicking their heels in the middle of the course particularly at London prices for accommodation and meals.

The second week dawned with us commencing the practical aspect of the course; the syllabus required that each student undertake a specified number of minutes underwater during the practical training, there was certainly enough time in the five days even when the course was full with ten students. The CSWIP auditors turned up on the third day, they went through the examination and quizzed our student as well as witnessing a dive. They audited the equipment checking that everything was in place for not only 3.1U but also 3.2U courses, at the end of the day, they sat me down and asked me a bunch of questions about my suitability to run the courses, they didn't find any problems, subsequently our courses were approved which was a big relief I can tell you. When I next saw Kevin, he made it clear that he was extremely pleased and could see a big future for me working with Interdive, this was good news, I was happy with the way things had gone.

Running the 3.1U and 3.2U was now a done deal but, I felt I would have a lot of work to do to be able to run 3.3U and 3.4U for Kevin; he didn't seem to worry about this and told me he was sure, we would cope! I was somewhat sceptical about this but of course was willing to do what I could. Interdive was not at all ready to employ me enough and for the first couple of years I was only getting about ten-days per month with them.

I was still managing to do part time work with Bovisand and in fact I was doing quite a lot of work with them; their training manager Peter Sieniewicz had managed to achieve a tie up with the Arab Academy for Science and Technology in Alexandria, Egypt. Bovisand was supplying instructors for ten-day Experienced Route Competence Assessments (ERCA) and first aid courses; Peter Sieniewicz asked whether I would be interested in running courses with him in Alexandria.

I of course said yes, luckily, I had a two-week window in February 1990 when nothing much was going on at Interdive and Peter had been able to organise an ERCA assessment for the Academy to be run in and around Alexandria. ERCA was a method for overseas experienced divers to gain a qualification equivalent to the UK Basic Air Diver or HSE Pt 1. So it was that we were on our way in early February via Heathrow, on arrival at the airport, I was stunned by Peter's bag it was huge and obviously very heavy! He told me he was taking a lot of things out that would be very difficult if not impossible to source in Egypt. His bag was in fact so large and heavy that there was a significant excess baggage bill but, apparently this was acceptable; Peter paid it and off we went.

We arrived in Cairo early evening, when we reached passport control and presented our passports we were rejected, it seemed that we hadn't purchased the required visa, the official pointed us to a tiny booth in the far left-hand corner. Where we joined the queue for the visa booth eventually arriving at the desk, we were sold visas with no questions other than did we have the correct fee, this would be ten US dollars or ten English Pounds? Well neither of us had US dollars so we both handed over ten-pound notes. So, there we were armed with visa's bought and paid for, we again approached passport control where we were ushered through. Next was baggage reclaim, as was my norm, I just had carry-on luggage but of course Peter had his humungous bag plus a smaller one for clothes.

Eventually all bags collected we headed for customs where we passed through the 'nothing to declare' route without any problems; we were then disgorged into bedlam. The arrivals hall was a mass of humanity, the noise level was immense, there were a lot of people running to and fro seemingly without any purpose. We fought our way through and outside to the taxi rank where we bagged a vehicle that looked vaguely roadworthy; we loaded all our bags into the boot, both climbing into the back seat and Peter showed the driver the address for our hotel in Alexandria.

The driver seemed to know where we were going so, we sat back and settled in for the journey; Cairo to Alexandria is served by a fairly well-maintained straight road that runs through the desert, it was apparently built by the British during the war. Egyptians drive on the right and it seemed that in Cairo traffic lights have an advisory status as it was not unusual for us to proceed straight through red lights together with everyone else; also, cars don't seem to be able to move without the driver keeping his finger on the horn! It was chaotic, I was glad I didn't have to drive; soon though we were out of Cairo and on the main Alexandria-road much of which was dual carriageway. Night had now fallen, the driver put his lights on, this just seemed normal to us we didn't even think about it as surely this was the norm when driving at night?

Well, after we had been driving for about an hour all of a sudden, our car swerved viciously, fishtailing alarmingly accompanied by a tirade of shouted Arabic from our driver; it seemed there had been another car driving on our side of the road but in the opposite direction, however they had been driving without the benefit of headlights.

We had it seemed missed each other by inches, I asked the driver whether this was something that happened often. He told us in his broken English that it was not all that unusual for drivers to join the dual carriageway but not wanting to travel in the correct direction especially if they didn't have far to travel. The problem was that as there was Armco fencing running down the central reservation, they couldn't easily get to the correct carriageway. So, instead they would just drive the wrong way until they came to a break in the Armco in the central reservation or alternatively reached their destination! He seemed to think this was considered acceptable; I was less certain by this and thought that surely, they should have their lights on, shouldn't they? He said that some of the older people thought that having their lights on would deplete the battery so they would only switch them on if they really needed them and because it was a moonlit night, he clearly didn't feel lights were necessary!

This was the start of a memorable trip for there were to be a lot of incidents; after about three hours we arrived at our hotel which was situated on the sea-front in Alexandria, it was a nice place and luckily, they sold beer which we both felt was needed after our trip from Cairo. The next day at seven o'clock in the morning we were picked up by Abanoub who was to be our main contact at the academy, Abanoub was an ex-Egyptian Naval officer who always seemed to have a cigarette on the go, over the next couple of years I got to know him and his deputy Mahmoud quite well as I was to make numerous trips to Alexandria teaching ERCA as well as First Aid, sub-sea inspection and air supervisor courses.

Abanoub drove us to the academy where we had a meeting with all their instructors who were due to be helping us with this course. The day was beautiful, with the sun beating down but there was a keen northerly wind that was keeping the temperature down; Abanoub drove us along the Corniche or sea-front towards the eastern end. The road was dual carriageway with central reservation separating the two lines of traffic. Although the central reservation didn't have Armco or any other crash protection, it consisted of a narrow-raised section made up of kerbstones laid in a line, generally it was about two feet wide.

The central reservation was however not continuous; there were some sections where for a hundred metres or so there would be no reservation at all. En-route Abanoub stopped at a roadside stall to purchase breakfast of falafel which were very nice, we ate these as Abanoub drove; when we arrived at the Academy he parked up in front of an impressive building. We followed him up to the first floor where his department had their offices. This was where we would meet the third member of the local team Saeed, he was to be assigned to us as our 'fixer', he proved to be a brilliant individual for this and it was thanks to him that we got any diving done at all.

The ERCA was aimed at experienced divers only, so they all should have the skills needed, the main aim of the ERCA was to carry out assessment of students for each of the significant duties required of offshore divers to prove this capability. Of course, this meant that there was a long list of required equipment. We ran through this list which had apparently been provided to the academy some months previously, Abanoub was very proud of the equipment they had managed to secure for the course; Peter and I felt we needed to go and see some of the bigger items to make sure all was as it should be.

Abanoub agreed and off we went to the yard to inspect the wet-bell and deck decompression chamber as well as the diving hats, umbilicals etc. When we arrived, we could see the wet-bell, this was a unit that had been leant to the academy by one of the local diving companies; it was the real thing and looked good, it was painted white and consisted of a steel base filled with concrete to give it the required ballast. There were four tubular uprights and at the top of these there was a steel dome where the diver's heads would be in a trapped air bubble, there were four fifty-litre air bottles for on-board gas attached to the outside in a frame, two each side. There were horns onto which the diver's umbilicals would be stored during launch and recovery; this all looked good; unfortunately, this was where the good news ended. I ducked my head under the dome expecting to find a panel with valves for the diver's air supply including options for changing over from gas supplied from the surface to on-board gas from the air bottles on the bell; there was no panel at all.

Additionally, when I asked Abanoub where the wet-bell's umbilical was, all I received was a puzzled expression; apparently the list had not specified that the wet-bell needed to be supplied with air from the surface; so, there was no umbilical or panel inside the bell.

This was a problem as a major part of the ERCA assessment at that time focused on the divers, use of wet-bell including switching to on-board gas and carrying out rescues from the bell; we decided we should go and see what the chamber looked like before we started on working out how we were going to put things right. Luckily the chamber was much better, it had again been supplied by an offshore diving company and had pretty much everything we would have expected of a chamber, not much would need to be done to this other than hooking it up to air and oxygen supplies.

The diver's hats, umbilicals, bail-out bottles, harnesses and all ancillary gear were also found to be acceptable, all we needed to do was check their certification, to make sure everything was serviceable and safe. Peter and I started to make lists of what needed to be done before delegating roles; Peter would go through all related paperwork to assess the level of certification for the equipment and I along with Saeed would go into town to purchase the necessary valves, gauges, pipework and hoses, to get the wet-bell up to a useable condition. Part of this involved a renegotiation of timings, it was agreed that we would stay for an extra three days in order to give us time readying the equipment, I wasn't sure we could do everything necessary in that timeframe but, well we would give it a go.

Abanoub gave Saeed a fist full of Egyptian Pounds and off we went, Saeed didn't drive so we were using taxis, I have no clue where we went other than we spent the whole day in hot, dusty bazars and souks in the middle of Alexandria; Saeed was a master negotiator and managed to find almost everything we needed. Unfortunately, we couldn't find metal pipe for the wet-bell panels so would have to make do with nylon push fit pipe, not ideal but it was all that was available. I was somewhat nervous of using this but, I thought that provided we limited the depth to which the wet-bell was used so that the divers could come to the surface using their bail-out bottles in an emergency it would be acceptable. Once we had all the kit needed for the wet-bell panels, we went looking for hose to make the main bell umbilical; this proved easier to find than I had been expecting, the very first place we went had everything we needed, good old Saeed.

However, when we first arrived, I was not very impressed by the place as it was an open yard with a dirt floor, the dust was awful and was being whipped up by a strengthening breeze. At the back of the yard there was a large corrugated iron shed, inside was a real Aladdin's cave; they had huge supplies of 'Gates' diving quality hose of the all sizes we needed and they had the required equipment to swage hose end fittings onto the hose as required. Before long Saeed had been able to pass on my requests to the foreman who assured him that all hoses would be cut, fitted with the required hose ends and delivered to the academy by the following morning.

When we left the yard Saeed told me that Abanoub would have a fit at how much all this was costing, I hoped that I hadn't got Saeed into any trouble. The time now was just after four o'clock in the afternoon and I asked where Saeed felt we could go to start building the wet-bell panels; he suggested we go to the big bosses, office where there were workshops, we could use. Off we went in our trusty taxi, it took us some three quarters of an hour to get there and as we started to unload all our purchases the boss came out to see us, his name was Bashir Al Mouti, he didn't speak to me much but spent a long time in what seemed a heated discussion with Saeed. Once this was over, they parted company all smiles, apparently my impression of the conversation being heated was incorrect, Arabic discussion just sounded heated to me.

Saeed led me through past Bashir's office to a room which Saeed announced was the workshop! It was not like any workshop I had seen before, there was no bench, vice or any tools in evidence. Apparently, all the engineers had their own equipment and would not leave it in the room in case it was stolen, whenever I was working away, I used to carry a small box of useful stuff, and in there I had a couple of crescent wrenches (adjustable spanners), a knife, pliers, a set of Allen keys, screwdrivers and rolls of self-amalgamating and PTFE tape; hopefully this would be enough. We worked away on the floor cutting the nylon tube to size and laying all valves etc., in place to get a visual idea of how the panel would go together. Once this was done, I started to put it all together using push-fit and compression fittings, while I did this Saeed asked whether I would like a drink; stupidly I said yes, I would love a beer please.

Saeed looked crestfallen; I had forgotten that I was in a Muslim country and so alcohol was only available in the hotels that catered for non-Muslims; I apologised and Saeed went off to find some soft drinks, Sprite for me and Orange for him. Building the panels took quite a bit of time but to be fair it went together fairly easily and by seven-thirty we had the makings of a useable panel; I had by now had enough of the day and suggested that we could finish off by taking the panel to the yard where we could fit it to the wet-bell in the morning.

Saeed agreed that this was a good plan but, he decided I should go back to the hotel and he would take the panel to the yard which was on his way home, he got no argument from me. I was very glad to get back to the hotel where Peter had a cold beer waiting for me, what a day.

The next day Abanoub picked us up again and following the obligatory stop for falafel we headed straight to the yard to continue our work. On arrival at the yard, Peter said that he had been presented with certificates for all the equipment meaning there was no need for us to pressure test the chamber or any of the umbilicals etc., this meant that the only equipment we would have to test fully would be the wet-bell umbilical and panels. The hoses had been delivered and were perfect for the bell umbilical, I set a couple of the divers who would be on the course to work binding them together with duct tape in just the same way I had been shown all those years ago at Oceaneering. Meanwhile Saeed and I set to work fitting the panels into the wet-bell; this all went well and by the end of the day we were able to pressure test everything successfully so that everything was ready for us to go diving the next day.

Day three started well with Abanoub again picking us up; today we would be starting the course and for this we needed some relatively shallow sheltered water; he told us he had managed to gain us access to the seawater pools at Montaza Palace, Montaza was on the coast at the extreme eastern end of Alexandria next to Abukir (Abu Qir) a promontory where in 1798 the Admiral Lord Nelson engaged with the French fleet in the battle of the Nile; Nelson's fleet was victorious and became dominant in the Mediterranean following the battle.

Cairo in high summer was not a place where the Egyptian royal family wanted to be as it was just too hot, they used to use Montaza palace as their summer palace until they were ousted in nineteen-fifty-two. Montaza was a beautiful if a little neglected palace and was a wonderful place for us to start the course; for this we didn't need the wet-bell or the chamber, all we needed was basic surface demand diving gear. We set up our dive control on a four-metre-wide wall that led from the beach out to the main seawall, we would be diving on the right-hand side of the wall into a tidal pool. This day was a very good shakedown for the group and the equipment, it went well and we could see that the majority of the guys were already proficient divers who knew their way around diving equipment.

After a few days of shallow work, we were ready to go a little deeper and to utilise the wet-bell, for this we relocated to Alexandria naval base just to the west of Alexandria. This area was a heavily restricted zone and we had to all be issued with permits before we would be allowed to enter. Even with the permits we would not be permitted to be in the base without being accompanied by a plain-clothed secret police presence, the guys who accompanied us just stood by and watched us all day from the moment we entered to when we left the restricted zone. Anyway, on arrival, we found that the bell was already on site together with a crane that would be used to lift the bell into and out of the water.

We started off by carrying out a lot of drills with the guys in the dry but by ten o'clock we were ready for the first two divers to enter the water in the bell; we knew the panel and umbilical worked so I wasn't unduly worried but it was of course the first time it had been used so there was a little apprehension on my part. Over the next few hours, we managed to cycle everyone through and they all performed well, this was their practice day tomorrow would be their assessment.

The day was a big success and I was chuffed that everything had worked as required, however, it was so cold, I must confess that I had not packed any heavy clothing as I thought that despite it being February, we were in Egypt so I had thought it would be reasonably warm, wrong! It was very cold, there was a northerly wind at about force five; we were on a jetty with nowhere to hide, both Peter and I felt freezing cold by mid-morning, by the end of the afternoon we were both miserable.

Adding insult to injury, we had ordered a packed lunch from the hotel that morning but, when I came to eat mine at lunchtime, I opened the box to find a lovely congealed mess of chicken and chips; of-course it was also cold and not in the least bit appetising!

We were all I think very happy when it came time to finish that day, Peter, Saeed and I piled into another taxi for the journey back to the hotel; luckily the driver seemed to also be feeling the cold and had the heater on full blast. As we were driving east along the dual carriageway sea-front road, it was as usual chocka-block with two lanes of nose to tail cars shuffling slowly in both directions.

We were in the outside lane next to the central reservation when I saw a white BMW coming towards us on the other side of the central reservation; he was about a hundred metres in front of us when he came to a point where there was a break in the central reservation of maybe fifty metres. Well, he was evidently in a big hurry so pulled into the middle of the road between the two lines of converging traffic, he accelerated towards us; unfortunately, he apparently hadn't seen that the break in the central reservation was only for a very short distance. The BMW was still accelerating towards us when the break in the reservation came to an end, there was now a double row of kerb stones between our row of traffic and the row going in the opposite direction. His car hit the kerb stones right in the centre of the car, his car jumped up onto the central reservation and with all wheels no longer in contact with the road his car passed us sliding along the kerb stones with sparks showering out from underneath. He travelled like this for maybe thirty or forty metres before toppling off into our lane behind us.

As we had passed him, I turned around together with Saeed and saw the BMW now stopped in our lane behind us; I saw his reversing lights come on and then off, but the car didn't move, he had surely broken something. Just as I was turning back, I saw a police motorbike come past us on the other side of the central reservation heading to the scene of the accident, he quickly arrived at the stricken BMW where he stopped and dismounted clearly going to have a word with the driver.

I turned to Saeed and asked him, "what do you think will happen to him?" Saeed replied, "oh it's very simple, the driver will be arrested, he will be taken to the police station where they will probably beat him up." He then went on to say, "once this has happened, they will make him agree he will never do this again and then they will let him go." I was stunned, but Saeed seemed to think this was an acceptable method of justice; it was a different world!

The next day we were back at the naval base diving the guys with the wet-bell again so that they could go through their actual assessment; I had been reflecting on last night's incident with the BMW and had some concerns about what we were doing now. I called Saeed over and asked him, "Saeed, what would happen if there was a problem with the wet-bell which led to one of the divers being hurt, especially given that I had built the panels in the bell?" Saeed spent a couple of minutes thinking through his answer before replying, "Well, the police would come and they would take you and Mr Peter back to the police station." I was thinking that this had a lot of similarities with how Saeed had thought the guy would be dealt with last night so I said; "and what would happen then?" He said, "they would ask you whether you had forced them to dive, and of course you haven't, they are diving of their own free will." "Does that make a difference?" Was my reply; to which he said, "yes of course, if they have dived of their own free will then it is the will of Allah." "OK, so what would they do to us then?" He said, "they would just let you go without penalty." Apparently, provided we hadn't forced them into the water we would not be penalised at all; while I was reassured by this, I have to say I was quite relieved when we had finished this assessment.

When the course was completed Abanoub and Bashir met with us, they were clearly very pleased with how things had gone and wanted to show us some of the sights in Cairo before we left the next day. They detailed Saeed to go with us to our hotel in Cairo; they had booked us into the Nile Hilton, this turned out to be a very plush hotel, we each had a suite of rooms which were exceptional. As soon as we were booked in and had left out bags in the rooms Saeed hailed a taxi and off we went to visit the Pyramids. I didn't really know how far we would need to travel but was somewhat stunned when after just a few minutes we turned a corner from a city street and there they were right in front of us; they were really on the edge of the city.

The Pyramids and Sphinx are situated on the Giza Plateau, which was as I say right on the edge of the city; beyond the Pyramids was just desert, it was so vast that people have been known to wander away from the Pyramids and get lost; there were sentries patrolling to stop people like us from doing just that.

We arrived about an hour before dusk which was great as this meant we would see everything both in daylight and would experience the light shows they use after dark. As we arrived in the car park the taxi was engulfed in hawkers and people trying to get us to buy the normal tat! I was very glad we had Saeed with us as he was able to shoo them away very effectively, after ten minutes or so we were left alone with Saeed to walk up to the first Pyramid. What a spectacle! They are immense, Saeed told us that they used to be faced in smooth stone but most of this had been removed to use as building material for Cairo over the years. The Sphinx was especially spectacular, and after dark the light show was impressive, Saeed told us that before the Sphinx was excavated all that had been visible was the head.

The face of the Sphinx is of course missing its nose, apparently in 1378 Sa'im al-Dahr a prominent Sufi Muslim was outraged when he noticed the local peasants making offerings to the Sphinx in order to gain help with the annual flood of the Nile thus hoping to increase their harvest. Sa'im al-Dahr defaced the Sphinx in the hope that this practice would stop. This didn't end well for Sa'im al-Dahr as he was later executed for this act of vandalism; the Pyramids and surrounding monuments and statues were a wonderful end to my first trip to Egypt.

Back in the UK I got back to work perfecting the Interdive inspection courses; and blending working with Interdive together with my other clients. Over the coming couple of years, I made several repeat trips to Alexandria teaching first-aid, inspection and air supervisor; by the summer things had moved on such that it was clear we would be very involved in training with the Arab Academy in the future. As far as Arabic was concerned though I learned a few phrases generally I needed an interpreter; this came in the form of Abanoub's daughter who spent several days working with me on the courses. This was my first experience of working through an interpreter and it soon became obvious that the theory part of the courses took almost twice as long as normal, this led to some very long days.

The first course she was enlisted to help me was a first aid course, one of the biggest problems with this was that some of the more devout students obviously felt that we were teaching them to get in the way of the will of Allah. Abanoub had an answer to this, he told his daughter to tell the course that if Allah had not wanted them to learn first aid, then he would not have allowed this infidel to come to Egypt! This seemed to work and the course became more attentive after this had been explained to them as apparently, I was carrying out the will of Allah; I was never very comfortable with this but I had to go with what Abanoub wanted.

Over the next couple of years, I was normally running one 3.1U or 3.2U course up in London every month, I was working away for eight to ten days per month; poor Chrissie was left at home bringing up our two boys pretty much on her own. When I wasn't in London, I managed to find extra work supervising diving operations for civil engineering companies and of course from time to time this included Fort Bovisand; I was very busy.

As I was spending a lot of time alone in hotel rooms while in London, I decided to write a course manual to be used as the textbook for both the 3.1U and 3.2U courses. My plan was that I would effectively write down all the words I normally used when teaching each of the lectures, I organised the book so that it ran completely to the programmes I was using; this would mean that students could follow the course page by page meaning they wouldn't need to be making loads of notes. I spent almost all the evenings holed up in my hotel room bashing away at the brand-new laptop computer I had bought for the job.

Laptops were very new and not very capable, the one I had was an Amstrad, it had what I thought at the time to be an enormous hard drive of twenty megabytes! I know this is tiny by today's standards but the programmes I was using at the time were all DOS based and so files were tiny compared to those produced by today's software. The computer was monochrome and although it could be carried easily as it folded up and had a handle it was quite heavy, so was not fun to carry very far.

When I first started the book it seemed a daunting prospect, there was a lot to do but, I took it a day and a subject at a time; I found I could normally complete a chapter during one or maybe two courses, of course I needed a great deal of in-depth knowledge about each subject which meant I was buried in books for a lot of this time. It might have been a little easier if the internet had been available then but as it was, I had to rely on textbooks and libraries, still it meant that I learned all the subjects to a much higher level than was needed to teach the courses.

By the end of the first year, I had completed the majority of the 3.1U subjects, I was pleased with what I had done but needed someone to edit the text; enter Chrissie again, the she was put to work correcting my numerous grammatical and spelling errors, in those days there was no such thing as in-programme spelling and grammar check. Between the two of us we managed to get the text to a level where it would be acceptable and I then moved on to the 3.2U subjects; I felt much more confident with MPI as I had gone through extensive training in the use of MPI already. I was not though so clued up on ultrasonic inspection so would need to research this subject, again, this took me about another year of London courses but eventually all of these subjects were also completed and ready for editing.

Next, I needed to add diagrams to the text, now again in those days the computer programmes I had access to didn't include drawing packages and so the only option I had was for me to draw all the pictures by hand. To help with this I used a Rotring technical drawing set to make a reasonable fist of the required pictures; however, the pictures were numerous and took me much longer than I had originally planned. Eventually, though all was done, I then had to cut the pictures to fit in with the arranged appropriate gaps I had left in the text for the pictures; I printed the whole book out. Then stuck the pictures into the book's text in the required places.

Chrissie had access to photocopying facilities at her work and had gained permission for us to copy everything which we did over one weekend; now we had a book with all text and pictures corresponding to my acetates for both 3.1U and 3.2U courses. I sent this finished document to CSWIP informing them that this would be the manual we would be using for our courses; they agreed that this was acceptable. During the next couple of courses using the book with the students following in their own copies was great, it made it so much easier for me and from the end of course comments it seemed the students agreed; there were just a few typos identified which I corrected for the second edition. I had done a deal with Kevin Salter that he would pay me a royalty for each student that used my book and associated paperwork, this was not a lot of money but would eventually pay for the time I had put into the project.

I continued to work with Interdive as a self-employed contractor for the next couple of years during which time Kevin had me teaching not only the inspection courses but also trainee air diving supervisor (TADS) and assistant life support technician (ALST) to the International Marine Contractors Association (IMCA) syllabi. I was very busy but at least the TADS and ALST were run in Plymouth meaning I could at least get home every evening during those courses.

In 1990 Kevin decided that he needed a full-time inspection manager and offered me the job, this was great as the salary reflected how much I had been earning as a contractor, additionally I was to be given sick pay if necessary and best of all paid holiday! We had always made a big effort to get away for a family holiday at least once a year even when we really couldn't afford it; I felt I needed this to be there for the kids as I was very often away and I missed them and I know they missed me, particularly as communications were not anything like as easy as they are today.

Since writing the original inspection manual computing had moved on and it was now possible for me to stop using Wordperfect, I moved over to using Microsoft Word six which was a much better package. In fact, in my view Word six was the best package and that some of the so-called advances applied since then have not really improved things. Word six had a lot of add-ons such as spell check and a basic drawing package that I found I could utilise. I had also now moved on to a much more capable Toshiba lap-top computer. Over the next couple of years, I redrew all the pictures and diagrams using the electronic drawing package; this made updating and editing everything so much easier although I spent a great deal of time again in hotel rooms hunched over the computer drawing.

During this time, we decided to commence 3.4U courses, Kevin asked me to look into producing the necessary paperwork such as exams, homework, programmes and all other associated material. Initially we decided to use the industry standard book that had been produced by a company called ORCA. The idea was to utilise this as our course manual so, I purchased a copy and started to teach myself the necessary. 3.4U was always something I was nervous of instructing as the qualification was aimed at very experienced personnel who I was sure would know as much if not more than I did about inspection offshore. While there were times when some individuals were clearly very capable, I didn't find myself significantly out of my depth as much as I had thought I would. On the day of the CSWIP audit for 3.4U all went very well with the result that we gained approval without the need of any significant alterations.

Interdive was now becoming a serious player in the field of training of advanced techniques for commercial divers; Kevin Salter had up to now always hired appropriate facilities as and when they were needed and so had minimal costs when no courses were being run. In 1991 this changed, Kevin started by building a large extension on his house; this would house the admin for the company and made perfect sense to me and to the other instructors. However, before this was fully completed, Kevin started looking for a building into which he could move the inspection courses and in addition commence basic air diver training. This was a big ask in my view, we spent a good-few-months, searching around Plymouth and the surrounding areas looking for somewhere that would have wharf access or at least be close to the water.

This in fact proved impossible to find, and ultimately, we ended up in an old print works in West Hoe Road, Plymouth; the place was in need of a tremendous amount of work to convert it into a useable facility for us. We had to install a tank very similar to the one I had been using in London, we had to build classrooms, store rooms, shower facilities and administration offices. Kevin felt we should do all the work ourselves; I think he felt this would keep the costs down, but as we were not tradesmen, I think we took much longer to do the work and certainly didn't complete it to such a high standard as they would have achieved.

In addition, while the instructors were refurbishing the facility in West Hoe Road, Interdive ceased running courses particularly inspection, supervisor and ALST although the DMT courses did still carry on the company's income was significantly reduced during this time which I felt was a mistake. I told Kevin I felt we should be continuing to run courses as before and use tradesmen to carry out the fit-out. I had stupidly told Kevin at some-time in the past that I had started my working life training to be a plumber; he clearly felt that this meant I was up to doing all the plumbing for the new place. We spent most of the summer working to make the new facility which was OK, I actually enjoyed most of the work although I didn't like some of the jobs. In particular the whole place needed painting which was OK but when it came to painting the newly installed dive tank I clearly didn't step back quickly enough as I got the job.

The paint being used was a two-part epoxy, once mixed this had to be used quickly, it also gave off very heady and probably toxic fumes. I needed breathing apparatus when I was applying the paint inside the tank; the only apparatus, we had available was underwater SCUBA equipment, so, there I was in the bottom of the tank with a SCUBA cylinder on my back, a half mask on my face with a SCUBA second stage regulator in my mouth. This was fine in so much as I was protected from the fumes but, I was extremely uncomfortable and hot in my overalls; it took hours to finish painting but at the end I have to say it looked rather good; the paint was a very light green, almost a pastel shade, it would be very good for inspection dives.

The water in the tank was going to be heated just the same as the tank in London; we installed a swimming pool gas boiler that would be perfect for the job. We had a qualified gas fitter install the boiler but then I was given the job of completing all the pipework to get the warm water into the tank. I organised for the boiler to become part of the filtration circuit so water would be taken out of the tank put through a circulation pump and swimming pool sand filter before being passed through the boiler where the temperature would be brought up to the required level, finally the water was brought back into the tank. This worked really well and once the tank was full of water, we saw the temperature came up to the required level within just three hours, perfect.

Sometime in late July we were still some way off completing the refurbishment of the facility when Kevin turned up and told us that he had bought a boat which would be perfect for running basic air diving courses from! This news was greeted by something of a stunned silence, especially when he told us how much work would be needed to bring the boat up to the necessary spec. I don't think I was the only one who thought this was going to end in tears; it turned out that the boat he had bought was totally inappropriate for teaching surface supplied air diving.

The boat was renamed 'Interdiver'; Kevin started to talk of it as his DSV, Diver Support Vessel; the boat had been previously used as a target towing boat; it used to tow targets that were then shot at by naval guns based at HMS Cambridge just outside Plymouth. There were a number of problems with the boat from my point of view; firstly, she was made of wood and therefore quite vulnerable to damage, it was also quite narrow and had virtually no working deck space. Kevin told us he had also bought an old hydraulic winch that had been used on a fishing trawler and he was going to have it refurbished so that it could be used as a winch for the wet-bell!

So, many plans without much thought as to how any of this was going to work; over the next couple of months a wet bell turned up for us to refurbish, a deck decompression chamber also arrived and this too needed complete refurbishment including hydrostatic testing!

As my work on the tank installation was now complete and I only had to help out with some of the pipework for the new low-pressure compressor that had been fitted into an outbuilding and fitting out the dive control. I set to work on the chamber while Ray Ives another ex-offshore diver concentrated on refurbishing the wet-bell. The chamber needed painting as it had been grit blasted down to bare metal; this took a few days. We then we refitted all new acrylic plastic view-ports checking their seals as we went; I fitted a couple of large diameter quarter turn valves into penetrators at the bottom of the chamber, one in each lock (it was a twin lock chamber), these would be used to drain the water out of the chamber once the test was complete.

All of the other threaded penetrators had blanks screwed into them apart from one right at the top of the chamber into which I threaded a gauge and a smaller quarter turn valve, this would be fitted with the pump that would be used to increase the pressure inside the chamber then we were ready for hydrostatic pressure testing. A Lloyds inspector had been organised to witness the pressure test. On the day, before he was due to arrive, we filled the chamber up with water. By filling the chamber with water, the test became much safer than it would have been if the chamber was full of air.

On the day of the test, we checked all was ready and then waited for the inspector; he arrived at nine o'clock in the morning and was keen to get on with the test as soon as possible. Kevin brought the inspector down to the main shop floor where everything was ready for him; he knew the chamber would already be filled with water and told us that was fine but that once the pressure test was complete, he would need to have a look inside. We got straight on with pressurising the chamber to its required maximum pressure of one point three times its working pressure; the chamber's maximum working pressure was six bar absolute so we needed to pressurise it to seven-point eight bar absolute.

As the chamber was full of water which is to all intents and purposes incompressible it didn't take long to bring the pressure up to the required level; the inspector took some notes, wandered around looking for any leaks; after the required time had lapsed, he gave us the thumbs up and we let the pressure out again. As soon as the chamber was back at atmospheric pressure, I made sure the inspector was happy and then opened the drain valves, there were clear plastic hoses attached to the valves the other end of which were already laid into the building's drain inspection pit. We watched water running through the hoses and quite soon the water level in the chamber had fallen to the point where we could open the door.

As soon as the door was open the inspector poked his head in and just made sure there was no significant corrosion pitting or any other problem visible; all was good and he headed off with Kevin to get the paperwork completed. We got into the chamber with towels to dry it as much as we could, then we left the door open to complete the drying process over-night. Over the next few days, we installed all necessary valves and fittings inside the chamber but left those that need to be attached outside until the chamber had been installed into the boat's hull. I wasn't involved with installing the chamber into the boat, this was done by my old friend Jim Walker and his son.

Meanwhile I continued with making the diving tank ready for inspection courses; we built a mezzanine across the top of the tank this was built using perforated deck plates. The idea was that divers would climb the ladder that was in the far corner of the tank, they would then come up to stand on the mezzanine where the water would drain harmlessly back into the tank. This worked very well and meant that although the divers would still be wet when they made their way to the shower room it was nowhere near as bad as it would have been if the mezzanine wasn't there.

We had already installed a gantry crane over the tank so that we could lower relatively large test-pieces into the tank as required, all was ready now except we didn't really have enough test-pieces, I had been spoiled for choice at City University but now we needed our own test-pieces. I put the word out detailing what we were looking for and quite soon an old friend called up, he had access to three large pieces of a rig that had fallen over in an offshore field some time ago. The rig was the 'Inter-Ocean 2', he sent us some photos and they seemed perfect to me so we bought them; they arrived by road a few days later and although they were quite large, they were just small enough so that we could swing them over the edge of the tank and into place. We set about painting them so that they would not corrode too much more than they already had and I inspected them to build up a set of staff-solutions.

Finally, the day came when we were ready to run our first inspection course in the new facility, this was a momentous occasion for us; I was excited to be able to run the courses in Plymouth as I felt the facility was very nice and would give us very high-quality courses. I was also able to go home every night which was a huge bonus for me. Being the first course in a new facility CSWIP needed to audit the facility; again, they were not due to come along until we were doing the practical part of the course in the second week. They were scheduled to arrive on the second day of diving, the course was a 3.1U and the first day of diving had gone very well with the guys all doing very well.

The tank was nicely up to temperature so the guys could dive in overalls just like in London. On the day of the audit, I arrived at seven-thirty to find that something had gone wrong with the boiler, it must have been heating all night, the tank temperature was far too high. It seemed the thermostat had somehow stuck, the fault was easily rectified but we still had a tank full of water that was far too warm to be able to put divers in. By eight-thirty we had everyone tearing around Plymouth picking up ice; luckily the fish quay on the Barbican had a large ice plant that we were able to make good use of; over the next couple of hours, I was throwing ice into the tank by the bucketful!

Thankfully by the time the auditors arrived the tank temperature while still being a little too warm had reduced to a point where we could safely put divers in the tank albeit I had to make sure they only stayed in the tank for a relatively short period of time! CSWIP were none the wiser thanks to the students playing their part and helping us by not making any reference to the temperature being too high; the audit went very well with the facility gaining approval, thank goodness.

My job now reverted to running inspection courses at least once and sometimes twice a month depending on numbers of applicants so I didn't really have much to do with readying the boat for the BAD courses. Gerry Mackenzie was the individual that Kevin had already used to run the HSE Part 2 courses with and Kevin had managed to convince him to also run the air diving courses for him.

By now my books had been translated into Arabic, both the inspection manual and trainee air diving supervisor manual were eventually translated which in some ways made the teaching a little better. Of course, I still could not speak Arabic; this was the first translation of my books but since then they have also been translated at least in part into Portuguese, Vietnamese, Spanish and Russian.

Most of the divers who wanted inspection courses were of course trying to work during the summer periods. This being the case I used to get involved with readying the boat during this period and then once the boat was complete, I would help running courses during the summer. I also would help whenever either Gerry wasn't available due to a Pt 2 course being run or maybe Gerry was on leave etc., during one of these occasions I was scheduled to run a twelve-week course from start to finish with help from a couple of other qualified divers.

On day one of the course, we used to put all applicants through an aptitude test part of which was to have them swim around in the tank. There was no way this was in any way as difficult as we had been made to do at Bovisand but it did give the instructors something of an idea as to how comfortable the people were in the water. On this day there were twelve applicants, we completed all necessary paperwork before taking them up to the tank where we told them what we needed them to do.

This was for them to just swim around in circles until told to stop. We put a rope onto each one in turn and watched them closely as they made their way down the ladder into the tank; all went well until one of the guys was clearly not happy at all; in fact, almost as soon as he let go of the ladder he started to panic. He was so bad that we had to put our standby diver in to rescue him; when he was again back on the mezzanine, I sat down with him to find out what was wrong, he proceeded to tell me that he couldn't swim! I was stunned, how did he think he was going to go through a diving course without needing to swim? He just said he thought he would be breathing from an air source and so could just climb down to the bottom and walk everywhere! Unfortunately, he didn't progress onto the main part of the course, I suppose that saved him some money at least because by now government funding had ceased meaning all the applicants were self-funded although some lucky individuals were funded by a company.

When we did eventually start the course there was one particular individual that gave me some cause for concern; this was Arjun, he was from India and seemed extremely nervous whenever we started to prepare for diving. One of the first things we used to do with the students was to take them through basic SCUBA drills, things like making sure their use of weights was correct, removing and replacing their second stage while underwater and of course mask clearing. Mask clearing was essential as it ensured two things, firstly when the student allowed the half mask to fill with water they didn't freak out and secondly, they mastered the skill of breathing out through their nose while pressing the top of the mask onto their forehead, this ensured they could empty the mask of water. On the day we were to take them through mask clearing I decided to pair myself with Arjun; first we clung on to the ladder in the tank at the surface.

I showed Arjun how to fill the mask with water by dipping my face underwater cracking the seal on the mask letting all the air out of the mask which of course then filled with water. I lifted my face out of the water so that Arjun could see the mask was full of water and then I pressed my finger to the top of the mask and breathed out through my nose thus evacuating all the water from the mask. I asked Arjun if he was happy to give it a go and he put his thumb up, he had several attempts which didn't go well; he just lost it as soon as there was any water in the mask! I told him to get out of the tank, we both climbed up onto the mezzanine area, where we broke down the kit and got dressed. Once we were both dry, I told Arjun that he would have to master this skill before he would be allowed to progress.

He confirmed he was keen to get it right; I took him into the kitchen where I filled a washing up bowl with warm water, we then went through the process of him allowing his mask to flood and then clearing the water. Eventually he seemed confident and happy with the process; I told him that we would try again in the tank that afternoon; meanwhile all the other students had completed most of their basic skills which I think put still more pressure on Arjun.

First thing in the afternoon we went through the same process of doing the mask clearing at the surface while hanging on to the ladder and he seemed to have actually mastered the procedure. Next, we had to go down the ladder to the bottom of the tank where he would need to do it again, he said he wanted to give it a try and so down we went. As soon as we were on the bottom, I again showed him how to do it and then indicated that it was his turn; he looked at me and all I could see in his mask were eyes that appeared huge it was like looking at a couple of dinner plates behind the face plate, he certainly didn't look relaxed.

We were at the bottom of the tank so at about four metres, I was facing Arjun when he started to let water into his mask; as soon as a little water had entered, he freaked! I could see he was panicking but couldn't really do much about it, he then just took off back towards the surface; we may have just been at four metres but I knew that if he held his breath, he was in danger of bursting his lungs. I grabbed his harness in my right hand and with my left I got hold of one of the rungs of the ladder, Arjun had inflated his stab-jacket (buoyancy device) and so would be on the way back to the surface super-fast. I held on with all my might, now I was holding the rung of the ladder with Arjun trying to pull me to the surface with him, I had to slow the ascent, I let go of the rung and managed to catch the next one up. And continued to do this all the way back to the surface, when we arrived, I was very relieved to see that Arjun was breathing without any signs of blood or real distress other than his panic.

We got him out of the water and dressed again; I then sat down with him where we had a full and frank discussion; I explained to him that if he couldn't master mask clearing in the nicely controlled conditions of our tank i.e., warm water and good visibility, he had no chance in the event of needing to do it for real in the sea. He agreed and decided to leave the course forthwith, I was sad to see him go and felt that I had somehow failed him but, in the end if he was not comfortable in the water perhaps diving was not a career for him; I thought we had seen the last of him.

However, this was not to be, four months later we were starting another course and who should walk through the door but Arjun! I was amazed to see him but even more stunned as he seemed to have got over his fears; he may never have been particularly comfortable with some of the drills but he did complete them all satisfactorily. When we had completed the mask clearing and were again dressed, I took him to one side and asked him how he had overcome his fears; his answer was a little unconventional. Apparently, he had two brothers who were both working divers, they told him he was being stupid, then dressed him in SCUBA gear on a beach they tied one of his hands to each brother put the second stage regulator in his mouth and told him, "If you spit that out you will die!" This was the beginning of his training by brother's, well, it might be unconventional but for Arjun it worked, he did eventually pass the course but I'm not sure he ever worked as a diver, I certainly never saw him again after the course.

At Interdive we used to train a lot of people from India, they were always cheerful and pleasant to be with. I got to know a few of them quite well as some of them used to come back again and again on various courses; it was their custom to always bring the instructor a present, usually this tended to be a bottle of 'Old Monk' rum, this was a dark rum which while a bit of an acquired taste was always appreciated. While I was training a lot of courses with Indians, I made the mistake of telling them that my wife was quite partial to the rum, I thought nothing of it until when the next course arrived, I was presented with two bottles, one for me and one for the Memsahib; I was accumulating a lot of bottles of rum.

When I was chatting to one group, I told them that I had noticed that almost whenever they were talking their heads would shake or wag from side to side; I said that I found this a bit odd. I said, "We English people nod our head if we mean 'yes' and shake our head from side to side when we meant 'no'". So, I asked "what does the constant wagging of heads mean for the normal Indian", one of them looked quizzically at me and said "Well, sometimes it may mean yes, and sometimes it may mean no!" As if this was the most natural thing in the world and why did this not make perfect sense to me?

Anyway, quite a lot of the Indians would already be working as divers and were being trained to carry out inspection or assistant life support technicians; if it was inspection then it would normally be to the Lloyd's diver inspector syllabus. On one of these courses, we had seven students who went through the whole course including theory very well; the last day of the course was always the examination as usual being witnessed by a Lloyd's examiner. On this occasion we were carrying out the examinations from our boat; we were tied up at Victoria Wharf in the Cattewater; as always, the examiner had brought his test-pieces with him and each diver was put on the bottom together with the test-pieces he was to inspect.

All went fine until, one of the divers wouldn't stop; I had turned off the MPI unit and told him to send the test-pieces back to the surface but he just wouldn't answer me; I knew he was alright as I could hear his breathing over the comms together with some muttered words that I couldn't understand. Eventually, it became clear he was not going to obey my instructions and I thought that maybe he wasn't understanding me? We always insisted that the courses were carried out in English and the students mostly had little problem with this but sometimes their level of comprehension was poor to say the least. I thought maybe I should have one of the other Indian divers talk to him and tell him he had to finish what he was doing and return to surface; the senior chap agreed, he came across the deck with a definite swagger in his step as his importance was clearly increased by this duty.

He took control of the comms; I stood back expecting to hear a fluent stream of Urdu or some other local dialect, instead he took a deep breath and said with exaggerated gravity, "You must stop what you are doing and come back to the surface." All delivered in highly accented English; I stared at him and said "I can tell him in English, I wanted you to tell him in his own language!" With a dead pan expression, he replied "None of us can speak his dialect." The examiner's face was a picture, eventually, we did get the diver back to the surface but unfortunately, he did not pass his exam which I suppose isn't surprising as he really didn't speak English; he must have spent the whole week just nodding or wagging his head at everything without understanding anything.

Another basic air diver course included a couple of brothers from India, Kabir and Jayesh they were a likeable couple of individuals, Jayesh took to diving like a duck to water, Kabir not so much. All was well until we were carrying out the deep dives, we were back at the victualling yard buoy in the Tamar River with the depth being something more than forty metres. On this particular day the weather was wonderful, it was a bright sunny day with almost no wind, the water was almost flat calm, we were just starting them on their flange task, on this day they were using just spanners as they hadn't progressed to hydraulic tools yet. I had been reunited with my good friend from Angola; Bart Bartholemew who had been taken on as our professional standby diver, we had spent a good-few-minutes catching up on news until we arrived on site, I was very glad to have Bart with us as I knew I could rely on him.

Some way through the day it was Kabir's turn to dive, all went well as he was dressed by his brother, he carried out all his pre-dive checks with confidence and we put him in the water. On this day we were using the diving basket so all the divers were being lowered to the bottom so I knew he couldn't get lost; when he told me he was on bottom, I took his depth with the pneumo, forty-two metres. I told him to start the task, I could hear some clanking over the comms so I thought he had started; after a few minutes though I heard him say "I am coming up." I immediately told him not to come straight up as he was already in need of some decompression stops, he just responded with "I am coming up."

I could see his depth was decreasing and it was clear that he was no longer in the dive basket; I called "jump the standby" this was the call for Bart to go in to fetch him. Bart was already dressed ready for the water except that he had his KMB10 in his lap, on hearing the call he was extremely quick at putting on his hat and telling me, "Ready for the water." I gave him the OK to jump and to follow Kabir's umbilical and off he went, he left surface and within a couple of minutes he had found Kabir, Bart quickly took control of the diver's buoyancy and brought him under control. Both diver's tenders then worked together to bring the divers up onto a lazy shot for their decompression; this was completed without further issue and everyone returned to surface safely.

Both Kabir and Jayesh did pass the course but when I saw Jayesh sometime later when he was attending a CSWIP diver inspector course he told me that Kabir had left diving and was working as a waiter in an Indian restaurant in Saltash, Cornwall; probably for the best.

Underwater searches were a big part of the diver training; we used to have the divers repeatedly practice circular searches, grid searches and Jackstay searches, the first thing I always said to them was that provided the divers search thoroughly the item will always be found! Now, clearly that isn't always the case but it is a good way to start when teaching divers search methods, the second thing I used to tell them was, always know what you're looking for. This might seem like an obvious thing to say but it's amazing how often people go searching for an item having just been told what they are looking for without actually being told what it looks like? Size of the object is very important as, if you are looking for a large truck then the search will be quite different to that needed if you are looking for a tiny item.

The final thing I used to tell them when they were looking for something small was to always look under the shot weight; certainly, for air diving the norm certainly for a circular search pattern would be to drop a weight attached to a rope. The weight used was often a 25-kilogramme weight and certainly when looking for something small looking under the weight was a logical first place to look; this was brought home to one of our courses in a very good way.

We were just over half-way through another twelve-week course when we were going to be diving in a location in the Tamar River called Barn-Pool, the depth there was some thirty-metres plus. The visibility was not good, maybe a metre or so, the first day we were there one of the students Raymond was the last student to dive, he was a Swedish Fire-Fighter and unfortunately on this dive he lost his watch. When he came back to the surface and realised the watch had gone, he was very upset as it had been a gift from his father just before he left home to come on the course. I told him not to worry as we would be in the same location in the morning and would search for it, we would clearly find it then. Before leaving the position I together with the course members took bearings on a number of fixed marks so that we could be certain to moor up in exactly the same place in the morning; it was clear there was a great deal of scepticism on the part of the team.

The next day, the team looked at the bearings we had taken and managed to moor up in exactly the same place, as soon as we were stable, we dropped the shot line onto the bottom, then we made ready for diving. The brief I gave the team was that we would carry out circular searches; each diver would leave surface and go down the shot line before organising themselves on the bottom to carry out their search. We spent the rest of the morning searching without any luck, I was not really that surprise as the visibility was very poor and the bottom was muddy but I had hoped we would find the watch; still there was only so much we could do.

When we broke down for lunch, the diver who had made the first dive came to me acting in a very conspiratorial way; when he was sure nobody could see him, with a flourish he produced the watch! He told me he found it under the shot and had then just gone through the motions of searching. But as we were planning on continuing searches with the rest of the crew including Raymond in the afternoon, we agreed that I would present the watch back to Raymond once the day's diving was complete.

When everyone had finished diving, Raymond was looking somewhat downhearted; I had the guys breaking down the equipment ready for it to be stowed for the night. As we were steaming back to the boat's overnight mooring and all the guys were congregated on deck behind the wheelhouse; I called them all in for a chat, as soon as they were all there, I beckoned the chap who had found the watch to join me and we presented Raymond's watch back to him. He was clearly very relieved to have his watch back; I had the diver who found it relate his tale and it was clear this was a great lesson learned.

In May 1994, late one afternoon Kevin Salter came to see Gerry and I, we met in the upstairs classroom. Kevin said that he wanted to give us an opportunity, Gerry and I exchanged glances but said nothing. Kevin invited us to buy the boat from Interdive and operate it as our own business, he would of course buy our time back so that the courses would continue to use the boat. There was no mention of cost at this time, he just wanted us to think about it and if we were interested then we would discuss finances etc., Kevin just left us with this and went home.

I stayed and chatted to Gerry, he was of the same opinion as me, in that we both thought Kevin needed an injection of money and saw this as a way to get it from us. I expressed the opinion that he would want a lot of money for the boat but, and as we both thought it was the wrong boat for the job anyway and that it had become abundantly clear that it was very soon going to need a lot of money spending on it. We both decided there and then that we should start looking for other jobs.

In fact, I had already started negotiations with Jim Sheppard; Jim had by this time left UCL and was now working for the welding institute (TWI) at their new facility up in Middlesbrough. Jim was in the process of moving, lock, stock and barrel up to Middlesbrough although at that time they had not actually found the right house. Jim was travelling from Plymouth up to Middlesbrough on a weekly basis until they could move so I had met with him a couple of times at his house in Plymstock. Jim told me that he had been impressed by how I had performed while we were working together at City University and wondered whether I was interested in working with him at TWI.

I told him that I would not move to Middlesbrough but was interested in working with TWI as a contractor, Jim seemed to think this would work, we agreed a day rate. Jim told me that the new facility in Middlesbrough was being specifically built for running CSWIP underwater examinations, he was to be the centre manager and was tasked with making the facility as cost effective as possible. To this end, he wanted to start running the full range of CSWIP underwater preparatory courses; Jim was already aware that the book I was using for teaching the 3.1U and 3.2U was mine and I confirmed that this could be made available for TWI's courses.

I told him that I would also be able to supply all the supplementary information and paperwork for the courses and would be interested in writing additional for the other courses as and when that became necessary. I came away from the last of these meetings, held in his garden on a lovely sunny Friday afternoon in early June with an agreement for me to become TWI's principle, instructor for underwater courses. Jim said the new centre had not been completed as yet but that he thought it should be ready to commence courses sometime in late September or early October, this suited me just fine as it gave me lots of time to complete the necessary additional paperwork.

As I've already said, we always tried to get away for a family holiday in the sun every year and 1994 was no exception. In mid-July we headed off to Rhodes for our two-week summer break, generally we had a lovely time although the hotel this time was not quite what we had been expecting. After the holiday we arrived home on the Saturday, Sunday was a very quiet day filled with catching up with post, washing clothes and all the other stuff that needs to be done on return home.

On the Monday morning, I made my way in to Plymouth to work, I was due to start a 3.1U course that morning, so, there I was letting myself into Interdive's building at just before eight o'clock. I wasn't expecting to see anyone there at that time of the morning and so was surprised to see Kevin when he arrived just a few minutes behind me; I didn't spend much time with him other than to respond to him that yes, we had had a great holiday.

The student's started arriving at eight-thirty and Kevin was clerking them in which again was very odd, where was our receptionist? I also couldn't find our storeman either as he hadn't turned up by nine o'clock when I started the course; it was strange.

At the end of the course's first day Kevin asked to see me before I went home; at four-thirty we were in his office where he and his wife Astrid were waiting for me; this didn't feel good at all. As it turned out I had been right to feel concerned as Kevin asked me to take a seat and proceeded to tell me that the company was being wound up, I was being made redundant. Interdive had taken on such a high level of debt that it could no longer service, creditors had called in their loans. It seemed that all the other staff had already gone but as we had the inspection course for the next couple of weeks Kevin asked that I complete it, this was fine by me as I was due a month's notice anyway.

I made my way home to break the news to Chrissie who was understandably upset by this but as she knew I had already been talking to TWI we both hoped it was not the end of the world. The main issue for me and my family was the short term, it was late July and the TWI work was unlikely to even be ready to start until the end of September. I spent the next two weeks running the course as I normally would but it did seem odd with nobody else in the facility, the students eventually got wind of what was happening and were very pleased that we were going to complete their course so that they would not be out of pocket.

On the second Friday of the course, the students were all done by three-thirty as was normal. Kevin then told me he had nothing else for me to do for the last two weeks of my notice period; he told me to go home. I didn't really say much other than to commiserate with him as it seemed he would lose his business and maybe even his home? As it turned out I don't think he did lose his home but maybe he did personally suffer financially I really don't know. I went home expecting one last pay check at the end of the month, unfortunately this never arrived so it seemed I had carried out that last 3.1U course for free.

I didn't receive any redundancy payment from Interdive although I did eventually get a somewhat reduced figure from the Government, oh well, I had to put it down to experience, but of course it meant there was even more pressure to find short-term work.

So, there I was, redundant with little prospect of work coming my way, I went looking for it; the following Monday off I went to Fort Bovisand again. Peter Sieniewicz seemed pleased to see me, he told me he would definitely have work for me and indeed offered me a few days that very week and indeed from then onwards he tended to offer me work whenever I needed it.

PHOTOS FROM MY TIME WORKING IN EGYPT

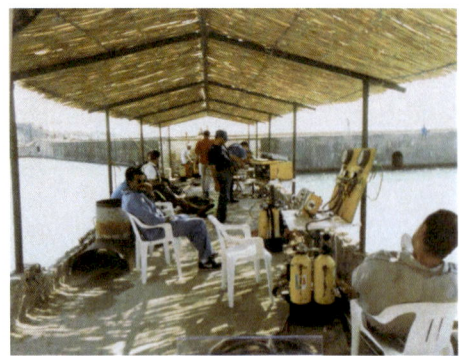

Dive site set up for the ERCA course at Montaza in Alexandria.

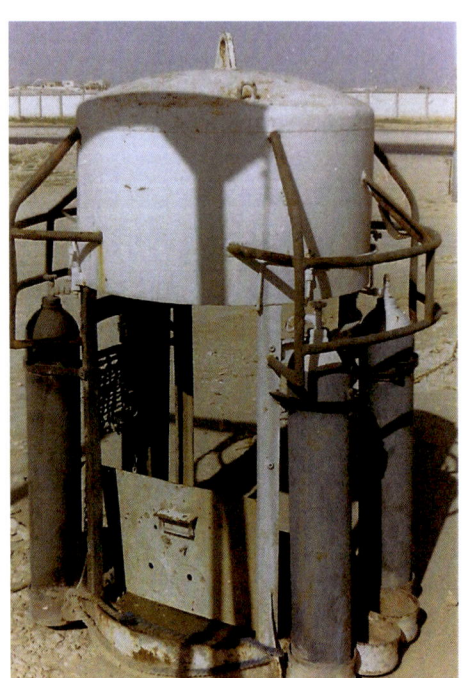

Wet bell when we arrived! Just a shell really.

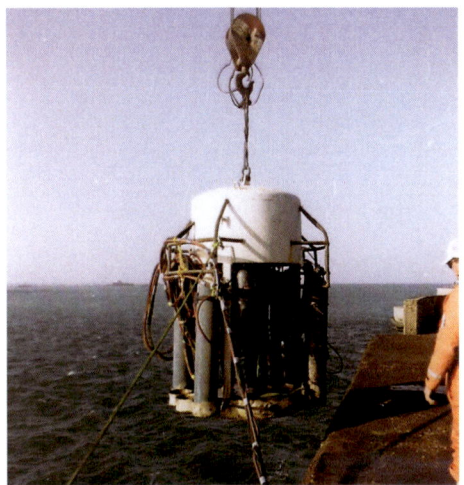

Wet bell entering the water following its refit.

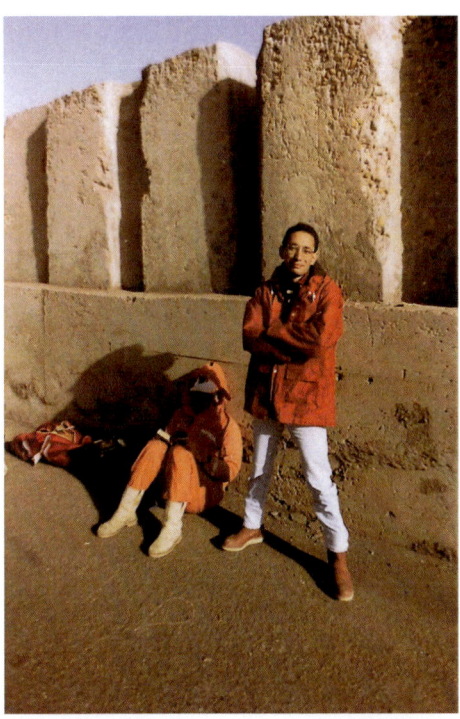

Two very cold instructors!

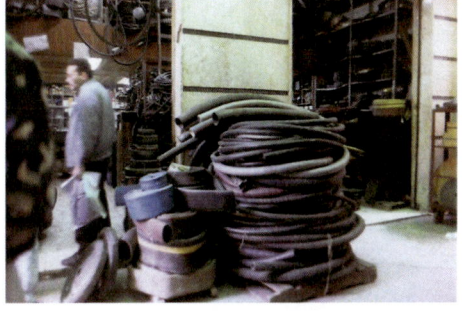

Ziad's key find where we were able to purchase all the hose we needed.

CHAPTER SEVENTEEN

Griffin Technology Ltd – 1994 to 2002

I was now faced with another decision; I had told TWI that I would be a contractor as I needed to make sure I was able to continue carrying out work for other companies; the way I saw it I could either go back to being self-employed or I could create a limited company. While I was researching the differences I started as self-employed but before too long, I realised that the limited company option was preferable when considering the future as when I undertook larger contracts this would limit my personal liabilities. Additionally, it was the route that would give the majority of clients confidence. My accountant also felt this was the correct route to take, so it was that Griffin Technology Ltd was created; again, I found myself on a fairly steep learning curve in order to ensure I ticked all necessary boxes.

I am convinced the limited company was the correct route to take and certainly, I did eventually gain significant contracts from large companies and local authorities who clearly expected the company to be limited. Anyway, in the short-term I was working again for Fort Bovisand; Peter put me to work as second instructor on Basic Air Diving courses. I found myself working alongside Tony Hillgrove and Paul Dart both of whom I knew from before, as second instructor my role was easy. It was my job to support the lead instructor and to keep an eye on the students; I very much enjoyed this role, there was really no responsibility on my head; the lead instructors did big me up to the students as ex-offshore diver though which meant they looked to me to provide real world experience. I continued in this role over the next couple of years; actually, I continued working with Bovisand from time to time whenever I could fit them in; this seemed to work well for all concerned and indeed, I found that Bovisand continued to want me pretty much whenever

I was free which was great.

Over the next few weeks, I was able to take days off here and there enabling me to complete all required paperwork for the TWI 3.1U and 3.2U course applications. Even though TWI was the company responsible for administering CSWIP examinations we still had to jump through all the required hoops to gain recognition of our courses; in fact, we had to be whiter than white as all the other schools would be sceptical of our gaining approval to run the courses. Jim Sheppard commenced the application with CSWIP and within a couple of months we were ready to run our first pilot courses. I was apprehensive about this application more than I had been for the Interdive ones, principally this was because I had been made very aware of the scrutiny we would be under, everything had to be right; I was not worried about the course really but, was worried that the CSWIP audit would be at a raised level than previous audits I had been through.

The course was due to commence on the Wednesday and would continue right through the weekend in exactly the same way I had run them at City University; so, on Tuesday the day before we were due to run the first course I bade my family goodbye, I would be away for another ten-days, I then made my way by car from Paignton up to Middlesbrough; this was about a five-hour journey. Jim had given me good directions of how to find TWI North, at their new facility, and it was on another nice sunny day that I turned off the A66 onto Riverside Park in Middlesbrough. Riverside Park was a fairly new industrial estate on the south bank of the river Tees; in the intervening years since I had last been to Middlesbrough with ICI there had been a lot of big changes.

Riverside Park had been built on the site of a slag heap in what was the 'Ironmasters' district but what I saw now was a nicely landscaped area boasting a large number of new buildings housing light industry. In the past Middlesbrough had been all about large heavy industry with Chemical plants, huge yards building offshore structures for the north-sea oilfields and of course steel works to name but a few. Now it seemed that although there were still some chemical works and construction yards, they had been scaled down significantly. As I cruised down Riverside Park Road, eventually turning left into Barton Road, there was a nice-looking two-story grey walled new building with red window frames on my right but not much else, directly in front of me was an area of scrubland between me and the river Tees, I could see across the river to a factory that I came to know was a chemical plant operated by BASF. Barton Road turned ninety degrees right, as I carried on along the road I saw a large TWI sign on the wall of the building, to the left of the door, it seemed I had arrived.

I parked in the car park just in front of the doors and made my way into a small reception area; in front of me there was a staircase leading up to the first floor, on my left was a small glass hatch where a receptionist was working. She noticed me and slid the hatch open, I introduced myself and told her that I was here to see Jim Sheppard, she said she would call him and I was to wait in reception for a few minutes.

After just a couple of minutes, Jim came bounding down the stairs sporting a wide welcoming smile, after a few pleasantries I followed him upstairs, when we arrived at the first floor, he turned right through a set of double doors into a large well-lit open area with windows looking out onto the car park, scrubland area, the Tees River and across to the chemical works. It was a nice outlook and seemed a welcoming environment, the whole area was carpeted in what looked to be new brown flecked carpet, Jim led me past two doors on the right that I could see from signage were toilets. Then he turned through a third door on the right which led into a large bright airy classroom that I was told would be mine for the duration of the course, it was again a step up from the magazines in Bovisand but also a lot better than the classrooms I had used with Interdive.

Jim told me to leave my bags in the classroom while he showed me the rest of the facility; the classroom had two doors along the left-hand wall, we left through the second one back into the large open area. Jim turned right and right again around the end of the classroom; we were faced with a door sporting a large yellow and black sign 'Danger deep water'; through the door there was another door on our right that Jim told me led to the diver's changing and showers. The flooring was a nice blue-grey non-slip surface that ran through the whole of this area, I followed Jim up a couple of steps immediately in front of us onto the deck alongside a large tank; this was a totally new building into which TWI had installed a large circular tank some seven metres wide, Jim told me it was six metres deep; at intervals around the rim of the tank there were vertical stanchions with chain looped between them to act as a safety barrier.

I looked into the tank and could see the water was beautifully clear. Jim told me the water wasn't heated but being inside a heated building would never be all that cold and given that the divers would wear dry-suits of which there were a large number in a variety of sizes, he felt there would be something for everyone. Adjacent to the ladder leading down the inner side of the tank there was a wooden bench on which there were two brand new Kirby Morgan Superlite seventeen helmets; each of these had its own hat mounted video camera and light, they were served by brand-new yellow, blue and red umbilicals. Jim said that we would be using all the same equipment as the exams utilised other than test-pieces, the exam structure was designed to be removed from the tank and was currently stored out of the way alongside the tank.

Above the tank was a large yellow gantry crane that could be rotated around the tank with a hook suspended from a dolly that could be moved to and fro as required, the crane could lift up to three tonnes and was actuated by means of a wireless handset; it was all state of the art as far as I was concerned. Jim walked half-way around the tank and leaning on the rail showed me a number of familiar looking nodes that were stored on the floor six metres below us alongside the tank. Jim said these were some of the nodes from City University and could be used as test-pieces for the courses, they would be perfect, I was very happy with the facility, it was great.

Turning back towards the entrance door, I saw a workbench on this level, on top of the bench there was a brand-new Bathycorrometer (CP meter) and Cygnus Digital Thickness Meter (DTM) together with stills cameras. Down the steps on the right-hand side was a nicely laid out dive control, it was set up with two separate diver's communications boxes, separate video recorders and TV monitors and all required valves for the divers. There were of course, no depth gauges as the depth of tank was known to be just six metres diver depth measurement was therefore completely unnecessary.

Jim then told me to go and make myself at home in the classroom while he got on with some work in his office that was through the first door on the right as we exited the tank room door. I spent the next hour or so setting up for the course, the facility was very good, there was a nice clean whiteboard with a variety of pens, a fairly new overhead projector, a TV and VCR on a stand, tables and chairs for the students and one for me at the front. I set up the tables in a semi-circle with each student having their own tablet of writing paper, TWI ruler and their own copy of my book; Jim had had the book printed off and each copy was in its own nice four-ring binder with a lovely photograph of a diver in the TWI tank on the cover.

I then went downstairs to make the acquaintance of the admin staff; the admin office was just off reception; as I descended the stairs back to reception I turned right through double doors and found the admin office through the first door on the left. Inside I introduced myself again and a nice lady who was sitting with her back to the window overlooking the car park at a desk immediately in front of me stood up and introduced herself as Helen. Helen had a nice welcoming smile and introduced herself as the office manager, she proceeded to offer any help I needed, I asked her whether there was a photocopier I could use as I needed to print off exams, homework sheets and some other bits and pieces for the course.

She told me to follow her and we went next door where there was a photocopier that would be more than up to my needs; she showed me how to use it and where to find additional paper should it run short. She then told me to let her know if I needed anything else and went back to her desk; I spent the next hour or so printing off sufficient paperwork so that each of the students would have their own set; I then thanked Helen and took all the paperwork back up to the classroom. Once this was done, I was pretty much ready so I went to find Jim and told him I was going to find somewhere to stay for the duration of the course.

In the days before the internet there was really no way to find hotels or guesthouses other than to drive around an area, so, off I went heading into the centre of Middlesbrough, I remembered from the last time I had been there that there were some cheap hotels along Marton Road so that's where I headed. Marton Road was a long, straight road that headed parallel to the A66, the area it went through was not what you would call a nice area by any stretch of the imagination but I was just looking for cheap digs.

I found a hotel that didn't look too bad, it was on the right-hand side of the road near the southern end of Marton Road; I parked up and went in to see whether they had a room for me. I was met by a harassed looking chap; he turned on a beaming smile and confirmed that he did indeed have a room that I could have for the full-ten days, the price was good and so I was in.

He asked whether I had a car, and when I confirmed that I did he told me that I should park it in the hotel's car park around the back; he said if I left it on the road overnight it would probably not be there in the morning! I thanked him, he said he would meet me out the back and I was to drive around there now; I would see him as I drove down the lane behind the hotel. I thought this was a bit odd, but of course that is what I did; as I turned into the lane behind the hotel, I saw him standing by a large door that he had opened for me. I turned into the car park and parked in a space near the gate, climbing out of the car I told him that I would need to be able to get out of the car park early each morning including Sunday, he said that wouldn't be a problem as he was always there.

I looked around the car park, there were six other cars; while I was unloading my bag from my car, he was closing the gate, there was a huge padlock and I could see barbed wire running along the top of the gate and all the walls bordering the car park, it looked like a prison compound.

While I wasn't particularly comfortable with this situation, I hoped all would be well, I made my way up to my room which was OK, it had an en-suite bathroom and both were at least clean. There was a double bed and a TV so it would do. When I was ready for some food, I made my way to the pub across the road, I made a call from the payphone to Chrissie and the boys and then had the perennial fish and chips, it was OK, well it filled a hole at least. That night I didn't get a lot of sleep as Marton Road was a bit of a race-track with cars racing up and down most of the night; this was punctuated by sirens and two-tone horns of police cars at intervals, and this had been Tuesday night, what was it going to be like at the weekend!

In the morning, I was served a hearty breakfast before making my way back to TWI, I arrived just before eight-thirty and spent a few minutes checking everything was ready. At nine o'clock I went down to pick up my students, Helen had corralled them in a waiting room across the corridor from her office, there were six students which I thought was a perfect number for our first course. The first five days were theory and went very well with the classroom and equipment performing brilliantly, TWI made filter coffee available to everyone whenever we wanted it and at lunchtime food was brought in by a jolly chef, the food was great, this took away something of the worry about me finding proper food for the evening at least.

The weekend was much quieter at TWI as there was really only us there although there was one security guard. On the fifth day the students did their theory exam and all passed with flying colours, this was a good result; day six was the first day of diving, I was introduced to the chap who was going to be assisting me and was the standby diver. I was very pleased to see it was Phil Bosten, I had taught Phil at Interdive when he underwent his initial basic air diving course and I knew him to be a very capable and nice guy.

The CSWIP audit took place on Wednesday of the second week and although they were as keen as always to see that the courses were being conducted properly; they seemed even more focussed on Jim and the management of ensuring the students had no access to the CSWIP test-pieces. They spent a good hour closeted with Jim and the on-site CSWIP examiners, when they eventually came out of that meeting it was clear that all was well, there were big smiles all round. Jim came to me when they had gone to let me know they were very happy with the course and as I thought the only slight concern, they had was that the students would get to see the CSWIP structure. This was a big result for us and although I hadn't been conscious of anxiety, I have to say I felt a weight had been lifted from my shoulders.

Over the next few months, I ran 3.1U and 3.2U courses every month so was spending ten days per month in Middlesbrough; I tried a lot of different hotels but they were either poor quality or too far away to be sensible. Luckily Jim and his wife Norma managed to find a nice house near Northallerton and they were nice enough to offer to put me up while I was running courses so I didn't have to spend all that much time in the hotels after all which was a big relief. I knew that Jim wanted to run 3.3U and 3.4U courses and he had mentioned that he also wanted to run Trainee Air Diving Supervisor (TADS) courses as well. These were to be run to the IMCA syllabi. I spent all my evenings and a good deal of the time at home preparing for all these courses.

My Diver's Guide to Underwater Inspection was being used for the 3.1U and 3.2U courses; I now worked to expand the book to cover the additional subjects for the 3.3U and 3.4U and I wrote a totally new manual to be used for TADS. By mid-way through 1995 I had finished the TADS manual, all the associated homework, exams and other required handouts so we were ready to start these courses.

On the first course we were to be audited by IMCA. I knew both of the auditors quite well, they were well aware of my background, the course was passed as fit for purpose with no requirements for change, this was almost unheard of at the time as they were known to always find something wrong!

This was great, for the first time since leaving Oceaneering I was associated with a very well-respected, well-funded and well-connected, company; TWI was recognised as a world leader in the field of underwater inspection training and examination. Over the coming months we were able to pool our knowledge and contacts to export our courses very successfully.

I had at least ten days per month working with TWI in Middlesbrough. Initially this was just teaching 3.1U and 3.2U courses but within the first year Jim told me he wanted to add IMCA Air Diving Supervisor, CSWIP 3.3U ROV Inspector and 3.4U Underwater

Inspection Controller both using my expanded Underwater Inspection Manual. In early 1996 work at TWI became even more involved with the advent of Alternating Current Field Measurement (ACFM) courses, I had already trained to be an ACFM operator and Jim had been working with Technical Software Consultants (TSC) who were the inventors and manufacturers of ACFM equipment. TWI became TSC's preferred training partner and of course this meant that I would do the majority of the training; a good deal of this training was done in Middlesbrough but, increasingly these courses were exported to Singapore, Thailand, Qatar, Canada, USA, Brazil, Vietnam and Australia; and although Jim and I shared the teaching of the ACFM courses pretty much everything else became my responsibility.

There were times when I would also be asked to carry out some work for Fort Bovisand, most of the time it would be as second instructor on BAD courses but occasionally I would be asked to lead a course, this would normally be a diving supervisor course or something that Bovisand didn't normally provide. Perhaps the most notable of these was one summer's day when I had been asked to run an air diving supervisor course for a group of Nigerian divers; when I arrived for the first day of the course, I was taken to one side by a chap who I vaguely recognised, his name was Brian and he used to work as a company rep for Shell UK.

I never did find out exactly what his relationship to the Nigerians was but he clearly had a vested interest in keeping them happy, it seemed this was the first of what could be a very lucrative contract for Bovisand. He told me not to worry too much about following the course syllabus as these individuals were very senior and clearly knew everything they needed to know anyway! He went on to tell me that I should basically give them whatever they wanted within reason; I was a bit taken aback by this and wasn't really sure what he meant? He gave me an example as he had been told that they were keen to be taken into Plymouth to go shopping sometime during this first day; so, it seemed I was to take them and shepherd them around Plymouth shopping centre. Oh well, it made no difference to me really and as he told me there would be no requirement for any of these guys to undertake any examinations, they could do whatever they wanted.

Brian introduced me to the three students, from Nigeria. Anyway, I started the course in the same way I normally would by talking about the physics of diving and while initially they seemed to be quite attentive but, when we broke for coffee at ten-thirty it was clear they had had enough. Their leader took me to one side and explained that they would like to go shopping; I tried to explain that we had a lot more to get through to which he replied, "We have the book so will teach ourselves tonight!" It was clear that nothing else was going to get done today; the crew all gathered their books together and told me they would meet me in the car park in ten minutes, well, that was me told!

I went down the hill to the top of the slipway leading down to the harbour and sat on the wall to wait, it was a warm pleasant day and I must say I wasn't at all sorry not to be cooped up in the classroom. When the three of them finally arrived we made our way to my car and off we went into Plymouth town centre; along the way they were all asking questions such as whether people owned the houses we were passing, what sort of people lived in houses like these and so on? I tried to answer as best I could but it was not easy as there were not really any right answers to the majority of their questions, well, none that I knew anyway. I decided to park up in the Charles Cross multi-storey car park; we then made our way down to ground level with a view to heading down through the centre of town, they all followed closely at first but I soon found I was talking to myself as I turned around to find I was all alone! Where had they gone? I saw one of them entering a branch of Littlewoods so I took off after him, when I caught up with him, I could see that the others were also in the same shop.

One of them had focused in on a display bin with cheap flip-flops, he picked up a pair and proceeded to the checkout where he started to barter with the cashier; well, I'm sure you can guess what happened next; the queue behind him started to get agitated and I thought all hell was going to break loose! I picked my way through the queue until I was right behind him and explained that bartering didn't work here, he looked completely nonplussed, threw the shoes on the checkout and walked out of the shop.

I followed him, we stopped just outside the shop, where I looked for the others, they were nowhere to be seen again; I eventually rounded them all up; I tried explaining a little of how shopping worked here in the UK but I could see nothing much of what I was saying was going in. We headed off again, moving down the hill, I decided to let them go in front of me so that I could keep an eye on them but this lasted no more than a couple of minutes. It was like a rehearsed starburst, each of them heading off in a different direction as something caught their eye; I didn't know which of them to follow so I decided to call them all back. This again took a few minutes but eventually we had a little huddle where I explained that they had an hour before we needed to be back at the car, I pointed to a bench where I told them I would meet them in forty-five minutes.

They all seemed to be on board with this course of action, we synchronised watches and I watched them all disappear into various shops; I bought myself a coffee and sat on the bench to wait. Over the course of the next three-quarters of an hour I saw all of them periodically, they would come past me becoming steadily more and more burdened with bags of goodness knows what! This went on for just over an hour, I had managed to grab two of them but the third had gone AWOL, after another fifteen minutes or so one of the guys spotted him plodding back towards us carrying a massive bean bag.

Back at the car we spent an interesting few minutes trying to get everyone and their random purchases into my small Datsun; the boot was full with everything from a plastic penguin to bottles of bleach, two of the guys were in the back seat with the bean bag and several bags of *Stuff!* The boss took his place in the front passenger seat, when everyone was installed, I climbed into the driver's seat and looking around found I couldn't see out the back window because of the bean bag and other bags on the rear parcel shelf; I could just about see across the bosses' bags so could see out of the passenger window, just. How on earth were they going to get all this stuff home on an aircraft? Off we went back to Bovisand, when we arrived it was just after two o'clock and I told them that they could have half an hour before I wanted to see them back in the classroom; they all just stared at me. They retrieved all their purchases from wherever they had been stowed and made their way back to their dorm; I decided to go and see whether I could get a sandwich in the café.

As I entered the café Brian was seated at one of the tables, when I had bought a sandwich I joined him, as soon as I was seated, he asked how things had gone this morning? I explained everything to which he treated me to a lopsided grin, saying that this was exactly what he had expected.

He asked what I had planned for the rest of the day, so I told him I had asked them to be back in the classroom in a few minutes; his expression told me he was sceptical about this and as it turned out he was right, just before I was due to head back to the classroom the boss poked his head around the door. He looked pleased to have found me and joined us at our table, he apologised but said that there would be no more teaching that day as they were too tired! I started to give my thoughts about this but Brian cut across me saying that it was fine and that we would recommence in the morning at nine o'clock! We did start again in the morning and to be fair we had a good day; they were all attentive and helpful but Wednesday was cancelled as they needed more shopping; they didn't need me as they had organised taxis to get into town.

Thursday and Friday were also cancelled and I was told not to worry or even go to Bovisand, I didn't mind really as I still got paid but, I don't think the guys really came for a course at all, they just wanted a shopping trip; as I say goodness knows how they got it all home!

At TWI we were now ready to tackle 3.4U; I had completed the updated manual and other paperwork and as was the norm, on the first course we underwent CSWIP audit, unexpectedly this went very well. The CSWIP auditor was an extremely experienced individual who wrote some very complimentary comments about my manual, paperwork and abilities in the classroom, this of course went down very well with Jim and TWI in general. 3.3U followed within a few months meaning we had the full house of underwater inspection courses under our belt; with these and the TADS and ACFM courses I found I was spending more like fifteen days per month in Middlesbrough which was making home life a little more difficult. TWI offered me a full-time job in Middlesbrough but I knew this would not work. I had already had a number of very attractive offers such as a two-year contract in Hawaii flying a subsea tourist submarine and a similar job in Malta; but Chrissie didn't want to move her family from Torbay. To be fair, I knew this when we married and so had accepted that commuting was to be the only option for me.

One of the advantages of working for myself was that I could take time off whenever I wanted too however, of course I would not be paid during time off so clearly, I had to temper my desire for time off with what we could afford. Mid-way through 1996 I decided to take a couple of months off in July and August; these were quite times as far as CSWIP courses were concerned anyway as most of the divers were trying to work during the summer months. I wanted to spend the summer with Steve and James, Steve was eleven and James was nine. I felt it would be great to be at home with them for the whole time they were on their school summer holiday; we had a wonderful summer windsurfing, swimming and generally playing, it was great. During this time, I also managed to rip out our tired old kitchen and replace it with a shiny new, white one, my doing the work saved us a good deal of money and I quite enjoyed doing it as well.

My skills soon became more in demand as I was offered more work as instructor on a rival's courses; at the time Wray Castle situated just outside Ambleside in Cumbria was the market leader in training of ROV pilots and to an extent 3.3U and 3.4U inspector training. Wray Castle was a stately home type property that had been built by the Gordon's Gin magnate sometime in the Victorian ear, it was a very impressive building set in wonderfully landscaped grounds leading down to the shores of lake Windemere. To date Wray Castle's inspection training had been done by an old friend of mine from Bovisand, Mel Baylis; Mel though had accepted a long-term job in Qatar and so would not be available for the foreseeable future, he advised them to contact me to take his place.

While in some ways I didn't need the work, I was conscious that I was very reliant on TWI and so thought it would be sensible to have more irons in the fire. I accepted the job on the same basis as TWI, the only difference was that they didn't want my books or paperwork, I again had to use the off-the-shelf manual as I had at Interdive; this was again 'A Hand-book for Underwater Inspectors', which had been produced for the Health and Safety Executive by 'OCRA'. I also had to use Wray Castle's exams etc., while this was OK, it did mean that in my view the training was not as polished as it was at TWI. I did several courses with Wray Castle, sometimes this involved my carrying out a ten-day course in Cumbria followed immediately by another set of courses sometimes fifteen days in Middlesbrough.

In April 1997, TWI provision of courses really went international, the first location was to be to Singapore; I flew again from Heathrow direct to Changi airport in Singapore. As soon as the door to the plane opened, I was again assaulted by that wonderful tropical fragrance together with high humidity and of course heat! As before, I loved it; I was met at the airport by David Lim who was a very nice, friendly Chinese Singaporean he was the senior manager for the company we had partnered with for provision of training, this was Metalock Underwater Maintenance (MUM).

On this my first trip out to Singapore I was to set up and run both an ACFM course and a Lloyd's diver inspector course in the tank they had; the tank was in fact a ship's hold that had been cut out of a ship and then setup in the yard at MUM's headquarters, the tank was huge and was certainly fit for purpose.

David picked me up from my hotel in the morning; I was not very happy with the location of the hotel as it was in a largely residential area with no restaurants or anything much else in the area, so David agreed to move me to a more central hotel. The new hotel was much better, it was the Hotel Bencoolen on Bencoolen Street which itself was just off Orchard Road, much more central and more to my taste. Anyway, David again picked me up and we made our way to MUM's yard; we parked up alongside a two-storey building that looked very like the accommodation block on an offshore structure, it was painted dark blue which was MUM's company colour.

The upper story were company offices with the lower floor being classrooms, David led the way up an external staircase and into the reception area where there was a bubbly and very helpful receptionist, also behind reception was Robert Chua, who was David's second in command. David turned left and went through the door facing him into his office, this was a relatively small room with a big desk which he sat behind, this was his kingdom, there were a number of mementos from his previous life in the Singapore military, there were caps, various small shields denoting events he had been part of as well as a number of photos with him shaking hands with dignitaries. It was a nice office and of course was air conditioned although in my view it was a little too cool, but this was how they seemed to like the temperature in their offices.

After all the introductions David asked Robert to show me around the facility; we left David in his office and made our way back outside into the heat and humidity. Robert took me around the building, we headed to the left through a busy yard with work going on refurbishing various offshore equipment; there was a subsea Christmas Tree, being painted bright red and a lot of other workers carrying out welding and work on other equipment. We walked past all this activity towards the dockside; as we walked, Robert explained the equipment we were passing, there were a number of sub-sea hydraulic ship's cleaning machines, he told me that Metalock's core business was ship maintenance with hull and propellor cleaning forming a key part of their business.

As we were returning back towards the classrooms, Robert stopped at a shipping container; he opened it up so that I could be reunited with all the inspection equipment I had last seen at Interdive. It seemed that David had attended the auction following Interdive's demise and had bought the lot, this included the digital thickness meter (DTM), Cathodic Potential Bathycorrometer (CP meter) and a lot of other diving and ancillary equipment. Possibly the best part of their purchase was that the lot included all the test pieces including the Inter-Ocean 2 nodes, this was great as it meant we would not need to fabricate more.

We spent the rest of the day setting up the diving equipment for the practical part of the course, this was relatively easy as David had bought all the Interdive dive equipment, this meant it was really just a case of putting everything together and testing. One of the main issues for me was the heat and humidity in dive control; the tank was already full of water. The dive control room was situated alongside the tank. The dive control room was accessed via a set of steps down behind the tank; as I entered, the right-hand wall contained a large window looking into the tank displaying the whole of the tank, this window was completely submerged and would be a great vantage point to view the divers at work.

The control room was brightly lit by fluorescent strip lights, as I reached the bottom of the steps, I was faced with a reasonable sized room with a good-sized desk towards the back wall on the left. This was where the dive control panel was situated together with the diver comms box; I thought it would work well. I started fitting the diver's umbilicals to the panel with the comms leads being fitted to the comms box; this took about fifteen minutes, by this time I was drenched in sweat! Working in the control room was like being in an oven, there was no air conditioning, Robert could see I was struggling a bit and disappeared off in search of fans. He returned with two large fans, when installed they did at least make the room bearable although keeping paperwork on the desk might be a struggle, still it could have been worse for sure.

At the end of the day David and Robert decided we needed to go to the military officer's club for sundowners; as I was to learn, this was a common event. Most days we would pop into the club on the way home where we all would have a few beers to round off the day it was very pleasant; the club was very much in the colonial style, with potted ferns next to large marble columns, marble floors and a huge bar area where officers of all ages congregated, some were in uniform but the majority were like David and Robert ex-officers, I think.

To cut a long story short the courses went off very well with all students again being awarded their Lloyd's diver inspector qualification or Lloyd's ACFM qualification depending on which course they had attended. Over the next few years, I travelled to Singapore two or three times per year and the courses became routine; on one of these courses, I was able to catch my wife out though.

I was conducting a course on September seventeenth (our wedding anniversary); I had already arranged for flowers to be delivered to her at work (this got me a bad rep with the males she worked with) and given the time difference between Singapore and home, I called Chrissie at what would be about seven AM UK time to wish her a happy anniversary only to get a grumpy, sleepy response, "what the hell are you calling me at this ungodly hour for." Turns out she had completely forgotten the significance of the date. She did get her own back in April the next year though; I was again conducting a course in Singapore on my birthday; I never made much of birthdays when I was at work but Chrissie took it on herself to call David to inform him of the significance of that date!

He came into the classroom and announced it to everyone on the course, I was then taken out for lunch to a very nice restaurant where we had to eat all the special delicacies like chicken's feet etc., this meant lunch took about an hour and a half instead of the normal half hour. We had to work late that day to catch up; still, there you go, it was nice in some ways although I was taken out again that evening and plied with far more beer than was prudent so had to go through the next day with an awful hangover!

Eating in the evenings in Singapore was not an issue, there were literally hundreds of restaurants to choose from, the Singaporeans all seemed to eat out much more than we in the UK did at that time. On one of these occasions, I remember watching a young couple arrive at their table and spend the whole evening just staring at their own mobile phones; they hardly spoke a word to each other. I thought this was a very strange thing to see a young couple do, I don't know whether they were dating or perhaps married, it just seemed odd to me. At this time in Europe mobile phone use was still very restricted as the costs were so high, obviously nowadays this would seem routine for England as well but not so much then.

I very soon got fed up with always eating in restaurants that were catering to Europeans or local professionals, the menu would have some Singaporean or Chinese dishes but, there were also a lot of European/American influenced dishes as well. I talked to David about this and he suggested I look for hawker's restaurants; these were restaurants where the local working people would eat and so were much more aimed at the local palate. I asked my friendly receptionist at the hotel and was directed to one close by, I found this very easily; there were about fifty plastic round tables with plastic chairs such as we might have on our patio at home. I chose a vacant table and sat down; it was great, the whole place was buzzing, there were almost exclusively Chinese people at the tables.

I didn't have to wait long before a waiter turned up and asked me what I wanted, luckily in Singapore everyone spoke English although sometimes the accent could make them quite difficult to understand; I asked to see a menu, he looked amazed and just turned to the rear of the restaurant where the kitchen was. He swept his arm across what looked almost like a self-service banquette, apparently, I was to go up there make my selection which I should indicate to the guys behind the counter they would then prepare it for the waiter to bring out to me.

At this time all the waiter really wanted was to know what I wanted to drink; I ordered a Singha beer and he toddled off. I made my way up to make my selection, where I was faced with glazed sections behind which were vats of various foods, I had no idea what any of them were so it was real pot-luck. The guy behind the counter caught my eye, he was clearly keen to get on so I selected a couple of likely looking candidates by pointing to them; he then pointed to rice and noodles, I selected boiled rice. He seemed happy with this and just turned on his heel, I was obviously dismissed, I made my way back to my table where my beer bottle was busy making condensation; almost before I had sat down my food arrived.

One of the selections I had made I could now see was chicken, there was half a chicken swimming around in this fragrant brown broth; great I thought, how do I eat that with chop sticks which were the only implements available? I beckoned the waiter over and asked him how I was to cut the chicken up, he said not to worry, he would do it for me! I didn't know what he meant, was he going to bring a knife and cut the chicken up like I might do for a child? Not a bit of it, he returned with a meat cleaver and much to the amusement of the other patrons proceeded to bash merry hell out of the chicken carcase; this was carried out on the plastic table which really was not up to the task. Obviously, it worked a treat and the chicken was soon reduced to manageable chunks; I thanked him, he twirled around to give the cleaver back to the chef and left me to it.

Now, the chicken might have been in manageable chunks but they were still adhered to small pieces of rib and other bones, in short it was not easy to eat with chop sticks and looking around I could see that everyone else was just picking their food up and chewing from their fingers. Of course, this would have been easier than trying to eat from chicken bones that had been annihilated with a cleaver. Oh well it was a learning experience; I spent a lot of evenings at these restaurants where the food was always very good and I never got ill from eating there; the one downside was that as soon as you were finished eating it was clear that the table had to be vacated, but it was very cheap to eat there and a great experience.

On another occasion I was conducting courses at Metalock in February, one of the courses spanned the Chinese New-Year and David invited me to a new year's celebration banquet; this was apparently a very big deal and there were certainly a lot of people there. There was a lot of pomp with Chinese dragons, dancing and a great deal of drinking! The main event was the traditional banquet, we sat down to a circular table of eight, everyone else was Chinese Singaporian and so knew the drill; nobody had told me anything about what this banquet consisted of though and as it turned out this would be to my detriment. The first couple of courses were pretty standard with prawns in their shells followed by a massive fish served on a platter in the centre of the table, everyone dug in taking what they wanted.

Now, I was thinking as an European and thought there would likely be another three maybe four courses maximum and was eating accordingly; this however, was not to be; as course seven arrived I leant across to David and asked him how many courses he was expecting; he calmly replied, "Oh, probably seventeen or so!" Oh, my goodness, where was I going to put it all? From the next course onwards, I just picked at the food making sure I always left a little on my plate to show I had had enough, as is the Chinese way, if you finish everything on your plate, they think you didn't get enough. By the time the final course arrived I was uncomfortably full and very glad when people started to get up from the table bidding goodbye to each other. The venue was not far from my hotel, I had always planned to walk back which I did but I took a very long route to try to relieve some of the discomfort; another lesson learned, what a great evening though.

Running courses overseas was always challenging but the main thing with Singapore was that everything was available and so most challenges could be solved by David going out to buy something. The other thing that was new to me was that they didn't want to work weekends, so, I had most weekends free and used them to visit tourist destinations. I spent one very nice weekend exploring Sentosa island which then was just beginning to become the go to recreational destination for both tourists and locals alike, it was very nice and gave me the opportunity to go to the southernmost point of Asia another box ticked.

On another weekend, Robert Chua took me out on his speed-boat, this was a great opportunity for me to see a bit more of the area, we drove east across the island to a marina in Loyang where Robert kept his boat. It was stored in a high-rise boat park which was another first for me; as we arrived the boat was being retrieved from its storage on the fifth level of a tubular steel structure. The boat was placed in the water alongside a pontoon for us to climb aboard; Robert's boat was a glass fibre dory shaped hull with an eighty horse power outboard motor on the transom. There was an awning covering most of the deck space which was great as it kept the sun off and although I like the sun, it did become quite oppressive, the shade was very welcome.

We made our way towards Palau Ubin island just off the Malaysian mainland where Robert knew of a Kelong (floating fish holding area) that we could visit. As we approached the Kelong all I could see were a mish-mash of floating pontoons with covered areas providing shade for the workers, it looked very dirty with almost no creature comforts in evidence. Robert told me that a number of men would spend weeks living on these pontoons looking after fish that were then sold to local markets or restaurants. As we came alongside Robert asked me to jump onto the pontoon with the bow line which I tied up to a handy cleat; once he had joined me on the pontoon, he chatted to one of the guys who had come to meet us and we were given the tour.

The pontoons had been arranged so that there were square areas of open water between them, when I looked into these areas, I could see that there was netting stretching down from the pontoons on all sides, this made a square netted pen, Robert told me that there would also be netting below meaning that live fish could be stored. The chap who had met us threw some food into the pen and the surface boiled with fish clamouring for food; some of these fish were huge, some tried to climb up the mesh alongside the pontoon, it was a spectacle for sure. We spent a nice hour on the Kelong before it was time for us to make our way back; I had a great day and never lost sight of the fact that I was privileged to have been taken out like this, Robert and David always went out of their way to make my time in Singapore memorable.

Late November ninety-seven was a very busy month for me, firstly I was overseeing a job on the marina in Torquay harbour, the main access walkway support had corroded to a point of becoming unsafe. My company was employed by the owner company, Marina Developments Ltd (MDL); I contracted a structural engineer to design the replacement supports and found a local company to carry out the fabrication. My main job was to be on site to ensure safety and to make sure the job was completed to specification and on time. During the time the work was being carried out the access ramp was out of action meaning the only access for boat owners was via a small tender that MDL put on as a ferry twenty-four hours a day.

Although the owners all seemed to take to this without much negativity clearly it was not an ideal situation meaning there was pressure to get the job done. Unfortunately, at the same time I had also been contracted by TWI to run an ACFM course in Perth, Australia for a company called Surespec. I organised for my good friend Malcolm Vale to oversee the MDL project while I was away; I was only going to be away for some seven days and off I went. The trip was via Heathrow airport with a two-hour layover in Singapore; I was flying Singapore airlines which I liked as although I was again in cattle-class they seemed to be a little more helpful most of the other airlines.

Altogether I was travelling for about twenty-two hours, when I arrived and made my way to passport control the officer clearly didn't believe I had come all this way to stay less than a week. He knew I had come to work but unfortunately, I only had a tourist visa; I was taken to one side and grilled about my purposes for visiting and why couldn't an Australian do the job. After a couple of hours where I had explained that the equipment was manufactured in the UK and had been sold to an Australian company with a week's training being included as part of the sale, they reluctantly agreed to let me enter the country.

When I eventually made my way into the arrival's hall luckily my contact Neil Pennison who was one of the owners of Surespec was still waiting for me, he was clearly very relieved to see me as they had eight of their employees set up for the training due to start on the Monday, I had a clear day to allow me some time to recover from jet-lag. Neil took me to pick up a hire car that I would have for the duration of my stay, he then drove ahead of me to show me where Surespec's facility was and subsequently on to my hotel via a bar where we ate dinner.

It was very nice, the temperature was very pleasant, the sun was shining and I for one was very glad to have finally arrived; after the meal and a couple of beers I was very glad to check in to my hotel get my head down. Neil told me that he would come by in the morning to show me around Perth which was nice of him; the next day having had an awful night's sleep due to jet-lag Neil arrived just as I was finishing my breakfast, we spent the day wandering around Perth and its suburbs; I particularly remember King's Park where there was a wonderful view across the Swan River, it was a lovely laid-back environment, what a place!

The following morning was not so good, I usually find that when I'm flying east the jet-lag is worse during the second night so, I had not been able to sleep much at all. Anyway, after breakfast I drove out to Surespec's facility, luckily, with Australia driving on the left just like the UK it wasn't too difficult and the route back to Surespec was easy to follow. The route took me past the famous WACA cricket ground which at that time was the primary international cricket venue in Western Australia; Perth is truly a lovely place although it is the most remote city in the world, being some three-thousand miles from its closest neighbour city; the climate was great and I was enjoying being there although I was not looking forward to being in the classroom that day.

That first day was a bit of a blur but we got through it somehow, the guys all seemed very keen; I knew one of the students (Reginald) quite well having taught him before; with all of them being existing welding inspectors they were already on top of most of the terminology. The course settled down to a good routine, when we took breaks, we would sit out on the lawn in front where we would be pestered by thousands of flies.

By the evening of the third day, I was beginning to feel almost human again I was now getting over the jet-lag; Reginald asked whether I would like to come to his house for dinner with him and his wife, I accepted and was looking forward to seeing a bit more of Perth. After the course was completed for the day, I went back to my hotel to freshen up before heading south of the Swan River to Reginald's home. On the way I wanted to find somewhere to buy a bottle of wine to take with me, this proved a little more difficult than I was expecting but, eventually I found a small store that was able to sell me a nice bottle of red wine. I found it a little strange to see their window adorned with spray of snow and Christmas decorations when the temperature was high twenties and I felt sorry for the Santa's I saw who were all wearing the traditional gear, dressed up for the cold northern winter but I suppose December is Christmas time so there you go. I was however, a bit shocked at the price of the Australian wine though as I could have bought the same bottle in UK for about half of what I was charged in Perth?

Reginald and his wife were perfect hosts, we had a lovely meal, after the meal Reginald suggested we wander down to McCallum Park which was just down the road from his house. The Park was beautiful, there was a spectacular view of Perth's skyline across the river, it was a lovely balmy evening just like a summer's evening in the Mediterranean, we spent a good hour strolling through the park trying to identify the Southern Cross and other constellations that were unfamiliar to me.

At the end of the week, I flew home, again with just a short layover in Singapore so when I landed in London again, I was feeling the effects of jet-lag on long-haul flights I religiously ensured I stayed hydrated, got up to stretch and walk about every two-hours and didn't sleep at all, but of course this meant I was worn out on landing.

As soon as I got home, I jumped in the car and went over to the job in Torquay to make sure all was progressing well; it was clear Malcolm had done a great job, everything was going very well, the job was going to plan and looked to be finishing on time, what a star. I had to be on the job every day for the next ten days though until it was completed, then I was back off up to Middlesbrough for the last course before Christmas that year, it was all go.

1998 dawned with my workload being much the same, I was back up to Middlesbrough early in January for routine courses and throughout the year this began to snowball with me spending at least fifteen days a month either in Middlesbrough or Ambleside or indeed both. This was coupled with more and more overseas courses including ACFM courses in Houston and Galveston, Texas; by now I had started to use KLM for the majority of my flights, the main reason for this was that they were one of the only airlines who awarded loyalty points for cattle class travel.

The points I was able to accrue were useful firstly as they could be used to purchase flights for private use; I used this facility to take Chrissie to Rome for a long weekend which was lovely. Secondly, points meant that I was rewarded with increased status to the point where I became a gold class traveller, meaning that I was allowed access to their lounges in the various airports this was a very nice perk. When in the lounges I had access to comfortable seating, free food and drinks with much less crowding, this was definitely worthwhile. One of the downsides to travelling with KLM at the time was that their hub was Schiphol airport in Amsterdam meaning that I always had an extra flight out and back to an UK airport normally Bristol in my case although from time to time I would fly from Middlesbrough to Schiphol.

The second problem was that they didn't seem to be able to marry baggage up with travellers very often; it was not at all unusual for me to arrive in Houston to find that my baggage had not made the trip with me. Frequently I would find that the ACFM equipment followed on a later flight, this always added a little to the stress of the trip but, I have to say though, they never actually failed to get the equipment to me in time for the start of the course. I would normally find the box waiting for me in reception of my hotel the next morning. So it was, that I would arrive in Houston without bags, therefore no change of clothes! I got to know the KLM staff quite well as I would head to their desk where they would normally give me fifty dollars to tide me over, ho-hum, such is life.

During February ninety-eight I was contracted to run a 3.4U course in Cumbria and directly from there to go to Middlesbrough to run a 3.2U followed by a supervisor course; twenty-days in total. When I was carrying out courses for Wray Castle, I used to stay at a lovely little guest house right in the middle of the Ambleside. The first few days were fine and were conducted as usual in the Castle, but, in the second week it started to snow to the point that I couldn't get up to the castle at all. The town was very quickly cut-off from the outside world; it was certainly very picturesque and the pubs became even more welcoming for sure. Luckily, all the students were also staying in Ambleside and as none of us could get up to the Castle we completed the course working in the dining room of my guest house, not ideal but it worked.

On the final day, while the snow was still in evidence, it had thawed enough so that I could finally get my car out and make my way across the Pennines to get to Middlesbrough. The trip was a little challenging but as luck would have it one of the students on the 3.4U course also needed to get to Middlesbrough so at least I wasn't alone.

At about this time it became clear that I was spending too much time at Jim's house I had to find somewhere else to stay; I was a little worried by this as I really didn't want to end up in guest houses again. Luckily, I was told to contact Phil Bosten, Phil had moved on from TWI by now but was still contactable. I explained my predicament and he said that his mum might be interested in taking me in as a part-time lodger, Phil was working offshore at the time but we arranged that as soon as he came home, I would meet him at this mum's house in Newton Aycliffe, near Darlington to discuss things.

I subsequently met with Mrs Bosten (Anna) who was a lovely Italian lady who I immediately got on with as I tried to use some of the Italian that I had learned when I was living in Sicily to break the ice, this seemed to work very well. Anyway, all was agreed, I would move in to her spare room whenever I was working in Middlesbrough; I think she enjoyed my being there, she certainly looked after me, cooking wonderful meals for me every evening.

The Russian's are coming: During June of ninety-eight I was due to run Lloyd's diver inspector courses at TWI; these were for a number of Russian divers who were working for Lukoil, Lukoil was the Russian national oil company and so this was a big deal. As was the norm on the first day of any course, I collected my students from the waiting room downstairs, there were six men and one woman, she immediately introduced herself as "I am Katerina, I will be your interpreter for the course."

It seemed that most of the course members didn't speak any English at all so Katerina would be essential, there were two course members who did speak reasonable English though they were Alexsandr Papov and Nikolai Sokolov, they would both become very useful for explaining the finer points to the others on the course. Nikolai was an especially valuable individual to my company as he used us to source and export equipment over the next few years, perhaps most notably we supplied light bulbs for the ROV that they used to try to locate the Kursk nuclear submarine following its sinking.

Katerina, was a striking individual, she was very tall, slim with dark hair. She certainly put the guys on the course in their place whenever she felt they were in her opinion getting out of hand! She wouldn't really be drawn as to how she learnt her English although over the two weeks she spent with us she let slip that she used to be on a Russian trawler cruising up and down the east coast of England.

The course went along very nicely with them all seeming to take on board all the necessary information, Katerina would explain everything in Russian and with the help of Alexsandr and Nikolai we seemed to get the necessary points across reasonably well. Some of the discussions we had over coffee and at lunch were interesting though; it seemed that vodka was an essential for them all; Alexsandr said that they used it as a bit of a cure-all, they certainly had no problem with using vodka and then going diving without any issues.

One of the evenings they invited me to go along to their hotel to take part in an evening of fun and drinking with them; I was nervous as I was sure I would not be able to keep up with them and I would need to be able to drive home afterwards. Anyway, there we all were, including Katerina in one of their rooms at the hotel; they had brought slabs of pig fat with them, there were two types. The first, was cured and the second, was raw salted; I was given a demonstration of how the ritual should go, we were to have a sliver of pig fat, whichever one we wanted, I chose the cured one.

We each had a glass of water and of course the obligatory glass of vodka; Alexsandr demonstrated by throwing the vodka down his throat as a shot, then taking the piece of pig fat and following this with a sip of water! As far as I could see, this was going to end up with everyone drunk before too long; I of course was next to go, I chose to have a small shot of vodka which went down burning my throat as it went, the pig fat was next, as I chewed it was not unpleasant but took me a lot longer than Alexsandr had taken then I finished off with quite a big swig of water. This raised a cheer from them and then everyone else got started; a significant part of the ritual seemed to be that each person had to make a toast before taking the vodka and these tended to get louder and lengthier as the evening progressed.

Before long it was clear that I was not going to be driving anywhere that evening; I resolved to bed down in one of their rooms which they were very happy about. It was a great evening, they were very good company, it remained good natured and convivial throughout. Katerina left us quite early as she felt worn out having been interpreting all day, I didn't blame her and certainly, the following morning I wished I had ducked out early as well, but at least my hangover was just a banging headache making the day's teaching a little challenging. I managed to stay in contact with most of the course members for a long time after the course by means of Facebook but eventually lost contact with all of them.

At this time when I was carrying out training in Thailand it would not be uncommon for me to spend three-weeks out there training a Lloyd's diver inspector (1-week), air supervisor (1-week) and ACFM (1-week).

For one of these planned periods, I had just carried out a ten-day stint in Middlesbrough and had to travel home on the Friday before being at Bristol airport on the Saturday to fly out to Thailand. It would have been better to just fly straight to Thailand from Middlesbrough, but I hadn't seen my family for two weeks and so felt I needed to see them before heading off to the far east. I was able to leave Middlesbrough at one o'clock in the afternoon and all went well until I hit traffic on the A1, everything was at a standstill, this didn't improve until I got to the M5 at Birmingham. The trip was an absolute nightmare taking me just over nine-hours, I got home at ten o'clock at night obviously a long time after the boys had gone to bed but at least was able to see them in the morning as I didn't need to be at Bristol until the evening of the Saturday; best laid plans of mice and men, and all that.

In September ninety-eight I was off to St John's Newfoundland, to conduct another ACFM course for a chap who used to work with Jim at UCL in London. I flew direct from London to St Johns which was actually not a very long flight, something less than four hours as I remember it. Newfoundland is the most eastern part of the north-American continent and so is actually not so far from UK, well, all went well with the flight, I checked in with a lot of luggage, I was taking my normal carry-on bag for clothes etc. But I also had to take an ACFM unit which at the time was a large box about sixty by fifty by forty centimetres and quite heavy; there were a lot of wires for the charger and probes, a steel calibration block and of course all my course notes etc. All of this was checked in with no problem and off I went to find my way to the gate; the flight was fine and all went well on arrival until I made my way to passport control; this is where things started to go a bit pear-shaped!

It seemed that TWI who had organised my visa for this trip had again only got me a tourist visa, the immigration officer was not happy with this as he didn't believe I had made the trip for holiday. I was not surprised as it would have been unusual to come all this way for just one week and also with me travelling on my own with all this kit. I thought, oh no here we go again, I had visions of Gabon all over again. I was taken to a small room by a Canadian immigration official who thankfully spoke English so at least I could make my case to him a little easier than had been the case in Gabon. It turned out that Canada didn't allow any work to be carried out by persons travelling on a tourist visa, this of course made sense.

He asked me to go with him to pick up my equipment luckily the ACFM unit and everything else had arrived safe and sound; once we had found everything, he proceeded to quiz me about what it was for, who owned the equipment, was it mine etc. I explained that I had been asked to carry out a training course for personnel at St Johns, university. He asked me for the name of my contact at the university, as soon as I showed him the letter of invitation everything changed, it seemed that St Johns was a very small town with everyone knowing everyone else; and he knew my contact personally. I was then taken through to the arrivals hall where I was greeted by a very relieved Ewan Garnett my contact; he had been waiting for the two hours it had taken me to be processed, Ewan and the immigration official were clearly old friends and after he had confirmed my story Ewan was told he had to take me to the department of works where they would issue me with the appropriate paperwork.

So, I was in, as we drove away from the airport I was struck by the windswept appearance of the land, it looked to be a cross between Dartmoor and Norway. As we drove into St Johns, he explained that it was a small and very friendly place; we passed through the main town on the way to his office, the appearance was that of a frontier town, everyone seemed to drive large pickup trucks and four-wheel drive vehicles. The place looked lovely, the weather was warm at about twenty-two degrees Celsius although it was a little overcast, Ewan told me that the majority of people worked in either fishing, the oilfield or shipping.

We drove to an industrial area some three miles out of town where my hotel was located, reception was welcoming just as every business hotel is, so, in we went, I checked in dropped off my bags then Ewan took me just a few hundred yards down the road to the unit where the course would be carried out. As we entered the unit, we were greeted by the receptionist who had me sign in, I was issued with the appropriate pass and told the routine for arrival and departure. I was shown the room to be used as my classroom and the area where practical work could be done, it was all fine, I was left on my own to set up, once I was happy Ewan took me back to the hotel where I settled in for my first night in Newfoundland. After a good night's sleep, I was up and breakfasted bright and early, I had told Ewan that I would just walk down to the unit in the morning and as the weather was again bright with a bit more sun today, out I went.

The hotel receptionist said goodbye to me as I left reception, I walked across the car park, on reaching the road I turned left and headed down the hill along the side of the road; within ten minutes I was back at the unit, checking in with my newly issued pass. There were lots of smiles and waves from the people I had met the previous day, I was shown where I could get myself a cup of coffee; at just before nine o'clock the students arrived, there were eight of them. Most of them were offshore inspection workers who were looking to increase their portfolio of inspection techniques with the addition of ACFM, this was great as it meant I didn't need to explain about welds and the basics of inspection to them.

The first and second days went very well, we would work all morning and then at lunchtime, I would be taken in one of their pickup trucks to the local shopping mall where in typical north American/Canadian fashion there was a massive food-hall selling everything from Submarine sandwiches to burgers, chili and everything in between. All the students were happy and very friendly, they called themselves 'Newfies' and again I thought they fit the bill as frontiers men, it was a pleasant few days.

The first couple of nights, I had eaten in the hotel but on the third evening I thought I would walk into town for a change. I always liked to walk following a day in the classroom; I spent most of my evenings when working alone in Alexandria just walking randomly, it was nice to be in the open air and I liked to mooch about the backstreets.

Anyway, there I was setting out from the hotel, I knew the town centre was about three miles away and having been driven out to the hotel away from town I thought I could find my way, I should be in town within the hour which would be fine. I didn't have a map and of course there was still no such thing as Google maps or even mobile phones, the first half-hour was really nice, I loved watching the birdlife flitting to and fro although I didn't see any larger animals. Eventually though it started occurring to me that I should be seeing some indication of town, I hadn't seen any signposts and by the time I had been walking for an hour I knew I had gone wrong somewhere.

I hadn't consciously turned off the major road but perhaps I should have done, by the time I had been walking for ninety minutes I decided I needed to ask someone; however, I hadn't seen a soul, nobody seemed to be walking and although I had passed a number of houses there hadn't been anyone about. I had seen a number of cars but short of leaping in front of one I didn't know whether any driver would stop for me; luckily, after about two hours a taxi hove into view coming towards me. There was nobody in the back of the car and so I thought they might stop for me, I raised my arm and waved to him, joy of joys he pulled over and wound his window down, we exchanged pleasantries and I explained that

I needed to get into the centre of St Johns.

He told me that although he had finished his shift, he didn't mind taking me and invited me to get in; it seemed I had missed the turning and was now some two miles past town. He was a really nice guy, we had a pleasant chat as he drove, he was quite passionate about St Johns having lived there all his life, he asked if I had been asked to 'kiss the cod' yet? I hadn't heard of this but he insisted this was something I should be introduced to, I told him I would ask my course members in the morning, he just sniggered! After fifteen minutes or so I started to recognise some familiar places that I had seen during my drive from the airport my driver told me we were driving down main street; he pointed out a few restaurants that were worthy of his recommendation. I thanked him and asked him how much I owed him, he said "Nah, don't worry I was going this way anyway;" he wouldn't take any money and deposited me outside his favourite watering hole, what a nice man!

The next day didn't go quite according to plan, as soon as I arrived at work the receptionist gave me a note; apparently my wife had been involved in a road traffic accident and could I call her? Straight away I asked to see the manager who was not very happy and didn't want to let me use the phone, however when I explained the reason for the call he changed completely and became very helpful. Within ten minutes I was talking to Chrissie who had collided with a bus just up the road from our house, her car was apparently an awful mess and was certainly undriveable; although she was a little shaken up, she was unhurt and neither of the children had been in the car so they were fine. I asked her whether she wanted me to come home early but she said that wasn't necessary as she would be fine; it was just another example of my not being at home when something went wrong!

The course exams were due to be held on the Friday, but on the Thursday evening the course wanted to take me into town to show me a good time and apparently this had to be done on the Thursday. The ring-leader was Harry, he set it all up, I was just told to be at a particular bar at seven o'clock in the evening; I had learned my lesson and so got a taxi into town. As soon as I arrived it was clear some of the guys had been in the bar for a considerable time, I was presented with a bottle of beer which went down very nicely.

Everyone was now up for a big night, this despite my reminding them all that they had an exam in the morning, of course but was told "how could this be a bad idea?" Harry, it seemed knew everyone in the bar and also knew a great night club that we could go on to; by now I was more than a bit drunk and was just going with the flow. We turned up at this so-called night club to find that it was actually a strip club; Harry sat us all down around the raised stage area and called one of the waitresses over to take our order for drinks.

More beers arrived and the floor show started, there was a procession of pretty girls shedding clothing while we all downed beers. This carried on until one of the girls who had just finished her show and was consequently stark naked shouted "Harry" from the stage; she then proceeded to bounce down from the stage only to deposit herself on Harry's lap where she wanted to be introduced to all of us. She was not in the least self-conscious at being without clothes and spent a good hour chatting to Harry and us before she had to go back to get on with her show. After this, I along with four of the other guys decided to call it a night, we said our goodnights and went off in search of a taxi, the guys knew where to find a cab and as one of the guys was living close to my hotel, we shared the cab, it was a good end to a nice evening.

To this day I have no idea who paid for all of this, I wasn't allowed to put a hand in my pocket at all, I hope they weren't expecting to sway my examination marking by this as that wasn't going to happen. The next day was Friday; examination day; six of the eight guys turned up on time with Harry and one other not arriving until the afternoon. Luckily for them my flight wasn't until the next day so I was able to organise for them to sit their exam in the afternoon; despite hangovers and lateness all passed much to my relief and the next day I was on my way back home.

Another time that I wasn't home for Chrissie was when I had to go to Haugesund in Norway; it was another ACFM job but this time we were carrying out a trial to see whether Remo a workclass ROV could carry out ACFM remotely. It was a good job and ultimately proved that Remo could work the kit, I was there for just over a week before returning home by sea; for this job I was working with TSC the manufacturers of ACFM, we had travelled from their base in Milton Keynes out to Haugesund in a Ford Transit van hired for the purpose. We crossed the north-sea from South Shields on the Tyne to Haugesund ferry, travelling via Stavanger, about a twenty-four-hour crossing; anyway, on the way back I thought I would try to call Chrissie using my brand-new mobile phone.

I had no signal until we were about an hour out of South Shields, as soon as I could I called; the phone was answered by Steven my eldest son who was fourteen at the time, he proceeded to tell me that mum had been savaged by an Alsatian dog! He then told me to hang on and he would get her; well after a few minutes she came on the line to tell me that her bosses' dog had bitten her left forearm quite badly but that she was basically OK. When I got home, I was pleased to see she had full movement of her hand but her arm was heavily bandaged, it was a very nasty bite which took a long time for her to get over; I of course have never been allowed to forget that I'm never there when needed!

Next was Thailand; my first trip to Thailand had been in October 1999 having never been there before I was quite looking forward to the prospect. I had a friend in Mark Shepherd who I had trained on CSWIP diver inspector courses, he was now working for Mermaid Maritime, this was a company located in Pattaya, Thailand; Mermaid's principle, business was in the sale and refurbishment of life-rafts for offshore ships and rigs but, according to Mark they were looking to diversify. Jim and myself had already identified that Indian divers would find it easier and cheaper to travel to Thailand than to UK. Lloyd's diver inspector courses were still very much in demand by Indian divers and so it was decided to work with Mark and Mermaid to set up Lloyd's diver inspector courses in Pattaya. Mark had already set up wet-welding courses with my old friend Mike Pett so I knew they already had a suitable tank for the Lloyd's course practical, I was assured they also had classrooms and everything else we would need.

For my first trip to Thailand, I took my seat in the economy 'cattle class,' section on a British Airways Boing 747 for the twelve-hour flight to Bangkok; the pilot was a bit of a comedian who had some choice lines for the PA system. One of these was when we were just commencing our descent into Bangkok airport; he came across the PA saying "good morning, this is pilot Pete again, we have now started our descent towards Bangkok, we're just getting the manuals down from the shelf so that we can work out how to land this thing, just sit back and enjoy the view". I had a seat on the right-hand side of the aircraft and as we descended into the airport it was clear that it was situated right in the centre of the city. We flew very low over ramshackle dwellings and roads packed with vehicles, the landing was routine with thankfully no excitement; as soon as we were off the runway pilot Pete came back over the PA with: "High again, this is Pilot Pete, you have now completed the safest part of your journey to Thailand, next is probably a taxi or bus on Bangkok's roads so good luck with that!"

Bangkok airport at that time was looking very tired, they were in the process of building a new airport on the edge of the city and so had not been doing much to spruce up this old one recently. I didn't care, it was wonderful to me, as I walked into the terminal it was great to be back in a hot, humid, tropical country again. Passport control was straightforward, I was issued with a three-month visa and was passed through to baggage reclaim. Unusually for me I had brought a suitcase with me this time, it was almost empty though as I had been advised, I would find very good quality and cheap clothes; I was planning on taking a lot of clothes back for all the family.

Customs was again just a formality as I had nothing with me really, as I entered the arrival's hall I was hit by a wall of sound! There were hundreds of people, most of them shouting and beckoning for any arrival to come and purchase whatever it was they were selling. The arrival's hall was not air conditioned and so was very hot, humid and fragrant! I had been told to turn right as soon as I entered the hall and to look for a sign advertising 'Limousine Hire'; almost as soon as I launched into the throng of people, I saw the sign and made my way towards the desk. I of course had absolutely no Thai language so the first thing I said to the chap behind the desk was "do you speak English", he smiled and said "yes of course."

I told him I needed to go to Pattaya he said that would be no problem and would cost one thousand Baht which at the time was about sixteen pounds. I paid the money and was given a piece of paper and told to take it to a guy who would be waiting for me at the exit rail; making my way through the crowd towards the exit I was greeted by another smiling face; he introduced himself but I'm afraid I didn't understand anything he said to me. I gave him the piece of paper I had been given, this seemed to do the job and we were off, I had already purchased a couple of bottles of water as I knew the journey would be at least a couple of hours.

As we came out of the terminal into bright sunshine the temperature took an immediate hike upwards, it was about thirty-two degrees in the shade and extremely humid, I loved it. The driver grabbed my suitcase and made it clear I was to follow him; we made our way to a rank where there were some eight or ten white Mercedes saloon cars. He stopped at the first one in line and opened the passenger door for me, my case was deposited in the boot and we were off. As soon as we were out of the airport traffic closed in around us, I had been advised to tell the driver to take the freeway, there was an extra cost for this but it apparently cut at least an hour off the journey time. The driver nodded that this was fine and headed east out of the city; the traffic was awful, there were tiny three wheeled tuk-tuks, hundreds of taxis, busses and coaches all billowing thick black diesel fumes and thousands of tiny motorcycles and mopeds; all trying to negotiate a two-lane highway.

There didn't seem to be any rules, at traffic lights the two-lanes became six or seven plus motorbikes pushing between wherever they saw a few centimetres of space. As had been the case in Egypt red lights seemed to be solely advisory with drivers inching forward and even driving through, if there was the slightest hint of a space someone (or maybe three) would fill it; I could see what pilot Pete had meant!

At the time the freeway running out of Bangkok was still under construction; for a few miles we were driving beneath raised sections of the new roadway that were yet to be completed. Eventually though we headed up a ramp where there were toll-booths; I paid the toll and we headed out onto an almost deserted motorway above the teeming hordes below. I asked the driver what the speed limit was for this road, he turned to me with a very amused expression on his face and said "how fast do you think this car can go?" It seemed there was no observable speed limit; oh joy! We headed along the raised section of the freeway which took us out of the city but then had to descend back to ground level as we had come to the end of the useable freeway.

From here on we were on two-lane road for the rest of the way. As I've said the road's rules were chaotic and on this two-hour journey I saw at least two accidents, one of these involved a large articulated truck that had run off the road into a ditch.

Still, the countryside was lovely, there were a lot of farmed ponds that I later learned housed shrimp, plus arable plots and a number of cows. Beyond the farms steep hills climbed into the sky, the exposed soil and rocks were deep red which contrasted very well with the tropical trees and foliage; after a couple of hours, night had fallen when we found ourselves entering Pattaya. Pattaya was originally a small fishing village until the Americans started fighting the Vietnam war, Pattaya then became the main place for US military personnel R&R; it must have expanded overnight and has never really looked back. My driver asked where my hotel was, well of course I had no idea, all I knew was that it was called the Weekender; the driver needed to ask someone so he stopped beside what I later found out was his office.

I was left in the car and told he would be a few minutes, while I was waiting, I spent the time watching the motorcycles, often the driver wasn't wearing a crash helmet but almost always he or she would be carrying one either looped around their handlebars or in a basket. The pillion was often not limited to one person, sometimes there would be a whole family behind and in front of the driver, it was crazy but great to see; after about fifteen minutes the driver came back and we were off again.

To this point we had been travelling through commercial districts with warehouses and shops on both sides of the road; but as we got closer to Pattaya proper I started to see bars on both sides of the road; there were hundreds of them, all were small shacks open to the weather. I couldn't see how so many bars could possibly make a living but the further we travelled the more densely packed they became, clearly there would be no problem finding somewhere to have a beer after work. We continued down what appeared to be the main throughfare of central Pattaya, until the driver turned left into a parking lot, in front of me I could see a neon illuminated sign advertising the Weekender hotel, well that is to say it was partially illuminated, several of the letters were no longer lit. The driver parked up right in front of the hotel's entrance, I climbed out and took back my case from him, he waved once and then was gone; I made my way up the steps into an open reception area.

This area was dimly lit, to my left there were a number of rattan easy chairs with drinks tables arranged somewhat haphazardly, to my right was the hotel's reception desk; behind the desk were three young Thai girls all of whom dashed to be the first to greet me. I was presented with a drink of papaya juice even before I had said a word; I told them who I was and after just a few minutes had been booked in and given a room key on an enormous key fob. I was directed towards my room which was past the swimming pool, as I walked past the pool that was behind the foyer and off to my left. I heard my name being called; someone was waving at me from in the pool, I wandered over to see who it was. Mike Pett was grinning up at me from the water, he told me that Mark had said I would be arriving this evening, he told me to put my bag in my room and come for a swim.

This seemed like a nice end to the day so I did just that; I dropped my bag and made a quick phone call to Chrissie just to let her know I had arrived safely; in those days, I would call as soon as I arrived and again just before leaving to go home, other than that we didn't really contact one another; she did of course know where I was if she really needed me. Anyway, after my call I changed into my swimming stuff and went out to join Mike, we had a nice swim for about half an hour before changing and heading to the restaurant for dinner. Mike told me that he was just finishing up a wet-welding course at Mermaid, he felt the facility was very good and that it would be perfect for my courses. Once we had finished dinner, we adjourned to the hotel bar which was alongside the swimming pool where we had a few beers and caught up on old times; before long I made my excuses and headed to bed.

I had not really looked much at my room when I dropped my bag off, now though I could see that it was also looking very tired! It was carpeted with an almost threadbare blue carpet, there was an enormous bed covered in just a sheet, two built-in bedside tables covered in very stained Formica and the noisiest air conditioner I had ever heard. It was though churning out cool air but it rattled and shook; I wasn't sure it would keep going all night. I did have an en-suite shower room but again it could do with some TLC for sure, it would do for this course but I resolved to look about and see whether I could find anything better for the next one.

The next morning, I was up and breakfasted early, I had not slept well due to jet lag but as I didn't have to work today that was not really a problem, Mark was due to pick me up at ten o'clock so that he could show me the facility. He arrived right on time, gave me a warm handshake and was clearly pleased to see me; we made our way out to the car park where he had left his pickup truck. He told me Mermaid's facility was situated in a bonded zone at the Laem Chabang Port about half an hour to the north, we set off with Mark giving me a running commentary of Thailand, Thai driving and everything we passed on the way.

It soon became clear that the area was poor, there were a lot of shanties with people obviously living hand to mouth, everywhere looked extremely run down, with the exception of the Buddhist temples we passed, these were all beautifully painted in bright colours and were very well kept. The other thing that was clear was the love of their King, there were photographs and paintings of him and his wife everywhere; Mark told me he was an extremely benevolent ruler who was loved by all the Thais, he was though quite old and it was not certain what would happen when he eventually died.

We eventually made it to the free-port area of Laem Chabang with Mark stopping at the guardhouse where he just acknowledged the guard and was waved through. He turned right at the first junction and then again right into Mermaid's yard; it was bustling with activity, there was a large building with huge roller shutter doors. There were a number of cars and pickups all parked in an orderly line; these spaces were all shaded by a bamboo canopy much the same as I had seen before in many Mediterranean towns. Mark parked his truck in a reserved space making sure it was shaded from the sun, we got out and started walking back towards one of the building's roller doors; as we entered, I saw the floor was painted light blue, towards the left-hand side there was a walkway delineated from the main floor by a painted red line. Mark told me that to the left of the line was for normal foot traffic but to the right special footwear must be worn; this was because life-rafts were being tested and repaired in that area and there must be no foreign objects introduced to them that could cause puncture.

We climbed a set of metal stairs leading up to the first floor where the offices were situated, at the top of the stairs we turned right walking along past the director's offices which were all on our left, to our right I could look down on life-rafts being laid out and checked. Ahead of us there was a door through which were more administration offices and the room I was to use as my classroom. The classroom was nice and bright, there was a window looking out over the car park, an air conditioner that was clearly a much newer version than the one in my hotel room. There was a clean whiteboard with pens, tables and chairs enough for twelve students, a table for me at the front together with a nice new overhead projector, in short everything I needed for the theory side of the course was there.

Mark then took me downstairs where he showed me the tank that was currently being used by Mike's course, we made our way into dive control where Mike was talking to his diver. Although dive control was not huge it was definitely more than good enough for my needs, all was good; Mark then led me through to his office which he shared with another ex-student of mine, Gareth Vickery. Gareth was Project Manager for Mermaid; this meant he managed diving projects for them, I didn't have a great deal to do with Gareth other than to meet up with him in the evenings from time to time.

My course was due to start the following day and Mark told me that he had arranged for a mini-bus to collect the students at my hotel; they were not all staying there but they would meet there to be picked up. This sounded great to me, I just needed to be in the car park at eight o'clock in the morning, simple. He then took me back to the hotel and left me to my own devices, I would see him in the morning at Mermaid; I decided to have a look around the streets by the hotel. I dropped my bag off in my room and headed out to explore, I stopped at the top of the steps in front of the hotel, immediately in front of me was the hotel's car park, beyond that was the road which at this point was a good forty feet across (12 metres). On the other side of the road were a number of bars, I decided to go and have a beer in one of them; I took my life in my hands as I crossed the road but it seems that rather than the European way where I could easily have been run down,; no, here it seemed that cars and motorbikes would turn to avoid me without any issue!

So, there I was on the other side of the road, as I looked at the many bars, I just chose the nearest one which was approached by a small flight of steps. As I walked up to the bar I saw that it was garish in its lighting, all bright reds and yellows, it had a rough wooden bar fronted by seven or eight bar stools; behind the bar there were four pretty young Thai girls who were either sitting chatting to customers of were huddled at the back of the bar eating from bowls of noodles.

Clearly, the bar had been open for some time but it was not busy; there were just three men sitting on bar stools, they all were deep in conversation with one of the barmaids and ignored me. I chose a bar stool on the right-hand side towards the other end of the bar counter; as soon as I sat down one of the bar girls came over and in broken English asked me what I would like. I ordered a local beer and settled down to watch the passers-by; she however was having none of that, she pulled a board game out from under the bar and proceeded to start a game with me?

I was told later that this was a ploy to get me to drink more and to perhaps invite her out with me; I know, I was again quite naïve but, I was new here. Anyway, I had a couple of beers with the game and then Mike turned up; he suggested going elsewhere, we jumped down from the bar onto the road where Mike raised a hand to a blue pickup truck; even though the truck was in the far lane it immediately braked pulling across the traffic to stop right beside us. Mike leaned in and paid the driver twenty Baht (about 30 pence), turning to me he told me to follow him, we went around to the rear of the truck where he climbed inside. I followed him, there were two wooden bench seats one running along each side of the pickup; I sat on the bench on the right with Mike sitting opposite. There were another four people in the back of the truck, three of them were locals and the fourth looked European; he immediately struck up a conversation with Mike, it seemed he had also just arrived but it was his fourth trip to Pattaya so he was an old hand.

The pickup truck was one of a large number that constantly circulate a fixed route, you paid a fixed rate and sat in the back until the truck came to the destination where you wanted to get off; once there you would press a bell push which rang a bell in the cab the driver would then pull in to the side of the road where you would jump off. Mike told me we were going to 'Walking Street', this was a part of the beachside road where there were a lot of bars and clubs; I sat back to enjoy the journey. It was quite an eye opener, there were a lot of young white men riding big motorcycles far too fast weaving in and out of the traffic, none of them were wearing crash helmets or any other protective clothing, I thought it was an accident waiting to happen. It seems I was right as Mike told me he had already seen a lot of bad accidents, apparently the bikes were hired, there were really no checks as to whether the hirers could actually ride a bike at all!

The pickup turned left down a fairly large side road and then left again onto Beach-road; night had fallen by now but I could see that there was a beach off to my right, we were travelling south alongside the beach. On the other side of the road were hundreds more bars and girlie clubs; there were hundreds of people, again it was chaotic; the majority appeared to be youngish Caucasian males but there were a lot of young Thai people as well, most of these were female. As we drove down Beach-road the bars were replaced by tourist shops and markets, they seemed to be selling 'T'-shirts, jeans and various bric-a-brac. I would later frequent these shops where I would buy a lot of 'T'-shirts for the family, they were obviously fake but nonetheless were of good quality and above all cheap! No-Fear shirts for one hundred Baht (£1.20); of course, there were also the fake Rolex, Pierre Cardin and the rest.

Very soon, we arrived at the extreme southern end of Beach-road where the pickup again turned left to take it back for the remaining part of its circuit; Mike pressed the bell and when the driver had stopped, we jumped off. Walking street is just that, it is a pedestrianised roadway where traffic is not supposed to be allowed of course this was Thailand and so there were always some cars, motorbikes and the inevitable tuk-tuk, but they all travelled very slowly and pedestrians were definitely in control. Walking street was a real eye opener for me, both sides of the street were lined with bars, some huge but the majority were just maybe five or six metres wide; they were thronged with customers, the place was heaving even though it was only just gone six-thirty in the evening!

As we walked down the road, we were constantly accosted by young Thai girls some of whom were stunning to look at, Mike told me that the really pretty ones were often not actually girls! He led me down to a bar on the left where he said we could sit and would be left alone by the prostitutes; apparently this bar was owned by an Australian woman who would not allow her customers to be harassed. So, we found a couple of bar stools and ordered beers; I turned to the street and just watched everything passing by; we spent a nice couple of hours catching up and of course putting the world to rights before making our way back to the hotel.

The first week had been a Trainee Air Diving Supervisor course, this had gone without any issues, all students passing with flying colours; the second week was to be a Lloyd's diver inspector course with six students so on the Friday afternoon I spent a couple of hours making sure everything was in place ready for the start of the course. The weekend was free for both Mike and I and Mark who was conscious that I had not been to Thailand before had planned some excursions for both of us. Saturday was another beautiful day, April was a nice time of year to be in Thailand; I met Mike for breakfast which was a leisurely affair taken in the thatched restaurant overlooking the pool; as you can imagine, it was hell!

Mark turned up at about ten o'clock, we all clambered into his truck and off we went, he told us that he was taking us to an elephant farm. When we arrived, I suppose it might be termed a farm but it had the appearance of being mainly a tourist attraction where the elephants were on display. Mark paid for a bunch of bananas each for Mike and I but almost as soon as he had handed my bunch to me one of the elephants started to show a great deal of interest in me. She put her trunk into my pockets and all around my torso looking for bananas; I gave her one but she wasn't going to leave me alone until I had given her the rest of the bunch! We all then took our place on tiered bench seating facing a large arena where we were treated to elephants playing football and other silly pursuits; when there was a pause in the proceedings a couple of elephants were encouraged by their handlers who were riding on the elephant's necks to step onto the benches between the spectators. They climbed up the tiers with their trunks searching out anyone who still had bananas, when they found some, they would grab them with their trunk and immediately pass them up to their handler who took them probably to re-sell to more punters.

When the show was finished, we were encouraged to wander onto the arena where one of the elephants was giving tourists a lift, Mark paid the handler and his elephant curled his trunk around my waist; he was extremely gentle and although he was gripping me, he did not squeeze me at all really. As soon as he had me in a comfortable clutch, he lifted me above his head, when he had put me gently back on the ground he moved over and repeated this for Mike; I must confess that I enjoyed this and the elephant was rewarded with bananas so I think he was reasonably happy as well.

We had spent a good couple of hours at the elephant farm before we got back into Mark's truck, next we were then taken to the 'biggest Buddha in Asia'; this in fact turned out to be an image of Buddha sitting cross-legged, with one hand resting on his knee and the other in his lap, the image had been engraved into the northern face of Khao Chi Chan. A solitary limestone hill to the South of Pattaya; the hill used to supply the local construction industry with materials. In 1996, in order to commemorate the King of Thailand's golden jubilee, there was a one-hundred-and-nine-metre tall, seventy-metre-wide image carved into the rock, the image was then etched in gold, as it was felt that and I quote the Thai tourist board; "otherwise it would be a total waste of a perfectly good and particularly beautiful mountain."

In the evening, we were joined by Mark's lovely Thai wife, we were taken to a particularly pleasant hotel some way south of Pattaya; here we dined on a raised wooden deck sitting over a calm sea with Khram Yai Island out in the distance; it was a lovely end to a great day.

When finally, the courses were finished, I was put into a taxi for the trip back to the airport, again as was the norm, I was to fly home in the evening of the final day so, I had done a full day with the course and was due to fly sometime close to midnight. I was deposited at the airport at about eight o'clock in the evening and started to make my way through the check-in and passport control to leave Thailand, unfortunately nobody had thought to mention that there was a tax of five-hundred Baht to be paid in order to be allowed to leave Thailand! Well, of course I had thought I was being very clever in that I had arrived at the airport with almost no local currency left.

The normal method of payment was via a vending machine positioned adjacent to the door between departures and the duty-free area; of course, these machines only accepted notes. I turned on my heal and looked for somewhere to buy some more Baht, there were a few currency exchange kiosks but the first three I found were all closed; I had to walk quite a distance before I found one that was open and by this time, I was getting close to the boarding time of my flight. Eventually I was able to purchase my leaving ticket and by running managed to get to the gate just as it was closing, that was close, still, another lesson learned; this requirement has now been dropped so nobody has to pay to leave any more.

Since I had been working with TWI from time to time, I would be asked to represent them at various events. TWI had joined the new inshore diving association this was the ADC, the Association of Diving Contractors. The ADC represented inshore and inland diving companies, it had no interest in offshore diving or companies so was much more relevant to TWI. ADC would meet quarterly and it was not unusual for me to be asked to go along, in May of 2000 I duly arrived in a hotel in Birmingham for their meeting. On arrival I found about twenty others, we were then told that we were all going to be invited to sit the pilot of their new Inland/Inshore Diving Supervisor examination. Well, I wasn't that keen but really couldn't say no, I was hoping that teaching the offshore version should prepare me quite well but you can never be sure of these things, can you? We sat through the normal meeting where the routine business was taken care of, then were given a bit of a brief as to what to expect.

We had some lunch after which we all sat down for the examination, now it really didn't matter at all whether I passed or not, other than they all knew what I did for a living. This meant that I felt a bit apprehensive and wanted to put on a good show, as soon as I turned over the page, I could see that it had been formulated in a similar way to the IMCA exams. The questions were all multiple-choice, I worked methodically through all of the questions finding them relatively straightforward, at least I thought so! As soon as we had all finished, the exams were to be marked with results being given to us before we would be leaving that afternoon. We all adjourned to another room where we had cups of coffee and of course the obligatory biscuit; after about half an hour Roger O'Kane came into the coffee room where he proceeded to tell us without any pre-amble or ceremony that we had all passed, what a relief! I was subsequently issued with my certification certificate number six.

One memorable trip to Thailand took place in April 2001; I was no longer staying in the Weekender hotel which was now in the throes of being torn down for redevelopment, instead I was staying in a much quieter and therefore in my view nicer hotel called the Sabai Lodge, this was situated not far from the Weekender down a side street between Beach Road and Pattayasaisong Road. My trip to Pattaya was no different from any of the other trips however on the Monday morning of the first week's course it was clear something was different, as before I was picked up by mini bus at my hotel, there was a difference though; even at this early time in the morning it was bedlam outside the hotel.

I was stunned as there were hundreds of people all throwing water over each other and indeed anyone and everyone; what was going on? Well, it turns out I was experiencing Songkran; this had originated as an Hindu festival marking the arrival of the new harvest season in ancient India. Nowadays though it is a week-long celebration marking the Buddhist-new-year; it was truly amazing, of course I had no clue as to what was going on at the time, but I climbed into the bus together with my students and we were driven out to Mermaid's base. All along the route there were pickup trucks with at least half a dozen people in the back armed with water soakers! Each truck had a water bowser or at least a large tank full of water in the back so that everyone could reload their water pistols; they would drive along soaking everyone they came across.

Everyone was in extremely high spirits including the people getting soaked beside the road, it was stunning to be witnessing this spectacle, I along with my students were treated to water being sprayed over our bus repeatedly, we were bemused. On arrival at Mermaid Mark cleared up what was happening for me which I then passed on to the rest of the course; what a laugh!

That evening, Mark told me we would wander down to walking street again to experience Songkran in all its glory. When the course had finished for the day, I went to Mark's office where he was sitting with Gareth who was somewhat less enthusiastic about Songkran; I suppose once you've experienced it maybe it can become somewhat tiresome to be soaked every time you set out of the office, house or anyplace else! He went on to tell me that this would go on for a full week and he for one couldn't wait for it to be over! In the mini bus on the way back to the hotel we were again treated to the full spectacle of hundreds of marauding pickups filled to bursting with super-soaker water pistols. At intervals along the road there were huge bowsers parked up where the pickups could replenish their water supplies, the whole thing clearly had official local support.

Mark came to my hotel at seven o'clock and we made our way to walking street where we found a bar (not hard), ordered beers and set about entering into the spirit of the event. The bar had enough super-soaker water pistols for all customers and there were a couple of huge bins full of water for replenishment; everyone who wandered past the bar was subjected to a barrage of water not only from us but from every other customer in all the bars along the way. We of course had been soaked from the moment we left the hotel I had left everything that I didn't want to get wet in my hotel room so there we were dripping wet having a ball! It was impossible to have anything approaching a conversation but who cared, it was great fun. As I say this went on for the whole week and I have to say that by the end of the week I was beginning to understand Gareth's point of view, I had tired a little of always being wet especially as it was quite difficult to transport my books and laptop computer to and from the hotel.

During August of 2001 we made what we felt may be the last family holiday with both our boys; Steven was by then seventeen years old and James was fifteen. Both Chrissie and I felt it was unlikely that they would both want to spend holidays with their parents for much longer, this being the case we had decided to do a real bucket list holiday. We were going to take them to Kenya where we would stay in a luxury hotel; during this time the boys could undergo SCUBA training and we would take a safari for a few days. We planned for a three-week trip and had booked a wonderful hotel, this was the Kaskazi Beach hotel on the outskirts of Mombasa; it was a beautiful hotel that had been recommended to us by Chrissie's boss and proved to be a great find.

On return from our epic holiday, I had to go back to work but it was a much-refreshed Peter who went back after this break. Over the coming few years, I made on average three trips per year to Thailand and a similar number to Singapore; it was while on my way home from one of these trips that I encountered what could have been a very significant problem. As was the norm, I was seated in cattle class again, this time I had an aisle seat which was nice as it meant I could stretch out a little more; after the meal was served and having had a couple of glasses of wine I settled down for the night. I should say that it was extremely unusual for me to be able to get any sleep on flights, this had nothing to do with anxiety, it was more about being unable to get comfortable.

This evening though I fell asleep before the end of the in-flight film and didn't wake up until several hours later when we were just starting our descent into London. On waking up I felt fine, it wasn't until I stood up and started walking off the plane that I noticed anything unusual; my right-leg felt heavy and full, it was like everything was a bit swollen? I didn't think much of it and hurried through passport control and baggage reclaim in a rush to get home; all went well, I was soon back on Reading railway station waiting for my train to carry me back to Devon. My leg was still feeling odd even when I got off the train in Newton Abbot, but again I didn't think too much about it. I had arrived home in the early afternoon on Saturday and was due to travel back to Middlesbrough on the following Tuesday; as was the norm I drove up to Middlesbrough arriving on Tuesday evening.

There was a 3.1U course starting on the Wednesday and all went fine until Friday, at the time I was a member of the British Institute of Non-Destructive Testing (BINDT); I used to attend their meetings when I was in Middlesbrough. On this Friday evening there had been a special event organised at NUTEC survival school; NUTEC ran survival courses for offshore personnel and the BINDT evening was to give our membership the chance to see something of what offshore workers had to go through. I went along with Jim, we were treated to a tour of their very impressive facility, there were of course classrooms with heaps of equipment such as scoop stretchers and the like.

Ultimately though we were shown into their pool area; this consisted of a very large swimming pool which was used for all types of survival scenarios. The pool area could generate wind, rain and significant wave action all of which could be in the dark when lights were extinguished, this made the scenarios that much more realistic and challenging. Luckily though we were going to attempt HUET, this was Helicopter Underwater Escape Training but with calm conditions that were lit very well. I had done this before and was looking forward to it as a bit of fun, but I could see that some of the guys were not looking so comfortable, I had always been very impressed by non-divers and sometimes non-swimmers who went through this training as it must have taken incredible guts.

Anyway, we were all lined up on the side of the pool, each dressed in a set of coveralls, we would not have any kind of face mask, first we were to watch a 'dry run' of the HUET simulator, the simulator was a mock-up of a helicopter fuselage; slowly it was lowered into the water. When it was completely submerged the operator pulled a lever causing the HUET to rotate until it was completely inverted, the instructor told us that we were to wait until the HUET had come to a complete stop then the person closest to the window should knock the window out and swim to the surface. This sounded fine to me, as I say those of us that were used to being underwater should have no problem but some of those that were not so comfortable might struggle a little; indeed, a couple of the older BINDT members decided to give it a miss at this point.

I was to be one of the first to have a go so six of us climbed into the HUET, there were two rows of three seats, I took my place in the middle seat and had made up my mind that I would head out of the left-hand window when the time came. There was a staff member sitting on a jump seat in front of us, he had a half mask on and had a SCUBA set so that he could offer help to any of us who needed it. We were to do two drops, for the first the HUET would not roll over, all we had to do was to wait for it to stop being lowered before swimming out to safety, this went very well with us all swimming to the side of the pool where we climbed out onto the side while the HUET was lifted back to its start position.

We then headed back in for the second go, this time the HUET would roll over simulating a helicopter ditching in the sea. As we had been briefed, as soon as we were all seated and had attached our seat belts I laid my arm across the back of the seat to my left, this meant that even if I became disoriented, I would know which way to swim, and could use the seat-back to pull myself towards the exit window; as the HUET was lowered I prepared to take a deep breath; the water started to flood into the HUET around our feet, it continued to be lowered with the water level rising.

Eventually as the water was almost to the ceiling of the HUET, I took my last breath and held it waiting for the HUET to come to a rest, I kept my eyes open so that I could keep track of proceedings, the operator on the surface pulled the lever allowing the HUET to rotate. After a short while we were completely inverted and came to a stop; I released my seat belt and waited for the guy to my left to knock the window out, I watched him climb out of the window leaving space for me to follow; it took me no time at all to pull myself through the open window and to swim up to the surface where of course I was again able to take another breath.

I think those of us who completed the exercise all enjoyed it as there were a lot of smiling faces, maybe that was relief at having finished it? We were then dismissed and headed for the changing room, when I peeled off my coveralls, I noticed that the veins on my right leg from thigh downwards had become black, very marked and solid to the touch. I wasn't sure what this meant but when I showed it to Jim, he felt that I should probably get it looked at; we drove back to Jim's house and I got straight into my car and headed to A&E at Northallerton hospital.

As always in A&E there were a lot of people in the waiting area when I entered; I waited at the reception window where my details were taken, as soon as I had described my symptoms I was told to sit down and wait to be seen. I thought I was likely to be waiting for quite some time but, within a few minutes a nurse approached me with a wheelchair; after confirming my name and date of birth she told me to get into the wheelchair. I protested that I could walk but she was having none of that making me sit in the chair, as soon as I was sitting, she pushed me through to cubicles where a doctor was waiting; I was now beginning to get a little worried as this seemed very unusual, I mean the doctor was waiting for me? I was told to take my trousers off and to get up onto the bed where the doctor inspected my leg, this took just a few seconds he then spun on his heel and beckoned the nurse to follow him.

They had a short conference outside the cubicle none of which I could hear, the nurse then returned and told me that I was going to be admitted for tests! What! I couldn't be admitted, I had a course to run tomorrow; she was adamant that I was going nowhere, apparently, I had a blood clot in my leg? I asked whether I could get up and make a phone call, I had to warn Jim, she told me that under no circumstances was I to get up off the bed and that she would get me a phone. Very soon a phone was wheeled in and I was told to make my call quickly; well, I was quite shaken at this point but I made the call, Jim was also shocked but he was extremely good about it all and told me not to worry as he would field the course for me.

Within the next hour I was seen by two more doctors who prescribed Heparin shots which a nurse administered, then I was taken up to a ward, all the time I was told not to move too much as apparently dislodging the clot could be fatal! Eventually, I found myself in a ward together with some nine other chaps all of whom seemed to be in varying degrees of consciousness, some were bright eyed and others were asleep. I was assigned a nurse to keep an eye on me, she was a very nice young Indian lady, I asked her whether she saw many people with blood clots, she told me she had never seen one until she came to England but now, she saw a lot of them. Most of them were suffered by long distance truck drivers or as was my case people who had been on long-haul flights; it seemed our lifestyle was the major contributor.

The time now was almost eleven o'clock when my nurse came over to tell me that my wife was on the phone; I made to get out of bed but was told to stay there and they would bring the phone to me; Jim had apparently called her to tell her what was going on, she was understandably upset. We had about a five-minute call during which she told me she would be coming up to see me the next day, Jim had offered for her to stay at their house; I was not in a good place and was wondering how long I would have to stay in hospital. After Chrissie's call I thought, the ward was starting to wind down for the night but Jim and his wife Norma turned up just to see how I was doing.

It was so nice of them to come to see me; I thanked them for calling Chrissie and agreeing to put her up. I was able to brief Jim on what the course would need from him over the next few days, he seemed quite happy to take this on, they bade me good night and left. I had a largely sleepless night, partly worry but mostly the ward was never quiet or dark really; anyway, at six o'clock we were 'woken' up to get us ready for the day; my nurse told me that I was scheduled for an ultrasonic check of my leg to see where the blood clot was and to formulate a plan of what to do about it.

So it was that at nine-thirty I was wheeled down to the ultrasound suite where a chap in a white coat proceeded to coat my leg in ultrasonic couplant gel, ran an ultrasonic probe up and down all the veins in my leg. I have to say that my leg already felt a lot better and the veins seemed to be less visible this morning so I was quite hopeful. He took only about twenty minutes to complete his examination and proclaimed me to be OK; I was very glad if a little surprised. I was then wheeled back up to the ward where I had to wait to be seen by a doctor; I spent the morning being bored with nothing to do, I had no books and the only magazines I could find on the ward seemed to be aimed more at women. I was told that the consultant's round would be late afternoon and after that they would decide what needed to be done with me.

At about four o'clock I saw Chrissie, Steven and James walking onto the ward; they had apparently managed to get a very early train; our reunion was a little tearful which seemed to confuse the boys but it was really nice to see them. Eventually, the doctor turned up and told me that the blood clot had apparently been broken up by the Heparin injections, he said that I should be fine to go home. I asked him about why he thought I had been affected like this, he was quite philosophical really, he said long-haul flights were not good for us; he told me that in future I should take seventy-five milligrams of Aspirin per day, wear flight socks for long-haul flights and not stay seated for more than two hours at a time on a flight. He also told me that I shouldn't carry my wallet in my back pocket as this could press on the vein in my rear end. He thought this could have caused a lowering of flow leading to the clot, he said that sometimes even a seam in the trousers could cause this to happen! We left the hospital and stayed at Jim and Norma's that night, Chrissie drove home the following day and I took the next couple of weeks off.

Between 1996 and 2002 I took on a number of inspection contracts for some of the larger projects in the southwest; these were great for me as it meant that I could work the project and still go home each day.

The first major project I took on was 'mothballing' of an elderly atomic submarine HMS Valiant; this submarine had been taken out of service and was lying alongside in one of the basins at Devonport Dockyard. My friend Mike Pett whose company Hydroweld had won the contract to produce the subsea welds; the contract required that a proportion of the produced welds would need to be inspected. Hydroweld was at the time by far and away the market leader in underwater wet-welding, they were able to produce welds that were almost as good as those produced in air on the surface. The welds needed visual inspection, photography and a percentage of the welds also needed to be subjected to scrutiny with MPI. With Mike's blessing my company won the contract as underwater inspection contractor, so it was that I arrived on site in April ninety-six armed with all required inspection equipment, computer generated datasheets and procedures.

I set to work checking everything was as it should be only to find that the principal contractor UTEC run by Brett Vardy was not prepared to pay me our agreed day rate for days when inspection wasn't being carried out. I was not happy with this as I had thought I was being employed at this enhanced rate for every day worked. Happily, once Brett realised that I was also a qualified diving supervisor he agreed to swap me onto the night shift as a diving supervisor at the enhanced rate for every day; the night shift was better with respect to inspection anyway so this worked out very well.

The main issue for me was that the night shift ran from eighteen hundred hours until 0-six hundred in the morning, I would then have to drive home and go to bed during the day. I actually preferred working night shifts when offshore as the cabins normally would be quiet and dark during the day, but the same could not be said for my house. It was hard to impress on the boys who were just eleven and nine at the time that they had to keep quiet so dad could sleep, this was particularly a problem at the weekends. Still, it all progressed well and the job was completed in good time with the submarine's ballast tanks and other assorted areas being sealed with welded plates as required.

In 1999 metalwork in harbours around the south-coast of UK was under attack from accelerated low water corrosion, this was an issue affecting steel, there was of course a great deal of steel used in the construction of harbours and the like. The issue was caused by sulphate-reducing-bacteria; these little bugs would take electrons from the steel so that they could use sulphates in the environment for nutrition; these bugs were especially prevalent at or around the extreme low water level. This resulted in steel at the extreme low water level corroding much more rapidly than the norm, holes started appearing which of course was not good.

My company won the contract to inspect welds produced during refurbishment of Brixham harbour, for this job my client was Torbay Council, I had met with the council engineers very early on in the project to discuss their options. They decided to use a company that would fit replacement plates over the affected areas, these plates would be fixed in location by welding. The plates would extend below the low water mark which meant that some of the welds would need to be welded below water level; the company that won the contract was not a diving company and did not plan to use divers at all. They were going to be using a 'Coffer Dam'.

The system they were using was quite ingenious. The coffer dam was U-shaped with the bottom end being contoured to fit around the shape of the Larson piling that made up the dock wall, the dam was some ten metres long, and was lowered into position with a crane, the crane then swung so that the sides of the U were against the dock wall; there was a rubber seal between the dam and the wall, this would produce a seal. Once the dam was in position pumps fitted to the bottom of the dam would be started, these would pump out the seawater from the coffer dam; as the water was sucked out of the coffer dam water pressure outside the dam would press the dam against the dock wall and inside the dam would be 'dry'. Well, I say dry but in fact the seals never completely sealed against the wall so there was always some leakage but, it was certainly dry enough for the plate to be lowered into place and to be welded using conventional welding procedures.

My job initially had been to advise the council on types of welds required and then levels of inspection appropriate; I was also able to advise them on methods of subsea corrosion protection that would be able to reduce if not stop a repeat of this problem. The system ultimately chosen was an Impressed Current system, this involved applying an electrical current to the metal from the surface, the level of current impressed on the metal would be dependant, on submerged surface area, environmental temperature and remaining paint coatings.

It was decided that I would be given a certain number of days for inspection; I would turn up unannounced to inspect plates randomly, this worked very well and I think resulted in a well-controlled repair.

As I say I had been given a certain number of days to be spread randomly throughout the contract, the company carrying out the work never knew when I would be coming and so, hopefully they would always carry out the work to specification. On the day that I turned up I would liaise with the harbour master whose office I would use to write my reports.

I would go down into the coffer dam to inspect any welds completed on that day. Inspecting inside the coffer dam was fine, I would be given the nod when the weld was complete and would climb down the metal ladder fixed to the inside of the coffer dam; as I say it was not really completely dry and I did get a little wet each time but not too bad really. The floor of the coffer dam was constructed using 'Texas Plate' similar to some of the offshore rigs, this allowed water to easily pass through the plate to the pumped out. I would climb down to meet with the welder where I would measure the weld and carry out visual inspection to check for any visual anomalies, if I found something I would point it out to the welder who would carry out repair there and then. This worked very well and the operation became quite slick; when I had completed the inspection, I would climb back out of the dam which they would then reposition for the next plate.

Unfortunately, before the job was completed the company operating the coffer dam system went into receivership and could not carry on; this left the council in a difficult position, after some considerable searching another company could not be found to continue using the coffer dam system. This left them with little choice but to look for a diving company to complete the remaining plates with wet-welding, I suggested Hydroweld but it seemed that the council were under some pressure to employ a local company. Eventually, the local company started work, I had a meeting with them to make sure they understood the quality and standards of weld expected. They had ruled out using Hydroweld's FS proven welding rods and had decided to use older technology, I was very sceptical of their being able to produce the required standard of weld using this technology but, they were given the go-ahead anyway. I was due to go on our annual two-week holiday while they were still going to be welding; the council were happy with this but I would have to inspect their welds on my return.

We had a great holiday on a Greek Island, Skopelos, where we were able to witness a partial eclipse of the sun, of course if we had stayed at home, it would have been an almost total eclipse in Devon. Anyway, as planned we returned home late on the Saturday afternoon two weeks hence; almost as soon as we arrived, I received a call from the owner of the diving company. He told me that they had virtually completed all welding and required me to attend for the necessary inspection; well as you can imagine I was not keen but, I had no choice so it was that at six-thirty in the evening I gathered up my equipment and made my way to Brixham harbour.

When I arrived, the team were working from a dumb barge (not powered) this was tied up alongside steps on the outside of the harbour, I was told that the welder was just finishing up and they would soon be ready for me to jump in and have a look. I sat alongside the supervisor and listened to what was going on, well, it sounded to me like things were not going well; I could tell by the way the generator was reacting that the welder was having trouble maintaining a steady arc. It was clear that the rod was sticking repeatedly, this normally would not produce a good weld but, we would see.

Well, it took a lot longer than I or I think anyone else was expecting and it was not until eleven-twenty-five that I eventually left surface; of course, by now it was fully dark but the hat I was using (KMB10) was fitted with a hat-light so I could see perfectly well. I made my way down the line to the work-site, the visibility was good, I could see about three metres which meant that when I arrived at the weld to be inspected, I could see it very well. What I saw stunned me! I was faced with a truly dreadful weld; it was so bad that I didn't know where to start with my report; before leaving for Greece, I had given the company authority to pack any root gap greater than two millimetres (separation between two pieces to be joined at the base of the weld) with thin strips of metal which they were then to weld over.

They had taken this to an extreme, I was looking at a section of square bar welded alongside the plate and when I say welded it was such a poor weld that I wasn't sure it would even seal the plate from ingress of seawater; it was truly awful. It was obvious that the welder had not been able to maintain a steady arc, there were big clumps of weld material sitting one on top of another, there was a lot of slag included in the weld, in short it was so bad that I couldn't find anything good to say about it. I stayed for no more than ten minutes and then told the supervisor I would be coming back to the surface; when on deck again, I explained the problem to the supervisor who was also the company owner.

He told me he would put the welder back in and make it right, I was not sure this was going to be possible but agreed they should try. I stayed with them until three-thirty in the morning when it was clear they were getting nowhere, I left them to it; the next day I wrote my report and sent it to the council engineer. I never did find out what they did about the weld as I was told my services were no longer required, this was a little disappointing but at least my conscience was clear, I have often wondered about these welds when I have been passing Brixham harbour, I imagine they must have been repaired by now.

Over the coming couple of years my company was employed as principle, inspection company for a number of large contracts such as welding repair of the Yonderberry fueling jetty on the southern bank of the Tamar River opposite Devonport Dockyard. Repair of a floating wave-screen again in Brixham harbour and many others, it was a very busy time. I found myself spending a lot of time on my jobs locally which normally required very long days and increasingly I was spending more and more time away from home servicing jobs for TWI both in Middlesbrough and overseas.

It was becoming a strain, not only for me but also for my family as I never seemed to have time for them; even when I was at home, I would often be writing reports or carrying out administration for the company. One thing that brought home to me the effect this was having on my family was when my youngest son James who is something of a talented artist made a drawing of me in my office. James was just twelve years old at the time but, clearly; he saw me as an angry man; the picture he drew was a caricature showing me staring over the top rim of my spectacles with steam coming out of my ears. It was a very good drawing which had a big effect on me; this all started to come to a head late in 1999. In November I had again been training in Middlesbrough for ten days and more or less immediately I had to make another one-week trip back to Perth in Australia to conduct another ACFM course at Surespec.

Same issues for me as before in that I had a very short layover in Singapore on the way out, meaning that I arrived in Perth feeling knackered this time though I had the correct visa so was not detained when I got to passport control in Perth. One thing that had changed was that they were now employing Beagle dogs to look for contraband in luggage, in baggage reclaim everyone's bags were subjected to scrutiny by this lovely little dog who climbed over everything sniffing out whatever he could; I didn't see that he found anything but by all accounts, this was a very effective deterrent.

Neil again met me at the airport and from there we went straight to have a bite to eat in a nice steakhouse; it was here that he told me that he had arranged for the course to start the following day. I was not keen, I normally had a day between arriving and starting the course, this would give me time to acclimatise a little but evidently this was not going to happen. We duly started the course the following day and all went well but I can tell you I found it a challenge with the effects of Jet-lag. I knew a few people in and around Perth by now and during the evenings I had some nice meals meeting up with old friends which was very nice; maybe the best of these was when I drove into Freemantle at the mouth of the Swan River just a few miles away from Perth. I had a lovely meal of kangaroo while sitting on a first-floor balcony in the old part of town, it was a very atmospheric vista reminiscent of how colonial Australia must have looked.

When I returned to UK, Christmas was imminent and as always this was a particularly hectic but pleasant time for me as I made a point of never taking on work over the Christmas or new year period. Obviously, this was a special year as it was the end of the millennium; we had planned millennium celebrations to be hosted at our house, Chrissie's sister and her family had all come over from the USA, there were five of them; we were also joined by Chrissie's mother and step-father; a big party was planned for New-Year's-Eve. At the time we lived in a lovely bungalow overlooking Torbay, we had a large wooden deck with a panoramic view across the bay, on that evening the weather was kind, it was clear but not too cold and it was dry so, as the clock struck twelve o'clock heralding the new millennium, everyone already had charged glasses ready. We all headed out onto the deck toasting the new year watching a tremendous firework display over the bay.

Over the previous few months there had been tremendous publicity around the so-called 'Millennium Bug' which we were told might stop all computers from working at the stroke of midnight on New-Year's-Eve 1999. All commercial aircraft were grounded, the world's financial institutions were primed for Armageddon and the rest of us held our breath and hoped our TV would still work in the morning! As it turned out, this was a great non-event and to my knowledge nothing major happened to computers at all that night.

January 2000 started pretty much in the same vein as the previous year had ended, I was off to Qatar in the Persian Gulf, to conduct another ACFM course I arrived in Doha the capital city of Qatar on the twentieth of January, this time again I had the correct visa and was admitted to the country without issue. As I was waiting for the ACFM equipment to be delivered to the baggage reclaim I caught sight of Mel Bayliss my old friend from Bovisand, he was working in Qatar and had been for some time. He told me that his wife Maria would be meeting him in the arrival's hall, he offered me a lift to my hotel which I was very happy to accept; as we entered the arrivals hall we were met by a very wet and somewhat bedraggled Maria. It seemed that in the time we had taken to get through baggage reclaim and the various immigration and customs checks the heavens had opened in biblical proportions! Maria told us that as she was parking up, she was caught in the torrential downpour and it was still going on.

As we made our way out of the terminal, night had fallen but I could see that where a few minutes before the concourse would have been a dry, dusty and hot expanse of tarmac, it was now awash; it was of course still hot and now very humid. We dashed to Mel's car which was a Jeep Renegade, and bundled ourselves and our luggage into the back as quickly as we could, still by the time I was settled into the rear seat I was drenched. Mel and Maria dropped me off at my hotel, before leaving they invited me to dinner on the Tuesday which was very nice, I was not going to be hiring a car so Mel told me he would come to pick me up.

Approaching the reception desk in the foyer of the hotel, I had to wade through puddles of water that had accumulated during the deluge, it was clear that they were not used to this level of rainfall. Indeed, when I eventually started to check-in to the hotel the receptionist told me that this was the first rain, they had seen for four years! Well, clearly anywhere that is suffering drought needed to pay for me to arrive! Qatar was a lovely place in those days, it was before the influx of high-profile sports events and the accompanying hype; the Corniche alongside the gulf was a very nice walk, and after that first night the sun came out and stayed that way all the time I was there.

The next couple of years were much the same and it was clear that to an extent we at TWI were victim's, of our own success; everyone wanted us all the time. Obviously, this was a nice state of affairs but it meant I was spending too much time away from home, meaning Chrissie was really left to bring up the kids and look after the house on her own. I didn't know what to do about it but clearly, I had to put some thought into it; my first thought was that I would need to perhaps push for more inspection work in Devon and Cornwall, we would see what could be worked out.

I decided to revisit local organisations that I had worked with before, unfortunately Fort Bovisand had gone to the wall by this time; this was a shame in a lot of ways as they had been my perennial go-to for work whenever I needed it. I had to look elsewhere and decided to see whether DDRC needed my skills as chamber operator or similar and to this end I made my way down to their facility which had now been relocated; they were now

392

in a brand-new purpose-built facility next door to Derriford hospital. On arrival, the first time I had been to this facility; I was faced with a very impressive red brick building with a sort of conservatory section directly in front of me. The windows and doors had dark red frames which tied in with their revised corporate image, I knew the building had only been completed in 1996 so was still fairly new.

My old co-conspirator Gerry Mackenzie who I had worked alongside at Interdive had in the meantime taken the job of Operations Director at DDRC and so I was hopeful he may want to help me get some work with them. I had worked with DDRC at intervals since I finished working offshore; I parked up in front of the building, and as I stepped out of my car, I was greeted by someone shouting my name from the door on the left of the car park area. This turned out to be the entrance to the chamber room and the owner of the voice was Jess Wade; Jess was a long-term DDRC team member who I had known since the early eighties. I had spent a long-time tutoring her when she was going through her IMCA life support technician qualification so we knew each other well.

We had a short chat about how things were going at DDRC, it seemed they were very busy treating both divers and NHS patients which I thought was very positive. She told me there had been very significant changes in the last couple of years; Dr Maurice Cross whose brainchild DDRC was, no longer worked with them at all. Similarly, Eddy Johnson who had been pivotal in getting the new building completed and the subsequent move of DDRC from its original base at Fort Bovisand had also gone! Wow, there was clearly a new regime in control I hoped this would not mean that they no longer needed the likes of me.

Once I had signed in as a visitor, I asked whether Gerry was available for a chat, he was and very soon joined me in reception, he greeted me enthusiastically which was nice. We walked along a nice shiny corridor into the patient's lounge where he made me a cup of coffee; we sat down for a chat I told him that I was looking to join their chamber bank team; I knew that DDRC had for years maintained a bank of staff who worked on a part time basis manning the chamber when required. He said he thought there would certainly be room for me to join the bank team; I thought this would be perfect as I could do this work whenever I was at home, certainly though at this time, I would still need to carry on with my TWI commitments.

Over the next few weeks, I went through their induction and chamber training; actually, I didn't need to do much of the training given my background, mostly I had to complete assessments. Within a month I was duly taken on to the chamber bank and became part of the team, I would be available to run the chamber when divers needed recompression, whenever I was going to be at home. I would give them my availability for the following month meaning they would then rota me in for a number of days or nights as appropriate. After doing this for a few months I moved up from chamber operator and attendant to chamber supervisor which suited me just fine; I was happy with this, it seemed the first step had been taken.

Early in 2001 I started to become aware of a medical problem that although I didn't know it at the time would eventually become life changing; as you know I liked to go out for walks after a long day in the classroom, it was during these walks that I found I started to limp. The first time I noticed this was when I was conducting courses at TWI in Middlesbrough, I was still staying in Newton-Aycliffe and had taken to going for long walks when I got home. I loved wandering around the lanes outside the town and would regularly walk for a couple of hours; I started to find that when I had been walking for an hour or so I would find it difficult to lift my right leg. If I kept on walking, I would end up dragging my foot very badly, clearly, something was wrong.

At the time I would also use gyms or swimming pools wherever I was and found that I couldn't keep up my normal training regime, on a trip to Crewe where I was teaching Bombardier staff ACFM to be used on railway rolling stock that they were either building or maintaining. Most evenings I would stop in at a gym on the way back to the hotel and I found that I couldn't use the running machine and even using the rowing machine wore me out; after just a short time rowing, I found I almost couldn't get back to my feet.

This all became especially noticeable during a subsequent trip to Pattaya, I was again walking in the evening when my leg started dragging after only a short distance, less than a couple of miles; it seemed that maybe the ambient temperature was enhancing the effect? I of course did nothing about this until during another set of courses in Middlesbrough; unusually I had a weekend off and had arranged to meet Chrissie in Manchester for the weekend. We had a very nice weekend and as was the norm for us rather than drive from the hotel when we went out for the evening we would walk. On the way back to the hotel Chrissie noticed my limp and challenged me about it; I of course had to own up to the fact that I had been noticing this for some months, she of course was horrified and resolved to get something done about it.

When I returned home at the end of the courses some ten-days later I was told that I needed to make an appointment to find out what was going on. The first step was to see my GP who identified there was an issue but was not sure of a diagnosis, he referred me to a neurologist but it seemed that on the NHS there were long waiting lists, something like eighteen months to two years.

We felt this was not acceptable as we both needed to know what was wrong, so, I made a private appointment at the Mount Stuart Hospital in Torquay; the appointment was with an eminent neurologist Professor John Zajicek. At my first appointment he did a very thorough neurological examination and came to the conclusion that not only my right leg but to a lesser extent the rest of my limbs were also affected; this shocked me as I had only been aware of the problem with my right-leg, he suggested I have an MRI to get to the bottom of the causes. I immediately organised this at a cost of nearly one-thousand Pounds for a full body MRI; I undertook the scan a couple of days later in a mobile unit situated in Mount Stuart's car park.

The following week Chrissie and I went to see the Prof again to hear his conclusions; as was the case with private consultations, we sat in a comfortable waiting area where we were offered tea or coffee. Neither of us felt like drinking anything at this stage but it was nice to be offered; after just a few minutes Prof Zajicek himself came around the corner to collect us; he led us into his small but tasteful consulting room where he invited us to sit. We sat in front of his desk as he took his seat behind the desk; on the wall behind him was a display on which there were MRI generated images of a brain which I assumed was mine.

Of course, I didn't know much about what I was looking at other than to know generally what it was. Zajicek stood and proceeded to point out a few small white spots on the image, he then sat back down and delivered the devastating news that these spots were indications that I was suffering from Multiple Sclerosis (MS). I have to say this hit me hard, at the time we had a good friend who had been suffering with MS for a number of years and I could not contemplate being affected in the same way! Zajicek was very good, he explained the various stages of the disease and painted a very much more positive picture than I was feeling at the time, clearly, there were going to have to be big changes to our lives.

Zajicek went on to explain that the disease cannot be categorised to any great extent, everybody was different, he told me that some fifty-percent of sufferers would still be walking unaided ten-years after diagnosis, it was important to put this in context and to not worry too much! Well, that was easy for him to say, I definitely didn't feel positive at all, what was I going to do? One thing that did come out of this was that I had been suffering from mild symptoms for possibly years already although I had been able to maintain a full offshore commercial diving medical part of which included a full neurological examination.

He told us that MS was not at all unusual, it was one of the most common neurological conditions, apparently it affected more women than men and normally would be diagnosed when the individual was in their twenties. Well, the last time I checked I was not a woman and at the time I was forty-five, so as always with me I didn't fit the profile. We thanked Zajicek and promised to make another appointment in four weeks to discuss treatment options of which it had sounded there were few to be had.

We left the hospital and adjourned to the nearest pub where I'm afraid I let my emotions get the better of me, I posed the impossible questions without expecting Chrissie to have any of the answers; when I had calmed down, we started to look at the problem more logically. I was at the time spending a great deal of time away from home, mostly with TWI in Middlesbrough and overseas in Thailand, Singapore, USA and Australia; would I be able to continue with this? At the time, while I knew I was affected it was not to the point where I couldn't do the job although Chrissie was not keen for me to continue overseas trips alone. I was due to travel to Thailand the following week and did not feel I could let Jim down this late in the day so we agreed I would do this trip and decide the future following that. During this trip I spent a lot of time on my own in the evenings analysing my condition and what if any changes needed to be made. Now, I don't want anyone to get the wrong impression here, yes, I was affected by my diagnosis but I was not going to let it dominate my life until I really had no choice. Generally, as I've said before throughout my life, I consider myself to have been extremely lucky, I have gone through life repeatedly being in the right place at the right time.

I could add to this that over the years, several times I have been extremely lucky not to have been seriously injured like the time they dropped a blow-out preventor on top of the diving bell I was sitting in at over four hundred and fifty feet! Generally, I felt that I am and have been a lucky chap, now why should that all change? As soon as I got home, I sat Chrissie down and explained that I had spent a lot of time analysing my predicament but, that I didn't want my diagnosis to rule my life; I was feeling much more positive and felt I should continue with my current commitments while I still could.

While this was going on I would look for something that I could move in to; perhaps carry out some retraining so that I could find something that paid a wage but that I could do from a wheelchair if necessary. I don't think Chrissie was completely on board with this but she was definitely happy to see me back with a more normal can-do attitude; I decided not to tell anyone outside of the family until I really had to. Chrissie was not going to let me get away with this, she wanted to be able to tell friends; I agreed to this but wasn't very happy with it as I didn't want people to feel they had to make allowances for me until there was really no option.

She was right, of course and all the friends we told were very supportive without going overboard; I didn't tell anyone at work though as in my view they didn't need to know at this time. Over the next few months, I started to change what I was doing in small ways to make it easier for me, perhaps I wouldn't carry so much equipment, I would enlist the help of students or work colleagues. People did though start to mention my limp, which was cause for concern but I was able to make light of it and certainly it didn't seem to alter their perception of me or the work I was doing.

The events of September eleventh 2001 are forever embedded in everyone's memory for all the wrong reasons, that of course was when Islamic extremists flew commercial airliners into the World Trade Centre in New York and the Pentagon in Washington. Air travel to the US was curtailed for a while after these events but eventually did resume and as was the norm in those days I had to make another trip out to Houston for an ACFM course. There was a tremendous increase in security for those flights which I found reassuring but when I took my seat on the flight, I was surprised by how empty the cabin was, normally every seat would be filled but, on this occasion, I had a whole row to myself!

The trip home from the US was even more difficult as the US airports were hyped up to a tremendous extent, they all but strip searched anyone who was the slightest bit out of the ordinary. They didn't like my laptop or all the course material I had with me, so, when I finally made my way onto the flight, I was very relieved.

I carried on with trips to TWI North in Middlesbrough in the same way as normal although I was happy that Jim took quite a few of the ACFM jobs in Brazil and Mexico which, I normally would have had to do.

Early in 2002 my working on the bank for DDRC meant that they were able to help me take the next step in my Life Support Technician role, I had completed my Assistant Life Support Technician (ALST) course while I was still at Interdive some time ago but had never been in a position to progress to finish off the qualification by taking the IMCA examination. Now that I was working with DDRC it seemed the right time to make an attempt at gaining this certification, as it turned out there were a couple of others at DDRC who also wanted to take this examination.

At the time one had to have gained 2,400 hours of 'Panel Time' following successful completion of the ALST course, I had by this time logged enough hours and together with my time in Sat with Oceaneering I was accepted as eligible. Geoffery Hardy DDRC's engineer was also accepted and we arranged to sit our exams on the same day; the venue was again Plymouth College of Further Education.

As was the case when I took my AODC air diving supervisor exam in 1988, we both turned up in the college's reception where we signed in, then we were shown into the hall just like before, the hall had been laid out with several rows of single desks with chairs. Again, we were to be in the same room with students taking their own different examinations.

I found a seat and was presented with my paper; the invigilator then again gave us the spiel about how long we would have for the exam; and what to do when we finished. I had suggested Geoff should buy the same metric converter calculator that I had and we also had a couple of pens each with us, the invigilator again gave us a few sheets of blank paper for calculations etc.

I turned over the paper, where I was again faced with eighty multiple-choice questions, I started with the calculations which for this qualification was a much larger part of the exam than had been the case with the diving supervisor. As I had been teaching ALST since 1988 I was used to working through the diving and mixed gas related physics questions, subsequently I found this section relatively straightforward; I hoped! I again finished the whole paper with time to spare, spent some time going over the paper to ensure I had not missed any questions before leaving my paper on the desk making my way out of the hall. As had been the case with the diving supervisor exam I only had to wait a short time before I was told that I had passed, in fact, we had both passed. Consequently, in March 2002 I became an IMCA qualified Life Support Technician (LST), my certificate number was 788/UK. I didn't know it at the time but this qualification was to become very important to me in the coming months.

In early 2002 my ability to be in the right place at the right time was again proven. I was at DDRC for a morning shift when Gerry came to see me and invited me to lunch; as I was due to finish my shift at twelve-thirty I agreed. We went to a local pub where Gerry ordered us food and a beer each; when we were settled, he told me that he was leaving DDRC to take up a position with the UAE Military in Abu Dhabi. I was a little shocked as I thought he was very comfortable at DDRC, it was clear that although he loved being at DDRC his long-term future lay elsewhere. I was now sure he had something else he wanted to tell me and I was not to be disappointed.

First, he told me more about his job, not only was he the Operations Director and Safety Manager for DDRC the charity but he apparently was also the managing director of the charity's trading arm DDRC Professional Services. He was concerned that his departure could and probably would leave the charity in a bad place as there were no other individuals currently employed with any real commercial diving expertise; he told me that he had already discussed this with their chief executive a Ms Karena Pring. He had apparently told her that he would be very difficult to replace as there were very few people with his skill set; he went on to tell me that he had suggested I be offered the job! This of course was very welcome news to me, we didn't discuss money or anything in detail that afternoon but, I told him I was interested and he suggested I have a meeting with Karena to see how we could make this happen.

My journey home to Paignton was carried out in a bit of a haze, I was very positive about this as I felt I could definitely do the job and was for a change actually qualified for it; when I told Chrissie she also was very enthusiastic about the prospects. The next day Gerry called me to tell me that Karena wanted to meet with me to discuss and wanted this to take place as soon as possible; I was due to do another morning shift the next day; Gerry thought this would be a perfect time for me to sit down with her. I now needed to know a bit about what was on offer, I was fairly well paid for the work I was doing with TWI, not only was I paid a good day rate for my time but I was also paid a royalty for each person using my books and other materials on the courses.

And that was without any of the other jobs I was doing; couple that with the tax benefits of running a limited company I was sure DDRC couldn't afford me! That being said, I needed to take into account the fact that it was difficult to see me continuing in my current role indefinitely and of course in the DDRC role I would be able to go home every night (well, as it turned out almost every night). Not only that but, in the DDRC job I would be entitled to paid holiday. Finally, Gerry's job was largely office based and I thought it was something that could be carried out, if necessary, from a wheelchair if the worst came to be.

Before my meeting with Karena, I managed to chat to Gerry who told me what he was being paid and although it would mean a significant pay cut it would certainly be manageable. When my shift was completed, we all sat down in Gerry's office overlooking the field on the other side of DDRC's car park, it was early April and the sun was again shining. Gerry kicked off the meeting describing his role and showing the similarities between his skill set and my own; to be fair to Karena, although we had met a few times she really didn't know me from Adam, it was clear though that she trusted Gerry's judgement.

After a good hour of debate some of it making clear to me that perhaps Karena was really not on board with this idea, she came to a decision, she offered me the job but, at a considerably lower salary than Gerry was on. I told her that I couldn't take the job at that rate, Gerry asked that I go and make myself a cup of tea while he chatted with Karena; off I went to the staff room, I was taking a big gamble as I did really want the job but felt that I was worth more than she was offering. I had finished my cup of tea by the time Karena came to get me; she was not smiling so I thought maybe I had blown it.

When we were back seated in Gerry's office Karena told me that having taken everything into account, she was happy to offer me the job at the same pay and conditions as Gerry was on. This was great, it meant I would be paid a reasonable salary certainly for a Devonshire based job; an additional incentive was that it came with five weeks paid holiday per year; this was a real result, I was chuffed. I actually had no commitment to give TWI any notice but as they had been so good to me over the years, I told Karena, I had to give TWI at least two months' notice which she readily agreed to, this meant that I would have to make two more trips to Middlesbrough but I felt this was the minimum I owed Jim.

The next day I needed to call Jim to tell him the news, I was really not looking forward to this call as he had treated me exceptionally well during the eight years of our association; even though I was an external contractor he routinely had increased my day rate in line with any raises TWI awarded their staff and he had of course been very helpful when I had suffered the blood clot episode etc. He was clearly upset as he hadn't seen it coming but he did understand and was very appreciative when I told him I could still do the next two months courses.

I was due in Middlesbrough the following week for the first of the courses, it was a strange feeling telling everyone about my new job, they were of course happy for me but would miss me which was very nice. I agreed with Jim that they could continue to use my books and materials provided they continued with the financial agreement and he agreed to this readily. This arrangement continued for some three years after I started at DDRC when they eventually took someone on who wanted to change things; this was fine by me as it was becoming difficult for me to keep updating things when I wasn't still working in that environment. I didn't know it at the time but my association with TWI would continue but in a different vein over the next few years when I needed to use their facilities training some of DDRC's students.

PHOTOS FROM MY TIME WORKING WITH TSC AND TWI

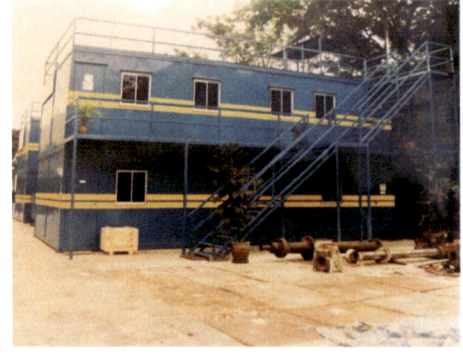

Office and classrooms at Metalock Underwater Maintenance, Singapore.

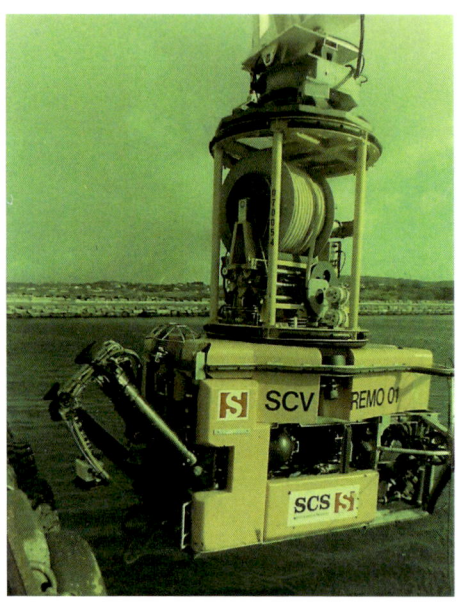

REMO work-class ROV during an ACFM trial in Haugusund, Norway.

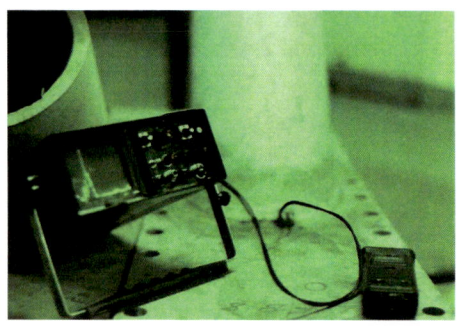

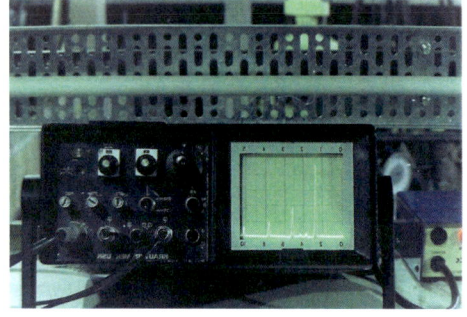

A-Scan set up for measuring steel thickness. Right photograph shows signals produced from a 25mm calibration block.

Part Six

CHAPTER EIGHTEEN

Diving Diseases Research Centre – 2002 to 2020

2002:

So it was that in early May 2002 I started what was to be my last paid job, I had been taken on in all of Gerry Mackenzie's roles. Principally I was DDRC's Operations Director, this entailed my being part of their senior management team (SMT); the team was made up of the Chief Executive Officer, Karena Pring (KP), the Medical Director, Dr James Hardwick (JH) and me. In addition, I also became registered at Companies House as the Managing Director of DDRC Professional Services Ltd (DDRC Pro-Services), the charity's trading arm, in this role I was responsible for ensuring DDRC provided training and consultancy services to outside organisations. In my role as the charity's Ops Director, I was also responsible for Health and Safety; this was something that I felt and still feel passionate about.

My first day in the role I spent most of the day walking around the site trying to get a feel for its current state, I have to say I was dismayed to see that there didn't seem to be any written risk assessments in evidence! In addition, I didn't feel the chamber training was being handled in a way that was repeatable; that's not to say staff were not well trained; they were, it's just that there was no written plan or pathway for an individual to follow showing steps necessary for progression; this meant that everyone carrying out training did so in their own way meaning some received better training than others; in short, there was a lot to do.

Towards the end of the day, I retired to Gerry's old office which of course was now mine; I liked this office, I felt it was the nicest in the building, it was on the north side of the building so in the summer it didn't become completely unbearably hot like the offices on the south side would. It had a nice bay window giving a view across the car park to a grassed area and onwards to the rest of the science park, it was a pleasant place to be. Over the next few days, I spent a lot of time getting to grips with finding where everything was in the office; this showed me that while Gerry was unquestionably very knowledgeable and capable, he hated paperwork with a passion! Probably the best example of this was the bottom drawer of one of the filing cabinets; it was labelled 'Certificates'.

When I first opened the drawer that is exactly what I found, there were hundreds of certificates but there was no order at all, they had all just been thrown into the drawer one on top of the other probably as they came in? Certificates relating to pressure systems are very important and need to be accessible, if we were to have a visit from the Health and Safety Executive (HSE) they would expect me to be able to put my finger on certificates for any of our plant and equipment. Now, I was reasonably sure they were all there but it would take a long time to identify and recover any particular one; I set about organising this by taking everything out of the drawer and grouping them into an order that made sense to me. I was still there at seven o'clock in the evening that first day, I had certificates all over the floor, on the desk and table, they were everywhere. By the time I left that night, I had piles relating to HP receivers, LP receivers, Chambers including one for their ports, Pipework, Gauges, Valves, electrical installations and various other miscellaneous items such as the building's passenger lift. This was a job well done and I felt much better having got a handle on where things were, over the coming days I filed everything in the office in a manner that made sense to me, however, it took me months to get it completely how I wanted it.

The next thing I needed to concentrate on was risk assessment, I knew that if there were to be an accident the HSE would ask to see our risk assessments relating to the process that had resulted in injury. At this time, I had no formal training in risk assessment so I set about finding an appropriate course which DDRC subsequently put me on. The first course I completed was a half-day risk assessment course carried out at Plymouth College of Further Education, this was a very good base from which to work and gave me the skills I needed to at least start risk assessing DDRC. Over the next few months, I undertook various courses culminating in my first Institution of Occupational Safety and Health (IOSH) course this was a five-day Managing Safely course again run at the same college. After successfully completing these courses, I was beginning to feel somewhat more comfortable and prepared for the job at DDRC.

Very early on in my job as operations director I had decided that DDRC being in the business of providing recompression for personnel inside hyperbaric chambers using of liquid oxygen was operating in a relatively high-risk world. While risk assessment was an imperative, they would not on their own be enough, I felt we needed a complete safety management system (SMS) written from the ground up; this would incorporate detailed methods for managing risks, recording incidents and all the other minutia needed to ensure a safe environment. I started looking for help and assistance and as luck would have it my old friend Peter Sieniewicz was now an HSE diving inspector, not only that but he was based in Plymouth. I contacted him and asked him to come up for a cup of coffee; Peter is a one-off individual who has always been very helpful to me, I like to think this is because he can see I always make every effort to do things properly.

Peter's visit went well and although he was not there in an official capacity, HSE inspectors are a little like policemen in that they are never really off duty; we had a walk around the building with me pointing out improvements I had already made and outlining my plans for the future. When we returned to my office, Peter was at pains to tell me that he was impressed with everything he had seen but was concerned that I didn't have sufficient back-up in the form of high-quality health and safety advice; he also questioned my level of qualification. I felt both these points were valid and when he left, I set about finding advice that I could lean on when required; I signed up for Jordan's Health and Safety.

Jordan's was a specialist Health and Safety advice service, I received a massive, thick, green, three-ring binder that was laid out with all required sections, it was relatively easy to navigate and gave me a helpline to call in the event I needed more help; I felt more in control by having this on my side. I also started to research higher levels of Health and Safety training; there were a number of routes I could have taken but ultimately, I decided to go the NVQ route for a number of reasons. Firstly, I could do the vast majority of the work during my normal working day. Secondly, while I was doing the work for my course, I could angle it towards facilitating the building of DDRC's safety management system; this way DDRC and I would both benefit. I started to look for a course provider, the most sensible organisation offering this training was again IOSH; the IOSH system would initially require me to attend a single day induction onto the course at their head office in Leicestershire.

Anyway, IOSH was for the future, over the following couple of weeks, I was back up to Middlesbrough for the last time to teach a CSWIP 3.1U course, the course went very well with the students who had been told it was to be my last course wishing me well for the future. Toward the end of the second week, Jim came into the classroom interrupting the lecture and told me I was needed outside in the common room; when I arrived, the place was full of staff, some of whom were not actually on shift that day. A party started with Jim presenting me with a very nice paperweight inscribed with "Good luck Pete, we will miss you". Al Wate the diving supervisor presented me with a silver hip flask inscribed with the Hartlepool monkey. The story goes that during the Napoleonic wars a monkey was caught in Hartlepool apparently none of the people of Hartlepool had ever seen either a Frenchman or a monkey, so the poor animal was convicted as a French spy and was hanged! Hartlepool residents became known as "monkey hangers" although this is not a popular term with them today. All of this was totally unexpected but made me feel quite humble, it was sad in a lot of ways to be leaving but it was definitely the right thing to do.

Returning to DDRC I started to get my head around their trading arm DDRC Professional Services Ltd, the company had been launched in 1989 under a slightly different name. To begin with the company had apparently been mismanaged. For reasons that I never fully understood, the company which was then and still remains a wholly owned subsidiary of the charity had been charged huge rents for everything it used or utilised regardless of how much use they made of them; this had resulted in the company amassing enormous debts to the charity.

When the charity's senior management changed in 1997 the way the company was charged for use of facilities was altered to a much more sustainable model, from this time onwards the company was only charged for equipment, personnel or facilities when they were using them at all other times the charity was free to utilise them. When Gerry had taken over running the company the company was relaunched under its current name, this took place in 1999. Gerry had inherited this huge debt; he of course set about reducing this and had managed to pay back a big chunk but when I took over there was still well over a quarter of a million pounds owed to the charity.

The charity's trustees were understandably nervous about Pro-Services current level of debt; the accountants had apparently been telling them for some time that they couldn't allow their trading arm to trade at a loss and so insolvent for a prolonged period; in addition, of course they didn't know me at all so their nerves were very evident when we first met. I was able to reassure them that I would continue the good work Gerry had commenced and hoped to be able to pay off the debt within the next few years. The key to making the company solvent lay in continuing to service contracts that Gerry had secured as well as others he had inherited; Gerry's main contract was with the United Arab Emirates (UAE) military.

Gerry had made a very important contact in the military who were now sending all their military and police divers to us for training as Diver Medic Technicians (DMT); this liaison had commenced with a number of UAE military personnel being sent to DDRC for six-months. During this time, they received comprehensive training on the running of a recompression facility; when they had completed the course, they returned to become senior personnel in the team running their chamber facility in Abu Dhabi. There had only been one of these initial six-month courses by the time I arrived and they remained an option for all the time I was there. Much more commonly, we ran refresher courses of four-weeks, these were required for each of the trained individuals every three years.

The other major contract was with the Hong Kong Fire Service (HKFS), DDRC had inherited this contract with the demise of Fort Bovisand, one of Bovisand's key instructors Paul Dart had come to work for DDRC and had brought the contract with him. This contract normally consisted of us training existing HKFS divers in the role of chamber supervisors, they would then return to Hong Kong to help with the running of their recompression facility. Their course consisted of four-weeks during which they received training as DMT, chamber supervisor and daily chamber maintenance; it was a nice course to run and everyone always seemed to enjoy it, this was true both of the students and staff alike.

Both of these contracts had to be maintained and if possible, added to for me to make a success of the company; luckily, Gerry had gone to work with the UAE military and was in a position to continue sending their personnel to us for training. It was though up to me to make the HKFS confident that the change in management of Pro-Services would not affect the quality of training; with this in mind I resolved to visit Hong Kong to meet the key players. I made this first trip in July 2002 my visit was scheduled to last four days and I was looking forward to it. I already knew some of the key players as I had taught them while at Bovisand; the main man I knew as Joey NG, he had moved up the ladder and was now quite senior in the HKFS. There were others and in fact when I eventually arrived in HK, I found there were quite a few who I remembered and who definitely knew me.

I landed in HK on the twenty-third of July. As I arrived in the arrival's hall, Joey was there waiting, it was a lovely welcome, it was just like being met by an old friend which I suppose in a way he was. Firstly, once we had made our way out to his car Joey told me he needed to visit the airport fire station for a few moments; this was fine by me, I was just glad to be there. This trip was a first for me, I was not there to run a course and my role was much more of a managerial/promotional one, I was there to impress the senior management in the HKFS, I was somewhat nervous about this though. The airport fire station was very impressive, I came to realise that HKFS was very well funded, they seemed to have everything they needed and then some. Joey's visit there took just fifteen minutes or so and then we were off to drive into the city; the airport was some thirty kilometres outside the city and our journey took about forty-five minutes with traffic causing most of the delay.

We drove to a club in Kowloon in the New Territories with a spectacular view across Victoria Harbour to Hong Kong Island where the skyline was dominated by huge skyscrapers all illuminated with advertising, it was very impressive. As we entered the bar another friend from Bovisand days Eric Kwan Kam-Wing greeted me and invited me to sit at a round table taking in the panoramic view of the harbour, so there I was in the bar with a cool beer and some snacks chatting to five HKFS officers I was definitely put at ease, they all knew of me and indeed I had taught three of them; I thought, I can do this.

After a couple of beers, it was time for Joey to take me to my hotel. I was up bright and early the next day although not very well rested, again this was due to jet-lag. I was waiting in the foyer of the hotel at eight o'clock ready for Joey who arrived on the dot of eight; he had parked illegally so we rushed out to his car and were very soon edging our way into the steady stream of traffic.

He drove straight to the HKFS head office which was just a couple of miles away in Tsim Sha Tsui, he parked in a dedicated staff car park and we made our way into the building;

Joey's boss Mike LI, had his office on the third floor, we climbed the stairs. Joey could see I was not comfortable but told me not to worry, all would be fine, this didn't really help as I was feeling out of my depth; anyway, I thought here we go. I didn't have long to wait, almost as soon as we arrived, I was ushered into Mike's office; we spent the first five minutes or so with the pleasantries of meeting, once this was out of the way we got down to business. It seemed that on the last course run at DDRC Gerry had managed to get the students through the Association of Diving Contractors (ADC) supervisor qualification at no extra cost to HKFS; I thought this would have been appreciated but evidently this was not the case at all. I was told in no uncertain terms that this was not to be repeated, the courses had to run to the approved programme with no alteration if we wanted to keep the contract; I of course agreed that we would make sure nothing like this happened again, how bizarre.

Towards the end of the meeting the frosty reception thawed and at the end it was clear all would be fine I was then invited to lunch by Mike but of course it was far too early. Joey suggested I visit their chamber facility before lunch which was agreed and off, we went; Joey told me when we were in the car that Mike was always like this and I was not to read too much into it; in truth I didn't care so long as we kept the contract.

Their chamber facility was a few miles from headquarters and at that time was almost a stand-alone facility however, since then, they have built their training school alongside so now it is part of a much bigger facility. Joey parked up in a small car park alongside an industrial building, inside was a very impressive chamber that had been built and installed by the German company Haux Engineering. Haux chambers were at the time definitely the market leaders in medical hyperbaric chambers, the system was far and away more modern and, in some ways, more capable than the one we had at DDRC.

The chamber was painted light green and consisted of three individual chamber locks; there were two treatment chambers capable of treating six persons seated in each, they were placed either side of a central entry lock. I was impressed and said so which raised smiles all round; we spent a good hour at the facility during which time I made a number of notes on equipment that I felt we could make good use of back at DDRC.

Returning to headquarters in time for lunch we had to wait a short while as soon as Mike was ready, we were marched at speed out of the headquarters building turning right along the road to a restaurant almost next door. It was obvious that reservations had been made as we were ushered to a large round table already prepared for us; we had a very nice lunch with almost no talk of work being raised; towards the end of the meal, I was asked whether I had plans for the next couple of days. I of course had no plans, and said so; it was decided that I would be assigned a guide for the following day who would take me across to Hong Kong Island and show me around.

This was very generous of them, as we were leaving Joey told me my guide would be Malcolm who was a junior firefighter on his watch; Malcolm would be at my hotel at nine o'clock in the morning to pick me up; I was then taken back to my hotel and left to my own devices for the rest of the day.

The next morning again my guide arrived spot on the allotted time; he had clearly been briefed and without further discussion we headed off on foot towards the Star Ferry terminal, the Star Ferry Pier was just a couple of kilometres from the hotel so within twenty minutes we had arrived. Malcolm had obviously been told not to let me pay for anything as he marched straight up to the kiosk and paid for two tickets to Wan Chai Ferry Pier on the island. As the ferry left its berth, I was again treated to that wonderful vista of Hong Kong Island's crowded waterfront consisting of large skyscrapers, staring at this I thought it was no less spectacular for being in daylight.

Malcolm was great, he showed me everything that day, first he took me up the peak using the furnicular railway which had been carrying passengers up to the upper levels of the peak since 1888; the view from the peak was spectacular I could see the whole of the north side of the island and across Victoria Harbour to Kowloon and the rest of the New Territories with their harbour complexes and industrial areas. Malcolm told me we were extremely lucky with the weather on the day as apparently it was not unusual for the peak to be shrouded in cloud which would have denied us the view, so there I was lucky again and what a view it was.

Next, I was taken back down to catch a double decker bus to Aberdeen; on the way we passed Happy Valley, the world-famous horse-racing venue which looked quite out of place amongst the high-rise buildings, it was a vivid splash of green with immense grandstands none of which would have been out of place in Ascot or Aintree but seemed at odds with where it actually was.

On we went to Aberdeen, this was a small fishing village on the south side of the island where tourists flocked for restaurants and to experience the bustling ambience. We spent a couple of hours in Aberdeen where we had lunch on a junk and walked along the dockside watching people buy fish directly from the fishing boats, it was a great day, I enjoyed it very much.

The next day I was summoned to headquarters, where I was told that I was to be taken out on the HKFS fire boat which doubled up as their dive boat, I was again looking forward to this very much. I was taken to the harbour in Joey's car, the fire boat was moored alongside; it was a very impressive ship painted bright fire engine red with white superstructure. As soon as I was onboard Joey showed me around, it was a very impressive ship featuring a wet-bell on the stern, with a plethora of shiny brand-new diving equipment, we spent the next couple of hours steaming around Victoria Harbour at speed. Joey pointed out all the significant districts and features as we passed them including the old Kai Tak airport that was at the time being converted into a cruise liner terminal and berthing area; they were justifiably proud of their ship it was impressive.

I again felt privileged to have this cruise, how many visitors to Hong Kong would be treated to this? When we eventually headed back to shore, I stumbled when getting off the ship, this was I'm sure to my not being as agile due to my MS but there were a lot of bodies who helped me so there was no real problem. Everyone congregated on the dockside where I congratulated Mike on the wonderful facilities they had at their disposal.

The next day, I was taken back to the airport where I was seen off by a number of the HKFS personnel which was nice. I boarded my flight home I was not absolutely certain but I felt the trip had gone reasonably well; as it turned out I was right and HKFS did continue to send their officers to us for training which was a great weight off my mind.

On return to DDRC I found there was an engineering issue that needed to be dealt with; at this time DDRC employed one engineer, he was a nice chap although his level of housekeeping used to drive me to distraction. His office was always a mess with equipment, tools, parts and manuals just left in piles, I never knew how he could work like that but he did manage somehow.

Later on in 2002, I as part of the senior management team of the charity, was called upon to go to meetings of the Trustee's board. The board's AGM was in October and was a big deal for me, I was required to report on my area of control within the charity but as I was also the MD of DDRC Pro-Services I needed to report on progress and future plans for the trading arm as well. In preparation for this I had produced a business plan laying out how I thought the business would progress through the next year with sections highlighting the company's strategy for the long-term.

On the evening of the meeting, we sat down in one of the training rooms upstairs at DDRC, there was Karena, James and me from the charity; facing us were six trustees, alongside Karena was the accountant and their assistant. Karena and James presented their reports, then it was my turn; I started off by giving my report on the operations within the charity, this took only a few minutes. I then handed bound copies of my business plan around to each of the attendees, there was a stunned silence; I was not sure what I had been expecting but anyway.

I launched into the status of the company together with the current level of debt showing that in the five months since I had taken over the business the debt had been reduced by some thirty-thousand pounds; when I had finished, I sat back and invited questions. The accountant sat forward and launched into what for him was a long speech; he started by saying he was pleased and reassured by the fact that I had produced a business plan; he could see that plans were in place to continue reducing the level of debt and that I should be congratulated.

I was stunned, it wasn't until after the meeting when Karena told me that both Gerry and his predecessor had steadfastly refused to produce any kind of business plan which had been a bone of contention for the trustees and accountants, this was especially true of the accountant; I didn't say anything but I think it might have been nice if someone had mentioned this before the meeting?

In my role as safety manager, I initiated monthly meetings with the chamber supervisors. These meetings gave us the chance to discuss issues facing us as a group, as the supervisors were key to safe working practice, I looked to this group to be DDRC's safety committee. We used to spend about an hour every month discussing issues of safety including implementation of any new standard operating procedures (SOPs). This was a very effective and potent group, by taking something to them at this meeting they would be properly briefed with the necessary information and then they would disseminate this efficiently to the rest of the team, this didn't always go to plan but over time it improved immensely.

When I had joined DDRC the main training expertise lay in training Diver Medic Technicians to the IMCA syllabus, I was not qualified to teach on these courses but, in any case, I felt I had moved away from teaching into a more managerial role. I was asked whether I felt DDRC should launch diver inspection courses but I was not keen for two main reasons; firstly, Interdive had tried and failed despite putting a tremendous effort into competing with a quality course and secondly, I felt that with TWI running courses and being the ones who hosted the examinations they would always be at a huge advantage.

We never did carry out inspection courses apart from a few for existing customers who wanted to add inspection to the package we already ran, this was true of the UAE military for instance but, whenever we ran inspection courses, we did so in partnership with TWI North thus taking advantage of their great facilities.

CHAPTER NINETEEN

2003

During 2003 I spent a lot of time working with the chamber team at DDRC, the charity maintained and indeed still maintains 24/7 availability; they were justifiably extremely proud that the charity had never been offline since they commenced diver recompression in the early eighties. This included the time when they were relocating from Fort Bovisand up to the new facility at Derriford, this was I think very impressive and I wanted to make sure this was maintained. When I had worked with DDRC as a bank worker I had been included in their chamber rota but, since taking the full-time job as Ops Director I was no longer expected to be part of the normal rota.

Having said that, I used to be floating to fill gaps created by illness, holidays or any other event that stopped one of the team being available. The result was that I tended to be on-call maybe three or four times per month, either as supervisor or chamber operator; this could be for a single night or perhaps a full weekend. In addition, I had never been much of one for going out to celebrate new-year's eve so normally I would choose to do both new-year's eve and new-year's day so that at least one of the team could properly enjoy themselves.

I found that working with the team I was able to maintain an idea for what they felt was right and what was wrong about how DDRC was run, this was extremely helpful in two ways. Firstly, I was able to use this knowledge to perhaps alter or at least to hone the direction taken by the senior management and secondly, I could float ideas about my plans to see whether the team had any views; this was particularly effective and ensured that whenever I made changes a lot of the team were already on board with them.

Over time I was refining chamber Standard Operating Procedures (SOPs), the aim was to make it easier for staff to do the job efficiently and of course safely; we needed to look at our systems and make sure they were laid out in a way that procedures could be written unambiguously. A big part of this revolved around our plant-room; the plant-room was where our compressors, air and gas storage and other equipment were located. The plant-room was in the basement below the chamber room, this ensured pipe runs were relatively short meaning high-pressure gas was not routed inappropriately.

DDRC's new building had been built from the ground up, I felt they had missed a trick with plant-room layout; unfortunately, the room was laid out by persons who knew the system intimately. While this should have made their job easy, I'm afraid that they didn't feel the need to make it simple; this resulted in relatively complex procedures having to be in place, for instance if we needed to route different gases into chambers such as Heliox mixtures instead of pure oxygen there was a relatively complex procedure which unfortunately relied on a significant understanding of the gas storage and pipework routing.

My main problem was that this reliance meant that training of new staff became complex and tended to be fraught with issues; I felt this could lead to problems and would be very difficult to defend if things went wrong. We needed proper, well labelled gas supply panels in the plant-room this would then make procedures much easier to follow and reduce the likelihood of error when setting up changes in gases etc. I and the other supervisors spent a long time writing down all gas supply requirements needed with the likely scenarios for routine dives, research dives, therapeutic diver treatments as well as allowing for gas mixing requirements.

Once we had this information, I used my offshore saturation system experience to map out designs for three panels in the plant-room; panel one was what came to be known as the 'HP gas distribution panel'. This panel allowed high-pressure gases, to be routed easily from and to various locations, this included supplying panel two the main 'chamber gas supply panel'; this panel was supplied with all required gases, selected via panel one; these gases could easily be routed to one or all of our chambers individually. This system actually allowed each of our chambers to run simultaneously using a wide variety of gas mixtures as required.

And finally, panel three known as the 'gas mixing panel' where gases could be routed allowing various bottles to be filled with gas mixes as required; this panel was fitted with a gas analyser capable of analysing helium and oxygen. These panels would be fully labelled and have properly numbered valves, gauges and regulators; there would be lines etched onto the face of the panels showing where gases were routed, the etching would also show any hidden valves such as non-return valves etc. Once installed these panels would be easy to follow, procedures could be written using the valve names and numbers, there would be much less chance of personnel making errors when setting up before any dive, ambiguity would be reduced dramatically and of course maintenance could be properly logged and scheduled for each numbered part.

One of my shortcomings at this time was that I had almost no medical training other than advanced first aid (DMT), therefore in April 2003 it was decided that I needed to attend a short course on hyperbaric oxygen therapy in the hope it would give me background knowledge of the subject. I agreed to attend and was then told that it would be held in Columbia, South Carolina, in the States. I would be travelling with an Australian doctor Dr Fiona Sharpe, Fiona worked as one of our bank doctors who I had met a number of times.

The course was primarily aimed at doctors and as such was completely over my head although Fiona was very good at translating the jargon for me so at the end of the course, I felt I had at least learned a few things. The course was run by an ex-north-sea-diver who I had not worked with but was an acquaintance; he had moved to America where he had been working on some very high-profile projects. He eventually found his way into provision of hyperbaric oxygen therapy and was running his own units, one of which was in the hospital in Columbia, it was a different world to DDRC, he had four Monoplace (single person) chambers which at the time of our visit were being utilised more or less continuously. As with all these courses and conferences there were some networking sessions organised, the one that I remember most was the one he hosted at his house.

He had a wonderful home right on the fairway of a spectacular golf course, it was a great evening where we spent a couple of hours reminiscing about diving in the north-sea.

On returning from Columbia, I threw myself back into production of procedures; for this to be done we needed to get the plant-room panels made and installed. Two companies agreed to quote, it soon became clear it was not going to be cheap; both quotes were around the same ball-park of about twenty-three thousand pounds. I then had to sell the idea to the rest of the SMT, this proved easier than I thought it would; it seemed that neither Karena nor James understood the plant-room pipework and both thought it had been made needlessly complicated. Karena thought the individuals concerned had made it that way as a way of protecting their jobs, I agreed that this was a definite possibility.

Having secured funding, I went back to both companies asking for installation lead times; unfortunately, one of the companies told me they were extremely busy with jobs for the MOD and couldn't see the job being completed before the end of the year, as it was just March, I felt this was unacceptable. I had no option than to award the project to the other company.

After a lot of delays and sometimes heated telephone conversations our panels did eventually arrive late August, I have to say, I was impressed with the panels. They were faced with bright blue plastic that had been etched with lines to show gas-flow, they looked great, I was looking forward to using them.

At four-thirty I went down to the plant-room to have a look at progress, all three panels were fixed in their final positions which was great progress, they really looked the part.

The next morning, when I arrived there was nobody working in the plant-room, I was not really concerned as I used to arrive at about seven-thirty and so maybe they would arrive later; by nine-thirty there was still no sign of them; I decided to call. They did eventually answer, I could hear they were in a car so thought maybe they were on their way in to us now; I thought OK, late start but maybe they would work late to make up for it. However, I was told they were instead on their way to Falmouth as they had another job to do which would take a couple of days!

I was livid; we had words but it was soon clear he would not be with us for the next couple of days; what could I do. They did eventually complete the job; the panels were a huge improvement and, in my opinion, made the system much safer; there was a much higher confidence in everyone's abilities to set up the chamber gas supply quickly and safely. We were able to at last produce proper, unambiguous plant-room checklists to be utilised for setting up various gas supplies for our chambers, it was a huge step forward; we did though never use that company again for any of our engineering work.

And so it was that on the eleventh of August 2003 we had a memorable day for the charity and truth be told for me as well; we held interviews for Chamber Superintendent and Centre Engineer both on the same day. We had three applicants for chamber superintendent and seven for engineer; the superintendent was an easy choice, Lawry Lawrence was an ex-naval warrant officer in the diving branch, he was head and shoulders above the other candidates and was offered the job the same day. Lawry became my right-hand man and really was the rock on which we built a lot of our procedures, he was a great addition to our team.

For me there was only one engineering applicant that I wanted, Ray Gibson again in my view was head and shoulders above the rest, he was again ex-navy but this time as an engineer, he was also qualified as a ship's diver so had a lot of what we needed. Again, we offered him the job on the day, he became pivotal in our new systems, he was great, he had a real can-do attitude and again I used to lean on him a great deal. With Ray coming on-board we at last had an engineer on staff who was capable of taking over the majority of jobs that we would have used outside contractors for in the past.

In August 2003 I attended my first European Underwater and Baromedical Society (EUBS) scientific meeting, these meetings were an annual affair where personnel from hyperbaric facilities throughout Europe and from the wider hyperbaric community worldwide would meet. There were several days of lectures highlighting advances, issues and problems associated with provision of Hyperbaric Oxygen Therapy (HBOT). In my role as operations director of DDRC I was required to attend these conferences most years; my first one was held in Copenhagen, Denmark in September of 2003. Generally, it was a real learning experience for me, I didn't know many people and of course almost nobody knew me; I spent the time learning about how other units provided HBOT and how this differed from the way we were doing it.

The hyperbaric system in Copenhagen was well put together and was run by ex-commercial divers, they certainly did things in a different way to us some of which I felt would not make me comfortable, but generally it was a well-run facility. I was travelling with three others from DDRC, this was evidently the norm for us, we all attended the lectures, a lot of which again went straight over my head but, I always picked up the odd nugget that was useful. The organising committee had arranged a number of networking sessions for the delegates, one on arrival, a second on the second evening and a final banquet on the final evening. A lot of wine was provided and everyone seemed to get along very well, I made a number of good contacts, some of whom I am still in contact with today.

On one of the evenings, we found ourselves at the Tivoli Gardens where there was a very famous wooden roller coaster; on the day we were there it was closed for maintenance though! We did however, find a nice hostelry in which to drown our sorrows.

The final evening was the banquet, while the weather had been kind to us for the whole time up to now, that was not to be the case this evening! The heavens opened, unfortunately, the banquet was to be hosted at Hamlet's castle on an island just offshore; we all arrived at the dockside and piled onto a small tourist boat, there were too many of us to all fit inside and so I and the others from DDRC were on the foredeck getting wet. During the journey out to the island we passed the famous statue of a mermaid that Copenhagen is famous for, the guy handling the public address on the boat was telling us about the history of Copenhagen as we passed various landmarks, he told us that the poor mermaid had been decapitated several times by vandals!

We eventually arrived at the island, all suitably informed but quite wet, we trudged from the dock up to the castle trying to avoid huge puddles along the way. On arrival we were presented with a glass of wine, the first of many and the food was very good, it was a good end to a very promising few days, generally I enjoyed it.

I had not really taken a great deal in during the conference but one thing that I did find interesting was a new body called the European Baromedical Association (EBAss), this organisation had been formed in 2002 and was specifically aimed at nurses and technicians working in the field of hyperbaric medicine. They seemed to be talking my language and I made up my mind to explore membership for both me individually and DDRC as a corporate entity.

Risk Assessment had been raised in Copenhagen as being absolutely imperative, this confirmed my view as to their importance, when I arrived at DDRC there had been very few risk assessments and this had been a timely reminder for me to make sure everything was properly risk assessed as soon as possible. I made sure that all the other chamber supervisors and managers were included in the push for continued risk assessment; they were all briefed and trained on methods of risk assessment, I had produced pro-forma risk assessment forms as well as hazard identification checklists etc. They all took this on board and went away to their individual areas to risk assess all processes and tasks, I was on hand to lend a hand but generally they all seemed to find the process straightforward.

By the end of 2003 I was confident that pretty much all work processes and tasks had been properly risk assessed, by a properly trained individual in collusion with members of the team who would normally carry out the assessed task. Each assessment was slated to be reviewed with an appropriate frequency, this meant that the majority were to be reviewed every three years but, some like fire risk assessment were to be reviewed annually.

All risk assessments were managed by an excel spreadsheet that I had set up with cells that were formatted to automatically change colour, normally they would be green but they would change to yellow when an assessment was within three-months of review and this cell would change to red if the assessment review had been missed. This meant that all I ever had to do was review the spreadsheet once a month to quickly be able to see which assessments were nearing review, I could then act accordingly; it was a good and simple system that I later applied to policies and procedures.

During this year I had also started to review all our current procedures, I had started with the plant-room but by the end of 2003 this review had been extended to most of the other procedures. It became evident to me that again, a lot of them had been written by individuals who assumed a high level of knowledge from the person who would be using the procedure. I felt this made them less useful particularly when they were being used for training new staff; I brought all supervisors and managers together; we divided up the procedures as appropriate to their individual speciality areas for instance chamber appropriate procedures to chamber supervisors etc., I briefed them as to how I felt procedures should be written. This went down like a lead balloon as a good number of the existing procedures had been written by them in the first place; I came in for a bit of flak but was adamant that in my words: "A well written procedure should allow anyone with minimal training to accomplish a complex task safely and competently."

This was the way I had always taught my students to write procedures during the CSWIP and IMCA courses and I truly believe it is the correct way to go. Policies can be very broad brush but in my view a procedure should be a step-by-step process. The aim should be to lead the individual logically through a process safely with the end result that the job is completed properly achieving the required end result with everyone going home safe and sound. Eventually, all procedures were rewritten to an acceptable level this resulted in our training becoming much more structured with newly qualified staff all learning the DDRC method of working.

Pro-Services continued to be on my mind, I wanted to focus on expanding the medical and clinical training we offered, this took years to fully accomplish but eventually we were able to offer Offshore Medic courses to the HSE syllabus, these courses trained existing nurses, paramedics or doctors in the skills allowing them to effectively become offshore GPs for want of a better description. Ultimately, we were able to offer training courses aimed at diving and hyperbaric physicians to the European Committee for Hyperbaric

Medicine (ECHM) and European Diving Technology Committee (EDTC) requirements.

By the time I retired in May 2020 DDRC, in the form of either the charity or Pro-Services were offering a comprehensive portfolio of medical training courses with help and support from hospitals and medical personnel throughout the southwest and beyond. That isn't to say I had done this all on my own, I had the support of the whole team including our doctors and nurses but, when I had started in 2002 there was no way we could even think we would be in a position to offer the majority of this training.

Another focus in 2003 as far as Pro-Services was concerned was maintaining the UAE military as a customer, they had for the past few years sent a group to DDRC for DMT renewal, they usually attended in July or August. This time of year, was chosen as during those months in UAE the temperatures were punishingly high; it was seen as a good time for their officers to attend overseas training. Gerry had left me in no doubt that they had very high standards and would go elsewhere if they didn't feel they were getting their money's worth, however, I had been given very scant instructions about how to price these or any other courses.

I worked backwards from what had been charged previously, I looked at what personnel and facilities were required to run the courses and eventually came up with a percentage figure that I felt could be applied to future course requirements. Anyway, the first group after I took over were due in early July. They kept us guessing right up to the last minute, we really didn't know if they were actually going to turn up until just a few days before arrival. This gave me significant headaches, I had to organise accommodation, personnel to run the course and all the other logistical requirements of a relatively complex four-week course. To say I had sleepless nights would be an understatement as the UAE contract was at that time key to being able to pay off the company's debt to the charity.

Eventually, they did arrive, I had to pick them up at Exeter airport one sunny Friday in early July; I was very nervous but as it turned out I was worrying about nothing! There were four students, I met them in the arrival's hall in the airport, they were all smiles and clearly very happy to be back in the UK, I had the company minibus with me so we all piled into the bus and off we went to Plymouth. I had booked them into student's accommodation with the University of Plymouth, this meant that they were all in a single unit and had cooking facilities which I felt would be ideal for them; by the time we had driven to Plymouth and checked them into their accommodation it was close to five o'clock in the evening.

I left them saying that they would be picked up by Paul Dart their chief instructor on the following Monday morning at nine o'clock, it was all smiles when I left them, great, job done, I was very relieved on my journey home that evening. Unfortunately, when I arrived at work on Monday Paul told me that all was not well, they hated their accommodation and wanted to move!

I didn't realise it at the time but this became something of a tradition, wherever we put them they would not like and always wanted to move; over time we found it best to check them into a hotel for the first three days during which time they would find their own accommodation. This of course was not always easy in July or August in Plymouth but we managed it somehow, over the course of my eighteen years working with them accommodation continued to be the single most contentious issue!

The next course for UAE personnel was to be run for their Naval officers, these guys were all experienced naval divers who needed to gain skills needed for salvage operations; our role in this was to provide them with diver inspector and welding qualifications. It had been decided that we would teach underwater inspection to the Lloyd's syllabus and my old friend Mike Pett of Hydroweld would teach them underwater wet-welding. For this the students would again come for four-weeks and I would first give them the theory of inspection during the first week which would be provided at DDRC in Plymouth.

We would all then travel up to TWI North in Middlesbrough for a week's practical inspection culminating in a Lloyd's witnessed examination. Following this they would have two weeks wet-welding and underwater oxy-arc cutting, the first week in Plymouth went very well and then off we went to Middlesbrough using the company's minibus. I had booked them into student accommodation at the Durham University's Queen's Campus which was just a couple of miles up-river from TWI's facility. I had told the students that this accommodation was the best that could be found in Middlesbrough and so they would have to stay put in there no matter what, to be fair, they were brilliant and made the most of the accommodation even to the point of asking me to eat with them from time to time. I had booked myself into a hotel in Stockton which was mid-way between TWI and the student's accommodation, it was fine for me.

For the practical side of the course, the guys had to dress into dry suits which was for some of them a completely new experience as they had never needed or used dry suits before but, one by one they made their way into the water. All went along very nicely for the practical side of the course with the Lloyds inspector turning up on the Friday to conduct their examinations, they all passed with flying colours.

The next two weeks were wet-welding, Mike turned up on the Monday morning and took control, I spent the time basically working on my Ops Director work from an office in Middlesbrough. While it was not as polished as it would be today, I managed to do most of the work necessary; Mike was an extremely patient and accomplished instructor who was able to get all the required theory drummed into them quite quickly. Then it was back into dry suits for them while Mike also jumped in the tank to show them how to weld. This again went very well and by the second day they were all producing welds on their own albeit not to the quality required, they just needed practice which is what they were given over the next eight days or so.

I was on dive-control one afternoon chatting to Mike when all of a sudden, the welder in the tank said that he had lost the arc? What was going on? Mike checked everything he could on dive-control where everything seemed to be as it should be; this just left the welding generator that was a diesel-powered unit on wheels outside the building, maybe it had run out of diesel. Mike ran down the staircase and out the door just in time to see his welding generator being hitched up to a van, it seemed that some unscrupulous individuals had decided to steal the generator while we were still using it; luckily Mike was in time. Although they had disconnected the cables running into our unit, they had not been able to hitch the generator to the van as yet so when Mike appeared they panicked and drove off leaving the generator.

We made sure there were wheel clamps fitted to the generator from then on and this was never a problem again. At this time in the early 2000's Middlesbrough had a fearsome reputation as the number one location for car theft and it seemed this also extended to generators, in short it seemed anything on wheels was fair game!

At the end of the four-week course the students had all passed everything which was a great relief to me and I'm sure to them, I dropped them off at Darlington railway station, where I saw them onto the train for London and was then free to make my way back home. On my journey home I reflected on my thinking that when I joined DDRC I would not be spending many nights away from home! Having just spent another three weeks in Middlesbrough, I imagine Chrissie was thinking things had returned to normal.

In January 2003 Gerry had sent me a request for two brand-new courses, it seemed the UAE military had a requirement for their personnel to be able to maintain their own diving equipment and chambers without the help of outside personnel or companies. We were to design and quote for technician's courses; I was invited to put together two different courses, the first would be for technicians who would be maintaining their diving equipment and the second would be for personnel maintaining their hyperbaric chambers.

I spent a lot of time looking into how we could provide these courses and while our resident staff could provide a reasonable amount of the required material, we certainly didn't have all the skills required in-house. In my view expecting their personnel to attain standards high enough to ensure they would be capable of carrying out this work during a relatively short course was a tall order; we were told the course attendees would be the same individuals who we had been teaching DMT to already and at least some of these were we knew not very practical individuals.

I eventually managed to find companies who were willing to work with us for these courses but I found it was turning into a major logistical endeavour, the diving equipment technician would be an eight-week course starting with one week in Aberdeen; weeks two and three they were near Blackpool learning how to test and maintain SCUBA systems; week four was booked for maintenance and servicing of a French re-breather set (Spiro Technique). Week five was high pressure compressor maintenance at a company in Middlesbrough; week six, they were back with us. We would need to fly a technician over from the USA to give the students training in maintenance of Draeger Lar-5 military re-breather units; week seven they were again with us learning day to day maintenance of chambers and week eight they stayed with us while we mopped up with single day visits from companies specialising in high pressure gas transfer pumps, pipework including gas regulators and finally, suit repair.

Re-breathers were units that at that time were mostly utilised by military forces around the world, they were very good for attack divers as they produced very few bubbles when they were being used as fully closed circuit, they were also largely silent in operation. These units had a 'lung' filled with the breathable mix, in some cases this would be pure oxygen but in others it could be nitrogen/oxygen or helium/oxygen mixes. The diver would breathe in and out from this 'lung'; their exhaled gas would be directed by a series of non-return valves through this closed system, the carbon dioxide (CO_2) would be 'scrubbed' from the mixture and oxygen (O_2) would be added to make up for the O_2 used by the diver. It was a simple system utilising the same processes as I had used in the JIM and Wasp suits. Nowadays, re-breathers are being used by an increasing number of recreational divers, allowing them to stay at depth for longer, dive deeper and because they do not have many exhaust bubbles, they can be excellent when used for photography or video.

The chamber maintenance course was slightly shorter at seven-weeks, the only real difference was the focus of training, they spent less time working with diving equipment and none at all on re-breathers and more time with chambers and associated support equipment. Both of these courses were high energy for us. I could not afford the time to be away shepherding the students for the amount of time they would be away from DDRC however it was imperative for someone from our company to be with them answering their questions and making sure everything went to plan.

So, I asked our trainers and maintenance technicians to accompany them instead. As I'm sure you can imagine these courses tended to be very expensive. Part of the issue for me was that we had to guarantee to pay the third-party companies regardless of whether the students turned up and most of these payments had to be up-front! This was a big risk for us as it was not at all uncommon for the UAE senior management to at the last minute tell us that the officers could not be spared due to operational commitments! I passed this on to Gerry who assured me that he could guarantee the officers would attend on the dates agreed, that at least meant I could perhaps bill them if they didn't turn up. We did run one of each of these courses in 2003 and thankfully they both went off more or less faultlessly; this was a tremendous relief to me, my stress levels both before and during these courses was again off the scale!

In fact, the summer of 2003 was bedlam, we ran two DMT refresher courses for the UAE and in addition we ran the two technician's courses and an inspection and wet-welding course. This all started in mid-May with the first diving technician's course; before this was completed the first DMT refresher course arrived in late June. The dive tech course finished on the twenty-seventh of June and the first chamber technician's course started the following Monday, thirtieth-June, the wet-welding course still had another two weeks to run at this time, as I say it was absolute bedlam and all my instructors were fully occupied and doing a tremendous job.

As part of the wet-welding course for the UAE we had to teach use of tools underwater, we were so stretched at this time that I had to take this part of the course. We were going to utilise a small tank in Portland for the wet part of this course, I accompanied the students and had booked rooms in a very nice hotel on top of Portland Bill. We had completed the first day's diving then made our way up to the hotel, when we arrived at the hotel in early evening on the tenth of July; we had a meal and then as it was such a lovely evening, the students and I went for a walk on the headland.

We had a very interesting discussion about which way they needed to be facing for prayer, I was always very careful and respectful of any student's religious requirements, so I had researched the direction for Muslim people to pray in UK. This is known as the Qibla direction; in England this is southeast (135⁰ degrees), now three out of the four students agreed with this but the fourth was not having any of it! He told me that he always prayed facing west, I tried to explain that this might be correct when he was in Abu Dhabi but it was not the same from here. He just wouldn't believe me or the other students until we found a map of the world in the hotel's reception and were able to explain the concept to him more pictorially; all was well in the end though and everyone went away happy.

The upshot of all this meant that by the end of 2003 we had reduced our debt to the charity to just under one-hundred thousand pounds making the trustees and accountants very happy.

As for the charity, by mid-way through 2003 the majority of operational procedures had been rewritten with a three-year review date set; I had also worked with the chamber superintendent and our training team to produce a comprehensive chamber team training schedule. This showed how an individual would be led through their training from a brand-new applicant right up to chamber supervisor; it showed timings, levels of training required, expected achievement and so on all the way through. In addition, it showed how persons with existing experience and skills could slot into the programme at the appropriate level.

Therefore, by the end of 2003 we had a system whereby certainly our chamber training leant on a tried and tested schedule using properly written procedures, from now on everyone would be trained in the same way to the same level regardless of who was carrying out the training. After we had been operating this system for a few years it came to the attention of the HSE and others who all were extremely positive; this and other reasons resulted in the HSE sending all new HSE diving inspectors to DDRC for a one-week diving induction. Although it was always something of a worrying time having HSE inspectors on site for a week at a time, I felt it was a vote of confidence that they sent their people to us for their induction into diving.

Eventually I got around to attending the induction day for my NVQ safety management course, I attended this day in late September 2003, the day was very well laid out and set the scene for all of us; following this day we would be invited to sign onto either level three or level four, at this time level four was the highest level available and I signed up for this. We were told we would have three years to complete all modules, level four consisted of twelve in all; we would be assigned a mentor who would be available to help us along the way. On completion of each module, it would be sent away for moderation by City and Guilds, the independent body, these modules were all stand alone and could be done in any order. This sounded a good way for me to learn, it was all about gathering evidence and together with help from my mentor I would build the effective safety management system that I felt DDRC so badly needed, driving home from the induction day I remember thinking, how hard can this be? I should be able to knock this out in a few months!

Well, quite frankly it was a lot more involved than I was expecting, I did manage to do my first few modules at a rate of about one per month but, unfortunately, other things inevitably started to get in the way; this was not always due to exceptional events it was often down to normal day to day work that made things very difficult. Having said that, I did manage to eventually finish everything in just over two years so not too bad really. So, it was that in August 2006 I was awarded Graduate Membership of IOSH (GradIOSH); I received this at a ceremony at Lincoln's Inn in London. The Honourable Society of Lincoln's Inn is one of the four Inns of Court in London to which barristers of England and Wales belong and where they are called to the Bar. This was an impressive ceremony where I was called up onto the stage to receive my qualification, Chrissie came with me, it was a lovely day but, more than that it meant that I now had the necessary qualifications for the job.

November 2003 found me on my way back to Thailand, I had for the past couple of months been liaising with Mark Shepherd with a view to organising DMT courses to be run in Thailand at Mermaid's facility in Pattaya. We were now to the point where it was time for me to visit in order to finalise everything, I arrived on the eleventh of November; I stayed in Bangkok for the first night as Mark had organised for us to see an Admiral in the Royal Thai Navy (RTN). The idea was that the navy wanted to train some of their medics as DMTs and they wanted a tie up with us to facilitate this.

It was a great idea and should work very well if we could iron out all the wrinkles; Mark had organised for us to meet with Dr Chakrii; he was at the time the surgeon general in the Royal Thai Navy (RTN); so, it was important that I impress him. I met with Mark in the morning and we drove to the RTN headquarters in Bangkok, we were admitted to the building and were ushered to Dr Chakrii's office. Right from the outset it was clear that he was on-side, he would be happy for us to use the chamber facilities both in Bangkok and also at the naval base in Sattahip, just south of Pattaya that would be much more convenient for us when running the courses in Pattaya. Our instructors and students would be given access to not only the hyperbaric chambers but also A&E and operating theatres if necessary; it was everything we needed and more. We agreed to allow four places on each course for RTN personnel free of charge and in exchange for this we would be given access to all these facilities also without charge, it was wonderful and more than I had any right to have hoped for.

With this in the bag we left Bangkok and travelled down to Pattaya, Mermaid had by now relocated to a massive new complex in Xhonburi just outside Pattaya; as we drove into the car park, I was faced with three large buildings, they were very large, light grey industrial units. Mark parked up in front of the building to the left of the site, this was the building housing Mermaid's training division, Mark's kingdom; as we entered Mark gave me a tour of the ground floor. In one corner there were rooms opening out onto a huge concrete tank which was wholly inside the building, Mark informed me that TWI were on board with them and would be carrying out CSWIP diver inspector exams in this tank.

It was a truly amazing facility, there were new Kirby Morgan Superlite 17s, new umbilicals and although the tank was empty at this time, I could see it was going to be a very impressive facility. Mark told me that CSWIP had come to the same conclusion as we had; it was becoming unacceptable to expect candidates to travel all the way to the UK, this new facility would attract people from Australasia, India and all of the far-east. I told him that we agreed and that was why we needed a base in Thailand; walking away from the tank area we went into a very nice dive control with everything required, it was even better than the Middlesbrough facility.

As we headed back to the foyer Mark showed me the classroom which also was perfect, white paint everywhere, new tables and chairs with multimedia projector fitted in the ceiling and brand-new large TV/VCR units; perfect. As we went upstairs to the admin department where all the offices were, Mark's was much larger than his old office.

We spent the rest of the day going through equipment requirements for DMT courses so that when IMCA came to audit the course everything would be there as required. Mark knew where we could purchase everything we needed, Pattaya had specialist shops with everything, some of the items for sale would not be available in the UK to anyone who was not medically qualified. By the end of the day, we had either purchased or knew where we could locate everything we needed; Mark dropped me off at my hotel and confirmed he would pick me up the next day when we had an appointment at the Sattahip Naval Base to view the facilities there.

The next morning, he arrived bright and early, I was just finishing up my breakfast and he joined me for a cup of coffee; we had an appointment at ten o'clock in the morning so there was really no hurry. Sattahip was on the coast some thirty kilometres south of Pattaya, it should take us about forty minutes by road; off we went arriving at nine-forty-five. We were admitted into the facility and met with the chamber supervisor and chief nurse; they had clearly been briefed and were keen to show us their facilities. These, were again very impressive and were at least as good as the ones we had been shown in Bangkok. They had another Haux Multiplace chamber with two locks, all set up to treat eight people seated in the main lock, for me it was perfect for our needs; we spent a couple of hours being shown around the hospital even to the point of being shown into an operating theatre while an operation was taking place! Everything was set for the course which I felt would be at least as good as the courses we were already running in the UK, sweet.

I left to travel home on the eighteenth of November feeling happy that we had found a perfect facility for our new courses; I would work with our instructors to make them happen as soon as possible.

CHAPTER TWENTY

2004

2004 dawned with the UAE asking for another DMT refresher course to be run in July, I duly prepared the required quotation and settled back to wait for the inevitable questions that would need answering before they would finally commit. This did eventually go ahead which again was a relief, we also conducted another inspection and wet-welding course commencing in June of that year as well as both dive technician and chamber technician courses. Meaning that the summer was again extremely busy with the first technicians arriving mid-June with wet-welding course running alongside from the end of June. Chamber technicians followed on so all in all things were looking good for Pro-Services.

In June I was contacted by an administrator at the Newcastle Royal Infirmary (NRI); evidently, they had a small chamber that Maurice Cross had lent to them for some research they were planning to do some years ago. Nobody currently at DDRC seemed to know anything about it but in any case, the NRI had decided they no-longer needed the chamber and as they were about to redevelop the building in which it was sited, they wanted it gone. Well, we decided we would like to have the chamber back and so I told them that I would come up to take a look at it with a view to working out organising the pick-up. I made my way up to Newcastle and found my way to the administration building where I was met by Nick one of their site managers; we made our way across to the building where our chamber was to be found.

Inside the building I was faced with something a little like an Aladdin's cave, there was loads of old equipment, in the centre was a familiar recompression chamber; it was another ex-Comex chamber painted off-white; this was very similar to the ones we had in Plymouth. In fact, as I climbed around the chamber, I found it was familiar, I remembered this chamber as it used to form part of the system when it had been set up at Bovisand. I had spent more than a few hours inside this chamber as a tender looking after divers being treated for DCI; the chamber I was looking at though was now showing signs of age and indeed was really too small to be of any real use to us now.

I was not sure what use we would be able to put this too but was sure we would find something to use it for; Nick and I chatted for a while and he asked me if there was anything else I felt would be of any use to us. I wandered around and selected a couple of large rotameters; these were clear graduated tubes inside of which were indicator weights. If the tube were to be fitted vertically and gas passed through the tube the flow of gas would support the weight, the amount of gas flow could be assessed from where the top of the weight was relative to the graduations on the tube. I thought we might have a use for this for one of our chambers so asked whether we could have both of them, Nick seemed delighted and we stowed them into our chamber; I said my farewells and told him we would arrange to have the chamber picked up over the next couple of weeks.

I had already worked with the haulage company IES, in Bristol, they had been very helpful to me in the past and I knew they would have no problem with organising for the pick-up and transport. When I returned to Plymouth, I contacted IES who as I thought, agreed to pick up the chamber and bring it back to us in Plymouth. When the chamber arrived back in Plymouth it sat in our garden for a few months before we were able to lend the it to the National Maritime Museum in Falmouth where it stayed for two years as the focal point of their static display of diving. Once the Maritime Museum decided they didn't want it any more, the chamber spent another couple of years in our garden before we donated it to Andark; a company near Southampton who wanted it. Their plan was to submerge it in their man-made lake as a feature for recreational divers to swim around and photograph.

As for Thailand, I had been in discussion with Dr Chakrii about other courses that could be run in Thailand; particularly he was interested in a form of DMT that could be offered to recreational divers, so with that in mind I travelled out to Bangkok again in early June. I met with Dr Chakrii and his manager who was a very helpful Australian, Nick Gillard; our meeting was in a waterside restaurant in Bangkok where we had a very nice meal. Although Dr Chakrii was still in the Royal Thai Navy, he was by then also running his own company BGH; primarily their business was operating Monoplace chambers offering recompression to divers in remote locations; he wanted to be able to run training courses with us; he aimed to offer advanced first aid courses to personnel working on dive boats operating holidays for recreational divers all around Thailand.

Before leaving Plymouth, I had discussed this with our instructors, we had come to the conclusion we could offer a one-week course along the same lines as the American DMT course, it would only result in DDRC certification but we felt that this would be acceptable. The first thing Dr Chakrii wanted was a catchy name for the courses, we put our heads together over the main course and came up with Remote Emergency Medical Technician (REMT), he liked it and felt we needed to promote the course at locations around Thailand. With this in mind it was agreed that Nick and I would make a road trip; although we weren't able to make it until the following year.

October 2004 saw me return to Pattaya as this was when we were due to run our first DMT course, I combined this with another trip to Singapore as Jack Pang an old friend of mine wanted to discuss us working together to again offer courses in Singapore. Unfortunately, when I arrived in Singapore Jack was not there and nobody seemed to know about his plans! I was left to tour a very impressive steel fabrication yard, I still to this day have no idea what Jack was after and I never heard from him again.

When I eventually arrived in Pattaya I met up again with Mark, everything was in place, I carried out an audit of the facility making sure that everything was as it should be then returned to the hotel to wait for my instructor Joe Allison.

I was waiting in the foyer of the hotel when Joe arrived looking very much in holiday mode, I got him checked in and then we met Mark for dinner to discuss the course. Joe had arrived with a day to spare before the course so we used this to familiarise him with the Mermaid and Sattahip facilities; on the first day of the course, I was there to welcome the students to our first course and then left Joe to carry on with the course. I stayed around for a couple of days just to help if necessary but, I wasn't needed and so decided to make my way home, Joe did a great job receiving perfect reviews from all the students.

We continued to run courses with Mermaid for another few years until Mermaid decided they weren't interested in training anymore; we then moved our DMT courses to the main RTN hospital in Bangkok where they've since flourished. Joe unfortunately left us when he secured a job at Plymouth University so the DMT courses particularly in Bangkok were taken over by an ex-police inspector Jon Parlour who did an excellent job right up until my retirement and beyond.

At the trustee's AGM in October 2004, I was able to declare that the company's loan to the charity had been paid off, this I'm sure you can understand was greeted with a good deal of smiling and congratulations. I have to say though that had it not been for Gerry continuing to send UAE personnel to us it would certainly have been a very different story. This certainly took the pressure off me somewhat, I was relieved to say the least, at least now we could start to make the charity money rather than just pay back what we owed.

DDRC had been trying to expand into south-Wales, we were already treating divers who had received DCI while diving in south-Wales and it had been highlighted that it would be a logical step for us to open a facility in Wales; this would allow us to treat not only divers but other patients as well. This had been going on since before I started but in the past few months, we had been told of a brand new Multiplace chamber that had been installed in Cardiff by an old acquaintance of mine.

He had been a trainee diver while I was working at Bovisand, I had been involved in his training; their chamber had finally been installed in a unit on an industrial estate in Pentwyn, Cardiff in mid-2004. Unfortunately for them, the expected influx of divers requiring treatment had not materialised, this had apparently resulted in them defaulting on loans with which they had purchased their chamber. They had in fact put together a very nice facility, there were all the required treatment rooms, equipment, offices and of course chamber with associated support equipment. They had purchased and installed a beautiful twelve-man Dutch, Hytech chamber, but of course without the expected income they wouldn't be able to service their loans, the chamber was subsequently repossessed by the finance company.

This had happened towards the end of 2004 and the finance company were now looking for a buyer, we were definitely in the market, Karena and I had an appointment with the finance company to view the chamber with a view to taking it on. Indeed, we were looking to see whether we could take over not just the chamber but the whole facility, it was quite exciting.

As I say the facility had clearly been put together with a high degree of quality, it was very nice, so much so that we agreed a price with the finance company who told us they would organise the necessary paperwork for transferring ownership to DDRC, we also started negotiations with the landlord of the building to see about making a deal to take on the unit. The building was locked up, alarmed and we thought secured so; off we went back to Plymouth to start the ball rolling with a view to opening up the facility in early 2005. I of course didn't know it at the time but, this would end up being a particularly distasteful time for all concerned!

2004 ended with the news of a dreadful Tsunami that had struck the eastern shore of mainland Thailand on December twenty-sixth of 2004; there had been terrible devastation all along that coast and the islands in the area as well, there were reputed to be thirty-metre waves hitting the beach resulting in some one hundred and seventy thousand deaths. We were to see evidence of some of the devastation when Chrissie and I holidayed on the island of Langkawi in Malaysia the following year.

CHAPTER TWENTY-ONE

2005

At the start of 2005 I had made contact with the European Baromedical Association (EBAss) with a view to joining. I was invited to attend the next EBAss board meeting that was due to take place in April at a hospital in Murnau, Germany; Murnau was a small town just to the south of Munich; I flew to Munich on Friday as the meeting was to take place on the Saturday, I continued my journey by train to Murnau. I had been advised of a suitable hotel close to the hospital where the meeting was to be held and duly booked myself in; I obviously didn't know anybody on the EBAss board although I had met the president while in Copenhagen.

In the morning of the meeting, I recognised the president at breakfast and introduced myself to him, he said he remembered me and proceeded to make me very welcome, he had driven from his home in Brussels and so offered me a lift to the hospital for the meeting. When I had arrived the day before it was already dark and so I hadn't been able to see much of Murnau, however, this morning as we drove to the hospital I was being taken through a lovely little town in the foothills of the alps; It was a lovely place, looking really peaceful and pleasant.

The hospital was a very impressive fairly new building, everything was extremely clean and well maintained, we were met by Andreas Kanstinger who was part of the chamber team. Andreas became a good friend and was always extremely helpful to me. The meeting was held in a small conference room where the board members gathered, there were eight of them and although I only knew a couple from my attendance at EUBS meetings, I soon came to know them all quite well. Board members were from Belgium (three), France (one), Switzerland (one), Greece (one), Italy (one) and of course one from Germany.

I was introduced as a prospective new board member, I had been asked to produce a short presentation as an introduction of both myself and DDRC, this went down quite well although some of the individuals were adamant that they didn't agree with the use of Monoplace chambers of which we had by this time one as well as our three Multiplace chambers. Once my presentation was complete, I was invited to stay for the rest of the meeting and of course that is what I chose to do, it was interesting. It seemed that EBAss had been involved in helping to produce a Resources Manual (RM), a document detailing training requirements and levels for hyperbaric staff, nurses, attendants and technicians. This document had recently been adopted as the key document for training across the whole European Union, I was glad to see that our (DDRC's) recently introduced training regime largely ran along the lines suggested in the RM.

At the end of the meeting, we were taken on a tour of the hospital's hyperbaric facility which was hugely impressive, they had a very new and large hyperbaric chamber in a beautifully set out chamber room; I took a lot of photographs and a fair few ideas back to DDRC.

When we got back to the hotel, I asked the receptionist to book me a taxi to take me to the train station in the morning; he looked nonplussed and replied to me "But it's Sunday tomorrow?" Evidently Murnau's taxi service didn't operate on Sunday mornings, this was a problem for me; because of my MS I couldn't walk all the way to the train station in the morning. Our president was still with me and bless his heart he told me he would get up and take me to the station in the morning, my train was early, leaving at seven o'clock so this was definitely above and beyond for him, I was though extremely grateful.

So, it was I had checked out at six-thirty the next morning and was driven to the station, as we parted, he told me he would see me at the next EUBS meeting to be held in Barcelona in September.

I made my way onto the platform, as I entered, I glanced at the station clock to see that I was five minutes early, there were a few individuals on the platform, looking around, I could see snow-capped peaks off to the south highlighted against a clear, blue sky with just a few fluffy, white clouds. Seven o'clock came and went with no train, five past seven, still no train; now, obviously being British I was used to waiting for late trains but I could see the others on the platform were not seeing this as acceptable.

By ten past seven there were a number of very bad-tempered individuals on the platform, some of them were berating an employee who scurried off, I was not sure whether he was going to hide or to find out the reason for the delay! The train eventually pulled into the station at just before seven-fifteen. I was by now a little concerned as the connection to my flight was quite tight but I needn't have worried as the train made up the delay and arrived back in Munich bang on time.

April the twenty-eighth 2005 was another memorable day to begin with it was my forty-nineth birthday but perhaps more significantly I was contacted by a tenant in one of the units adjacent to our new chamber unit in Pentwyn. It seemed that the boss of the original company had broken into our unit and was currently engaged in removing equipment; as soon as I put the phone down, I called the police in Cardiff who told me they would send someone along to the unit.

I informed the rest of SMT and drove straight up to Cardiff. When I arrived, I could see the door to the unit was open, there were a number of men carrying items out of the building; as I was driving in through the gates to the industrial-park I had failed to notice that only one gate was open; I collided with the second gate which luckily was quite a flimsy affair, it gave way and I drove through. I saw the landlord and a police car both of whom were sitting in their cars across the road from the unit, I parked alongside them and proceeded to ask them what they had seen.

They had been watching for an hour or so and had seen a number of individuals removing equipment which I could see was now being stacked on the driveway in front of the unit; I told them I would go and see what was going on. As I approached the door to the unit accompanied by the policeman, we were met by the owner of the company who proceeded to tell us he was just taking back what was rightfully his, he disputed that the finance company now owned the chamber and other equipment. Eventually, I managed to talk him down and he agreed that he would put all the equipment back while we would enter discussions between him, the finance company and us to see how we could move on with this issue.

However, he was adamant that DDRC couldn't purchase the chamber although he was very angry that any charity could have squirreled away enough money to be able to purchase the chamber anyway. I felt this was not going to end well; I couldn't see how we could manage the building and keep the equipment safe when we were faced with an individual who had already shown that he would break in through the roof of the building! I left that evening having agreed with him that he would give us a week to sort things out, the police had promised to increase patrols in the area which I felt was the best we could hope for. Certainly, this was not how I had thought I would be spending my birthday!

I felt that our chamber was at risk if left in the building in Pentwyn; the next day I called an extraordinary SMT meeting with Karena and James. I went into detail of what had happened the previous day, they were both horrified to say the least; I felt we had no option other than to move the chamber system out of the building as I didn't think it would ever be safe where it was. They both agreed, so my next job was to organise removal and storage of the chamber in a safe facility. I had already been in contact with an extremely helpful chap in a big haulage firm, Tim Patten of IES in Bristol.

Tim had previously helped us to relocate our old chamber from Newcastle and had proven to be very much a can-do individual as were the company generally; as soon as he picked up the phone he was on board with the project. I explained what we needed together with the urgency and he was great, he said he could not see this being a problem; we agreed to meet at the unit so that he could get a feel for what was required, off I went back to Cardiff. Just after lunch I met with Tim at the unit, I showed him what needed to be moved and was able to give him most of the weights for the various pieces of equipment; we agreed that he would organise craneage, trucks and manpower and would let me know as soon as this could be done. When he left, I felt reassured, he was treating it as just another job and exuded confidence; I locked up the unit and made my way home.

Next day Tim called me at eleven o'clock to tell me everything was organised for the following day but the chamber and other equipment needed to be in a state whereby it could all be moved as soon as they arrived which he told me would be nine o'clock tomorrow morning! Wow, this was great although I now had another problem as the whole system was currently set up ready to dive; I needed to get everything disconnected ready for the move in the morning. Enter our engineer Ray, I went down to see him to discuss how we could achieve this, he was great, there was never any negativity, he just started making a list of tools needed.

I of course would be there to help but we needed another hand at least; at the time Ray had a part-time support engineer, Trevor Burnett, Trevor was an ex-submariner, who was also very much another can-do individual. I had always kept both of them appraised of the situation in Cardiff and they were very much on board with developments. I explained that we needed to disconnect the whole system and this would need to be done before nine the next morning; neither of them showed any unease with this and agreed they would work through the night to get the job done; they were a couple of absolute stars!

I left them to get their tools together and headed back up to Pentwyn to meet up with the landlord, Ray and Trevor would follow in the company minibus later. When I arrived, the landlord was already there and had opened up the building, he was not at all happy with the situation as he was now losing his tenant but he completely understood our point of view. As it turned out within a couple of months of us moving out, he had a new tenant who was servicing Jaguar cars and to my knowledge they are still there so it all worked out well for the landlord in the end.

As soon as I had finished discussions with the landlord, I started to look at dismantling the chamber system, this was not something new to me as I had been involved with lots of demobilisation of chamber systems while working offshore. I started with identifying where hoses, pipework and cables ran so that I could point Ray and Trevor in the right direction when they arrived, it was a well laid out system that had been installed by Hytech; I knew the boss of Hytech well and had been confident that everything would have been laid out sensibly. Unfortunately, while looking around the dive control section I noticed that the computer required to run the chamber system was missing, I don't know to this day what happened to it but I can make an educated guess. This would be a problem when we came to reinstall the chamber somewhere else but I was confident that Hytech would help us with this when the time came.

Ray and Trevor arrived early afternoon and immediately we all met to discuss what needed to be done; we divided up the tasks between us and got to work; I was by now suffering a little more with mobility due to my MS so I was left to dismantle the peripherals on the chamber. I set to work dismantling the CCTV cameras, the comms systems and removing the chamber side panels, these panels were hiding pipework and made the chamber look very sleek and pretty.

By six o'clock I had finished removing all the parts assigned to me, I had stacked the side plates inside the main lock of the chamber and had tidied up the dive control panel with all cables being coiled up inside. While I had been doing this Ray and Trevor had disconnected the HP air bank, the compressors and the fire suppression system. All was going well so I went off to get food and drinks for us from the local McDonalds; we sat outside the unit to eat our meal and noticed that we were being watched by two men in a grey van parked opposite one of the empty units just down the road from us.

We were a little unnerved by this, I'm sure we were all over-thinking this wondering what they might be planning, I called Tim to let him know about this development but he just told me there would be a lot of burly, young men with us tomorrow so bring it on! Anyway, we went back to work and to be fair never saw or heard from anyone all night, so perhaps the guys in the van were just taking a break and watching the show? We had been making great headway so far but that was because we had done the easy bits; the majority of the pipework for the chamber was flexible pipe, this had all been disconnected and coiled up. All of these were labelled and stacked in the front corner of the unit ready for shipping tomorrow; similarly, the majority of cabling had also been labelled and coiled.

Next, we had to strip down the HP air bank, this consisted of fifty, fifty-litre bottles; arranged in racks along the back wall of the unit. The bottles were plumbed together with hard pipework which all had to be removed, this took quite a long time as it needed to be done carefully, I labelled everything as it came off so that putting it all back together would be simpler. We eventually finished dismantling everything we could by half past two in the morning, we were all ready for the morning; we didn't have any bedding or anything much to lie on at all really so we all just got our heads down on a piece of floor and tried to get some sleep. I had chosen a carpeted office as my bedroom, and while I did doze a little, I don't think I actually slept at all; I was up making coffee for us all at seven in the morning, I was soon joined by Ray and Trevor who both looked bleary eyed so I'm sure nobody slept any more than I had.

At nine o'clock on the dot a Ford Transit van sporting the IES logo turned up with Tim in the driver's seat, as it came to a halt the side door opened and five large men leapt out stretching themselves and making ready to get to work. Tim and I went inside with Ray and Trevor to explain what we had achieved over night; Tim beckoned to one of his guys who he said was the foreman. We spent a few minutes looking at the chamber and how we could get it outside; the chamber could not be lifted from its current position, and would need to be slid outside; I wasn't sure how this could be done but of course Tim had no such worries this was all in a day's work for him. The chamber was sitting in a shallow pit about thirty centimetres deep.

Tim explained how they were going to jack it up out of the pit and then they would settle it onto small dolly trucks; the chamber could then be wheeled out onto the forecourt where the crane would be able to lift it easily. Ray, Trevor and I stood back to watch, it was like watching a well-oiled machine; within just an hour or so the chamber was out of the pit, on the dollies and slid out of the building.

We then discussed loadings for the crane and it was decided that the crane was more than capable of lifting the chamber with enough capacity to be able to cope with us putting the various hoses, cables and other ancillaries inside. This made things much simpler as it reduced the number of lifts dramatically; the crane turned up at eleven o'clock together with a low-loader truck and another panel van; everything was loaded onto the various trucks over the next couple of hours and by two o'clock I was waving them away. We had arranged for the system to be stored in IES's secure facility at Avonmouth until we could find an appropriate location for our Welsh unit.

Ray and Trevor climbed into the firm's minibus and after I had secured the building again, I handed the keys back to the landlord and followed in my car; we all headed to IES's facility to witness the offloading and storage. Tim and the rest of the team completed everything very quickly and by four o'clock the chamber was sitting in its new temporary home, I told Tim that I would keep him updated with when and where we would be taking the chamber. I didn't know it at the time but things wouldn't go to plan at all as far as this chamber was concerned, we never did find a site for a Multiplace chamber in Wales resulting in us selling it again through Hytech.

Korea:

Out of the blue in May I was contacted by a Korean chap by the name of Kai Park (Soo), he was working with a Korean diving company and the Korean Government; it seemed that the Korean government had realised that most of the diving being carried out in Korea was currently being done by overseas personnel. They wanted to put a diving school together and they wanted divers leaving this school to have their qualifications recognised by the UK HSE; Kai realised that they needed help to achieve this and this was where DDRC came in. Initially, contact was via email which led to phone conversations.

I needed to find out exactly what they were planning so that we could put a plan together for them; the list I was eventually provided with was extensive, in short, they wanted everything! They were looking for consultancy from us to advise them on saturation diving systems, they had already purchased a small saturation system which they were about to install on an old pipe-lay barge. This all sounded promising but fell short of giving me a full picture. At this time, they seemed to be focusing more on saturation diving with not much emphasis on the route to qualifying personnel in air diving which certainly in the view of the HSE would be an essential first step. Before long it was suggested I should travel out to their diving school to get a first-hand look at what facilities they currently had and what still needed to be done.

I got to work on what would be needed for the Korean school, I called my contacts in the HSE who were very helpful; they pointed out that the HSE were no longer able to actually accredit diving schools outside of the UK. All they could do would be to add them to the list of recognised diver qualifications, this listed overseas diving courses that trained to HSE standards. He went on to explain that for this school to be accepted as providing recognised training they would need their training to be audited annually by a recognised UK training establishment. I of course asked him what constituted a recognised UK establishment; it seemed that this establishment should have membership of IMCA or an equivalent organisation, with staff who had experience in the relevant diving disciplines; they would need to be able to show a proven background in training of divers; he agreed that DDRC would fit comfortably into this category.

July arrived; Chrissie and I had planned another of our bucket list holidays, when we had first found each other, Chrissie had recently met a lady while on holiday. This lady had holidayed in Bali where she had reputedly seen dolphins frolicking in the sea just offshore of her hotel's beach. Chrissie had always wanted to experience this and this was the year when that was to take place. We planned a three-week holiday starting off in Bali for a week then on to Kuala Lumpur where her dad had been stationed and finishing off on the tiny Malaysian island of Langkawi; well, this was a wonderful trip although the dolphins didn't play ball, we did see some lovely sights in Bali though. KL was also great we spent a lot of time in the older colonial areas where Chrissie could feel she was walking streets where her dad had been.

DDRC's summer again consisted of servicing UAE DMT refresher, wet-welding as well as dive equipment and chamber technician courses all running at the same time; again, the instructors, engineers and all the chamber team handled all these courses brilliantly, they were all stars. When we were running courses for the UAE it was always full on, generally, I used to get on very well with the students, they almost all had a great sense of humour and were fun to be with; on one of the first courses, I ran for them this was made very clear to me. We were half way through a lecture on diving physics when I could see I had lost them; they were all staring out the window, I couldn't see what they were looking at as to me it just looked like an awful day weatherwise, it was raining cats and dogs.

I asked them whether they wanted to take a break, they all leapt up and almost ran out the door into the car park; where they just stood in the rain looking up getting soaking wet. When they came back in, I asked what that was all about; it seemed that for them rain was really something special, as they saw rain so infrequently when they did see it, they liked to properly experience it. This cleared things up for me and made it obvious why they liked to come to the UK in our summer where they were bound to see lots of rain.

In September we were again off to EUBS, this time I was to be delivering a presentation to the full conference which I have to say was making me nervous; this year the conference was in Barcelona. I was travelling with Dr Hardwick, Gary Smerdon and a couple of others. Gary had recently come on board at DDRC following external appraisal of DDRC's research activity, it had been decided to create a part time position for a Research Director and in August Gary had arrived from his previous role in marine research. Gary would turn out to be a great colleague and travelling companion and we would work together right up until my retirement.

We were all booked into the conference hotel which made things easier as far as transport was concerned. My presentation would detail the training of hyperbaric personnel, I was to lay out the new EBAss/ECHM system that detailed who should be trained and to what levels etc. This was due to take place in the afternoon of the first day but before that I had to take my place at the associated EBAss poster in order to field questions. When I was on my way back down to the conference room to get ready for my presentation, I was descending in the lift when suddenly it stopped between floors! Who would have credited it, of all the times for this to happen, I pushed the alarm button but nothing, there was no response? Eventually I used my mobile phone to call Gary who was sitting listening to presentations in the conference room. He managed to raise the alarm and get staff to release me from the lift just in time for me to dash to the podium to deliver my presentation.

While I was quite comfortable presenting to classrooms full of students, this was a different ball game completely. As I arrived at the lectern, I heard my name over the PA as my lecture was being introduced; as I had only just been released from the lift and although I wasn't late, I did only just get to the stage in time so, I was somewhat out of breath. I had to pull myself together, as I looked out over the conference floor, I was faced with a couple of hundred faces all looking up at me. I had to remember that they were all here to listen to what I had to say and would not be critical of me or my presentation; this is easy to say sitting here but I can assure you it wasn't very reassuring to me on the day.

I had notes to follow and of course a PowerPoint presentation was displayed on the large screen behind me as well as on the screen in front of me. I took a deep breath and started with my introduction, I was extremely nervous and found it somewhat difficult to breathe to begin with. Very soon though as I clicked the mouse to advance into the main presentation my nerves disappeared and I was off; I had twenty-minutes to fill which was really not enough to cover the subject but hopefully I was able to lay out the basics and pique their interest.

At the end of the presentation, I told them all that I would be available for questions during the rest of the conference; that was the end and I was free to leave the stage, I can tell you I was very relieved when this was over and I could find my way back to my seat. Over the coming days it became clear that some delegates had been listening and wanted more information which I was glad to be able to supply for them.

The second day I was due to attend the EBAss board meeting where I would be co-opted onto the board; the meeting was not scheduled to be in the main hotel, rather it was in a small room in a building on the edge of the harbour. The existing board members and I traipsed down to the venue where again there were the eight existing board members and me; there was a good deal of business to get through before we arrived at the point where I would be invited to come onto the board though. Eventually, we got there and I was duly invited to take up a position on the board, I was pleased about this as I felt I could be of use to them although I was not so pleased with the next development.

It seemed the current treasurer a French lady was retiring from the board and so would no longer be treasurer and yes, you've guessed it I was asked whether I would take this on! I have to tell you, I was not keen, I had no clue what was involved and would have preferred to have a role to do with safety or chamber operations; it just got worse though, when after the meeting I sat with her who had two thick folders with all the documentation. She didn't really speak much English and I certainly didn't speak enough French; everything was in French the bank was in Belgium and she couldn't really explain much to me.

This nightmare was not going away though, I took the folders with me and made my way back to the hotel where I found the EBAss president; I explained that I didn't see how I could be treasurer when everything was in French. He saw my point but didn't seem to feel it was as bad as I was making out, eventually he agreed to help whenever I found a problem that I couldn't solve; this it seemed was going to be all I could expect and I would just have to get on with it. I did operate as EBAss treasurer for the coming year but towards the end was able to convince him that treasurer was not for me and he did eventually agree to take the role from me.

In early November following discussion with James Hardwick and Karena I was given the opportunity to undergo a course of hyperbaric oxygen treatment (HBOT). I had been reading a lot of articles relating to treatment of MS using HBOT, there were a few trials that seemed to show there could be a benefit but there were more showing that HBOT would show no benefit. Well, I was keen to at least give it a go and thought that given where I worked, I should try it. Before I started the course of treatment, I underwent a series of exercises so that any improvement following the treatments could be gauged accurately. I then carried out a six-week course where I had a ninety-minute treatment at twelve metres five days per week in our Monoplace chamber.

It was very nice to be allowed to effectively have an hour and a half lie down in the middle of the day, initially I thought there might be some benefit and a few of my colleagues seemed to feel my walking improved. However, once the course of treatment was complete, I underwent the same exercises as I had done before I started the treatment and it became clear that I really had not experienced any marked improvement; it was a shame but I was not really surprised; I was however very grateful to the management for letting me go through this treatment, as I would have always felt it might have helped if I had not done this trial.

Back to Korea, my trip had taken a long time to organise, South Korea was not the easiest place to visit in those days, I eventually made my way to Seoul, in late November 2005. Soo met me in the arrival's hall at Incheon airport, following introductions we made our way out of the airport to his car; Seoul was of course the capital city of South Korea, it was situated on the west coast but the diving school was on the east coast so we had to make our way across South Korea to Goseong on the east coast. This turned out to be about a five-hour trip along a well-built motorway system, by the time we arrived it was mid-evening so Soo took me straight to the hotel where I checked in; he then told me he would pick me up in the morning and take me to the school.

In the morning, I was just finishing my breakfast when Soo turned up; the school was not far from the hotel so after just a few minutes we drove in through the gates, I was pleasantly surprised by their yard. I could see there were recompression chambers, a diving bell together with a wet-bell, various hoses and umbilicals; around the perimeter of the yard there were several buildings. Soo parked up and we made our way through the door to the building on the left, inside we immediately turned right and climbed metal steps, on reaching the top of the steps, we emerged onto a deck alongside their diving tank. I had a feeling of Déjà vu, I was transported back to TWI in Middlesbrough, it was almost a carbon copy although here it was a rectangular tank; there were Superlite-17s and all the other equipment necessary for diving. It was very impressive, I also saw topside equipment from Hydroweld, Soo told me that Mike Pett had already run some wet-welding courses for them.

After our tour it was time to meet with the Director of the Korean Government Human Resources Department; this meeting was to be conducted in the school's main administration building, which was on the other side of the yard. As we entered the administration building Soo led me upstairs to the first floor where the Director was already waiting for us; we went through the routine required whenever people in Korea meet for a business meeting. Following this we sat on comfortable seating arranged in a semi-circle so that we could all be facing one another easily; unfortunately, the director didn't speak any English and of course I had no Korean language at all. Soo was going to be interpreting for me; I had produced a PowerPoint presentation but of course it was in English and was virtually useless other than as a prompt for me.

I explained how we could work together with initial audits of their facilities followed by annual audits of the facilities together with assessment of student attainment etc., I showed them what the HSE had told me about their expectations; they seemed to take this all on board but I wasn't really certain. They agreed that they would make it a priority to join IMCA and I agreed to help with their application; we would see where everything went from there.

Next on their agenda was lunch; apparently, I had to be taken to lunch at a posh and very traditional restaurant; so off we all went; the restaurant was not far from the school, I was taken down small, semi-rural roads in Soo's car towards the restaurant which was right on the sea and very picturesque. When we arrived four other men joined the party, as is the tradition everyone removed their footwear, we were then taken into a small room with a very low table; around the table were blue cushions for us to sit on.

Now, by this time my MS was beginning to affect my abilities, I found it very difficult to sit on or in anything that had no back; I could not sit cross legged at all and this looked as though it might be an issue! However, they were great and very understanding; the table was rearranged so that I could rest against the wall and have my right leg laid out straight in front of me, this took a good fifteen minutes but eventually we were all sitting and while I can't say I was comfortable I at least was stable. We were then served by Korean ladies wearing traditional Korean dress, they brought a large quantity of dishes that were placed onto the table, none of these dishes seemed to contain anything that was remotely recognisable from an European idea of what food should look like; oh well here we go, another voyage of discovery.

I don't to this day know much about what we were fed that day and while some of it was very tasty; some of the other dishes were in my humble opinion not actually food! Some of them contained black goo that was extremely bitter containing gelatinous lumps! I have no idea what this was or what the lumps consisted of, there were some dishes that were clearly local delicacies that I was told I just had to try; some of these were nice but again some were not. I sampled them all and made the appropriate noises and faces to show my appreciation; that being said it was a nice lunch and Soo was at pains to tell me that they were all very appreciative of my coming all this way to meet with them and to offer our help.

After lunch the majority of the guys left us to return to whatever they were supposed to be doing and Soo and I went off to have a look at the barge that they were planning to use for the open water diving part of the courses. For this we headed north along the coast road that ran along the coast of the Sea of Japan; we were heading towards Goseong although the barge was in a small harbour on the coast some way past the village. When we arrived; Soo parked up and we walked towards the harbour, off to our left there was a concrete wall which I could see was topped by some fortifications.

There were several guards with rifles and a fixed gun that could have been an anti-aircraft battery (I'm guessing there though), we were joined by some of the guards who walked behind us down towards the jetty. Soo told me we were close to the demilitarised zone (DMZ) so, the guards were interested in anything going on that they hadn't been told about in advance; while they were all smiles for Soo, they were clearly nervous of me.

Anyway, all of us wandered down to the harbour where there was a large barge, while it was certainly large enough and had a big flat area on which work could be carried out,

I couldn't see any evidence of diving equipment. Soo told me that they hadn't started the conversion but that over the next three months it would be transformed with all the equipment I had seen in the yard at the school being installed on the barge. Well, if that were the case then it would make a very good platform for the school to operate from.

This was the end of my visit and Soo took me back to Seoul where we met with his boss, his main focus seemed to be on where to eat that evening and thankfully he chose a bar-b-que restaurant. We, made our way across town to a very modern looking restaurant where they had bar-b-que pits in the centre of each table. This was great, although again the seating was similar to lunchtime in that the table with the bar-b-que in the centre was very low, around this table there were five or six large cushions for us to sit on. I had a seat where I could lean back against the wall and I got to cook my own food; what's not to like? We were asked what meat we would like and I chose beef steak, this was supplied in very finely sliced portions which took almost no time at all to cook, now I would never claim to be a good cook but bar-b-que of thinly sliced beef was within my capabilities so we had a lovely meal being supplied with a baked jacket potato each and some nicely cooked vegetables to go with our meat.

After this meal it was almost time for me to leave as I had an early flight in the morning, Soo took me to an airport hotel where I checked in. The hotel was a little strange from an European viewpoint, it was more of a suites hotel as you might find in the USA or Australia in that when I got to my room it was quite large, there was a nice big lounge with seating area and a huge bed, there was a kitchen with all the mod cons you would expect and of course an ensuite bathroom. This room was approached by riding up in the lift to the sixth floor where I found myself on a concrete walkway around a large central atrium, as I peered over the balustrade downwards, I could see the reception area on the ground floor, all the different levels rising from there had rooms arranged around the outside of the atrium well.

Around each level were a large number of doors which I assumed led into similar units to the one I had been assigned. It all looked very futuristic; I made my way back into my room which was again white painted. I had not seen any restaurant or bar area but was in need of something to drink, I decided to have a look outside the hotel to see whether I could find a shop. As I exited the foyer and turned right along the outside wall of the hotel, I came across a small general store, inside it felt as though I had been transported to the USA, it was reminiscent of an American seven-eleven, I was able to purchase a bottle of water and something for breakfast the following day.

The next morning, I caught the courtesy bus that would take me to the airport, this was available every fifteen minutes and was free, much better than the service available from London hotels where you always had to pay for courtesy buses. My journey home was fine with nothing exceptional in any way. I did continue to work with the Korean school but we never did carry out any audits so I assume they decided to not go with having their courses recognised by the HSE, ah, well you can't win them all.

CHAPTER TWENTY-TWO

2006

2006 was another memorable year both for me and for the charity; in January and February it was becoming clear that the Care Standards Commission who were at the time responsible for ensuring care was being administered appropriately (the Care Standards Commission began to morph into the Care Quality Commission (CQC) which became active on the 1st April 2009), were likely to be paying us a visit sometime in the near future. While we were not overly concerned by this it was becoming clear that their audit team were extremely heavy handed and of course they had the power to close down facilities should they feel the need.

At one of our fortnightly senior management team (SMT) meetings I suggested the charity should gain a quality standard which would I thought go a long way to reassuring any interested party. Following lengthy discussion, it was decided that I should look at appropriate routes for the charity; I was given two months to formulate a plan, I would then present a budgeted plan to SMT. Consequently, I presented my findings at a meeting in early May, my view was that the charity should become ISO 9001 registered, the cost of this was not high in monetary terms with the majority of the work being carried out in-house. I suggested we purchase an off the shelf product called 'ISO in a Box', this product provided the framework for an effective quality management system that could be adapted to our specific requirements; this was given the thumbs up and I was told to get on with it.

The company marketing ISO in a Box were of course were very happy to help us; I was assigned an auditor and mentor; Jonathan Lea. Jonathan would be available to provide specific assistance and would carry out the required internal audit of our system immediately before we went for ISO accreditation. ISO in a Box was provided to me on a CD, there was virtually no associated paperwork but there was an introductory file that explained things well; on the disk there was a complete Quality Management System (QMS) but of course it was generic and had to be tailored to our specific needs.

I set to work learning what was required starting with the ISO 9001 document that laid out everything that would be expected of our system at audit. Luckily the pack we had purchased allowed for Jonathan to come to us to carry out some training for me; he spent two days with me initially during which time we formulated a plan. There were supplied electronic pro-forma documents for almost everything we would need but, I had to go through them and assign specific information regards where the documents would be stored, I had to assign version numbers, date of first issue, logos and in some instances signatures.

This was all quite exhaustive and although most of the documents were supplied; they all had to be individually altered to suit our facility; this process was not limited to altering the supplied documents from ISO in a Box but also all our existing Policies, Procedures and Risk Assessments had to be altered to show issue dates, version numbers and specific information to make it easy for everyone to find and be assured they were using the correct version. This took me a couple of months, by the first of July I was ready, or at least I thought I was ready for our first audit.

During the last couple of months, I had enlisted the help of the other senior management as the ethos of a good QMS should come from the top down to all levels of the organisation. The middle managers or department heads also had key parts to play and luckily were all on board with the process although not all of them were totally convinced of its value at this time. And, of course all the 'coal-face' workers were involved as they had to know their part of the process. They would be quizzed by the auditor to ensure they knew things such as which specific set of procedures they should be using etc.

The last step before going for the official external audit was for Jonathan to perform a full dress-rehearsal audit of our system; this took place in late July and perhaps unsurprisingly he was not able to find any major issues. There are two levels of non-conformance that could be raised during audit, these were 'area of concern' and 'major non-conformance'. We had no major non-conformances identified and only one area of concern which was very minor, I was very happy and so was Jonathan, he declared us to be ready for the full external audit.

I duly organised this with the company who would finally issue us with ISO 9001 accreditation, I hoped! The company charged with this was EQUAS, my contact was Henry Gough who would be carrying out our initial audit in early August; this was a really big deal for us and I was nervous; Jonathan had of course passed us but I was not sure EQUAS would be so lenient with us.

On the day of the audit Henry turned up with a second auditor Kim Rowse; they first wanted to review our system by carrying out a paperwork exercise. I explained that we did not have a printed paper copy of our quality manual as we were working with an electronic version, this was absolutely fine with them, Phew I was relieved as having to print everything would have taken hours. I sat down with them in one of our training rooms, I supplied them with a lap-top computer that was logged on to our system; they spent a couple of hours working through our system; they were already au-fait with the ISO in a Box system and so were quickly able to identify the significant points.

Following this, Henry came with me to interview the senior management; meanwhile, I had previously arranged for Lawry to handle Kim, Lawry had been briefed to take the auditor around our system to show that all SOPs and other paperwork had the correct version numbers and issue dates etc., this also included him introducing the auditor to our team members so that he could see how the system had been rolled out to all our staff. This audit made it a long day for me and the team; as this was the initial audit the auditors quite rightly wanted to see everything; as it turned out I needn't have worried, it seemed Jonathan was far more pedantic than the EQUAS auditors were which, I feel was exactly the right way for things to be. At the end of the day the auditors declared we had passed with no non-conformances or indeed any areas of concern, a completely clean bill of health; DDRC were now to be registered as ISO 9001 accredited.

Of course, everyone was very relieved that we had gone through this process and achieved the desired result, I certainly was extremely happy driving home that day. Over the coming months this was borne out by discussions we had with the likes of the Care Standards Commission, our NHS commissioners and other auditors such as IMCA and HSE who were tasked with routinely auditing us for various reasons. Each time we had a visit from any of these auditors who all would have heaps of forms and paperwork to complete, as they came to the quality part of their forms the fact, we had achieved ISO 9001 was good enough for them resulting in ticks going in all the appropriate boxes!

As I said before, August 2006 was when I finally passed my ISOH qualification and was awarded GradIOSH status; this was very important for me but also gave DDRC the safety qualified individual in the senior management that they had never had in the past but which in my view had always been necessary.

With both the ISO accreditation and my health and safety qualification DDRC became of more use to the likes of the police and other bodies. We were subsequently contracted by the Police Service Northern Ireland (PSNI) and the local Devon and Cornwall forces to carry out investigations of diving equipment that had been recovered from recreational divers who had died. We had to test gases in the bottles, download dive computers and carry out function tests of equipment; I would then write reports that would be used as evidence in coroner's courts. This would mean that I could be called as an expert witness at Coroner's Court; one time this happened I was summoned to appear at the Coroner's Court in Brighton.

While I didn't mind the work, I found appearing in the court where I would describe our findings to be somewhat unnerving, the friends and family of the deceased would be in court and of course wanted to find out more about why their loved one had died. While I could give results and findings, often this didn't really go very far towards proving what actually happened, I was not really sorry when the HSE decided they would take on this duty as I felt it should have been their job in the first place.

The EUBS conference this year was to take place in Bergen, Norway, it was this year to take place in late August; this time DDRC sent three of us, there was Dr James Hardwick, Dr Gary Smerdon and me. I was not scheduled to present this time, the conference went well with a number of the great and good of hyperbaric worldwide presenting the latest advances in the field, again, we all sat through these lectures and I did gain some good insight that I felt could be put to good use back in Plymouth.

The associated EBAss meetings went as well as could be expected. One evening after the conference had finished for the day our EBAss president and I found a small bar where we could sit down; I wanted to discuss things and how my role in EBAss should progress. As I said before, EBAss had been involved in the production of the EBAss/ECHM Resources Manual (RM), I started our chat stating how important I felt this had been but that I was worried EBAss needed a new role. I felt that if we didn't have an active role our membership would dwindle as the members needed to see a purpose for EBAss, it was clear that he agreed to some extent. I went on to describe my thoughts; in my view the RM though fundamental to full and proper training across all the European member states it did nothing to ensure staff had actually achieved the required standards.

My plan was that EBAss launch an independently accredited examination system; EBAss would accredit schools who would then teach individuals according to the RM requirements. Individuals who achieved a pass from these accredited schools would be eligible to sit the EBAss examination at the appropriate level; I went on to suggest these examinations could be carried out on-line, meaning the candidates would not need to travel to an examination centre. I also felt that without too much trouble the examinations could be carried out in the student's language; I have to say though, that I hadn't realised how hard this would be but that was initially the plan anyway.

I had explained that if adopted my system would be very similar to the system currently in place in the USA, under the umbrella of the National Board of Diving and Hyperbaric Medical Technologists (NBDHMT). I have to say he took some convincing, he said that he could see the need for something like this but wasn't sure EBAss was the right body to provide it, he felt there would be a lot of work and couldn't see who would do the work. I had already raised all of this with DDRC's Senior Management so was able to reassure him that as one of DDRC's charitable aims were to provide training to diving and hyperbaric personnel they were happy to allow me the time to put this in place provided EBAss were on board with the project.

Well, he couldn't really say no to this, he did I think see how a system such as this had to be in place if we wanted the training to be accepted as we all hoped it would be. We left the bar with me having been tasked with putting a plan together as to how this could be delivered. I told him I would do this over the next few months and would lay the plan out to the full board at the next board meeting in April 2007. It was clear that the EBAss board working with ECHM had done a great job already in finalising the Resources Manual for training and I was sure that we together would be able to take this to the next level with the proposed examination system.

Perhaps the highlight of the Bergen conference was a trip out on a large tall-ship; as we set out from the quay alongside the Bergen Maritime Museum into the outer harbour and from there out into the surrounding fjords, we passed the offshore survival school where there were several life-boats including at least one free-fall boat. We carried on out into the roads between islands and the mainland where we turned to port passing under the Vestland bridge where there was not much clearance for our very tall masts. Meanwhile we were plied with food and drink late into the evening, it was very pleasant.

2006 also saw DDRC finally realise the dream of opening an hyperbaric unit in south-Wales; since the debacle of the Hytech chamber in Pentwyn we had been looking hard for a hospital that would allow us to open a unit on their site. We had several promising leads and very nearly managed with the Heath hospital in Cardiff; we found an almost perfect site with plenty of room and went a long way with negotiations but at the final hurdle that fell through. We then found a doctor working at Llantrisant hospital who was very keen; again, we met with hospital administrators who made all the right noises but it just never happened. I seemed to spend a great deal of my time driving up to Cardiff just to have our hopes dashed at the last moment.

After Llantrisant we were finding most doors closed to us and were almost at the point of giving up when at last we found a private hospital run by nuns in Newport. St Joseph's was a small private hospital who did seem to be keen to add a hyperbaric facility to their site, Karena and I met with their hospital manager Patrick Raeburn; he was a real breath of fresh air. They had a small room that we could rent at a reasonable rate, they were happy for us to install a liquid oxygen (LOX) tank and wanted this to happen as quickly as possible. We had already taken on a manager for the unit some months before so just needed to find a nurse; the manager was Chris Walsh who came to us from the Rambler's Association, he was now tasked with organising the new centre which was to be called 'DDRC South-Wales Hyperbaric Centre'. We already had an HYOX Monoplace chamber earmarked for the facility, I worked with Chris and Patrick to organise installation of the chamber and LOX systems.

We had some time ago made the decision that we would not treat emergency patients or divers inside Monoplace chambers. Although there are companies doing these treatments in Monoplace chambers our medical director didn't feel it was appropriate; this meant that all divers and emergency patients would still be treated in Plymouth.

By November the unit was ready and opened with articles in the local newspapers and local dignitaries visiting; it was a good day, one that DDRC had been working towards for years; the unit worked well accepting its first patient to great fanfare. Unfortunately, it soon became obvious that a unit with just one chamber treating a maximum of four patients per day would not be economic; whilst this was not really an issue for DDRC as it was one of their charitable aims it clearly as far as sustainability was concerned would be much more defensible if the unit at least broke even in the longer-term.

CHAPTER TWENTY-THREE

2007

2007 started with an ISO internal audit in January, this again went well with Jonathan finding no non-conformances but did highlight a couple of areas of concern that were easily put right.

Cannabis! Early in 2007 I was contacted by my MS consultant Professor John Zajicek, as you may remember he had originally diagnosed my MS in 2001/2 and I had been visiting him roughly once per year since then. In 2007 he called me asking me to come to see him to discuss a clinical trial he was organising; I was keen to be involved in trials as I felt they were the only way I was ever likely to find something that could help my condition.

When we met John laid out his plans for the CUPID trial; this was to be a randomised, double blinded, placebo-controlled trial. John was the lead for the trial which was being run in collaboration with some twenty-seven neurology centres throughout the UK, there were eventually four-hundred and ninety-eight patients randomly assigned treatment on this trial. Some seventy-three of the participants were assigned to the placebo arm but all the others received some level of cannabis administered via pills. As the trial was double-blinded none of the participants were made aware of whether they were on the active drug or the placebo and neither were the trial operatives who were administering the trial. In effect nobody other than the senior physicians knew who was taking the active drug this meant that the likelihood of any resulting benefits or outcomes being less likely to be slewed in any way.

Once I was accepted as fitting the criteria for the trial, I had to go through a number of tests to establish a baseline set of data as to my condition prior to starting the trial. This involved me undergoing a number of simple tests to establish my short-term memory, coordination, walking etc. In addition, I had to have another MRI scan which this time I undertook at Derriford Hospital in Plymouth and didn't have to pay for; once all of the tests had been completed, I was issued with pills, were they cannabis or placebo? I didn't know although it wasn't long before it became clear to me that I was indeed in the active arm of the trial, I was taking cannabis! The trial duration was to be three years for each participant so, I would be on cannabis for the next three-years. During this time, I had to maintain a diary detailing any effects and to attend a clinic in Plymouth (luckily this clinic was run on the Science Park just across the road from DDRC) once a month where they would repeat the same tests again to assess any changes in our cognitive awareness or walking abilities; additionally, every six-months we would all undergo another MRI scan.

We had been told that the active ingredient of cannabis that would normally give the effects of getting high had been removed; so much so that we were not banned from driving while on the trial; sounds fine, doesn't it? I was still working with DDRC in my roles as before so had a responsible job for which I needed to be very much on my game. I was not worried about this as after all we had been told we would not be high when taking the drug. DDRC being a research establishment were fully on-board with my participation in the trial but of course they had every right to expect me to still be able to carry out my job effectively.

Initially, I had been told to take four tablets twice per day, four in the morning and another four in the evening so this was exactly what I did; on the first day I popped the pills in the morning and off I went to work, of course this involved me driving the thirty odd miles from my home to DDRC in Plymouth. This was no problem as they had assured me all would be OK right, I felt no effects from the drug, did this mean I was on the placebo? Well, the drive took about forty-five minutes and as I say I felt fine, however at ten o'clock I took myself off to attend the routine senior management team (SMT) meeting, this was now some two and a half hours after taking the pills.

As usual I sat at the table in the CEO's office together with Karena Pring and James Hardwick and we got down to the business of the meeting, I then started to feel a little strange; well, that is to say I started to feel stoned. I was in a dreamworld, it was a very nice feeling but, I found that although I could hear and understand everything that was said by either Karena or James, I was not really there in mind at all! This was brought home to me when I suddenly realised, they were both looking at me with quizzical looks on their faces, I had evidently been asked a question or at least I was expected to contribute in some way? Oh dear, although I had heard every word spoken, I just had no idea what had been said and certainly had no idea what was expected of me, luckily, they both seemed happy to repeat the question and I was able to fumble my way through the rest of the meeting. Clearly, I was on the active arm of the trial and not on the placebo; the meeting went on for another hour or so with me doing my best to concentrate on the matters being discussed although I'm sure they must have both been aware something was wrong with me, neither of them mentioned anything.

When the meeting was over, I retired to my office where I sat with a cup of coffee wondering how I was going to function for the next three-years! Over the next few days, I was able to work out how the drug affected me, it seemed that about two hours after taking the pills I would effectively be out of it for the following couple of hours. Once I knew this, I discussed my predicament with Karena and James who were incredibly understanding and supportive, between us we were able to work out a compromise that would allow me to continue working effectively.

Daily, I would take the second four pills with my supper at maybe six-thirty PM, I would then sit in my chair watching TV for the evening although I don't remember seeing much and certainly, I never seemed to see the end of programmes, I was effectively away with the fairies for most of the evening!

I put up with this situation for the first month but when I returned to the clinic for my monthly consultation, I raised this with the nurse who told me that he would talk to the trial administrator and let me know what they said. A few days later I received a call where they told me to reduce the number of tablets I took in the morning; I was worried that this would nullify the effectiveness of the drug but was reassured that they really didn't know much about what would be an appropriate dose anyway! Over the next few days, I reduced the number of pills I took in the morning to two, I found that at this dose although I was still affected and had mild symptoms, they were not so bad that I couldn't work effectively.

I continued to take four pills in the evening as the effects didn't matter so much in the evening; I suppose I could say that I was effectively stoned for three years but still managed to hold down a responsible job, not bad eh! Sounds great but I have to say that looking back I feel I really lost three years as being constantly stoned does not allow for much productivity!

In March I was due to take off again on a bit of a tour of the far-east, I was worried about travelling to the far-east while carrying cannabis pills. I again discussed this with the trial nurse who this time was a female nurse, she told me she would have the administrator write a letter explaining that I was a participant on a clinical trial and that the pills were required for the trial; I have to say that although I was reassured this would be fine, I was not altogether convinced. Anyway, I started my trip in Hong Kong visiting the HKFS again, this time I was met at the airport by Patrick and Joey; I was immediately taken to see Mike and Eric at headquarters. It seemed they wanted us to put together doctor's courses; this was definitely something I was keen to discuss.

We met with their Dr Chow who was super keen for us to run two courses for his doctors in Hong Kong, I was asked to produce a costed proposal. I only spent a couple of days in HK before heading off to Thailand again. Here I was asked to meet with the Royal Thai

Navy again but this time to discuss doctor's courses, I couldn't believe it, we had been struggling to find any interest in physician's courses for some years and all of a sudden everyone seemed to want them!

During this trip Nick and I finally got around to making our road trip to promote the REMT courses in Thailand, we were just a couple of years later than initially thought, anyway, the trip for me started in Phuket on the west coast, I arrived from Bangkok at six o'clock in the evening, to be met by Nick who took me straight to my first presentation; this was for some twenty-five dive masters; the presentation took about two hours during which they all seemed to be quite attentive but didn't actually sign up for anything. We then travelled by road down the west coast presenting at various locations promoting the REMT courses.

The first night Nick had booked me into a very small, rustic place, it was absolutely in the middle of nowhere although Nick told me he lived just down the road; I was shown into my room; well, I say room, it was a stand-alone hut with a bedroom, shower room and thank goodness air conditioning. We had arrived after dark so I hadn't been able to see much when we arrived, however, in the morning I woke to find I was in a delightful little development of tiny thatched huts, I seemed to be the only guest though. I had been told to walk across to the reception building where breakfast would be served; it was great, I was sitting in the middle of the Thai jungle sipping fruit juice and eating an omelette accompanied by a pot of reasonable coffee.

Nick picked me up again at nine o'clock and we continued down the west coast, at intervals Nick pointed out signs for Tsunami zone, these had been put up following 2004's terrible Tsunami that had caused so much damage and death in this area. Nick showed me some large vessels that had been washed a long way inland, it must have been truly horrific. My second presentation was in Krabi, this was a beautiful little village where I presented to twenty-nine people who again appeared very interested but didn't actually commit to anything! The next day we were back on the road we crossed to the east coast where we boarded a ferry to Koh Samui, this was a real holiday island. However, we didn't present on Koh Samui, it was just a staging post to get to Koh Tao for the final location, Koh Tao was a tiny island that had become something of a Mecca for recreational divers, there were literally hundreds of live-aboard dive boats operating out of Koh Tao.

The ferry we were travelling on was a basic but fast hydrofoil; we were delivered to Koh Tao at Mae Haad Pier. Nick told me this was Koh Tao's main port. Well, it wasn't much of a port, as we approached a ramshackle wooden pier, I could see hundreds of people both on the pier and along the waterfront; the waterfront was predominantly made up of small bars and some shops, all were made of wood with corrugated iron roofs. The hydrofoil bumped alongside the pier and was quickly tied up, we then became part of the traditional free-for-all that seemed to ensue whenever disembarkation took place from any vessel in that part of the world. Nick had an associate on the island who had organised a pickup truck to take us to our hotel; we climbed on board with our bags and immediately took off.

As we drove through the town, I could see that there were quite a number of white faces, although predominantly the place was populated by Thai's, there were of course a number of holiday makers. We of course hoped for rich pickings from the boats servicing these holiday makers; as far as I could see the town consisted of just one road running parallel to the beach, it was lined with small restaurants and of course bars, it was terrifically noisy.

Nick had booked me into a nice hotel right on the beach, when we arrived, we both wandered into reception where he checked me in and I was shown to a room on the ground floor, it was a nice enough room with double bed, en-suite shower and air conditioning. This was fine for me but I wasn't keen on sharing a double bed with Nick; I raised the issue with him and he told me that he would be staying elsewhere at the home of his local agent. I was going to be on my own then, this was fine by me; Nick told me that the presentation was scheduled for seven o'clock that evening so he would pick me up at five and we could get a bite to eat beforehand. It was just after eleven in the morning so I had the whole afternoon to myself; I spent the time heading to the beach where I just chilled in a local bar, I went for a swim and had a lovely chilled afternoon.

As promised Nick turned up at five, we then found a small restaurant where I had a lovely green curry together with a couple of beers, following this we wandered around the corner to a large bar where the presentation would take place, the bar was extremely busy. Nick told me that the music would be turned off while I gave my presentation and that this would be OK as most of the patrons were from the boats anyway. Nick had previously told me that the dive masters from the live-aboard boats worked extremely hard, they only really got one evening off a week at most and sometimes it would be just one evening every two weeks.

I told him I thought they would just want to be getting on with partying and would not be up for listening to me surely; he thought they would be attentive but I was not convinced. Anyway, at seven-thirty the music stopped and I was on, I put my pitch across to thirty-four people telling them that they really needed an advanced first aid qualification such as the REMT that we were offering.

I think it went as well as could be expected but, by eight-thirty the music was back and I was not aware of anyone asking follow up questions, at all. About eleven I was back at my hotel and was glad to be stepping onto a nice cool air-conditioned room; unfortunately, this was short-lived, at midnight the air conditioner stopped working; I thought it was a power cut but when I saw Nick the next morning, he told me the whole island only had electricity from eight in the morning until midnight. So, no air conditioning at night, perfect!

I was due to travel to Pattaya again that day, I had a flight from Koh Samui to Bangkok and from there I would go by road as usual, we arrived at the airport on Koh Samui a good three hours before the flight so Nick and I took up residence in a bar across the road. Over a couple of beers, we discussed our next moves in promoting the courses, he was keen to do other road trips but I told him it would not be me although I would supply an instructor to do them with him. Nick and I parted company at the check-in queue with Nick going back to the mainland via ferry to pick up his car again.

The airport on Koh Samui was tiny, the check-in desks were in an open area covered by a thatched roof, I was quickly able to make my way through into the departure lounge where I sat down to wait for the flight. This was the nicest departure lounge I had ever been in, there were no windows with the walls being only waist high; the thatched roof was shading us very nicely but it was hot! After an hour or so, the beer was beginning to make its presence felt, I needed to pee; however, I couldn't see any signs for toilets or indeed anything much else, there were no restaurants or any other vendors. I eventually found a member of staff to ask and she told me there were no toilets in the departure lounge, this was not good news, I had never been particularly good at holding on for a long time anyway but unfortunately MS doesn't help in this regard.

By the time my flight was called I was getting a little desperate, luckily here the fact that I was walking with the aid of a stick came to the attention of one of the staff, a lovely Thai lady who took pity on me, clearly, she could see I was uncomfortable; she probably thought this was due to my not being able to walk very well! She took me by the hand and pulled me towards the departure gate which had just been announced; she shooed the attendants away before taking me through the door and down to the tarmac where she beckoned an electric golf cart across.

The driver was given instructions to take me straight to the plane and make sure I was settled on board; she gave me a lovely smile, a wave and off we went; the driver took me straight to the plane and helped me up the steps. The stewardess showed me to a seat very near the front and told me to just sit down while the other passengers arrived, as soon as she turned her back, I was up and, in the toilet, ahh, what a relief.

After some half-hour the rest of the passengers arrived having been ferried out to the plane in a normal coach, not like my VIP passage at all. I really don't think this whole trip had been worth the expense or my time but sometimes you have to try these things. We did run REMT courses with BGH though, we ran at least two a year; these normally ran either before or after DMT courses and these courses were reasonably well attended so maybe it had been worthwhile after all.

In Pattaya I met with Mark for dinner to discuss our meeting with the RTN next day, where we discussed their ongoing requirements, they seemed to want everything but didn't really want to pay for anything. They wanted to trade places on courses for the use of facilities, this worked well with the DMT but never did get off the ground for physician courses, oh well, we tried. Having crossed numerous international borders on my trip I was relieved that although I had a significant number of cannabis pills with me, I was never quizzed about them and never had to test the validity of my letter.

On return to UK, I was contacted by John Mitchel of the Guernsey Harbour Board (GHB), they had two requests; the first was for chamber operator courses as they were going to be expected to run a recompression chamber about to be installed and the second was for someone to write them a set of diving rules. I decided I should visit to discuss: my trip took place in May, I was met at the airport by John, we went straight to the harbour where the harbour divers had a unit. I had a good look at their equipment which I could see was very well maintained and in good nick, most of it seemed relatively new; we discussed the types of diving they undertook and what he felt they needed.

All commercial diving companies had to by law have their own diving rules; laying out how diving operations would be conducted, routine diving decompression arrangements and emergency procedures to be utilised should things not go to plan. At this time GHB had none of these things; that's not to say they didn't have procedures and decompression tables they operated to it was just that they had no specific document tying all this together. He went on to tell me about their recompression availability, again, all commercial diving companies must have procedures in place for recompression of their divers in the event of decompression illness. At the time Guernsey's recompression facility was run by an individual who was about to retire; John told me the chamber was very old and would no longer be available once this individual went.

I felt it would be helpful to have a look at the chamber to see what we were faced with so off we went; the chamber was housed in the St John's ambulance facility in St Peter Port and as soon as we arrived, I could see there were issues. The chamber was very small, it was jammed into a tiny room adjacent to the main entrance, I could see that although it seemed to have been maintained I couldn't see any evidence of testing of the depth gauges. Maybe it had been maintained but, there were no stickers giving dates etc., and I couldn't see any certification so, not ideal. Anyway, by today's standards it was too small, when we left, we chatted about this and it seemed I was just confirming what John already knew; they needed a new chamber and somewhere to put it. This should really be close to a hospital, ideally this would be the main hospital, of course this would need significant negotiation; John was tasked with this by his bosses, I told him, I and DDRC would help wherever we could.

After a couple of days on Guernsey I flew home and got to work pulling their diving rules together; this didn't take long, I was able to send the first draft through to John by mid-way through the following week. There were very few alterations necessary; these rules were officially adopted by GHB, everyone was happy. Still though when the chamber at St John's became unavailable GHB would have to stop diving as they were diving to UK regulations which require there to be a chamber within six-hours of the dive site.

While Guernsey is within six-hours of DDRC provided weather conditions were reasonable, there would be times when a diver would not be able to get to us within the timescale required. This meant that GHB needed a chamber installed pronto; as a stop gap, they were to hire a containerised chamber from another old friend of mine Howard Kelsall of Searchwise in Ellon north of Aberdeen. We trained a couple of GHB divers in chamber operation this allowed them to continue diving until they did eventually get a very nice new chamber installed at their hospital.

During 2006 and 2007 I had been working with Martin Cridge to put the EBAss on-line examinations package together, this was a much bigger commitment than I had envisaged. First there were the questions and answers (they were all multi-choice) then there were the systems to put in place to allow candidates access under controlled conditions; finally, there was the translation of all questions and general information into the various languages, this turned out to be a very major undertaking to be sure.

By September we were getting there but still had a heap of work to do before the system would be ready for launch. I headed off to EUBS which this year was in Sharm el-Sheik, Egypt; Sharm was a tourist mecca but other than the proximity of the red sea there was not much there. We were again staying in the conference hotel where we all sat through another few days of lectures, I was not scheduled to present but had organised several meetings with the EBAss board to discuss the on-line examination system. This although became fraught but we did in the end agree on an acceptable path.

The main talking point of the conference was a Bedouin experience where we were all taken into the desert at night to find out how the Bedouin live. It was a great experience with no lights making the sky beautiful and very memorable; I decided not to partake of the supplied food as I thought it was questionable as to how it had been cooked to say the least and I thought the levels of hygiene were suspect. Anyway, the following day my reticence was proven to have been sensible as the majority of people who did partake missed the conference due to stomach upsets.

Our trip home was marred by a six-hour delay at the airport due to non-arrival of our plane, there were no facilities to purchase drinks or food so it was a very relieved party who eventually boarded the plane; it was always such fun going on these trips or so I was told by some of DDRC's staff who didn't get to go, those of us who did go though, felt they were always extremely hard work and not always so much fun.

CHAPTER TWENTY-FOUR

2008

After running the Welsh unit in Newport for two years we started negotiations with Patrick to move the unit to a room that would be large enough for us to site two Monoplace chambers. We had worked out that two chambers could be run with the same number of staff and would make a slight profit provided we had sufficient patients. Again, unfortunately the only room St Joseph's could offer us was really not appropriate so we again started looking elsewhere; we had lowered our aspirations from our previous search as we were now only looking for somewhere to site two Monoplace chambers. We did eventually find a perfect location this was in the Spire private hospital in Cardiff; spookily it was just down the road from the unit where the original Hytech chamber had been installed. So, we were on our way back to Pentwyn, the Spire Cardiff hospital chief executive was a real breath of fresh air, she made everything we needed available, she was a real joy to work with. Again, we had to install another LOX system but within a couple of months we had moved the whole kit and kaboodle out of St Joseph's and into Spire adding the necessary second Monoplace.

2008 was unfortunately a year of significant staff unrest at DDRC, to this day I don't know what caused it but even the staff who were normally calm and collected seemed to find themselves upset about something this year. I spent a lot of the year firefighting staff issues; probably the most significant of these were that Karena Pring our chief executive and I thought a firm friend in terms of management of the charity and James Hardwick our medical director fell out big time. This resulted in James being signed off with workplace stress for a large part of the year and Karena becoming more and more affected, this resulted in my taking on most of the management for the charity as well as the trading arm. In turn I found myself relying on Gary Smerdon our Research Director for support, at the time Gary worked four days per week for us; he was a tremendous help to me during this period.

With James being off we had to engage the services of another doctor to act as medical director, initially we utilised the services of a very experienced Dutch diving doctor. This worked OK but was far from ideal as of course he had to come up to speed with our procedures very quickly, I think he felt caught between a rock and a hard place as he of course had some affinity with a fellow doctor but had to show the management a degree of loyalty.

At this time, we also had our first visit from the Care Standards Commission, we had received no notification of the visit and unfortunately on the day of the visit, our medical director, CEO and also our nurse manager were not on site, James was still off sick, Karena was working away from the site as was Ali Bishop our nurse manager. So, it fell to me to handle the visit, I was very nervous of this duty as I am not clinical or medical so would normally have relied on others to handle the technical questions in those areas.

The first I knew of the visit was when the inspectors turned up in reception at nine o'clock; our receptionist phoned me asking me to come down to meet with them; so, started a very stressful day. The first impression was not good at all; I made my way into reception where I was faced with two stern looking middle aged women, I of course introduced myself with name and job title, they asked whether the medical director was available, now while we did have an interim medical director, I didn't feel it was fair of me to throw him to the wolves so to speak. Although, I would involve him later in the day when they needed to discuss medical issues. I asked them to sign in which they immediately took issue with; I was stunned by this as I was under the impression that I was within my rights to ask all persons to sign in to comply with fire regulations.

The lead inspector proceeded to put me in my place by telling me they didn't need to sign in as they had access by law to every part of the premises and I couldn't stop them, indeed, she told me that if I were to try, she would "Put my big boots on and march straight in!" Well, after this I decided to let them dictate where they wanted to go and to just try to help them carry out their inspection with the least amount of fuss.

Ultimately all went well, I was able to field the majority of their questions with the help of our interim Medical Director and our nurses, the inspectors clearly didn't know much about hyperbaric chambers or the operation of HBOT. Our ISO accreditation really came good on the day as it answered a great number of the questions on their forms. Eventually they seemed to thaw a little and by the end of the day they went away seemingly happy with our unit but I felt completely wrung out on my drive home at the end of the day.

The second significant issue for this year was with our finance manager went completely off the deep end; he decided to have a number of huge rants during any and all meetings he attended; he seemed to be blaming Karena and I for everything that he saw as wrong with the world! Again, it all came to a head with him being sent home; both Karena and I were subjected to a number of very unpleasant hand written letters from him where he laid out our shortcomings in stark detail showing how we were ruining his life; this went on for well over a year with the situation constantly deteriorating to the point we were getting ready for law-suits.

We had recently taken on a new employment lawyer on a part time basis, Jon Loney was another breath of fresh air to both Karena and I, he started to show us how we could take back control of the situation and to stop the, in his words "Tail wagging the dog!"

To this day I have no real idea as to why so many people felt stressed at DDRC, in my view it was a relatively low stress environment; maybe that was part of the problem? As we were to an extent an emergency service, we had to have a relatively high number of staff on the books at any time, this resulted in them having a lot of time on their hands; nobody had to work to deadlines unless a diver was due imminently. This seemed to result in staff having a lot of time to sit drinking tea or coffee, there used to be huddles of people where conversation would cease whenever I arrived. I think they perceived many more issues than actually existed, they constantly felt we were hiding things from them when in fact, all we didn't share was the mountain of mundane crap we had to deal with to keep up with the demands of the Care Standards Commission, HSE, commissioners and the like.

Anyway, for whatever reason DDRC was an unhappy place for a lot of our staff; up to this point I had been used to staff coming to me in my office to pour out their woes but, now this didn't seem to be happening anymore? I tried to get to the bottom of it a number of times but whenever we had a meeting where they were invited to discuss their issues nobody would speak up. Right from day one in my job I had operated an open-door policy, they all knew they could come to me to discuss issues; in the past this had worked very well but for some reason it had stopped. As part of our quality system, we had instigated an Improvement Log system where anyone could raise issues anonymously if necessary but, again, nobody did! I found out later that there were a couple of bad eggs who were stirring everyone up and telling them that if they were to raise an issue they would be out! I really don't know how they were able to convince anyone of this as certainly in my time at DDRC nobody had ever been penalised for raising even the thorniest of issues. By August this was wearing me down and I resolved to make something happen to push things which I hoped would lead to resolution one way or another.

Of course, the world continued to turn during this time and we had to get on with the business of running both the charity and Pro-Services. In September I was again required to attend the EUBS conference which this year was held in September in Graz, Austria. Again I attended this with Gary Smerdon and a couple of others from the team, Graz was and I'm sure still is a wonderful city with a great deal of history; we again sat through a couple of days of presentations by eminent personnel extolling the virtues of HBOT, this was the first year that I was invited to attend the EUBS executive committee, I was just there as an help with understanding for the new EBAss president who was Italian, although she did speak English she would sometimes struggle with technical language so I was there to help; it was certainly interesting to meet these individuals and to become part of their inner sanctum albeit only on the periphery at this time.

The EBAss board meeting was interesting that year as it was the first year where everyone was brought up to date with our plans as regards the EBAss examinations. I thought our President had been keeping everyone in the loop but apparently not, there were some significant discussions resulting in difficult questioning. However, the net result was that everyone seemed to see the benefit to both EBAss and the wider hyperbaric community of the proposed EBAss independent examinations; this was a great relief to me as I and Martin Cridge had already put a huge amount of work into bringing this to fruition.

As I think all would agree it was accepted that the normal first aid for divers suffering Decompression Illness (DCI) following a dive would be to have them breathe pure oxygen. This would normally be administered by them breathing from an oxygen bottle via a demand valve; however, in the normal state of affairs recreational dive boats would not be able to carry large quantities of oxygen; resulting in it not being unusual for a diver to only have enough oxygen on board to facilitate breathing oxygen for just a few minutes following an incidence of DCI which was not an ideal state of affairs.

At the EUBS conference in Egypt the previous year I had met with the inventors of the 'Wenoll' medical oxygen re-breather system, this in my view was a huge step forward in diver safety. This unit was very nicely presented inside a bright yellow 'Pelican' style box, there was a one litre bottle of oxygen with the system allowing the diver to breathe from a closed loop, he/she would re-breathe from this loop with the exhaled CO_2 being scrubbed out of the loop by passing the gas through a soda-lime canister. This system would allow a single diver to breath one-hundred percent pure oxygen for about seven-hours from this one small bottle; this should allow for the diver to get to a hyperbaric chamber while continuously breathing pure oxygen.

In March of 2008 I flew to Germany to meet with their management and the Wenoll inventors. It was an excellent piece of kit that they were manufacturing in Germany; he had of course heard of DDRC and wanted to tie up with us to promote Wenoll in the UK; this was exactly what I was hoping, quite quickly we came to a deal whereby DDRC Pro-Services Ltd., became the sole UK importer for this equipment. This was something of a coup for us and, I hoped would lead to big things; the Wenoll system was being carried on some airlines and I was sure we would be able to have very promising discussions with the larger UK international airlines.

The first year of our association we were able to demonstrate the units to a lot of diving companies, recreational dive boat skippers and the MOD. The main obstacle was the cost of the units, at about one-thousand pounds in 2008 this was some way outside the range of a lot of the recreational market although the MOD were keen though. The MOD subsequentially made a ruling that all diving taking place from small boats or remote locations must have access to at least one Wenoll unit.

The Care Standards Commission had come in for some flak over the past couple of years, the end result was that it was to be replaced by the Care Quality Commission (CQC); to be established as a single, integrated regulator for England's health and adult social care services. This was achieved by introduction of the Health and Social Care Act 2008. The commission was created on 1 October 2008 and came into force on 1 April 2009; we of course had to comply with the new act from its inception. Ultimately, we managed to comply and the new act did make things more streamlined which I think was helpful.

CHAPTER TWENTY-FIVE

2009

In March 2009 I was contacted by an individual from a prestigious racehorse stables in Newmarket; they were one of the leading racing stables where the horses were treated extremely well and had the benefit of any and all possible aids to training. This included unparalleled efforts to look after the horse's health and medical needs, including having the use of hyperbaric oxygen therapy; this was used to help horses recover from the extreme exertion of racing. Unfortunately, during one of these HBOT sessions there had been an explosion inside the chamber, this killed the horse and hurt a couple of the attending personnel. The safety manager had searched for someone to help with improving safety at their facility, he called me to discuss and we agreed that initially it would be sensible for me to travel to their facility in Newmarket to have a look at their facilities.

They apparently also wanted to discuss research so I suggested that I bring our research director with me, he immediately agreed to this and the trip was on. Gary and I made our way up to Newmarket on another sunny day in April, we had been booked into a nice hotel in Newmarket for the night before the visit.

On the day we presented ourselves at the gate of the racing stable, the place was very impressive, the gatehouse was manned by security and had the feel of a military establishment. We were invited to sit in our car and wait for the safety manager to arrive so that he could escort us, within a few minutes he turned up and following introductions we followed his car. As we drove into the facility, it was immaculate, everything was beautifully kept, the hedges were trimmed to perfection as were the acres of grass which were wonderfully green with not a single blade out of place. As we drove along the road we passed a number of pristine buildings, there were a lot of staff who were engaged in keeping the place looking perfect, eventually, he parked up and beckoned for us to park alongside him.

We complimented him on the facility and he told us that 'the boss' was justifiably proud of the facility, nothing was too much trouble for the horses, we had to agree, it looked wonderful. He then explained what had happened as we walked around the corner into one of the pristine buildings, none of this looked like anywhere I had seen before, there were no piles of muck or anything else to indicate horses were here at all. As we walked into the building, we were faced with one of their chambers it was a white painted vertically oriented tube with a large door in the side through which a horse would enter and exit the chamber. There were a few acrylic ports for personnel to view the horse inside; the top of the cylinder was closed with a dome into which there were a number of large diameter pipes welded.

It was an impressive chamber, it looked to be very well maintained and had been installed to a very high standard, we were told that this was one of two chambers they had, it was exactly the same as the one where the event had taken place.

He took us around the back of the facility where the affected chamber was stored; this was a different world, here was the chamber we had come to see; it was clear there had been a significant fiery event inside the chamber, the chamber had been pressurised using pure oxygen which of course always gave rise to significant safety concerns. It seemed that while the chamber was under pressure with a horse inside, the horse had become spooked and had kicked out at the wall of the chamber causing a spark which then led to the fire killing the horse, of course this had to be a one-off event that couldn't be allowed to happen again. We spent a few hours inspecting the chamber and discussing the accident before adjourning to his office to look at their procedures etc., at the end of which it was decided that their team had insufficient training and that this had possibly contributed to the failure.

He then told us that he would give us a bit more of a tour and we all jumped into his car; he drove around the site showing us the horses swimming pool, hospital facility and finally the gallops where the horses were exercised on a daily basis. The whole place was perfect, there was no point where we saw anything out of place, He told us that the boss spent a fortune on keeping the place perfect, it was his hobby and he didn't mind lavishing money on it. Lastly, we met with one of the senior Management who was particularly interested in research; Gary our research director and I had tea with her while the prospects for research were discussed.

As we left to travel home, we had agreed that Pro-Services would put together a set of rules for the chamber, this would include pre and post-dive checklists as well as a maintenance regime. It had been agreed that we would provide training for a number of their staff to teach them safe chamber operation so that every possible step could be taken to avoid a repetition of this problem. Over the coming months we wrote the chamber rules and all associated checklists we then provided courses for his team; this all went very well but, in the end the boss decided he didn't want to risk his horses in the chamber anymore and I don't think they used them again.

EUBS meeting this year was to be in Aberdeen in August but I was on holiday in Norway and couldn't attend, I was not really sorry as I felt I had spent enough time in Aberdeen over the years and so didn't worry about missing it. I produced reports detailing progress on the EBAss examinations; Martin Cridge had done a tremendous job utilising the Moodle package and some of the EBAss board had supplied various questions which I had now integrated into the system. I had written some three-hundred questions and now felt we had finished the majority of the required questions. In short, we were nearly there; I felt we were ready to trial the site which I was planning on doing over the coming months.

Throughout 2009 HR issues continued, I was plagued by a couple of admin staff who were quite happy to lie through their teeth just to get their way. One in particular took this to extreme levels, she was apparently very happy to lie to my face about a conversation we had had, this was done in the presence of a union rep. DDRC didn't recognise any unions but she had a friend who was an union rep and so wangled a way for her to accompany her to the meetings. It would have been laughable if it hadn't been so serious, but what can you do about people like that; ultimately, she left with a pay-out much to my chagrin!

As a way to show staff how good they had it working for DDRC we decided to organise a trip to a local factory, this factory was part of a huge multinational company. The visit was well attended as it was carried out during the working day with us still paying everyone during the visit; they spent a whole morning at the factory and it was clearly something of an eye opener for a lot of the staff. On their return I met with them all to be told that they couldn't believe some of the things that went on there, apparently staff were required to clock on and off and if they arrived more than fifteen minutes late for their shift, they would be docked a full hour's pay, staff on the production line were only allowed three minutes for a toilet break, they were only allowed one tea break of fifteen minutes in the morning and the same in the afternoon! This had been a great project for us, they were buzzing about how much better conditions at DDRC were, this was music to my ears; this continued well into the following year so it was very well worth our while for sure.

CHAPTER TWENTY-SIX

2010

Towards the end of 2009 things were becoming very strained between all of the senior management, James was continually off sick or on reduced duties and Karena Pring seemed to be offloading everything she didn't want to be bothered with onto me. I really felt that my position was now that of caretaker manager which was not a comfortable place to be; the trustees had asked me to produce a report on specific qualities, qualifications and capabilities needed for a medical director at a hyperbaric facility. To do this I researched using the HSE website, CQC guidance and the European Code of Good Practice for the operation of hyperbaric units (ECGP) as well as the American Undersea and Hyperbaric Medical Society (UHMS) guidance.

In February, I could tell Karena was not coping very well I decided to see whether I could get to the bottom of what was wrong and poked my head around her office door to ask her; the answer she gave shook me. It seemed that she felt undermined and unsupported by all at DDRC and that included me; I was astonished as I thought I had been going out of my way to support her, clearly that hadn't worked.

Karena had been DDRC's Care Standards Commission and latterly CQC Registered Manager since she had taken on the role of chief executive before I joined; in discussion with the trustees, it was decided that Karena should step back from this role and that I should take it on! While I was not against this, I was nervous about it as I had very little background in medical or clinical issues, on discussion with our new chair of trustees who had been part of the Care Standards Commission for several years. He told me that it was an advantage to not have medical or clinical background as the role was principally there to police the CQC rules and regulations; he said that they would all have to convince me they were doing the job properly and this would tie in very well with my quality background.

I agreed to take this on and we started the process. It turned out this was not a quick process at all, I had to complete a significant number of forms, supply a heap of evidence of my qualifications, references and even my birth certificate. After all of this had been vetted the last step was an interview with one of the senior inspectors who grilled me for over an hour, finally though I was accepted as DDRC's CQC Registered Manager, phew!

March 2010 signified the end of my involvement in the CUPID trial, I had continued taking the tablets for the whole three years and had attended the clinic religiously every month as well as undertaking the required MRI scans every six-months. I can tell you I was not sorry to be able to cease taking the drug, it might seem like a wonderful situation to be able to take a drug that gave you a big high every day for three-years but I was not a fan of the effect, I feel that really, I lost three-years of my life to the drug.

It was not until some twelve months after the last trialist had completed the trial that results were published, unfortunately, when they were eventually published the results showed that there appeared to be no overall effect on the progression of MS. I was not really surprised as my experience was that I didn't feel any significant alteration to my symptoms; this of course was a great shame but as they say nothing ventured, nothing gained. If the results had shown an improvement, then I would have been one of the first to benefit.

April 2010 saw me travelling to Athens for one of our regular EBAss meetings, this was a particularly important one as it was the last one before we were to launch the EBAss accreditation scheme. There were a few alterations required to the paperwork relating to the scheme but we left the meeting with agreement to go live and launch which I felt was a wonderful result. Chrissie had accompanied me to Athens, where we were planning to stay on for a few days to take in the sights, initially she accompanied me to the routine end-of-meeting meal; this meal was the norm for EBAss, we all went out for dinner to a local restaurant on the last day of our meetings.

Chrissie came along and I think began to realise why I always used to return from these meetings worn out; even though the official work was complete I spent the whole evening being quizzed about the accreditation scheme ensuring I didn't really enjoy the evening. The next few days though were wonderful, we did all the touristy things like visiting the Acropolis and associated museums, being April, the weather was wonderful, lots of sun but not too hot and there were not too many people, great.

In August of 2010 we were invited to tender to provide chamber operator training on board a superyacht, this was a first for us and although we didn't know it at the time would eventually become a significant new income stream for Pro-Services. All of these yachts were owned by mega rich individuals who used them as playthings, they were as you can imagine extremely well equipped, they had everything a rich playboy or girl could want ranging from helicopters to jet-skis and everything in between. They were all equipped with diving kit and because they would inevitably be in far-away locations where access to healthcare might be limited most of them had very well-equipped sick bays and often a recompression chamber.

We were asked to provide not only chamber operator training but also REMT training to their crew, funnily enough I had absolutely no problem finding personnel to take on this training as even the crew's quarters were always very comfortable and as I say were normally in lovely locations. The first course took place in the Caribbean on one of the ships owned by a Saudi prince, it went very well and would become a regular thing as the crews didn't seem to stay for very long. In fact, the crew from one ship would almost inevitably cycle through to another similar superyacht so it was not long before we were catering for the training needs of several of these ships.

September was EUBS again, this time the venue was Istanbul; what a place, incredibly busy and hot; again, I was not scheduled to speak so spent the time listening to presentations that largely went over my head, nothing new there then. Istanbul though was great, we managed to get out to visit the Blue Mosque and found some wonderful restaurants. A good part of my time was spent with EBAss, as 2010 had seen the official launch of the accreditation system; I was now EBAss' President of Accreditation. We spent a lot of time talking to individuals about how their staff could and should enrol in the system etc., it all seemed to go very well and I definitely thought the system was being well received.

We had also managed to tie up with the European College of Baromedicine (ECB), this was a real triumph for EBAss, I worked closely with Alessandro (Sandro) Marroni of the Diver's Alert Network (DAN). ECB was a more established entity and therefore carried much more credibility which of course it lent to our certification; this was a huge step forward in gaining acceptance of our system. I had known Sandro for several years and he had been completely on board with our system right from the word go, he had helped me tremendously in ironing out specific procedures. Now anyone who achieved a pass in the EBAss on-line examinations would be awarded an ECB certificate this was again much better as the ECB certificate would be seen as much more credible.

For the first time hyperbaric personnel from any country in the European Union could be trained to universal standards and then undertake independently accredited examinations which if successful would lead to them being issued with a certification that would be recognised throughout Europe. Now of course in the first instance there were a large number of personnel who had been working in the hyperbaric field for many years who also wanted to gain the recognition of our certification. For these people we had a 'Grandfathering' clause in the scheme. This proved to be extremely attractive and resulted in nearly two-hundred certified individuals in the first year. This was much better than I had anticipated and indeed over the next few years our system became attractive to personnel outside Europe with applicants from Australia/New Zealand, the far east, middle east, south America, there were even some from Africa: it was becoming not just European, more like a worldwide qualification.

Towards the end of the year, DDRC's management issues came to a head. The Trustees decided that they wanted the roles of CEO and Medical Director to be combined; there was I'm sure a great deal of discussion regards whether either of the current incumbents would be appropriate for the joint role but, in the end, we were told that it was felt that neither would be suited for the joint role. This decision resulted in both Karena Pring and James Hardwick being made redundant. This meant that with regards the Senior Management Team I was now the only one left standing so, therefore by default I became the acting Chief Executive Officer (CEO) and Gary would join me as a full member of the SMT, which was an enormous help to me.

In my roles as Operations Director, Safety Manager, CQC Registered Manager and Managing Director of Pro-Services I felt I had enough to be keeping me occupied anyway. The trustees agreed with my decision and commenced the task of looking for both a new permanent medical director and CEO.

Gary Smerdon and I discussed the joint CEO/MD idea at length and came to the conclusion that it would be a big mistake, of course the trustee's decision prevailed.

Advertisements were produced and circulated in relevant publications and of course on our website; at the time our interim medical director, was a Rumanian doctor Michaela Ignatescu who was a very capable individual. She became one of our candidates, as it turned out the only other was a female doctor who had been with us before but was currently managing an unit in Perth, Australia; we did have a third shortlisted candidate but unfortunately he dropped out before we even got to interview. The trustees took on the task of organising interviews for these individuals.

CHAPTER TWENTY-SEVEN

2011

Early in January 2011 we had our first CQC inspection, this went very well with them being extremely impressed with our facilities and procedures. I was very happy with this, especially when they told us they were happy for us to treat any disease provided we documented outcomes, this was a huge change of policy for them and was very welcome.

The date was set for MD/CEO interviews as twenty-fourth and twenty-fifth of January; the two candidates, had agreed to attend. I was not at all comfortable that we would end up with someone who would be good for the charity but as there had been so little interest in the job we felt we would have to appoint and make do with whatever resulted. So, it was we ended up with a combined CEO and Medical Director. By this time, I had been acting CEO for about two-years.

Anyway, work carried on, this year we again continued training UAE officers and personnel from Hong Kong as well as running courses in Thailand and equine courses; this meant all was going along beautifully as far as Pro-Services was concerned.

In April, I travelled to Stockholm for the EBAss meeting where I was able to relate very favourable figures for the accreditation scheme; examination questions had by now been translated into Italian and German so these languages would soon be added to the scheme.

EUBS this year was held in August in Gdansk, Poland, it was nice to meet with my EBAss colleagues as well as Sandro Marroni who was very happy with the way the EBAss/ECB accreditation scheme was progressing. Gdansk is a wonderful city which had been lovingly restored to its former glory following the Soviet era occupation that had seen many buildings fall into disrepair apparently.

CHAPTER TWENTY-EIGHT

2012

In April off I was to Rome for the first of two scheduled EBAss meetings this year. I arrived at Leonardo da Vinci International Airport which was at the time somewhat rundown, I always liked to visit Rome as it was such a great place although at this time EBAss meetings were quite fraught as there was still so much to be done as far as the accreditation system was concerned. I was staying at the Villa Torolonia Hotel, a nice little family run place that was close to the Policlinico Umberto I hospital where the meeting was to be held. On arrival I headed out to a small restaurant just up the road where I had a delightful meal with a couple of glasses of nice house wine, the next day I set off to walk the short distance to the hospital. Before long I turned left from the road into the main entrance of the hospital and walked up to the main reception desk where there were three ladies, of course I didn't speak much Italian so asked whether any of them spoke English (I could at least ask this in Italian); nobody could though.

Eventually I was able to explain that I needed the Hyperbaric chamber, they seemed to understand and sent me back out the main door where I had been told to turn left, immediately in front of me across a small internal roadway was a steep slope running downwards. I had been told to walk down the slope which I could see was a dead end, when I reached the bottom of the slope there was a dark green painted door on my left, I knocked on the door, eventually it was opened by a guy wearing theatre scrubs, he seemed to be expecting me and beckoned me in. Immediately, I could see I was in the right place, there was another light green painted hyperbaric system consisting of three chambers situated right in front of me. I could see the EBAss Italian representative entering the back of the room.

She greeted me with the usual kisses and hugs and told me that some of the others had already arrived, I followed her through a door at the back of the chamber room and along corridors until we entered a classroom. The room was set up with tables and chairs in a formal classroom style. The EBAss president was there already as were five others; I started to set up my computer as I knew I would be expected to minute the meeting. The meeting went well, we were getting things done but only very slowly, we did however have a nice visit where I agreed that the German and Italian examinations should be uploaded before the end of the year. At the end of the day, we decamped to a very busy restaurant where we had a lovely meal although again most of the talk were extensions to the subjects we had been covering during the day.

On my return from Rome, I was able to set my mind to my own professional development. For the last six years I been working as a Graduate Member of IOSH, following the successful completion of my NVQ qualification; I was very comfortable with this but, was keen to take the next step. This would be for me to achieve Chartered Membership of IOSH; in early February I took the first step by attending a day's training in Bristol where I was shown the necessary steps. It seemed that completion of the NVQ had resulted in my having done the majority of the required work and as I had been a graduate member for six years; there were only a few bits and pieces left for me to complete; I set about working on these, I was ready in just a few weeks.

The final step would be for me to undertake a peer review, this consisted of an interview with the IOSH panel; for the interview I was required to produce a PowerPoint presentation. This presentation had to detail my working life to date with particular emphasis on health and safety and how I had managed risks in the past. Following this I would be quizzed by the panel on issues of health and safety; when the date came through for me to attend my interview, it was to be in early May; again, this would take place in Bristol at a building on the Aztec business park.

On the day of the interview, I arrived in good time in fact I was a few minutes early, I made my way to the room where the interviews were to take place. I knocked on the door and went in, only to be asked to wait outside until they were ready for me, oops, I wondered whether I should have waited outside until the actual time of the interview? Well, in any case after a short delay I was invited back into the room; the panel consisted of three individuals all of whom were either chartered members or IOSH fellows. They did all they could to put me at ease with their introductions; I was invited to take a seat at the large conference table, I handed over a memory stick containing my presentation, the file was subsequently loaded up with the first slide of my presentation being displayed on the screen to my left. The three personnel of the panel were seated to my right with a good view of the screen and I was invited to start, so I was off and running.

I had been told to keep the presentation short, just ten to fifteen minutes, it covered my life as an offshore diver showing my progression to being diving supervisor. From there I went on to show how I had operated my own company finally finishing off with how I had built DDRC's safety management system from the ground up etc. When I finished talking, I was asked a few questions relating to the safety management system, this allowed me to explain my pivotal role in gaining ISO 9001 for DDRC etc. The whole thing took about an hour, I was then told they would be in touch with the result in a couple of weeks; I wasn't really sure whether it had gone well but felt reasonably confident.

Almost exactly two weeks later I received notification that I had been successful and was duly awarded chartered status on the eleventh of June 2012; this was great for me and also, I thought for DDRC, they now had a fully qualified and chartered member of IOSH as a key member of their staff.

In July it became clear that I would be required to make a trip to Saudi Arabia; I had over the years been working and liaising with Mark Jennings who at the time was working for Algosabi Diving and Marine Services (ADAMS) who were based in Bahrain. Mark was working with the Saudi Military who in turn were in the process of setting up hyperbaric chambers at a number of locations, we were being asked by Mark to organise and run chamber operator and DMT courses to be conducted at various locations inside Saudi Arabia. I duly gained my Saudi Arabian visa and was all ready to go when everything came to a halt, so much so that my visa expired meaning I had to apply for a second visa before I could travel to Saudi; as it turned out this didn't actually take place until January 2013.

In September I travelled to EUBS again, this time it was again held in Belgrade, Serbia. It was a very useful meeting of minds where I was again able to promote the EBAss/ECB accreditation system, the system was now becoming well recognised throughout Europe. It was very nice to meet up with friends again and to be taken to lovely locations for banquets and the like although in Belgrade the tour guides seemed to be most proud of showing us buildings with bullet holes in them from the recent war!

In November I was off for the second EBAss meeting of the year, this time the location was Amsterdam, another of my favourite destinations, the Dutch are always fun to be with. I was staying outside Amsterdam in a small hotel close to the hospital where the meeting was to be held; at the meeting I was able to report that the German and Italian examinations had now been uploaded, tested and launched. This was a real weight off my mind, the news was very well received. The numbers of certified personnel were also looking good so it was all good news from my point of view. Following the meeting we ventured into the centre of Amsterdam where the local representative had organised for us to eat at a small restaurant in the old town.

This restaurant also doubled as a theatre venue, following the starters we were all ushered upstairs one floor where there was a small venue; at the front was a low stage with some thirty seats for the audience arranged in rows facing the stage. We all found a seat and were treated to a short twenty-minute comedy show; it was I'm sure great but, as a lot of it was conducted in Dutch, I must admit I didn't understand much of it; the atmosphere was great though. Following the show, we all made our way back downstairs for the main course accompanied by more wine and chat. It was a nice evening but most of the conversation was again work of course, this was really the only thing most of us had in common. After the meal I found my way back out to the hotel via the excellent rail network, very thankful for my bed that evening you can be sure.

Immediately before I left for Amsterdam, I had met with two of our trustees, the trustees were an old friend Jon Loney the employment lawyer who had helped us tremendously in the past, he was joined by the ex CQC inspector trustee who had been inspirational to me with respect to the CQC and my responsibilities; as I said previously, he also felt that in my place he would feel nervous about how I was being treated.

I was dismayed that the meeting didn't go as well as I had hoped, I was left in no doubt that in a straight fight between the Medical Director and myself there would only ever be one winner, I would lose. It was clear to me that this was mainly due to the fact that the Medical Director's role would be very much more difficult to fill than mine.

I travelled home from this meeting very depressed; that evening I discussed all of this with my wife and we came to the conclusion that it was not worth the hassle and that I should resign and look for another job.

I felt that as I was now a Chartered member of IOSH, I should be able to find something reasonably easily. Indeed, the very next week I responded to an advertisement for a Health and Safety officer for Torbay council. I had actually missed the closing date but following a phone call with a council official I was assured that my application would be accepted, he encouraged me to apply, he seemed very keen on me and accepted that given my qualifications my application would be welcomed. This being the case I applied.

The very next day I met with Gary in my office; where I tendered my resignation and was very surprised by his response; he absolutely did not want to accept my leaving he told me he felt a huge amount of sympathy with my issues and concerns most of which he shared.

Gary set the scene for a new structure that he and the chair of trustees had come up with. It had become clear that combining the roles of Chief Executive and Medical Director had created a role too stressful to be dealt with, and that being the case the Trustees decided the role should again be split with Gary being offered the role of Chief Executive which he accepted.

We spent a long time discussing my role and agreed that I would resign as CQC registered manager a role that Gary would take on; he also felt I should step down as Managing Director of DDRC Pro-Services Ltd, I have to say that I was less happy with this but could see that it was a necessary step. Gary told me he would be taking on MD of Pro-Services; finally, it was agreed that with my giving up these roles my job would reduce dramatically; therefore, I would reduce my hours from the full five days down to three days per week. This would commence as of the first of January 2013; I felt that although this timescale would be tight it would be doable and should allow sufficient time to properly implement the necessary changes. I would of course be required to take a reduction in salary. It was agreed that this would be on a pro-rata basis; I would be paid three-fifths of my full-time salary; as it turned out this was still more than the offer from Torbay council for a five-day full-time job.

We agreed that I would continue as a full member of the senior management team, as I was adamant that safety management should come from the top level; I would also continue as Operations Director, Gary was keen for me to remain DDRC Safety Officer making use of my diving and safety expertise; he also wanted me to stay on as Quality Manager. Additionally, I would continue as President of Accreditation Committee for European Baromedical Association. Gary wanted to know whether I was prepared to continue as technical representative for the British Hyperbaric Association (BHA) committee; which I agreed to do. I also agreed to carry on as Chamber Supervisor and Operator for as long as my health would allow. So, there I was effectively semi-retiring at the age of fifty-seven!

CHAPTER TWENTY-NINE

2013

First of January 2013 I started in my much-reduced role, three days per week was strange for me as I had never had so much time to myself before. I was though prepared to try very hard to make things work in support for Gary and DDRC in general.

As it turned out though I never had much time to get bored, I started to look for extra work on the two days a week when I was not working for DDRC and found there was a lot of work available, I was contacted by another old friend George Gradon who at the time was in the process of setting up a brand-new commercial diver training school in Fowey. This was the Commercial Diver Training school (CDT); George was working with another acquaintance Warren (Sal) Sallis; they asked me to help with putting together their HSE submission. This involved designing and producing all required paperwork for the course, things like pre and post dive checklists, dive logs, work plans, programmes, examinations; in short everything!

This was a big job; both Sal and George were very competent and had already done a lot of the preparatory work; most of the diving would be carried out from an old RN Fleet Tender, this was a self-propelled boat that could carry everything they needed and was much more sensible than the old boat Interdive had tried to use.

I set to work producing the required paperwork and from time to time would meet up with both George and Sal so that they could review and proof read the documents; this went very well and by mid-June 2013 the submission was ready. My involvement was over as soon as the submission had been made but it was very nice to hear that they did gain approval and from then on have been running courses very successfully from their boat. CDT has since gained an exemplary reputation for high quality diver training, this has been mostly down to their excellent attitude, abilities and investment in quality equipment.

There were for me other short-term contracts which generally I enjoyed, these topped up some of the lost income I was experiencing from my reduced weekly days for DDRC. I continued to carry out these ad-hoc contracts for the next couple of years but eventually decided I couldn't really do the necessary site work anymore, so stopped all but very sporadic paperwork exercises other than DDRC's three days.

On the fifteenth of January 2013 I did finally make my first (and as it turned out only) trip to Saudi Arabia, I flew in to Dhahran international airport where I had been told to look out for a local 'fixer' who would help me through passport control and customs. As I made my way onto the concourse in front of passport control, I was met by a thin wiry individual who appeared extremely agitated. He confirmed my name and although he was clearly happy to see me, he hadn't been briefed about my walking ability as he just took off telling me to follow him! Well, I just couldn't keep up which seemed to irritate him, he kept stopping and gesticulating to me to 'come on'; well, when we did eventually reach passport control, we found ourselves at the back of several very long queues of passengers already there.

My fixer was having none of this though, he pulled me straight to the front of the nearest queue where he barged in front, he proceeded to speak very loudly and to my ears aggressively to the passport officer. I thought this was a risky thing to do as surely, we had to be nice to these people didn't, we? As soon as my passport was presented the official got his head down and although he did give me a cursory glance, he obviously had been given his orders, my passport was stamped and I was ushered through in no time at all. Mr fixer then bade me goodbye and disappeared pointing me towards the arrival's hall; I again only had carry-on luggage so didn't need to pick up any other bags. I found my way into the arrival's hall where immediately I saw my name being displayed prominently on a board.

The board was being held by Mark Jennings, my contact; it was nice to finally meet him as up to now we had just been meeting via email and phone conversations, he greeted me like a long-lost friend and off we went to his car. Mark was a Brit who had been working in Saudi for a number of years and so knew his way around. As soon as we were in his car, we made our way towards Bahrain, this involved travelling over the King Fahd Causeway, the causeway was some forty kilometres long and was in my opinion quite a spectacle in its own right. We entered Bahrain via customs some halfway across the causeway; it was a nice trip.

It would have been a lot easier for me to fly directly into Bahrain but at that time the initial entry point into Saudi to verify my visa had to be made via a limited number of entry points, these were all inside Saudi Arabia and therefore the causeway was not an acceptable entry point although once you had landed into Saudi you then could exit to

Bahrain and re-enter via the causeway!

Bahrain was extremely built up with high-rise buildings everywhere, it was reminiscent of Singapore; I was taken straight to Algosabi's offices where I was introduced to Ahmed Algosabi, Ahmed was a family member of the Algosabi clan and was the main boss who luckily spoke good English. He was a very nice man who was extremely interested in our project; I had been told to prepare a presentation for Ahmed to let him know our plans; Mark took me into their conference room where we prepared the presentation. When we were ready with the first slide being projected on the screen, Ahmed took a seat; I went through my presentation highlighting other projects DDRC Pro-Services had been involved in such as training on super-yachts and training other military personnel.

Although this was very well received; pretty much as soon as I was finished Ahmed was off; Mark told me this was just the way he was, he would not be in the office for long so we were lucky to have been able to have even this amount of time with him.

After this we left the office with Mark taking me on a whistle-stop tour of the island, he showed me the F1 Grand Prix circuit and other areas of interest although we didn't spend much time at any of them. Towards the end of the day, he stopped off at the local bar where Algosabi personnel would congregate at the end of the working day. Although Saudi Arabia was a 'dry' state where alcohol was not allowed, Bahrain was not 'dry', alcohol was widely available and subsequently there were a lot of bars and restaurants serving alcoholic beverages. Mark told me that a lot of Saudi nationals would make the crossing to Bahrain every weekend to take advantage of the laxer rules; as we walked into the bar. I was met by Sam Abbott who at the time was Algosabi's general manager; I had been liaising with him for many years although again we had never actually met. Sam used to be my main contact when liaising with Algosabi with respect to Lloyd's diver inspector courses right back to my days with Interdive.

After a couple of hours and a good-few-beers, Mark finally took me to my hotel and told me that I would be picked up in the morning to travel back to Saudi where we would see the facility where our training would be carried out.

Early the next morning Mark picked me up and off we went back to Dhahran where we went through scrupulous security checks to be allowed onto the air base where the hyperbaric facility was situated, this took over an hour to complete but eventually we were in. We were welcomed into the facility and shown a wonderfully appointed system, it was brand-new and had everything required for treating both divers and other patients. Mark had big plans and showed me where new classrooms and practical training areas were to be built: Mark told me he was also in talks with TWI for them to carry out inspection and welder training at this facility too. All the staff I met were similarly keen and seemed very committed, I was sure all would go very well here. Unfortunately, things didn't go the way we were thinking and although the training did go ahead it was on a much smaller scale than was at the time being planned.

In the afternoon Mark left me with George Marshall ADAMS technical services assistant manager, we would be staying in a hotel in Dhahran that evening and George would take me to see some other big-wigs in the morning. The hotel we were staying in was extremely plush and very well appointed, I did however find it a little odd to be sitting in a restaurant where food from all around the world was available but where you couldn't order a beer or glass of wine! Soft drinks all round then; the next day George took me to meet senior military and local coastguard personnel where we discussed their training requirements, once this was done George took me back to the airport and my first trip to Saudi was over.

I did enjoy the trip but it was very clear from my discussions with both Mark and George that Saudi Arabia although extremely rich had some significant issues that they were struggling to deal with. They generally had a large number of young adults who were it seemed not very keen on working; a very large amount of the actual work was being carried out by ex-pats mostly from UK, USA, Germany as well as India and the far east.

Back at DDRC I was properly into my three days per week, this should have been easy but, it had quite soon become clear that our calculation of time required had been incorrect. I was finding that three days were not really enough to keep on top of everything particularly the quality system, review/renewal of policies, procedures and risk assessments was exhaustive and took up a great deal of my time. Some weeks there would be times when my three days became extremely long but, with help from our nursing and the administration teams we were able to make it work most of the time. Now that I was no longer the CQC registered manager my stress levels reduced hugely, I was no longer under threat of prosecution for anything by them. As I was no longer the Managing Director of Pro-Services, I had no legal responsibilities there either, although I was still heavily involved in management and preparation of courses particularly for overseas contracts however, the responsibilities were all Gary's.

Home life was now also set for a big change; for the previous twenty years we had been very happily living in a four-bedroom bungalow with a wonderful view out over Torbay, it was a tremendous place to bring up kids and we loved it. Unfortunately, the garden was quite large, because of my MS I found I was no longer able to manage it. We had for the last couple of years been paying gardeners but quite honestly had not found anyone who really took pride in their work, it left me feeling frustrated as whenever they left, I felt I had to try to finish what they had started! I knew I was only going to get worse so Chrissie and I agreed that we should look for somewhere that would be easier to look after; so, some mid-way through 2012 we had started looking for a smaller bungalow but, although we viewed a good few none of them were what we were looking for. We broadened our search looking for local flats and yes, we found and looked at a few but again, nothing really ticked all the boxes. This had been going on for months until January of this year.

Chrissie came upon a set of particulars for a new-build flat in Paignton, it was less than a mile from our bungalow, situated lower down the hill and although it would not have the panoramic views of the bay it was a lot closer to town. Chrissie wanted to go and have a look but, I was really not keen, I told her "It's a new-build, the rooms will be tiny, there won't be anywhere to store anything, I'm not going!" Having put my foot down firmly, we of course went to see it the next day!

As soon as we turned up, I could see that Chrissie was right, the flat (apparently, I was to term it an apartment) was ground floor, it was entered via its own dedicated entrance not shared with anyone else; the flat benefitted from ownership of a large pitched roofed double garage with an electronic roller shutter door, there was also a small private garden area that was laid to gravel with shrubs. This was very promising, but what would the inside be like?

The estate agent opened the door onto a beautiful, large entrance hallway with engineered oak, wood flooring; the flat was empty as nobody had lived there as yet; the first door on the left led to an open plan lounge-dining room and kitchen; the room was huge. There were two bedrooms, one with ensuite shower room; there was a second family bathroom, there was a very good size utility room and another room leading to a back door. In short, all the rooms were good size, the whole development consisted of just three flats set over three floors; the development was freehold with each flat owning one third of the freehold, it was perfect. We made an offer there and then, this was accepted so, now we had to work out how we were going to pay for it; we were not in a position to buy it for cash until we had sold our bungalow, but the developer was not willing to take the flat off the market until we had made a financial commitment.

I set out to find a way; we had no mortgage on our bungalow and it quickly became evident that we could re-mortgage our bungalow for part of the sum needed as a buy-to-let and raise the rest with a small mortgage on the flat. We were advised that there would be no problem renting the bungalow and the monthly rental would easily cover both mortgages; we were able to move this ahead very quickly and moved into the flat on the first of March 2013. On the day, the move went well and within a month we had a paying tenant installed in the bungalow so all was perfect; the flat was exactly the right move for us and at the time of writing we had lived there very happily for some ten years.

Travel to overseas locations reduced for me as I was no longer required to travel much to drum up business or to ensure overseas locations were appropriate however, I still was required to travel for EBAss and EUBS commitments. My next overseas trip was in April, I was again off to Murnau in Germany for EBAss duties, this time I was able to report that I had been asked by a Dutch company whether the examinations could be translated into Dutch. The company concerned had evidently been contracted to train a large number of Dutch personnel as the Dutch government had started to make the EBAss/ECB certification a requirement for all chamber staff; this was another huge step forward for our qualification system. It was agreed that a translator would be found and that this would become a priority for us this year.

I spent the next few months beavering away at DDRC keeping the safety and quality management systems running along nicely; I still had to get involved in some of the HR issues but I found them easier to deal with as I was not so overwhelmed by other issues. The perennial problem was always communication, although the staff member(s) concerned would never admit they could easily have just asked someone!

EUBS that year was on the French island of La Reunion in the Indian Ocean, I was asked to attend but I felt the costs were too high, also our medical director and one of our training instructors were scheduled to go and I felt this would be enough for the charity to fund. My EBAss colleagues also didn't want to fund travel there and in fact the only person to go from EBAss was the president of EBAss whose trip was funded by EBAss.

We did have another EBAss meeting in October but this was done via Skype in order to keep costs down. I had not been able to have the examinations translated into Dutch but there was now a translator who had been given the go ahead for the job so hopefully everything could be rolled out early in the new year.

CHAPTER THIRTY

2014

2014 started pretty much in the same way that 2013 had finished, I was kept very busy with management of the safety and quality systems.

EUBS this year was held in Wiesbaden, Germany, Wiesbaden is again a beautiful city and we were treated to some nice trips around the sights. The most significant thing for me was that the EBAss president and I had a very successful meeting with ECHM Executive Board where it was decided that Monoplace (single person chambers) personnel should have their own dedicated EBAss/ECB certification. We were asked to submit revisions to the ECHM/EBAss Resources Manual (RM) showing separation of Monoplace training for ratification by ECHM. ECB also indicated that they would support Monoplace certification, this being the case on my return I started producing an examination for European Certified Hyperbaric Chamber Operator Monoplace (ECHCOM). The EBAss/ECB system really seemed to be gaining recognition by all interested parties.

No sooner had I returned from Wiesbaden than I had to fly off to Stockholm for the annual general meeting of the EBAss board. Stockholm is a lovely place if a bit expensive! Our Swedish representative at the time was Peter Kronlund who was a good friend of mine, we always looked forward to grabbing a few beers together whenever we met up. Peter was working at the Karolinska hospital where they had a huge hyperbaric chamber, it was truly immense and was set up to handle intensive care patients including having the facility to lock in ventilators and all the other necessary equipment; the system was very impressive. We at DDRC could also handle intensive care patients including ventilated patients but our ventilator was nowhere near as state of the art as the ones Karolinska were using. I spent my time there updating on the accreditation system including our meeting at EUBS, all of this was very well received.

During the winter of 2014 our youngest son James was working as a manager of ski lodges in La Plagne in France, I had never been skiing and given my continuing issues with MS was very unlikely to manage skiing at all. This being the case we had not planned on taking a holiday in the snowy alps but as James was now managing ski lodges, we felt it would be a nice thing to experience even if neither of us would ski. We had a tremendous week staying in a lovely ski lodge with a bunch of people we had never met before who had come to enjoy the skiing, the evenings were great and we made a lot of new friends.

James and his partner Ali made us very welcome and gave us a great week sampling all the local delicacies, it was a lot of fun and the alpine scenery was stunning, it made me wish I had made more of an effort to try skiing when I was more able, still, such is life, live every day as though it's your last.

When the winter season finished James and Ali took a job with the same company for a summer season at a resort on Lake Garda, Italy. We decided to travel out to see them which we did in August, a great time was had by all.

CHAPTER THIRTY-ONE

2015

The first of two EBAss meetings this year was held in March via Skype; again, I reported on the accreditation system and was extremely happy to be able to report the examinations had been translated into Dutch and were ready to be launched. This was of course very well received.

The exams were eventually launched in May and very soon after this we had several students take the tests; most of them passed but a couple of them failed to meet the expected pass mark. There were a number of complaints relating to the translation, in fact all of the candidates made comment about the Dutch being unconventional which made the questions harder to understand. I took this feedback back to the EBAss board where it was not well received, a couple of the board members felt that the translation was good but that as the individuals concerned were from the north of the country their normal conversational Dutch was somewhat colloquial and that this may have led to the problems. Our Belgian representative told us he would have a journalist friend of his look at it and where necessary correct the translation; she would ensure that the language used was the generally accepted 'Royal Dutch' being accepted as the correct form of Dutch language.

This would take another few months and I agreed to take the Dutch exams down making them unavailable until this check had been completed. This was the first time we had found problems with any of our translations, it seemed this could be put down to the fact that there are a very large number of colloquial variations around the Netherlands.

Early May Paul Dart came into my office smirking, he looked like the cat that got the cream; I asked him "What's tickled you?" He proceeded to tell me that he had a chap on his course who was convinced I had died! We both thought this was amusing as I was fairly certain I was still alive I went with Paul down to the patient lounge where his course was taking coffee. When we entered Paul showed me which of the students had made the comment, he was sitting with his back to me so I wandered over and tapped him on his shoulder. He turned around and I recognised him as George, I had taught him on a CSWIP course some years before, I said something along the lines of "Hello George, I believe you were under the impression I was dead!" Evidently, the offshore world had misinterpreted the fact that I had somewhat disappeared from public life by having moved away from front-line teaching and once the rumour mill had started up on this it had morphed into my having died. Everyone in the lounge fell about as they all seemed to accept that perhaps George had got it wrong.

EUBS this year was again in late September, it was held in Amsterdam, I again made the trip with Gary and a couple of others from DDRC. As before I enjoyed visiting the Dutch city, it was a wonderful place, the locals were very friendly and I like the architecture especially the houses alongside the many canals. A lot of the buildings seem to be leaning towards you as you walk along the pavements; this is not an optical illusion as the property taxes were based on the footprint of the house. This meant that a lot of the buildings have upper floors that are wider or deeper than the ground floor, I suppose this makes perfect sense but does make the buildings look a little top-heavy.

The main conference was another gathering of the hyperbaric great and good, I now knew a lot of them and found it easy to interact with them, EBAss was gaining a much-improved level of acceptance which was of course nice to see. Of course, the fact that the EBAss/ECB examinations were again available in Dutch was very well received at the conference and showed we were making good on our promise to make the exams available to people in their own languages where possible.

The obligatory grand banquet was this year held on the roof of the NEMO Science Museum. The evening was well attended and as was the norm there was plenty of beer and wine available, the weather was balmy with clear skies enhancing the panoramic views across the canals and downtown Amsterdam.

While I enjoyed this event, I have to say I was finding it harder and harder to manage these trips given that my MS was now making mobility much harder.

The second EBAss meeting was this time held in November in Geneva which again is a lovely city, I have never been anywhere cleaner except perhaps Singapore but Geneva was different from Singapore in that it was extremely costly by comparison. However, I was amazed to find that on arrival at the airport all visitors were invited to print out a bus pass that was valid on all busses and public transport for the duration of your stay; this was completely free! That sort of thing would never happen in the UK now would it. Again, at the meeting I reported on the accreditation scheme and was pleased to be able to report that the revised Dutch translation now appeared to have cured the reported issues. This was definitely a big improvement but I'm afraid we never managed to iron out all of the translation problems for the Dutch exams and I think this is one of those things that owing to the large variations of language in the various Dutch regions it may never be perfect!

CHAPTER THIRTY-TWO

2016

By this time MS was really affecting my mobility the rate and distance I could walk was now becoming a real problem, I decided that it was no longer safe for me to be supervising chamber operations as in the event of any kind of emergency I would not be able to react as required. Similarly, I did not feel confident that I would be a safe bet for being on call; together with the others on the SMT I reluctantly decided I had to take myself off duty as chamber supervisor. I conveyed this to the other supervisors at our regular monthly meeting in February, the news was I think expected and was met with a sombre mood; but I explained that as safety officer I would expect anyone who was affected such as I was to make the right decision and that was to hang up my supervisor overalls. I was of course not happy about this as I felt being a supervisor had allowed me to keep my finger on the pulse as far as the team was concerned, from now onwards I would be relying on others to keep me up to date, but there you go, it was inevitable and looking back I had been diagnosed for some fourteen years so in a lot of ways it could have been worse.

The first EBAss meeting this year was held in March via Skype as had now become the norm; the meeting was very useful we had completed the update of the Resources Manual including not only Monoplace but also Safety Manager as well, this detailed updates to training requirements bringing the manual in line with current best practice. It was hoped that these revisions could be ratified at the next ECHM meeting to be held during the EUBS conference.

EUBS was held again in September, in Geneva; I again travelled with our CEO Gary Smerdon and this time Tim Mockridge one of DDRC's chamber supervisors also came along. By now my mobility had become poor enough that I had bought a mobility scooter which I had been assured would be acceptable for taking on flights. Gary drove a van and agreed to pick me up at my house so that I could take the scooter with me, this all went fine, we turned up at Heathrow where we were to catch our flight. We were flying with British Airways and so off we went to check in, all went well until they realised, I wanted to take the electric scooter; there was then a lot of head scratching and phone calls. I had already checked the BA website which was very clear that the scooter qualified to be eligible for carriage on their flights.

Eventually, someone senior enough to make a decision arrived, I had all the specs of the scooter therefore could answer all their questions until they got to the point of "can the batteries be removed?" Well, no they can't but on the BA website the text said that either the batteries had to be removed or there had to be a key that could be removed; my scooter had a key. Eventually they agreed to take the scooter and I was told to take it with me to the departure gate where it would be taken from me and loaded into the hold; this was fine and I have to say I was more than a little relieved!

When we arrived at the departure gate, I was met by two staff members who again asked all the same questions, eventually they were satisfied, they then asked me to put the scooter in neutral so that they could wheel it easily and off it went.

On arrival in Geneva, I was very relieved to find the scooter had also been delivered so all was well, off we went into Geneva by public transport all of which was geared up to accept mobility scooters although I didn't see any others all the time we were there. The conference went well with the obligatory tours and banquet, ECHM did ratify the alterations to the Resource Manual (RM) accepting our suggestions of a new category of personnel, this being Hyperbaric Safety Manager; this meant that the RM was now ready for reissue.

At the end of the conference, we were due to catch an evening flight home, on arrival at the check-in desk for BA they took exception to my scooter! They told me that it could not fly on a BA flight as it did not conform to the allowed criteria, we all explained that BA had carried the scooter from Heathrow to Geneva just a few days ago. To begin with they refused to believe this as they told us they definitely couldn't handle something of the weight of the scooter. They were adamant that it would not fly, they tried to come up with all sorts of reasons such as it was too heavy and they didn't have any way to load it onto the flight anyway it couldn't fly with batteries installed! This went on for some half-hour before they managed to find a senior individual who took one look at the scooter and said, "that's fine, it can fly." It's amazing, but I suppose the front-line staff don't feel empowered to make a decision, anyway, it all worked out OK in the end but, I could do without all the angst!

On arrival at Heathrow, I was told to sit at the front of the plane and await help to disembark, this was not unusual and had never caused any issue in the past. This time however, was different, the BA crew were shutting down the plane for the night, this took about another half-hour by which time the stewardesses were getting concerned as nobody had come to collect me. When the captain was ready to leave, he was horrified to see me still seated on the plane and insisted that I be taken to the terminal in the crew-bus with them.

I was quite happy with this and indeed it was nice to chat with the captain in the bus, he was a very nice chap who was interested in what I did for a living and why I had been in Geneva. The crew obviously knew each other very well as there was a lot of banter between them as we drove to the terminal. On arrival at the terminal, we obviously entered via the crew door which was unmanned, I had to walk a little way which wasn't a problem for me, but we then ascended an escalator to the arrivals level where it became clear there was a good bit more walking necessary.

The captain could see that I was finding this difficult and told me to sit down while he went off to find a wheelchair! He was gone five minutes or so and returned with a traditional self-powered wheelchair, I of course thanked him and sat down in the chair, I thought he would then leave me to it but no, he took the handles and started pushing me. The rest of the crew also seemed to find this a little surprising but it seemed he had decided to take control of my entry into the UK; he dismissed the rest of the crew who all made off to collect their bags etc. When we arrived at passport control, the captain wasn't going to stand in line with me so we both went through the lane for air-crew, there was no issue and very soon we were entering the baggage reclaim area.

The captain asked me whether I had any bags to collect which of course I didn't but I did need to find my scooter; I tried to tell him that I was sure I could cope from here on but he was having none of that. He pushed me all around the baggage hall but the scooter was not there. He then got on his phone, I could hear that although he was talking to someone senior, he was making it clear he was not happy with the situation and how I had been treated; he made it clear he would be finding out who was to blame for my being left on the plane. After some five minutes of discussion, he was evidently told that the scooter would be found and brought to the baggage hall. Hanging up, he turned to me with apologies, he was great and had nothing to apologise for, I couldn't remember being so well looked after albeit not by the persons I should have been with.

Sure enough some ten minutes later one of the large doors alongside the carrousel where our flight's baggage had been delivered opened and there was my scooter being wheeled by two very apologetic ground staff. I then thanked the captain, (unfortunately, I never did get his name); when he was completely sure the scooter was working and that I was OK we shook hands and off he went. What a gent he was great, he took me under his wing and made sure I was OK before he would even think of leaving me.

Motoring out of the baggage hall I found Gary and Tim waiting in the arrival's hall, we loaded the scooter back into Gary's van and made our way back to Paignton where we arrived at about two in the morning. I have never attempted to take the scooter on a flight again as I feel we were very lucky that time but I could see that it could so easily have gone the other way meaning I would be stranded unable to get the scooter home. I always felt this was not worth the risk and so resorted to taking my self-propelled wheelchair with me on future trips.

Our first holiday this year was Iceland, we had always wanted to visit Iceland and this year we opted for a fly-drive where we would take a week to do a full circuit of the island. We had a wonderful week revelling in visiting geysers in the morning and glaciers in the afternoon we spent the week visiting wonderful waterfalls, spectacular glaciers and geysers that erupted regularly creating a startling spectacle.

The year's second EBAss meeting was in Rome again; this time as my walking was poor as I've said although I didn't want to risk my mobility scooter, I decided to take my self-propelled wheelchair, all went fine at Heathrow, I checked my wheelchair in as luggage and the ground-staff organised one of their own wheelchairs together with a young chap to push me.

This was my first experience of being taken through passport control and on to the departure gate like this; I have to say it was very easy for me, my helper took my passport and rather than wait in line we were ushered through in double quick time, sweet! I was then given priority boarding so was onto the plane at the same time as business class passengers, this was nice as it gave me time to find my seat and stow my bag in the overhead locker before the hoard started to board.

Once we arrived in Rome a very nice member of ground staff was waiting for me at the door to the aircraft, she was an extremely nice young lady who had a wheelchair with her, I was invited to sit and off we went to baggage reclaim where I was reunited with my own wheelchair.

At this point I thanked the young lady and told her I would be able to manage from here but she was also not having that! She pushed me all the way to the train station where she helped me purchase the correct ticket to take me into the city; I again shook her hand and thanked her, I offered her a tip but she wouldn't take anything, I then made my way along the platform looking for a door that would give me access to the carriage. When I came to the door there was quite a big step and I was struggling with my wheelchair and carry-on bag when suddenly I found myself being assisted onto the train, she had seen I was having difficulty and had come to my aid again; what a lovely lady. I found a seat and was transported to the city terminus station, here things started to go wrong, I was propelling myself down a slope to get a taxi to the hotel when an apparent taxi driver offered to carry my case for me, he was over friendly which should have rung bells but I just went along with it.

When we got to his car which was sporting taxi signs on the door and roof, he just threw my bag into the back seat and took my wheelchair which went into the boot, he left me to get into the back seat after my bag. As soon as I was in, he drove off very fast we went all over the place but, not the way I was expecting. After about twenty minutes he pulled up on a quiet street and told me we had arrived, now I had booked myself into the Villa Torolonia Hotel as before so I knew this wasn't the right place. I told him I had been to the hotel before and knew I was in the wrong place, I explained this to him and he got quite shirty telling me I was wrong! He took me up the road a short way and pointed up an overgrown path which he told me led to the hotel!

I just knew he was playing a fast one he then told me that I owed him thirty Euros which was far more than the fare should have been; we argued for a while and he made to leave with my bag and wheelchair still in his car so, I decided I had no option other than to pay him as by then he was becoming quite aggressive.

He then drove off with spinning wheels and a cloud of tyre smoke and diesel fumes, looking around I found myself on a quiet residential street not knowing where I was, I strapped my case to the back of the wheelchair and sat down. I started to make my way to somewhere but I didn't know where! I had no cash left so was looking for an ATM, after about fifteen minutes, I found a small arcade of shops and thankfully an ATM. I was able to get some more money and then started to look for another cab, there were a few women walking along who I think could see I was lost and asked if I needed any help; luckily one of them spoke good English and when I told her what had happened, she was extremely helpful; she called me a cab using her mobile phone, this time the taxi was a real one. He then took me straight to my hotel where I was very happy to pay him his eight Euro fee, even experienced travellers get conned sometimes.

During the October half-term Chrissie had two weeks where we planned holiday in Sri Lanka; we flew with Sri Lankan Airlines and it is a wonderful place and we had a great couple of weeks before having to get back to work.

CHAPTER THIRTY-THREE

2017

March saw the first of two EBAss meetings, again this was held via Skype and went off without issue, the main point was that at last year's EUBS conference it had been agreed with ECHM that there needed to be an examination added to the EBAss portfolio, this new exam would be for Hyperbaric Safety Managers (ECHSM). I tabled the final draft laying out the spread of questions appropriate for the Safety Manager examination. We discussed whether the new examination would need to be translated into languages other than English and it was agreed that no, it would only be available in English certainly in the short term. I then agreed to have the examination ready for launch within the next month.

I had previously asked the board to forward any questions they felt needed to be included in the exam so I was confident the examination would reflect all of the board's thoughts. I agreed that the examination would be launched and trialled before our next face to face meeting in Porto in October. We also agreed to advertise our first EBAss Hyperbaric Safety Manager's course to be held immediately before the meeting in October; I agreed to present a number of subjects on the course.

EUBS this year was in Ravenna, Italy; during September, I travelled again with Gary I again took my self-propelled wheelchair with me, so mobility shouldn't be a huge issue for me. We flew from Heathrow to Bologna and from there we were to take a train on to Ravenna, all went fine until we arrived in Bologna where we were told my wheelchair had not arrived with us and may not have even been on the flight! This was a problem for me obviously but after the ground-staff had spent a few extra minutes looking for it we decided we just had to leave in order to catch our train; I left them our hotel's address in Ravenna and my mobile phone number asking them to let me know when the wheelchair arrived.

Once outside the terminal we quickly found a taxi and all piled in hoping we would still be in time to catch our train; in fact, we had plenty of time so I was confident there would not be a problem. We were just driving towards the exit of the airport when I received a call from the ground-staff who had found my wheelchair; they asked that I come back to collect it.

We asked the taxi driver to take us back to the terminal which he did with some haste, clearly telling an Italian taxi driver you're in a hurry is taken very seriously! When we arrived back at the terminal there was another problem, it was impossible for us to re-enter the terminal and although we could see a staff member with my wheelchair just the other side of the glass doors, we couldn't get to them. Gary jumped out of the taxi and worked with the Alitalia staff member who launched the wheelchair through the doors inside and as the outer doors opened Gary was able to rush in and grab it, what a star. The wheelchair was subsequently loaded into the taxi and off we went at speed to get to the train station, we were able to purchase tickets and board the train in plenty of time, whew!

When we arrived at the hotel it was a nice three-star hotel but unfortunately was not geared up for wheelchair users. True there was a lift to take me up to the floor to get to my room but in order to enter the hotel I had to climb steps as there was no ramp and getting to the lift, I had to negotiate more steps, just as well I could still walk some distance. Anyway, such is life travelling with a disability; you just have to get used to it and cope as best you can, I was very lucky to be travelling with Gary as he was extremely helpful all the time making my life much more manageable.

The conference was as usual, I sat in on the majority of presentations at times when I wasn't required for EBAss or ECHM duties; we were treated again to evening receptions and at one of these I unfortunately had a bit of a mishap. The reception was in a piazza venue fairly close to our hotel so Gary was happy to walk and push my wheelchair; we had a good time networking as was the norm at these events. I stood at the bar talking with Gary and other UK based personnel for some hours, at about eleven o'clock I had had enough and decided to make my way back to the hotel; Gary also agreed and we started to make our way home.

I had left my wheelchair about ten metres away next to the wall behind the bar so I started to walk over to it, I was using a couple of sticks which normally made me quite stable but unfortunately, the piazza was paved with cobbles which I was finding quite difficult as my sticks were tending to slip on them. When I arrived at my wheelchair, I pulled it away from the wall and started to turn around so that I could sit into the chair however, I slipped and fell, I landed on my right hand bending back the fingers unnaturally. I found myself sitting on the ground with a very painful right hand, I wasn't on the ground long as there were soon many hands helping me up and dusting me off.

When I was finally seated in the wheelchair, I assessed my situation and found that my hand was extremely painful, so much so that I just couldn't grip the wheel to push the chair forward at all; enter Gary, he took up the duty of pushing me back to the hotel while I nursed my hand.

The next morning my hand had swollen dramatically, I certainly couldn't make a fist or grip my wheelchair wheel so I had to rely on Gary again; he never complained telling anyone who asked that we were the 'A' team, but I'm sure there must have been times when he wanted to join another team.

Gary and I stayed until the end of the conference when we travelled home as planned, again, people used to tell us we were lucky to be able to undertake these jollies. But I have to say, these trips were extremely hard work and although we went to some lovely locations and were treated to good food and drink, I was not at all sorry when I was able to stop travelling to them.

August saw Chrissie and I undertaking another holiday, this time we were taking a Danube River cruise and it was wonderful I can certainly recommend it.

Later in September of 2017, I, as the EBAss president of Accreditation had been invited to speak at the International Committee for Hyperbaric Medicine (ICHM), the meeting was to be held in Belgrade, Serbia. ICHM were paying my travel and accommodation costs so I was able to stay in the hotel where the conference was being held which was a big help for me as I always found using the self-propelled wheelchair difficult as my upper body strength had largely reduced due to my being unable to keep fit or work-out due to my illness. I was due to speak just before lunch on the first day of the conference; the theme of my presentation was training of hyperbaric staff, a subject dear to my heart and had been the main driver for me and I think EBAss in general. I did not need to concentrate on doctor training as this was already covered quite well and indeed my audience were medical directors from all around Europe who would not, I thought take kindly to me lecturing them on how to train their doctors!

I had prepared a presentation using PowerPoint where I was able to demonstrate the positives of properly organised training. I concentrated on introducing the ECHM/EBAss Resources Manual and how this laid out subjects to be covered and levels of training required. I tried to show how training carried out to the ECHM/EBAss Resources Manual requirements would ensure all staff would have a high level of proven training regardless of where they were working in Europe. I then went on to give the converse point of view laying out the negatives of not training staff properly. I went on to bring them up to date with regards the EBAss/ECB examination system; explaining that the EBAss/ECB system was a facility that would allow staff to carry out independent examination without their needing to travel and that the examinations were provided in a number of different languages.

I finished off by reinforcing my belief that our system would provide independent proof of the candidate's understanding, with successful candidates gaining certification issued by ECB. I pointed out my own experience of how this system had been received very positively by commissioners, insurance companies and regulatory bodies in the UK. I'm not sure they all took this on board but the more times we put it out there the more it would become accepted, at least that was my view.

In October I was off to the second EBAss meeting of the year, this time the meeting was to be held in Porto, Portugal. I was met at the airport by the Portuguese EBAss representative Manuel Preto, he was an extremely enthusiastic individual who had been working in the hyperbaric field for a number of years as well as running a business, teaching recreational divers, I felt he would be a wonderful addition to the EBAss board. We left the airport with Manuel pushing my wheelchair, out we went to Manuel's car, he then took me on a bit of a tour of Porto ending up on the seafront watching surfers riding very impressive waves.

Prior to the EBAss meeting as planned we held the first EBAss Hyperbaric Safety Manager's course; this was conducted over three days Tuesday, Wednesday and Thursday with the EBAss board meeting taking place on the Friday and Saturday.

The course went very well. Manuel was tasked with photocopying all the PowerPoint slides so that each student had a copy; this would allow them to concentrate on the lectures without having to make copious notes. All students passed the end of course examination with good marks; qualifying them to sit the EBAss safety manager examination that I had trialled and launched just the previous month.

During the course the evenings were not busy for the instructors so we spent them visiting various hostelries; one evening Manuel took us for a visit to a couple of Port warehouses where we were able to sample their wares. The names of a lot of the warehouses were very familiar to me with Croft, Sandeman, Taylors and others that were common names in the UK. Porto at that time of the year was a very pleasant place to be with the weather warm and sunny although there was a constant breeze which Manuel told me was almost always present. On Sunday morning Manuel had agreed to take me back to the airport, I had a flight booked for four o'clock in the afternoon so Manuel took me down to the seafront where we had a bite to eat, this was extremely pleasant; we sat outside in a warm sunny spot it was great. Manuel then took me to the airport where I found the flight time had been changed and was now set as three o'clock, luckily although it would be tight when I checked in for the flight the ground-staff moved exceptionally quickly arranging for someone to push me to the departure gate just in time, again, phew!

My mobility had by now become a big issue and Chrissie told me that she was fed up with watching me struggle with the self-propelled wheelchair, it was true I found use of the wheelchair hard but also, I felt I was making myself a burden to other people especially when travelling. Anyway, she told me to find a powered wheelchair pronto or she would! Well quite honestly, I didn't start looking immediately well evidently not immediately enough for Chrissie because within two days she had found one from a company in Malaysia!

This was a lightweight chair that would fold and was sold as being perfect for taking on flights; it was constructed from aircraft grade alloys giving it great strength and lightness, it even came with a canvas bag into which it could be placed for when it would be taken on a plane. It was powered by lithium-ion batteries that could easily be removed again for carriage on planes; I have to admit it looked pretty much perfect for me so I decided to go for it I ordered the Wheelchair 88 PW-1,000XL; it was ordered on-line and within three days it had been delivered to my door. It was just as described, very easy to put up, fold again and very easy to control, great.

CHAPTER THIRTY-FOUR

2018

March saw us achieve another milestone in the EBAss story; since its inception in 2002 EBAss had been a Belgian not-for-profit organisation. It was registered to an individual the former EBAss president with the registered address being his private home address; he had now retired I had argued that EBAss needed to become a registered charity. The board had agreed early in 2017, of course nobody wanted to take on the work but I was lucky in that DDRC saw my work with EBAss as part of their charitable aims and so were happy for me to carry out the work during my normal working hours, therefore, I had been happy to take this forward.

There was a great deal of work, in fact I had not realised how much was needed in fact it took up a great deal of my time, I had to ensure all required paperwork was in order, we had trustees in place; I was the chair of trustees with Angeliki Chandrinou of Greece and Manuel Preto of Portugal being the others. We established the EBAss charitable aims and ensured there were systems in place to enable them to be adhered too. This had all taken until March before I finally managed to get EBAss accepted as a UK registered charity. On the seventeenth March 2018 the European Baromedical Association EBAss finally became registered with the UK Charities Commission. This, I felt was a great asset for EBAss, EBAss was now a legally secure body with a proper constitution and all the other required governance documents, it had been a long slog but eventually we got there and I was very pleased. This meant that when I did eventually leave my position EBAss would still have a proper legal footing, DDRC Healthcare had agreed to continue to maintain EBAss the charity as part of their own charitable aims which was again a great reassurance.

March again saw the first of two EBAss meetings, this was held via Skype and went off without issue, I reported the progress of the examinations again adding the numbers of people who had successfully attempted the European Hyperbaric Safety Manager's (ECHSM) examinations. Of course, the major news was that EBAss was now a registered UK charity which everyone seemed to be very happy about, all was going well and it seemed there were no other big issues for us to deal with; we agreed to meet up face to face in Barcelona in October.

April of this year saw Chrissie and I heading off to another of our bucket list destinations for a two-week holiday, we were going to India. Specifically, we were taking a tour of the Golden Triangle; we would be touring New Delhi, Agra and Jaipur with some other detours to find tigers and the like. We were again travelling with our very good friends the Caunters. We were flying from Heathrow again but this time I was going to be taking my new powered wheelchair, we arrived at the BA check-in desk; again, I was prepared with answers to all the questions I could think they would ask, that is until they asked whether the batteries could be removed.

Now I knew they could but stupidly I had not actually explored how easy this was going to be; John and I exchanged nervous glances before bending down to have a look at the batteries. I put my hand under the battery rack and felt for a clip or something, there was a sort of flap protruding from the battery and I found that if I pulled on this the battery unclipped and slid easily out of the rack, there were a couple of leads to unscrew but it was not going to be a problem. We stood back up with relieved expressions on our faces and proceeded with the check in process; I was able to take the chair to the departure gate which meant we would not be escorted through passport control but you can't have everything. This was another brilliant holiday with the Taj Mahal being the stand out memory.

2018 was a year of holidays for us, in August we took our whole family, both sons, with their partner/wife together with our grandchildren to a villa in Tuscany for two weeks. Although we had a brilliant week, my wheelchair kept letting me down as it would for no apparent reason just stop!

On my return home I contacted Wheelchair 88 to discuss the issues I was having with the wheelchair as it was still under guarantee; they were very helpful indeed they were falling over themselves to help. After I had explained the situation and sent them a video of the chair showing the fault, they told me they would send me some new cables and connections for the batteries. I was reassured by their response and hoped the parts would finally fix the problems. True to form the parts arrived within a couple of days and of course I fitted them immediately, we would see whether these would cure the issues over the next few days.

EUBS this year was not in Europe at all, this time it was a meeting encompassing the European, Australian and South African Hyperbaric communities, this was the second time these bodies had collaborated, the previous time was when the meeting was held on La Reunion Island five years ago. These meetings were labelled as TRICON meetings and it was planned that there would be a TRICON every five years. This time the meeting was to be held in Durban, South Africa in September; again, I travelled with my faithful friend Gary, this time though we were the only two attending the conference as our new medical director Doug Watts had booked onto a training course also in South Africa just a couple of weeks before and didn't want to spend any more time away.

At the time there were no direct flights from London to Durban so we chose BA flights via Dubai, this turned out to be a night flight meaning we touched down in Dubai for a three-hour layover starting at about two in the morning. All in all, I have been to Dubai four times but have never left the airport, I staged there twice when travelling to Qatar and twice again on this trip to and from Durban, one day maybe I will actually get to see the sights of Dubai but it certainly wasn't going to happen on this trip.

This was the first work trip where I would be using my new powered wheelchair, again, Gary drove us up to Heathrow where we made our way to the BA desk. There was absolutely no issue raised with me taking the wheelchair onboard, they of course asked me the normal questions about its weight, types of battery etc., I had all the answers for them and this went down very well, they were quite happy with me taking it to the gate where I would put it into its bag for a baggage handler to put into the hold; I was much more practiced with putting the chair into its bag by now thank goodness, what a difference from when I was trying to take my scooter on a flight, of course this was a tremendous relief! I was constantly expecting the chair to stop but, luckily it didn't at all so perhaps the problems had been resolved?

On arrival in Durban, we found our way to the hotel's courtesy bus which deposited us at the hotel with no fuss whatsoever; the hotel was right on the beach with just a road between us and the promenade. At check-in we were told in no uncertain terms that we should not walk across the road to the beach as it was not safe! Evidently, the colour of our skin made us a target and we were assured that there was a high probability of us being mugged if we were to ignore their advice! This was not the image of Durban I had in my mind; before we arrived, I had been told by a good friend who used to work in Losotho a small country only some three hundred and fifty Kilometres from Durban. The country of Lesotho was wholly surrounded by South Africa, Durban was seen as a great place for rest and recuperation when he was working there some twenty-five years before. Clearly things had changed since then if what we were being told was to be believed; this was confirmed by other locals we spoke to during our stay which is of course a very sad state of affairs.

Durban must have been a wonderful place before the current troubles and unrest came about, although we couldn't spend much time getting out and about, we did have one afternoon to ourselves, Gary and I resolved to make the most of it. We asked at the hotel's reception whether there was anywhere that we could go reasonably safely to get some idea of the locality; after some deliberation it was decided we should get a taxi to a downtown market area where they thought we should be OK. They duly organised a taxi giving the driver specific instructions on where to drop us, how long to leave us there and to then pick us up again to bring us back to the hotel. We were taken to the proposed location where the taxi driver told us he would pick us up after one hour; as we watched him drive away, we saw that we had been dropped right in the centre of a busy market square.

It was buzzing, there were merchants in their colourful clothing shouting, yes everyone was shouting! I climbed into my wheelchair and off we went along the street stopping to see the various items on sale, this was not a tourist market so there was none of the traditional tat, rather it was general fare that you would find in any traditional market in Africa. There were clothes stalls, butchers, fishmongers although they were working largely without refrigeration. There were shops for hardware, cafes and of course bars. It was great, as we wandered around, Gary noticed that my wheelchair was attracting attention, it seemed nobody had seen anything like it before; although there where hundreds of people in the market we never felt threatened in the least. In fact, everyone was exceptionally happy and we enjoyed banter with some of them because they all spoke English to some extent; we had a lovely if a little warm hour just wandering around until it was time to get back in the taxi to be taken back to the hotel. It was a shame that we couldn't spend more time but that is the problem with work trips, they kept expecting us to work!

During my time in Durban, I met with my EBAss colleagues, specifically Angeliki Chandrinou (Kelly). I told her that I was going to be retiring soon and that I would no longer be able to maintain my EBAss commitments. She was understandably concerned by this and asked whether I would consider staying on for at least another year; we chatted for some time during which time I tried to reassure her that all would be well. DDRC had made a commitment to EBAss and that would continue after I had gone, my replacement at DDRC would also become my replacement on the EBAss board and DDRC would not desert EBAss. While she seemed reassured by this, I don't think she was happy but I didn't think there was anything more I could do to help EBAss.

In October I was again off to the EBAss board meeting, this time the meeting was in Barcelona; I had been to Barcelona several times before and liked it very much. There was of course the influence of Gaudi the architect responsible for the Sagrada Família the huge basilica but there are numerous smaller items on view. In fact, it seems that around almost every corner there was something either of Gaudi's work or at least something influenced by him. As was the norm with EBAss trips I was travelling alone which had never bothered me and given my new powered wheelchair I was feeling upbeat about the trip although given the previous issues with reliability remained a little nervous. All went well to start with, I caught the train from Newton Abbot station and settled in for the trip to London, when we arrived a Paddington station, I unloaded the wheelchair and my bag from the train.

I prepared the chair by opening it up, putting the motors in gear then climbed aboard, switched the power on, all the expected lights glowed and off I went, then, all stopped! It was a repeat of the previous issues, the chair was completely dead, the lights had all gone out and nothing seemed to be working at all; I got out of the chair, went around to the back to check all the connections, they all seemed to be OK, I undid them all and remade them. The lights came back on and everything seemed fine, off I went to catch the Heathrow express train; this was no problem and in fact this was the first time I had been able to use a proper wheelchair friendly train, I just drove on and back off again when I arrived at the correct terminal, great.

As I was heading up to the check-in desk though the chair again stopped? Again, I pulled all the connections apart, remade them and things were back to normal, I really wasn't sure where the fault was, I was now wondering whether it was the cables at all? I thought maybe I could resolve it by exploring a little more when I arrived at my hotel. All went well with check-in, packing my wheelchair into its bag for the flight, when we arrived in Barcelona my chair was waiting for me so great, things were all good except that when I had put the batteries back in and was ready to go, I only managed a couple of feet before all stopped again! Clearly this was not going to get any better until I found the real problem; each time the chair stopped I was able to get it going again by fiddling with the cables but understandably I was very nervous of it.

This continued until I reached my hotel, I then spent a couple of hours really stripping all the connections apart, cleaning everything and trying to see whether there was any kind of loose connection; I found nothing that appeared out of place at all, I put everything back together and made my way down to have some supper. For the rest of the evening the chair performed fine, it didn't stop again although I really didn't go far, I was hoping maybe I had cured the problem?

The next morning, I made my way to the hospital Creu Roja where the hyperbaric centre was located; this facility was run by one of the senior individuals in EUBS, he was revered in the hyperbaric world so I was looking forward to seeing his establishment. As I was powering up the hill towards the hospital's entrance the chair again stopped! Oh no, I clearly hadn't solved the problem, I spent the next ten minutes fiddling with the connections, with people walking either side of me; not a soul stopped to ask whether I needed any help but well, I suppose I was only a disabled individual entering a hospital having problems with a wheelchair!

I did eventually get it working again and made my way into the hospital, where I found my way to the meeting room, I met up with the other EBAss board members without any further issues. The other members of the board had run another safety manager's (SM) course during the previous three days, I had not been involved as I felt that these courses should be run by EBAss accredited schools and not the board members.

In fact, we at DDRC did eventually run the first SM course to be conducted by a school the following year, this I felt was how things should be run, the schools had much more experience with running courses properly than the EBAss board did. Anyway, apparently their course had gone well with everyone passing the end of course test; this did not change my view on the board continuing to run SM courses though.

We spent the next couple of days immersed in EBAss business, I gave updates on the accreditation system, we were steadily increasing the number of accredited personnel, things were still going in the right direction. On Friday evening at the end of the board meeting we all headed off to La(s) Ramblas; La Ramblas is a large boulevard running through the heart of the city centre. It is filled with Barcelona action at its best; there are many bars, restaurants with heaps of atmosphere; I had been there before and knew that not only was it a great tourist destination but also hosted a lot of pick-pockets and other non-desirable types. However, we were guided by our Spanish colleagues who took us to a small tapas bar, we were soon seated at the bar and were treated to a wonderful selection of tapas; it was great.

We had a very nice evening before heading back to our hotels, I got back to my hotel by eleven o'clock and was very glad to have made it back with the wheelchair not letting me down again. Over the next couple of days, we finished off our work and I made my way home on Sunday, my wheelchair would stop working from time to time but, each time I was able to get it working again by fiddling with the connections.

On returning from Spain, I again contacted Wheelchair88 telling them that I had completely lost confidence in the wheelchair and that I was not at all happy with the situation. To be fair to them, they again responded with excellent service for a company that at the time didn't have any UK based servicing facilities.

They agreed to provide a completely new replacement electronics package which duly arrived within a couple of days; I had to fit this myself but it was extremely easy given the way it had been manufactured. All it took was a couple of Allen keys and a bit of time, there were two main parts provided, the first was the main control box that held all the required processors and relays, replacement of this just required removal of the old one and replacement with the new one. Next was replacement of all cabling, this again was very easy and just involved replacing one cable at a time making sure the routing was the same as original. Finally, they had given me a new control module; including the joystick for controlling the motors, the main power on/off switch, speed regulator switches and all indicator lights that gave indication of battery condition. In all it probably took about an hour to switch this over, I'm sure an able-bodied individual would have been much quicker but of course I was more concerned with getting it right rather than being quick!

Once complete I took the chair out for an extended trial ride, and joy of joy, it performed perfectly; hopefully all would now be fixed; we would see over the next couple of months.

This was just in time for another of our bucket list holidays; I had always wanted to transit the Panama Canal, this trip commenced for us starting in late October when we flew to

Panama. Spent a night in a hotel before boarding the Silver Cloud in Colon, the port at the eastern end of the canal; Silver Cloud was one of the Silver-Seas fleet. She was very well turned out and the crew made us very welcome from the start, our trip was a real once in a lifetime opportunity; the ship was great, it was quite small but with plenty of room for all passengers of which there were only about two-hundred and fifty.

We were able to visit five countries in central and south America all of which were absolutely brilliant.

CHAPTER THIRTY-FIVE

2019

January of 2019 saw me return to my work at DDRC for the usual three days per week but, it was becoming clear to me that my health was continuing to decline. It was not that I couldn't do the work and indeed although I always used my wheelchair when I was travelling, I never felt the need to use it when I was working in Plymouth. However, I found that at the end of each day after the drive home I was absolutely shattered; given my position as safety officer and operations director I was now beginning to worry that I would miss something that could lead to a real safety issue. I was not sure what to do, I had already told Gary and the trustees that I would retire in October 2021 but I was really not sure I would be able to continue until then.

I had been paying into private pensions since the age of twenty-three albeit probably not as much as I should have been; I felt I had a reasonable pot of money but of course how much is enough? Recently I had started to work with an independent financial advisor who was new to me, specifically I wanted to make sure my private pensions were being managed properly, I thought maybe this was the correct time to meet up to discuss things. Calling him up, telling him my thoughts we agreed to meet in early April.

When we did meet, he had done a lot of work showing financial projections making various assumptions, he was very good at explaining his thinking and I could see he had carefully considered all the variables as much as it was possible for anyone to look into the future. He showed me that it would be possible for me to start drawing my pension earlier than originally planned without too much detriment. He showed me that it was likely that the pot I had should be able to provide a reasonable pension to me for at least the next twenty years or so, after which time I would probably not be wanting to holiday in far flung locations and so would be able to exist with a much smaller pension. I agreed to consider the options he had laid out and that I would get back to him with my decision.

I sat down with Chrissie that evening and we agreed that I would bring my retirement date forward; I still wanted to do the best for DDRC and although I only had to give three-month's notice I decided I would give them a full year.

I had now been a member of DDRC's permanent staff sitting on the Senior Management Team for seventeen years when I sat down with the rest of the team at our routine SMT meeting on Monday 29th April 2019 to tell them of my decision to retire on the first of May 2020. I don't think this came as too much of a shock to them but both Gary and Doug said all the right things and I was sure they really did feel they would miss me. I told them that I would make sure that the transition to whoever took my role was as seamless as I could make it; I would be writing a detailed task-book breaking my role down into manageable chunks detailing what I did as much as possible.

I think this reassured them to an extent, although there was a short discussion about how my role would be covered in the future, I left the specifics to be worked out between them over the next few weeks. I was at pains to tell them that I didn't want this to be secretive in any way and that my decision should be relayed to all staff at the appropriate meetings as soon as possible.

Following this meeting I got to work on the task-book, in fact there were two, the first was the most extensive as it was aimed at whoever took over my role. The second was for our administrator Nicola Aindow who had recently started to take on a lot of the routine administration of my roles including keeping an eye on when SOPs, Risk Assessments and other routine documents required review; she was also keeping an eye on when EBAss accredited staff renewal was coming due.

As I started to write these books, I broke my role down into weekly, monthly, quarterly, bi-annual and annual tasks; once I had these headings, I put procedures together detailing specifically how the tasks were done currently and where the necessary information could be found on our systems. Over the coming year, I kept coming back to the books filling in the blanks as tasks I had either forgotten or which I had not put enough information into.

The first task-book eventually ran to over sixty pages. I was happy that I had done all I could to give the staff left behind at least a start in carrying on with my role. A lot would depend on who finally got the job, without being too immodest I felt the individual they were looking for would need to have a similar background to mine. I didn't think it would be easy and would not have been surprised if they decided to break my role down and assign parts of it to different people. As it turned out when the role was initially advertised there were not many takers and some of them were completely wrong for the job, although I was not excluded from the process I was quite rightly not in the forefront. Eventually, it was decided to offer the job to our engineering manager Chris Bryan, Chris had already taken on the role of chamber superintendent when Lawry left; another engineer had been taken on to assist Chris which had freed him up for his new duties.

I was very happy that Chris would be taking on my role as I had worked with him for over ten years and knew he would make a good fist of it. Some three months before I was due to go, Chris started to work alongside me; he took to the tasks like a duck to water and together with my assistance and the task-book he seemed to be handling things pretty well. There were some significant holes in Chris' qualifications as he only had minimal health and safety training, this meant he would need to enrol in advanced training as soon as possible, he did this and as quickly as was possible he was working towards the required qualifications although this would not be completed before I left.

I was able to work with Chris during audits for the quality system, introducing him to the auditors who in turn were extremely helpful in leading him through their requirements. Chris also agreed to take on my roles with EBAss and in turn Gary reinforced DDRC's commitment to continue supporting this role; I therefore was able to resign as trustee of EBAss before I retired from DDRC and Chris took up as trustee seamlessly.

By late 2019 Chris was already carrying out my roles very well. Before long, our weekly chats became much less about the routine job and more about unusual events that maybe hadn't been fully expounded in the task-book.

Chrissie and I headed off for another major holiday in April of 2019, we were going to visit Hong Kong and China; initially we arrived in Hong Kong, Chrissie had never been to HK before and I was keen to show her the sights. Last year we had had an HKFS crew at DDRC for training, during their stay I had told them that we were planning on visiting both HK and mainland China the following year. Immediately, I was told that they would be very keen to meet up with us and they would then help us as much as they could, one of the younger lads took it on himself to tell me to call him personally, this was Maverick and as it turned out he was extremely helpful during our trip.

As we entered the arrival's hall Maverick was there, he was holding a big sign with my name on it. I was in my powered wheelchair and so rolled straight up to him, I climbed out of the chair to be greeted again like a long-lost friend; I introduced him to Chrissie and off we went to his car. Well, I say car, it was actually a crew-cab pickup so there was plenty of space for our bags, my wheelchair and both of us; as soon as we were all on board, we were off with Maverick and to a lesser extent me giving Chrissie a commentary during our trip into the centre of Hong Kong.

For our holiday trip we would be staying in a much nicer hotel than when I had been there for working trips; we were in the Crowne Plaza Causeway Bay hotel, this was a very nice hotel actually on the island of Hong Kong. This would be our base for the time we were in HK, Maverick dropped us off at the hotel but then had to go back to work which was fine, it was very nice of him to put himself out to pick us up. He told me that he was arranging a meal out for us at a local fish restaurant for the following evening when we would meet up with a few of the lads I knew. This was great, we had a lovely meal with a lot of the guys I had worked with, maybe the only slight downside was that Chrissie was not keen on picking a live fish that was then killed so that she could eat it.

Other than that, the whole trip was memorable with Beijing, the great wall and then on to Xi-an to see the Terracotta warriors wonderful.

2019 saw the normal routine as far as EBAss board meetings were concerned with the first one being held via Skype in May with the second being face-to-face in November, the November meeting was to be held on Gozo a small island just off the western tip of Malta.

This year EUBS was to be held in Tel Aviv, Israel; again, this is not in Europe but it seems that Israel has almost been adopted as part of Europe certainly as far as EUBS and indeed Eurovision were concerned? The EUBS conference was again in September; this time it was just the European Society, both the Australian and South African societies did their own thing that year. This year the special focus of the conference was on traumatic brain injury; this was a subject that fitted in with DDRC's expansion plans, as part of our new building was occupied by the Plymouth University new Brain Research and Imaging Centre (BRIC). The planned collaborative expansion of DDRC's building included the space to install a three Tesla Magnetic Resonance Imaging (MRI) scanner for brain research; this was one part that had attracted the University.

Dr Stephen Hall was the university's lead; his particular interest was in research into brain injury and so the EUBS conference was right up his street this year. Therefore, I travelled with both Gary and Stephen, I had not met Stephen before but he was a very nice chap who was easy to talk to and was a welcome addition to the team. Gary again picked me up at my home and drove us up to Heathrow; our flight was not until the following morning so we had decided he would pick me up at about lunchtime.

Before he arrived, I decided to have my lunch, there were some bread rolls which I proceeded to cut using a brand-new bread knife we had just purchased as part of a set of kitchen knives. I obviously wasn't paying attention as I managed to slice the end of my thumb off! There was blood everywhere; I managed to pack a bunch of kitchen roll around the wound, this was then held together with Elastoplast tape; what a mess! No sooner had I finished this than Gary and Stephen arrived, my wheelchair and carry-on bag were loaded into the back of the car and off we went with blood continuing to seep through the kitchen roll. By the time we arrived at our hotel in Heathrow the seepage had almost ceased, I had brought enough kit with me so that I could redress it which I did as soon as I made it to my room. When we met up for dinner, I asked the waiter whether they had a rubber of plastic glove I could buy; he didn't know but disappeared to ask in the kitchen.

A few minutes later he came back with a couple of latex gloves which he told me I could have, these were perfect, I cut the thumb off one of them and was able to tape that over my thumb including the dressing; this provided much more robust wound protection.

The next day we made our way to check-in at the BA desk again, this time again my wheelchair was accepted without question which I was obviously very happy about. More to the point, the chair had not let me down again since I had changed all the electronics so hopefully all would continue to be good. Our flight was fine, we arrived in Tel Aviv on time, transitioning to the hotel without a problem as well; this time we were not staying in the conference hotel, we had decided to book into a cheaper hotel some mile or so along the coast from the conference. Tel Aviv beach was lined with a beautiful brick-built promenade, this would make a pleasant stroll or in my case motor to the conference in the morning and of course home again in the evening.

The morning was beautiful, bright sunshine with almost no breeze, after a great breakfast we made our way south along the promenade towards the InterContinental David which was the conference hotel. We were accompanied along the way by joggers, skateboarders and locals out for a walk; we passed outdoor gyms and exercise facilities; it reminded me of Venice Beach in California. This was a very pleasant way to start the day and indeed it turned out to be pleasant both ends of the day as we tended to return only after we had had our evening meal at one of the hostelries.

Overall, the conference was again much the same as previous years but with a lot of the lectures focusing on brain injury, quite frankly these lectures went even further over my head than previous years but I think Stephen and Gary got a lot from them. As this was to be my last EUBS I spent a lot of time at the network sessions saying my goodbyes to people I had come to know as friends over the years, in some ways it was quite emotional although of course I didn't tell anyone that. Angeliki Chandrinou (Kelly) was quite sad that I would be leaving EBAss but I reinforced that although I would be gone, I now knew that Chris Bryan would be taking my place so was able to reassure her that I was very confident he would continue where I left off.

Over the next few days, we were treated to some very pleasant meals and visits with some people taking time out to visit Jerusalem although I didn't do that as I felt I had too much networking to do and couldn't afford the time. At the end of the conference when we returned to the airport for our trip home, I was extremely glad that the wheelchair had performed perfectly, this gave me a lot more confidence.

In November my very last overseas work trip was to be the EBAss board meeting on Gozo, this again started off with my travelling on my own to Heathrow, I made my way to the airport by train. Following my recent successful journey to Tel Aviv I was reasonably confident that my wheelchair would perform properly so settled back to enjoy the trip.

The flight took me to the Malta International Airport at Luqa near Valetta on Malta, on arrival I was reunited with my wheelchair at the airport's door, happily it had survived and as soon as I had replaced the batteries, I was able to power it up and make my way to passport control, result! I had never been to Malta before and was looking forward to seeing how it compared to Sicily where I had spent four months back in 1981, Sicily was after all only a short ferry ride away. I made my way through passport control and customs without any drama.

Before leaving the UK, I had organised a taxi to both pick me up at the airport to take me across the island to the ferry-port where I would ride across to Gozo once there, they were to take me to my hotel, I had also booked for them to bring me back to the airport at the end of the trip. As I entered the arrival's hall, I was confronted by a bunch of people waving boards with people's names on them and luckily my name was on one of them being brandished by a middle-aged Maltese chap. As I made myself known to him, he beckoned me to follow him; we were soon outside the airport terminal where he led me to his car; it was a reasonably respectable vehicle if a little beige.

My driver was a jovial chap who helped me collapse the wheelchair which he then lifted into the boot as though it were light as a feather, he also stowed my carry-on bag and off we went for our trip across Malta. We were off to Marfa Bay where Comino Ferries operated a ferry across to Gozo; the trip confirmed that Malta was very similar to Sicily other than the fact that on Malta they drive on the left and there was a very British feel to the spread of vehicles on the road. My driver Sam, was easy to talk to and proceeded to tell me all about Malta including a good deal of its history, including as he said, Malta had been invaded by 'everybody'. As we drove, he pointed out areas of interest including the Popeye Village where they shot the film where Robin Williams portrayed the famous cartoon character. As we continued, he seemed to drive without much consideration of the road or other road users. Indeed, at one point he was leaning around to chat to me as I was sitting in the back when I saw that we were on the wrong side of the road and a car had come around a corner ahead; we were on a collision course, I pointed this out to him; he turned back around and swerved back onto the right side of the road before telling me he thought this part of the road was one-way!

Eventually, we arrived at the ferry terminal and although it was a car ferry, he told me that I had to go on as a foot passenger, apparently, I would be picked up on the other side by another taxi to take me on to the hotel. This seemed a bit odd but clearly there was a cost issue to taking the car on the ferry which had not been factored into the equation. The ferry terminal was wheelchair friendly and so I easily made my way up to the main concourse where I purchased my ticket, I was told I had to buy a return ticket as one way were not even available. When I had been issued with my ticket, I started to make my way toward the departure gate only to see that the ferry was already leaving!

At the gate there was a staff member who could see my confusion and told me that there would be another ferry along in half an hour; this was fine but, I told her that I had a taxi waiting for me on the other side. She said that would not be a problem and she would call to tell the taxi driver to wait for me as I would be on the next ferry, off she went to find a telephone; she didn't ask my name or any details so I was not sure this would work. A few minutes later she returned telling me the taxi driver would wait for me, well, we would see, wouldn't we?

Darkness had fallen by now so all I could see of Gozo was a line of lights off in the near distance, Gozo was only five Kilometres from Malta after all. As promised the ferry returned right on time and I was able to board together with about a dozen other passengers, we all made our way to a lounge on board where there were seats for the passengers and a small café although I couldn't see many people were going to be using their services with a ferry journey lasting only a few minutes.

The sea was flat calm making the crossing easy and before long I was motoring down the ramp from the terminal, in Mgarr on Gozo; at the bottom of the ramp, I was greeted by a young, heavily pregnant lady. She had clearly been briefed as to who to look for as she came right up to me, we shook hands and she told me to follow her; she led me around the corner where her taxi was parked. The taxi was a Toyota Hi-Ace with a sliding side door, I could see another woman sitting in the front passenger seat and as we approached, she opened the door and got out. This second lady was much older and looked a little frail, I was introduced to her and learned that she was my taxi driver's mother who I think was probably there in case labour came calling.

Now of course my wheelchair weighed twenty-eight kilos and although I could at a push lift it, I certainly didn't relish this as the bed of the van was quite high, we discussed this and I told my driver that I didn't think she should be lifting it either and mum certainly wasn't up to it! The driver didn't seem at all perturbed by this, she just turned on her heel and beckoned to a random chap who was walking past; a quick conversation took place and he wandered off, I was not sure what had been said or what was happening. After a minute or so the chap returned with two other men and without a word, they picked up my wheelchair that I had already folded, they placed it straight into the rear of the van; then waved over their shoulders as they sauntered off; job done.

My driver told me to hop in, and off we went to the hotel; I was staying in the Grand Hotel which she said was no problem she knew exactly where it was, I had no idea how far away the hotel was so settled in to enjoy the trip. As it turned out the trip was short! She pulled out of the ferry terminal turned left to drive along the harbour before turning right after just a hundred metres or so up a fairly steep hill also running alongside the harbour. We drove up the hill for about another hundred metres, before she turned left into the hotel's drop off parking lot, all in all we were no more than two hundred metres from the ferry terminal, I could have easily made the trip in the wheelchair although obviously I hadn't known that to be the case. We decamped with the hotel porter helping to get the wheelchair out of the van, my driver and her mum then bade me farewell telling me that they would be back to pick me up on Sunday morning for the return journey.

As I had paid up front there was no need for money to change hands and she waved away my offer of a tip, I watched her drive off up the hill, she didn't come back on Sunday so maybe she'd had her baby?

I checked into my hotel which was very pleasant, I had a nice meal in their restaurant and then organised for a taxi to pick me up in the morning to take me to the hospital where the hyperbaric facility was located. The next morning, I had a couple of hours before my taxi was due so I took my wheelchair and headed up the hill to have a bit of a look around the town. It was a very sleepy town with nice quiet squares with shade trees and small bars, but nothing much was going on even though it was Friday morning, it seemed the place was asleep. I had to be at the hospital for my meeting at midday, the taxi was to pick me up at eleven-thirty, the driver arrived spot on eleven-thirty, he loaded my chair into the boot and off we went.

Gozo is a tiny island and although the hospital was in a town in the centre of the island the trip only took about ten minutes, almost as soon as I had settled in the seat I was getting back out again. I made my way into the hospital following the signs for the hyperbaric unit where I met an old friend Dr Mario Saliba; Mario was the medical director of the facility. I and DDRC had helped him with procuring a new chamber for his facility some four or five years ago; I also used to meet him at various EUBS conferences over the past few years.

Mario was justifiably very proud of his facility and while the chamber was quite small it was beautifully clean and well maintained. The whole facility was excellent; after a few minutes of chatting with Mario I made my way to the room where the EBAss meeting was to take place. Most of the crew were already there as they had again been running another safety manager's course over the past three days, there was the usual hearty catch up chat for a few minutes before we got down to the business of the meeting. There was a lot to get through as this was to be my last face-to-face meeting with them, they were understandably a little concerned about the future but, I think I was able to reassure them about how Chris would be a very capable replacement for me. I gave an update on the new UK Registered charity status, all was now in place and working perfectly; we had UK bank accounts and all the funds had been transferred, EBAss PayPal account had been transferred over to the new charity so, in short all was good.

I was very happy that I had been able to get this completed before I retired as EBAss being a proper legal entity would continue regardless of any future changes in personnel; they all seemed reassured and as happy as they could be.

That evening we made our way back to our respective hotels agreeing to meet up for a meal later in the evening, we had agreed to meet at one of the restaurants along the Mgarr harbourside, this was good for me as it meant I could get there using my wheelchair. I waited at the first restaurant I came to and called our Swiss board member Miguel who told me that they were already in the restaurant, it was called Sicilia Bella, an Italian restaurant some way along the harbourside; he told me to wait where I was, he would come along to get me. After just a few moments we both made our way to the restaurant which was tiny, there was just room for me to get my folded wheelchair in alongside the table where all the crew were already seated. We had a lovely evening with very good food and quite a lot of wine and beer, at the end of the evening I was a little sad that this would be my last time but I had had some fifteen years of working with them and it was definitely time for me to pass the reins over to Chris.

We met up again for the second day which turned out to be quite a long day but then we all went off to our respective hotels, some of them were actually staying on Malta so would not meet up again in the evening. I had a quiet meal in a nice little restaurant and an early night back at my hotel.

The next day my taxi arrived promptly to take me back to the ferry terminal, before long I was again on the Maltese side where I sat down to wait for my ongoing taxi, I was not concerned as I had plenty of time before my flight. However, no taxi arrived, I waited for half an hour before I called the number, I had for the company I had booked through. Eventually I was told that the taxi was on its way but had been held up, he would be with me shortly; well shortly turned into another three quarters of an hour, I was now becoming a little concerned about missing my flight.

When he did eventually turn up the car was not looking particularly roadworthy although the engine was running it was not sounding good; when the car pulled up at the terminal it was accompanied by a cloud of blue smoke emanating from under the bonnet! The driver climbed out and came around to me where he confirmed he was my ride to take me to the airport. Between the two of us we managed to load my wheelchair into the boot but this was only possible once we had moved a spare wheel and tools onto the back seat to make space for it. I was to be seated in the front passenger seat and was keen to fix my seat belt but I think I might have been the first to want to use one in a very long time, although the belt was there it was extremely dusty and when I pulled the belt out, I could hear graunching noises from the inertia mechanism!

Oh well, off we went, with the engine coughing and spluttering repeatedly, I am sure it was not making use of all its cylinders but at least we were on our way. Over the next hour we had several near misses as the brakes seemed a little unreliable and certainly made a lot of noise when applied; we did though arrive at the airport in reasonable time, I was very glad to get out of that car in one piece though. I made my way to check-in and managed to catch my flight which was a big relief, the rest of the journey home went without a hitch. I picked up my car from Newton Abbot railway station before driving home reflecting on all the years I had been making trips like this and although I would miss some things about them, I was definitely ready to only travel for fun from now on.

Towards the end of 2019 we started to hear about a new virus termed COVID-19 it had originated in China; I was not really concerned as I had been in Hong Kong when the SARS virus was about, I thought this would be another one of those that would eventually just peter out; got that wrong didn't I!

CHAPTER THIRTY-SIX

2020

2020 started with me continuing to make ready for my retirement, I was putting the finishing touches to the two task-books and trying to make sure everything was up to date so that I would not be leaving a great deal of unfinished work for Chris to take over. Chris and I worked together very closely over the first four months of 2020 with Nicola also continuing to take over a good deal of my routine admin work, it was all going along very well.

I had no trips planned and indeed it soon became clear that due to COVID-19 trips may well not be happening for the foreseeable future, indeed EUBS was cancelled for 2020 and the EBAss board meetings would be held via Skype until things improved.

My retirement date was to be the first of May 2020 but on the twenty-third of March the Prime Minister announced the first lockdown instructing everyone to stay at home, these measures achieved Royal Assent on the twenty-fifth of March and became law on the twenty-sixth. Well, that was it, I worked from home for the last six weeks of my working life, I was quite used to working from home but, I have to say this was not how I had seen my working life ending. On the thirtieth of April, I signed off from the DDRC system for the last time and entered retirement. It was a bit of an anti-climax as I had planned a leaving do which now unfortunately could not take place so there were a lot of people who I had really not been able to say goodbye to. Still my problems were nothing compared to a lot of others, it was really weird to think I would never have to get up for work again if I didn't want to, hmm, there had been a lot of times where I didn't think I would make it to this point but here I was.

PHOTOS FROM MY TIME WITH DDRC

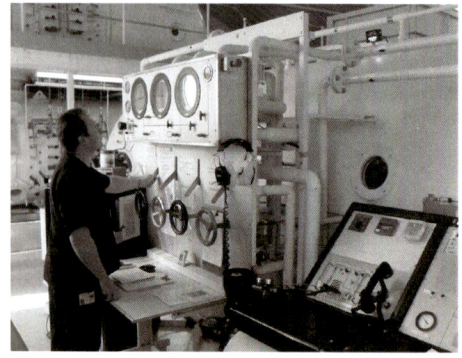

Chamber dive control at DDRC.

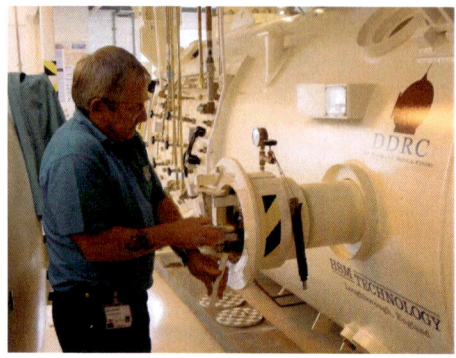

Medical lock on one of DDRC's Comex chambers.

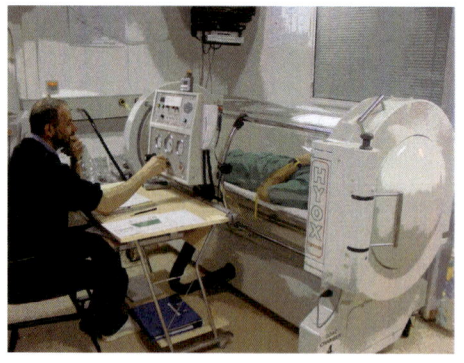

HYOX Monoplace chamber at DDRC.

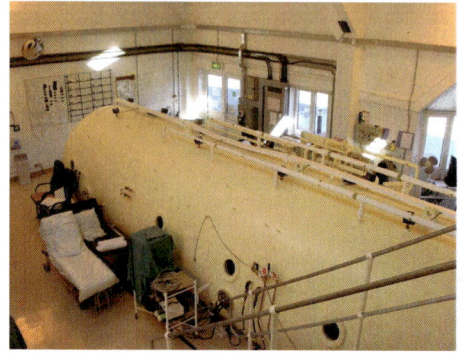

General view of DDRC chamber room.

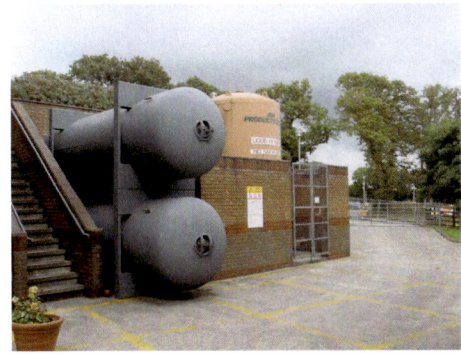

Air and Liquid Oxygen (LOX) storage at DDRC in Plymouth.

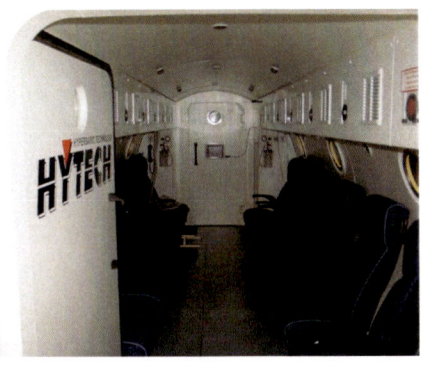

View inside the Hytech Hyperbaric Oxygen Therapy (HBO) chamber, Cardiff.

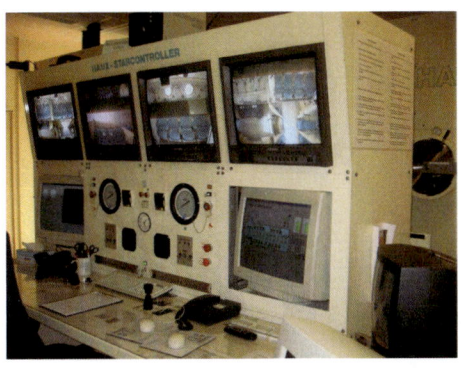

HBO dive control

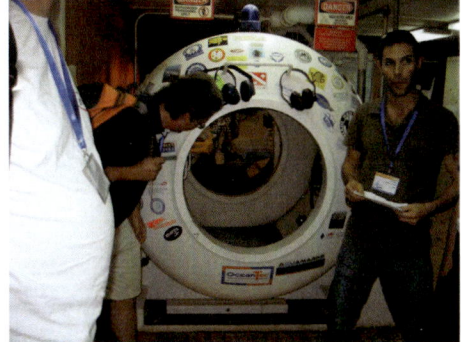

Recompression chamber in Sharm El-Sheik, Egypt.

CHAPTER THIRTY-SEVEN

Retirement

Retirement, well, I had a plan; I had resolved to do nothing much at all for the first six months following my retirement effectively taking the summer off. This was great as the weather was brilliant, we had a lovely warm, sunny summer which despite COVID lockdown I enjoyed immensely, I read lots of books and did a lot of gardening; I think the plants would have preferred me to leave them alone though as I seemed to have found a talent for killing them!

I did continue with chatting to Chris Bryan every week and indeed in the early days perhaps a few more times during the week when he couldn't find something; I enjoyed helping him and was glad when a few months had gone by it became clear that we were just having a social chat. We eventually let the calls lapse and then only chatted every month or so, I'm glad to say that even today some eighteen months after I retired Chris still calls me from time to time though.

I think the weirdest thing I found about retirement was getting to grips with never having to go to work again, this was obviously completely alien to me and although it was nice, even now, I sometimes have to pinch myself; reminding myself that Sunday evening is no longer all that significant for me. At the end of October, I decided I had to get on with something and started to digitise all my old photographs, I had thousands of pictures from the pre-digital era of photography. Some of these were holidays, some were kids growing up, days out, weekends away and not a small number from work trips over the years.

The project was a little daunting, but as with any big job the hardest part was starting; once I had started it just became a job to me. I had bought a scanner that would copy both negatives and positives onto an SD card; in the morning I would open up either a box of slides or a folder or album of prints and would either photograph them or scan the negatives. Eventually, after some six-months I had finished the initial job of copying them all although it was clear there was still a tremendous amount to do to make useable slide shows from them. So, all the pre-digital pictures were now copied as digital files; I had stored them on hard drives (there were two just in case). All that was left now was to organise them so that duplicates were weeded out, well I say all, even after a further couple of years this is still an ongoing job!

Chrissie and I had big plans for holidays this year and the next, firstly we had planned a trip to the USA to see Chrissie's sister who lived in Chicago; this was due to happen in August. Well of course by August nobody was allowed to travel anywhere especially to or from the US due to COVID restrictions so that never happened, luckily, we were able to secure a full refund so didn't lose any money; but of course, it was sad particularly for Chrissie as she really missed seeing her sister and the rest of their family.

Secondly, we were planning a major trip to New Zealand and Australia for March 2021; my dad was born in New Zealand but I had never actually managed to get over there to see where he came from; I really wanted to see where my roots were. Chrissie had never been to Australia and wanted to see Sydney and other sites; I was keen to snorkel on the Great Barrier reef and although I had been to Australia a couple of times, I had only been to Perth which I am told is not indicative of the rest of Oz.

This trip was a planned thirty-day duration, with stops on the way out and back in Dubai where I was planning to meet up with some of my Arab friends. This was a big deal for us and was the typical retirement binge of a holiday; we had spent a great deal of time planning hotels, tours and the like with a great and exceptionally helpful company called Travelbag. All of this was ready and in place for March-April 2021, we had paid for it all up-front, over fifteen-thousand pounds in all for both trips; I felt that it was certain that by March 21 everything would be back to normal; wrong! This holiday also was cancelled; I am very glad to be able to report that Travelbag were exceptional, they refunded every penny and all without me having to threaten anything! So, although we had lost our trips, we didn't lose any money which was something at least, we were gutted with losing the trips but all in all I think we got off lightly.

Following completion of digitising the photographs I decided I would finish the book about my life that you have now struggled through, I had initially started writing this some twenty-five years ago but what with career, family and life in general had never been able to find the time to research and put things down on paper so to speak. Now though given my retirement I had the time and resolved to get it done! Even with lots of time though, I found I could not concentrate for long periods maybe this was due to my MS or maybe it was just age related. This meant I would sit down in the morning and do two to three hours at a time before I would need to sit back and do something else for a while.

In reality I probably managed four or five, three-hour sessions per week and even then, I would not manage this every week. In short it still took a long time before I was happy that I had written everything into the book that I wanted too; I hope you've found it entertaining and not too boring as I would like you to go away from this with the understanding that as I have said a few times in the text; I feel privileged and feel I have been extraordinarily lucky to be in the right place at the right time to take advantage of some wonderful opportunities. I have been lucky enough to travel widely around the world with someone else paying, I've been able to 'play' (my dear wife's words) with heaps of very expensive kit and experience things that very few others have managed. My luck has enabled me to take advantage of government funding for my diver's course, leading on to employment with the leading offshore diving company at that time.

I also feel fortunate that I have survived relatively unscathed despite riding motorcycles for some forty years. There have been several times when I have had heavy weights dropped on me like the time in France when they dropped the BOP on the bell I was sitting inside, in short, I think I must have used up at least five or six of my nine lives! This luck then continued when I decided to stop diving offshore, I was able to find relatively well paid and interesting employment ashore. I feel my luck even extended to my diagnosis of MS, clearly, I was not lucky to have contracted the disease but, as it turns out the disease has progressed relatively slowly with deterioration in my abilities not becoming a huge issue until recently; I was able to continue working in a high powered, stressful and rewarding job for nearly twenty-years after diagnosis.

The future: Well, as much as anyone can predict the future, I hope to be able to continue to contribute usefully in some way. To this end I have been accepted onto the governing body of a local special school in Paignton the Medical Tuition Service; I hope to be able to help them by giving them the benefit of my health and safety experience. I have also been invited onto the board of trustees of the charity DDRC Healthcare where I will continue my association with them as I still feel very committed to their cause and am sure I still have something to give to them.

Perhaps I should mention regrets, there are many but, as you know we cannot change the past and although I have done some (a lot!) of stupid things and have from time-to-time upset people by my actions, I have tried to minimise this and hope that I have not really hurt anyone by my actions. I have two real regrets though I would have loved to be able to play a musical instrument but never got around to it. Certainly, at school my musical capabilities were recognised as being miniscule and indeed I was thrown out of the choir for being tone-deaf so maybe I couldn't have learned an instrument anyway but I feel I should at least have tried. The second regret has to be that I would have liked to learn a second language although I keep getting told I haven't really mastered English yet so maybe again this would not have been possible for me. I will though give it a go I think, maybe I will continue with French because I do at least already have a smattering of understanding.

Anyway, finally, thank you for taking the time to read my book and hopefully it will have given you a couple of chuckles along the way; here's to the next thirty years.